New Frontiers in
Geriatrics Research

New Frontiers in Geriatrics Research

An Agenda for Surgical and Related Medical Specialties

David H. Solomon, MD, MACP, Editor

Joseph LoCicero III, MD, FACS, Associate Editor

Ronnie Ann Rosenthal, MD, FACS, Associate Editor

A Project of
The American Geriatrics Society
and
The John A. Hartford Foundation

PUBLISHED BY THE AMERICAN GERIATRICS SOCIETY
New York, NY, USA

This publication was prepared by the American Geriatrics Society as a service to health care providers involved in the care of older persons. Funding provided by The John A. Hartford Foundation made the development of this publication possible.

New Frontiers in Geriatrics Research is independently prepared and published. All decisions regarding its content are solely the responsibility of the authors and editors. Their decisions are not subject to any form of approval by other interests or organizations.

Citation: Solomon DH, LoCicero J 3rd, Rosenthal RA, eds.
New Frontiers in Geriatrics Research:
An Agenda for Surgical and Related Medical Specialties. 2004.

ISBN 1–886775–11–7
Printed in the U.S.A.

**To our older patients
and to those dedicated to providing the best care for them**

CONTENTS

ACKNOWLEDGMENTS

THE JOHN A. HARTFORD FOUNDATION

We are indebted to The John A. Hartford Foundation for their unswerving commitment to "improving the quality and financing of health care and assisting the health care system to accommodate the nation's aging population." The innovative programs developed with their support will provide better health care for current and future generations of older adults.

We are grateful for the wisdom and guidance provided by Laura A. Robbins, Senior Program Officer for the Increasing Geriatrics Expertise in Surgical and Related Medical Specialties (Geriatrics for Specialists) project from its inception through October 2003.

We thank the members of the Board of Trustees and Cory H. Rieder, EdD, Donna Regenstreif, PhD, Christopher A. Langston, PhD, and the rest of the staff at The John A. Hartford Foundation for their continuing guidance and support of our efforts to improve the care provided to older adults by surgical and related medical specialists.

For additional information about The John A. Hartford Foundation, located in New York City, please visit their Web site at http://www.jhartfound.org/

PROJECT PARTICIPANTS

Many talented and knowledgeable people have collaborated to make this publication possible. Each has made a substantial contribution to the development of the research agenda, and we thank the following people for dedicating their time and effort to complete the tasks that made this volume possible:

Anesthesiology

David J. Cook, MD, *Content Expert*
Associate Professor of Anesthesiology
Mayo Clinic and Foundation
Rochester, MN

G. Alec Rooke, MD, PhD, *Senior Writer*
Professor of Anesthesiology
University of Washington School of Medicine
Veterans Affairs Puget Sound Health Care System
Seattle, WA

Jerry Reves, MD, *At-large Leader*
VP for Medical Affairs and Dean, College of Medicine
Medical University of South Carolina
Charleston, SC

Jeffrey H. Silverstein, MD, *At-large Leader*
Associate Professor of Anesthesiology, Surgery, and Geriatrics & Adult Development
Associate Dean for Research
Mount Sinai School of Medicine
Vice Chairman for Research
Department of Anesthesiology
New York, NY

Emergency Medicine

Scott T. Wilber, MD, FACEP, *Content Expert*
Assistant Professor of Emergency Medicine
Northeastern Ohio Universities College of Medicine
Rootstown, OH
Associate Director
Emergency Medicine Research Center
Summa Health System
Akron, OH

Lowell W. Gerson, PhD, *Senior Writer*
Professor of Epidemiology and Associate Director
Division of Community Health Sciences
Northeastern Ohio University College of Medicine
Rootstown, OH

Stephen W. Meldon, MD, *At-large Leader*
Associate Professor
CWRU Department of Emergency Medicine at MetroHealth Medical Center
Cleveland, OH

Arthur B. Sanders, MD, *At-large Leader*
Professor, Department of Emergency Medicine
University of Arizona College of Medicine
Tucson, AZ

General Surgery

Walter E. Pofahl II, MD, FACS, *Content Expert*
Associate Professor
Chief, Division of General Surgery
Brody School of Medicine
East Carolina University
Greenville, NC

Walter J. Pories, MD, FACS, *Senior Writer*
Professor of Surgery and Biochemistry
East Carolina University
Department of Surgery
Greenville, NC

J. Patrick O'Leary, MD, *At-large Leader*
The Isidore Cohn Jr. Professor and Chairman
Department of Surgery
Louisiana State University School of Medicine
New Orleans, LA

Ronnie Ann Rosenthal, MD, FACS, *At-large Leader and Associate-Editor*
Associate Professor of Surgery
Yale University School of Medicine
Chief, Surgical Service, Veterans Affairs Connecticut Healthcare System
New Haven, CT

Geriatrics

John R. Burton, MD, *Consultant to Orthopedic Surgery*
Project Co-Director 1998-2003, Project Director 2003-2005
Mason F. Lord Professor of Medicine
Division of Geriatric Medicine and Gerontology
Johns Hopkins University School of Medicine
Baltimore, MD

Colleen Christmas, MD, *Consultant to Anesthesiology*
Director, Hip Fracture and Geriatric Consultation Service
Assistant Professor of Medicine
Division of Geriatric Medicine
Johns Hopkins University
Baltimore, MD

Evelyn C. Granieri, MD, MPH, MSEd, *Consultant to Gynecology*
Associate Professor of Geriatric Medicine
Mount Sinai School of Medicine
Chief, Geriatrics Services
Bronx Veterans Affairs Medical Center
Bronx, NY

Dennis W. Jahnigen, MD *(deceased, Project Director 1994-1998)*
Goodstein Professor of Geriatric Medicine
Director of the Center on Aging
University of Colorado Health Sciences Center (UCHSC)
Denver, CO

Paul R. Katz, MD, *Consultant to General Surgery*
Professor of Medicine
University of Rochester School of Medicine and Dentistry
Medical Director, Monroe Community Hospital
Rochester, NY

Brenda K. Keller, MD, *Consultant to Ophthalmology*
Assistant Professor
Section of Geriatrics and Gerontology
University of Nebraska Medical Center
Omaha, NE

C. Seth Landefeld, MD, *Consultant to Emergency Medicine*
Professor of Medicine and Epidemiology and Biostatistics
Chief, Division of Geriatrics
University of California San Francisco
Associate Chief of Staff
Geriatrics and Extended Care
San Francisco Veterans Affairs Medical Center
San Francisco, CA

Douglas K. Miller, MD, *Consultant to Thoracic Surgery*
Richard M. Fairbanks Chair in Aging Research
Associate Director, Indiana University Center for Aging Research
Scientist, Regenstrief Institute, Inc
Indiana University School of Medicine
Indianapolis, IN

Myron Miller, MD, *Consultant to Physical Medicine and Rehabilitation*
Professor, Department of Medicine
Johns Hopkins University School of Medicine
Academic Director, Division of Geriatric Medicine
Department of Medicine
Sinai Hospital of Baltimore
Baltimore, MD

Joseph G. Ouslander, MD, *Consultant to Urology*
Professor of Medicine and Nursing
Director, Division of Geriatric Medicine and Gerontology
Chief Medical Officer, Wesley Woods Center of Emory University
Director, Emory Center for Health in Aging
Research Scientist, Birmingham/Atlanta Veterans Affairs GRECC
Atlanta, GA

David H. Solomon, MD, MACP, *Consultant to Otolaryngology and Editor*
Project Director 1997-2003
Professor Emeritus of Medicine/Geriatrics
David Geffen School of Medicine at UCLA
Los Angeles, CA

Gynecology

Karen L. Miller, MD, *Content Expert*
Assistant Professor, Department of Obstetrics and Gynecology
University of Utah Health Sciences Center
Salt Lake City, UT

Morton A. Stenchever, MD, *Senior Writer*
Professor and Chairman Emeritus
Department of Obstetrics and Gynecology
University of Washington School of Medicine
Seattle, WA

William C. Andrews, MD, FACOG, FRCOG, *At-large Leader*
Professor Emeritus of Obstetrics and Gynecology
Eastern Virginia Medical School
Norfolk, VA

Holly E. Richter, PhD, MD, *At-large Leader*
Associate Professor
Medical Surgical Gynecology
University of Alabama at Birmingham
Birmingham, AL

Ophthalmology

Anne Louise Coleman, MD, PhD, *Content Expert and Senior Writer*
Professor of Ophthalmology
Jules Stein Eye Institute
University of California
Los Angeles, CA

Andrew G. Lee, MD, *Content Expert and Senior Writer*
Associate Professor of Ophthalmology, Neurology, and Neurosurgery
University of Iowa Hospitals and Clinics
Iowa City, IA

Richard Alan Lewis, MD, MS, *At-large Leader*
Professor, Departments of Ophthalmology, Medicine, Pediatrics, and Molecular and
    Human Genetics
Faculty Associate, Huffington Center on Aging
Houston, TX

Gwen K. Sterns, MD, *At-large Leader*
Clinical Professor, Department of Ophthalmology
University of Rochester School of Medicine and Dentistry
Chief, Department of Ophthalmology
Rochester General Hospital
Medical Director
Association for the Blind and Visually Impaired—Goodwill
Rochester, NY

Orthopedic Surgery

Susan Day, MD, *Content Expert*
Clinical Instructor, Michigan State University
Grand Rapids Orthopaedic Residency Program
Grand Rapids, MI

Robert Karpman, MD, MBA, *Senior Writer*
Phoenix, AZ

E. Dennis Lyne, MD, *At-large Leader*
Pediatric Orthopaedics
Program Director
Orthopaedic Surgery
Professor, Surgery and Pediatrics
Chief, Division of Orthopaedics
Michigan State University Department of Surgery
MSU-Kalamazoo Center for Medical Studies
Kalamazoo, MI

Charles Weiss, MD, *At-large Leader*
Chairman Emeritus
Department of Orthopaedics and Rehabilitation
Mount Sinai Medical Center
Miami Beach, FL
Clinical Professor of Orthopaedics
University of Miami School of Medicine
Coral Gables, FL

Otolaryngology

Hinrich Staecker, MD, PhD, *Content Expert*
Associate Professor of Otolaryngology, Head and Neck Surgery
University of Maryland School of Medicine
Baltimore, MD

Steven M. Parnes, MD, *Senior Writer*
Chairman of Otolaryngology–Head and Neck Surgery
Albany Medical College
Albany, NY

Ara A. Chalian, MD, FACS, *At-large Leader*
Associate Professor
Department of Otorhinolaryngology–Head and Neck Surgery
University of Pennsylvania
Philadelphia, PA

Physical Medicine and Rehabilitation

Helen Hoenig, MD, MPH, *Content Expert*
Associate Professor of Medicine
Division of Geriatrics, Department of Medicine
Center for the Study of Aging and Human Development
Duke University Medical Center
Chief, Physical Medicine and Rehabilitation Service
Durham Veterans Affairs Medical Center
Durham, NC

Hilary C. Siebens, MD, *Senior Writer*
Professor of Clinical Medicine
Professor of Clinical Physical Medicine and Rehabilitation
University of California, Irvine, College of Medicine
Irvine, CA

Arlene S. Bierman, MD, MS, *Consultant*
Senior Research Physician *(2001)*
Center for Outcomes and Effectiveness Research
Agency for Healthcare Research and Quality (AHRQ)
Rockville, MD
Ontario Women's Health Council Chair (*August 1, 2003*)
Women's Health University of Toronto
Inner City Health Research Unit
St. Michaels Hospital
Toronto, ON, Canada

Gary S. Clark, MD, CPE, *At-large Leader*
Professor and Chair
Department of Physical Medicine and Rehabilitation
Case Western Reserve University School of Medicine
MetroHealth Medical Center
Cleveland, OH

Gerald Felsenthal, MD, *At-large Leader*
Chairman Emeritus Department of Rehabilitation Medicine
Sinai Hospital of Baltimore
Clinical Professor Department of Epidemiology and Preventive Medicine
University of Maryland School of Medicine
Baltimore, MD

Thoracic Surgery

Nicola Francalancia, MD, *Content Expert*
Associate Professor of Surgery
Department of Surgery
Division of Cardiothoracic Surgery
University of Massachusetts Medical School
Worcester, MA

John Yee, MD, *Content Expert*
Assistant Professor of Surgery
University of Michigan Medical Center
Section of Thoracic Surgery
Ann Arbor, MI

Joseph LoCicero III, MD, FACS, *Senior Writer and Associate Editor*
The Point Clear Charities Professor
Chair of Surgery
Director, Center for Clinical Oncology
Director, Center for Interventional Technologies
The University of South Alabama
Mobile, AL

John R. Benfield, MD, FACS, *At-large Leader*
Professor of Surgery Emeritus
David Geffen School of Medicine at UCLA
University of California, Davis
Los Angeles, CA

T. Bruce Ferguson, Jr., MD, *At-large Leader*
Professor
Departments of Surgery and Physiology
LSU HSC Cardiovascular Outcomes Research Group
New Orleans, LA

David A. Fullerton, MD, *At-large Leader*
Professor of Surgery
Chief, Cardiothoracic Surgery
University of Colorado Health Sciences Center
Denver, CO

Nicholas T. Kouchoukos, MD, *At-large Leader*
Division of Cardiovascular and Thoracic Surgery
Missouri Baptist Medical Center, BJC Healthcare
St. Louis, MO

Urology

Tomas L. Griebling, MD, *Content Expert*
Assistant Professor of Urology
Assistant Scientist, Center on Aging
The University of Kansas
Kansas City, KS

George W. Drach, MD, *Senior Writer*
Professor of Urology
University of Pennsylvania
Philadelphia, PA

M. Craig Hall, MD, *At-large Leader*
Associate Professor and Director of Urologic Oncology
Department of Urology and Comprehensive Cancer Center
Wake Forest University Medical Center
Winston-Salem, NC

Pat Duane O'Donnell, MD, *At-large Leader*
Director of Oklahoma Incontinence Center
Urologic Specialists of Oklahoma
Tulsa, OK

Cross-Cutting Issues Chapter

Marion Danis, MD, *Contributor*
Head, Section on Ethics and Health Policy
Department of Clinical Bioethics
National Institutes of Health
Bethesda, MD

Laura C. Hanson, MD, MPH, *Contributor*
Associate Professor of Medicine
Division of Geriatric Medicine
University of North Carolina at Chapel Hill
Chapel Hill, NC

National Institutes of Health, National Institute on Aging

Evan C. Hadley, MD, *Conference Observer*
Associate Director (Geriatrics and Clinical Gerontology)
National Institute on Aging, NIH
Bethesda, MD

Stanley L. Slater, MD, *Conference Observer*
Deputy Associate Director for Geriatrics and Clinical Gerontology
National Institute on Aging
Bethesda, MD

RAND Health, RAND Corporation

Paul G. Shekelle, MD, PhD, *Advisor and Facilitator at Content Experts meeting,
    February 2001*
Senior Natural Scientist
Santa Monica, CA

Catherine H. MacLean, MD, PhD, *Advisor and Facilitator at Content Experts meeting,
    February 2001*
Natural Scientist
Santa Monica, CA

Roberta Shanman, MLS, *Literature Reviews Consultant*
Senior Librarian
Santa Monica, CA

Amy Atchison, JD, MLIS, *Literature Reviews Consultant*
Senior Librarian
Santa Monica, CA

Patricia Smith, *Meeting Planner, Technical Assistance*
Administrative Assistant
Santa Monica, CA

Publications Consultants

Sue Radcliff, *Research Consultant*
Denver, CO

Barbara B. Reitt, PhD, ELS(D), *Medical Editor*
Reitt Editing Services
Northampton, MA

L. Pilar Wyman, *Indexer*
Wyman Indexing
Annapolis, MD

American Geriatrics Society

Janis Eisner, *Project Manager, Geriatrics for Specialists*
American Geriatrics Society
The Empire State Building
New York, NY

Nancy Lundebjerg, MPA, *Associate Vice President for Professional Education and Special Projects*
American Geriatrics Society
The Empire State Building
New York, NY

Marina Shaykevich, MS, *Health Coordinator*
American Geriatrics Society
The Empire State Building
New York, NY

Amy Tam-Liao, *Health Coordinator*
American Geriatrics Society
The Empire State Building
New York, NY

AGENCY FOR HEALTHCARE RESEARCH AND QUALITY (AHRQ)

We thank the Agency for Healthcare Research and Quality (AHRQ) for co-sponsoring the conference on a research agenda in Potomac, Maryland, in November 2001. We especially thank Dr. Arlene Bierman for making the local arrangements for the meeting.

AGS COUNCIL OF THE SECTION ON SURGICAL AND RELATED MEDICAL SPECIALTIES

We thank the members of the Council (formerly the Interdisciplinary Leadership Group) for their wise guidance of the overall Geriatrics for Specialists project. Members in 2001:

American Academy of Ophthalmology (AAO)
Andrew G. Lee, MD
Thomas J. Liesegang, MD

American Academy of Orthopaedic Surgeons (AAOS)
Kenneth J. Koval, MD
Charles Weiss, MD

American Academy of Otolaryngology-Head and Neck Surgery (AAO-H&NS)
Steven M. Parnes, MD
Allan M. Rubin, MD

American Academy of Physical Medicine and Rehabilitation (AAPM&R)
Hilary C. Siebens, MD
Dale C. Strasser, MD

American College of Emergency Physicians (ACEP)
Richard S. Slevinski, MD

American College of Obstetricians and Gynecologists (ACOG)
Gerald Holzman, MD
Luella Klein, MD

American Society of Anesthesiologists (ASA)
J.G. Reves, MD
Alan D. Sessler, MD

American Urological Association (AUA)
George W. Drach, MD
Martin I. Resnick, MD

Association of Program Directors in Surgery (APDS)
J. Patrick O'Leary, MD
Walter J. Pories, MD

Society of Thoracic Surgeons (STS)
Mark B. Orringer, MD
Joseph LoCicero III, MD, FACS

Society for Academic Emergency Medicine (SAEM)
Lowell W. Gerson, PhD

1

INTRODUCTION

David H. Solomon, MD, MACP; Joseph LoCicero III, MD, FACS;
Ronnie Ann Rosenthal, MD, FACS*

Welcome to the first attempt in the history of geriatrics to develop a research agenda specifically aimed at enhancing the quality of care of the elderly patients who are cared for by specialists in surgical disciplines and related medical fields. We hope this volume will be useful to the many specialists who are interested in helping to create an up-to-date base of evidence in support of geriatrics aspects of clinical practice in their respective disciplines.

To a certain extent, it is presumptuous to put forth a research agenda. Doing so could be interpreted as claiming to know all there is to know about what research most needs to be done. We therefore hasten to clarify that what is presented here is just *one* research agenda. A different team would probably come up with a different agenda. Our only assertion is that the agenda we propose has behind it substantial reviews of the existing state of knowledge in each of the disciplines and that therefore it is firmly based on three objectives: to fill obvious gaps in knowledge in each specialty area covered, to clarify inconsistencies in the existing literature, and to point to possible resolutions of ongoing controversies.

THE SCOPE OF THIS RESEARCH AGENDA

The ten specialties addressed in this volume include five surgical specialties: general surgery, orthopedic surgery, otolaryngology, thoracic surgery, and urology. Two other specialties are included that are predominantly surgical but have a significant element of medical practice: gynecology and ophthalmology. In addition, three related medical specialties are included: anesthesiology, emergency medicine, and physical medicine and rehabilitation (physiatry). Altogether, these ten specialties encompass the full course of most surgical patients. An elderly patient with an acute illness might well present to the emergency department of a hospital where an emergency medicine physician would stabilize the patient, make at least a tentative diagnosis, and refer the patient, if indicated, to one of the surgical specialties for treatment. The anesthesiologist would then join with the surgeon in preoperative assessment and management and in carrying out intraoperative and immediate postoperative care. The surgeon would perform the operation and be responsible for postoperative care and discharge planning. In many circumstances, such as cardiac, abdominal, and orthopedic surgery, crucial assistance in recovery would be provided by the physiatrist.

Each chapter presents research agenda items focused on clinical research in selected topics in the specialty; the agenda items in each topic are based on the descriptions of the status of relevant clinical research concerning current practice in caring for the elderly

---

* Solomon: Professor Emeritus of Medicine/Geriatrics, David Geffen School of Medicine at UCLA, Los Angeles, CA; LoCicero: The Point Clear Charities Professor, Chair of Surgery, Director of the Center for Clinical Oncology, and Director of the Center for Interventional Technologies, The University of South Alabama, Mobile, AL; Rosenthal: Associate Professor of Surgery, Yale University School of Medicine, and Chief, Surgical Service, VA Connecticut Healthcare System, New Haven, CT.

patient. The text is based on extensive, systematic reviews of the literature summarizing the findings of recent research. In some instances, research has begun to fill in the gaps, but usually much more work remains to be done. Eleven chapters report the literature reviews and propose research agenda items in the ten specialties. The eleventh chapter emerged when it became clear that the literature base for cardiac surgery and that for general thoracic surgery are so divergent as to require splitting the coverage of thoracic surgery into two separate chapters. A twelfth chapter deals with the literature and research agenda for cross-cutting issues that are important to the practice of most specialties.

THE AGS–HARTFORD FOUNDATION PROJECT

OVERVIEW

How did this book happen? To answer that question, we need to recount a bit of history. In the early 1990s, Dr. Dennis Jahnigen, Chief of Geriatrics at the University of Colorado School of Medicine and a widely respected leader in academic geriatrics, advanced the then revolutionary idea that the next frontier for improving health care for older adults would lie in the subspecialties of internal medicine and in surgery and certain related medical specialties. Geriatrics, first named and identified as a special field of knowledge in 1909, had lain dormant through most of the twentieth century. A renaissance began in the mid-1970s and gained strength throughout the late 1970s and the next decade. This renaissance, however, was limited to the care of older patients within internal medicine, family medicine, psychiatry, and neurology.

Dr. Jahnigen sought to spark a similar change in other specialties that accounted for a large, crucial segment of the care of older patients. Spurred by Dr. Jahnigen, the American Geriatrics Society (AGS) and the John A. Hartford Foundation joined forces to create the project entitled Increasing Geriatrics Expertise in the Non-Primary Care Specialties, later changed to Increasing Geriatrics Expertise in Surgical and Related Medical Specialties and often shortened to simply the Geriatrics for Specialists project.

The project began in 1992 with a planning grant. The Phase 1 grant ran from 1994 to 1997. It was renewed for Phase 2 from 1997 to 2001 and again for Phase 3 from 2001 to 2005. In Phase 3, the annual budget rose to almost $1.5 million, and several new programs were introduced. Leadership of the project has changed.* When Dr. Jahnigen developed a fatal illness, Dr. David H. Solomon was appointed as co-director of the project, and when Dr. Jahnigen died, Dr. Solomon became the director. A year later, Dr. John R. Burton became co-director. Recently, Dr. Solomon retired as co-director and Dr. Burton became the sole director.

The mission of the Hartford-funded Geriatrics for Specialists project is to improve the health care of elderly Americans by enhancing specialists' knowledge of geriatrics. Its specific objectives are to improve the amount and quality of geriatrics education received by residents in the surgical and related medical specialties, to identify and support specialty faculty in promoting geriatrics training and research within their own professional disciplines, and to assist certifying bodies and professional societies in improving the ability of their constituencies to care for elderly patients.

* Hereinafter, individuals who have participated in the project are identified at first mention by name alone; their titles and affiliations are given in the list of participants in the Acknowledgments.

PROJECT ACCOMPLISHMENTS

The project has accomplished a great deal in the 10 years since its inception. The following list describes the high spots and indicates the breadth of its reach:

- It established working relationships with leaders in all ten of the selected specialties.

- It funded new educational efforts in the geriatrics aspects of all specialties. These have included symposia at national meetings of societies, associations, and academies; the formation of committees, task forces, and special interest groups on aging; the publication of teaching articles in journals; the development of lecture slides, lecture outlines, or other educational tools; the creation of model curricula for residency training in most of the specialties; the establishment of mini-fellowships for research or visits to geriatrics centers; and awards for research presented at national meetings of the societies.

- It organized an Interdisciplinary Leadership Group (ILG) in 1998, which has met annually. It was originally made up of one, and later two, leaders in each specialty, along with Drs. Burton and Solomon and six additional geriatricians who were appointed as deputy directors of the project: Drs. Paul R. Katz, Douglas K. Miller, Myron Miller, Joseph G. Ouslander, Peter Pompei, and Jane F. Potter. Dr. Ouslander retired from this position in 2001 and was replaced by Dr. Evelyn C. Granieri.

- It responded to ideas advanced by members of the ILG at its 1999 meeting by incorporating them into an ambitious, markedly expanded project that began at the onset of Phase 3 in 2001.

- It published a Statement of Principles promoting the development of studies in and the practice of geriatrics in the specialties in the *Journal of the American Geriatrics Society* and in a variety of specialty journals. The Statement often was accompanied by an editorial.

- At the behest of the ILG and with the concurrence of the AGS, it created a Section for Surgical and Related Medical Specialties in the AGS. The Section meets annually as part of the AGS annual meeting. Concomitantly, the ILG was transformed into the governing Council of the Section. Subsequently, all ten of the specialties became official participants in the Council and the Section, and the component societies contribute to meet the costs of maintaining the Section and the movement for geriatrics for specialists.

- Official relationships have been cemented between the AGS, the John A. Hartford Foundation, and the following specialty societies (listed in alphabetical order): American Academy of Ophthalmology (AAO), American Academy of Orthopaedic Surgeons (AAOS), American Academy of Otolaryngology–Head and Neck Surgery (AAO–H&NS), American Academy of Physical Medicine and Rehabilitation (AAPM&R), American College of Emergency Medicine (ACEP), American College of Obstetricians and Gynecologists (ACOG), American Society of Anesthesiologists (ASA), American Urological Association (AUA), Association of Program Directors in Surgery (APDS), Society for Academic Emergency Medicine (SAEM), Society for the Advancement of Geriatric Anesthesia (SAGA), Society of Thoracic Surgeons

(STS), Society of University Urologists (SUU), and Thoracic Surgery Directors Associations (TSDA).

■ It is currently negotiating with the American College of Surgeons (ACS), which in 2001 established an Office of Evidence-Based Surgery. The ACS is in a liaison relationship with the AGS-Hartford project and is exploring ways in which it may participate actively in the Section for Surgical and Related Medical Specialties.

■ It offered the Jahnigen Career Development Awards of $100,000 per year for 2 years to support junior faculty in the specialties while they undertake research training and geriatrics education under joint mentorship of a faculty member in the specialty and one in geriatrics. The first cohort of Jahnigen Award recipients began their studies in July 2002. A second cohort began work in July 2003, and ten Jahnigen Award recipients will be appointed each year for the next several years. The Jahnigen Career Development Award program is funded by The John A. Hartford Foundation and The Atlantic Philanthropies.

■ It offered grants to support experiments in geriatrics education for specialty residents in training sites all over the country. From 1998 to 2001, representatives of 21 programs in 19 institutions participated in the Faculty Development and Residency Training Outreach Program, a precursor to the Geriatrics Education for Specialty Residents (GESR) program. The GESR has provided grants for 29 programs, awards that were based on competitive applications.

■ It has published a concise, groundbreaking *Geriatrics Syllabus for Specialists* (2002), which has been favorably reviewed.

■ And, pertinent to this volume, it has carried out a research agenda–setting process that has culminated in the publication of this book.

THE RESEARCH AGENDA–SETTING PROJECT

MISSION

The mission of the Research Agenda–Setting Project (RASP) is to help develop the area of clinical science that would lead to improved care and outcomes for older patients receiving specialty care. The first step was to review the current state of knowledge—or ignorance—in each discipline and in the cross-cutting issues. The focus of the review was on the ways that the diagnosis and treatment of older patients may differ from that of younger patients, on the geriatric syndromes as they occur in the course of surgery and postoperatively, and on the clinical picture that older patients present to anesthesiologists, emergency medicine physicians, and physiatrists. In developing a research agenda that highlights the importance of geriatric syndromes in complicating the surgical care of older patients, we hope to point researchers in the specialties in directions that ultimately produce better results for specialists and better outcomes for their older patients.

We hope that the publication of this book will lead to increased research activity; attract new researchers to study the unique requirements of the older patient in the surgical and related medical specialties; increase the number of grant applications for such research, thereby leading to increased funding by the National Institutes of Health, the Department of Veterans Affairs, and other agencies; and ensure greater attention to the well-being of older patients in specialty care.

This book may also provide a framework for developing an evidence base for the practice of geriatric surgery. In turn, this may assist the quality-improvement work of the Office of Evidence-Based Surgery of the American College of Surgeons, described recently by Jones and Richards. [1]

HISTORY OF THE PROJECT

The RASP began in 2001 with selection of faculty members, one in each specialty, to serve as content experts. Their assignment was to review the present state of research on the geriatrics aspects of each specialty. A Senior Writing Group (SWG), consisting of one senior leader in each of the ten specialties, was also appointed. The senior writer in each field was charged with assisting and guiding the content expert in conducting the literature review. The SWG also was responsible for identifying the cross-cutting issues and writing a first draft of that chapter.

The content experts met at the RAND Corporation in Santa Monica in February of 2001 to receive instruction in how to conduct a systematic literature review and how to classify research by type of study design. They developed preliminary search strategies, assisted by RAND librarians Roberta Shanman and Amy Atchison. During this process, many of the content experts, in consultation with the librarians, revised their search strategy and created new lists of titles, abstracts, and full papers. In a few instances, the content experts expanded their search independently. In all cases, reference lists from papers were searched for additional relevant earlier publications.

Content experts submitted drafts of literature reviews to the editors, who guided them in making revisions. These revised chapters formed the basis for a working conference in Potomac, MD, in November 2001, which was cosponsored by the Agency for Healthcare Research and Quality (AHRQ). We invited five-person teams in each specialty to attend; each team was made up of the content expert, the senior writer, two at-large leaders in the specialty, and one geriatrician. Each content expert presented the major findings of the literature search, and Dr. Joseph LoCicero presented an early version of the chapter on cross-cutting issues. The specialty teams then met to critique the literature review and start to create the research agenda. Preliminary research agendas were presented to the conference in plenary session, and considerable time was spent reorganizing the topics being covered in the cross-cutting issues chapter. There were no face-to-face meetings after November of 2001. Since then, project participants and leaders have been occupied by some updating of research reviews, further refinement of the chapters, and refinement and coordination of the research agenda items, followed by the final editing and production of this book.

USING THIS BOOK

CHAPTER STRUCTURE

The text in each chapter presents the key elements of the literature review for that specialty or for the cross-cutting issues. The reports discussed are listed in the references section at the end of each chapter (in Chapter 13, they are listed at the ends of sections). Chapters are organized in sections, each on a major clinical topic. Each section ends with the pertinent research agenda items; each item has a unique number to facilitate cross-referencing and citation. Each specialty chapter ends with a discussion of the issues of greatest concern in the care of older patients by practitioners in the discipline. Three key research questions are identified, that is, those having the highest priority in the opinion of the experts participating in the project, and examples of hypothesis-generating and hypothesis-testing research needed to address each key question are provided.

THE LITERATURE REVIEWS

The basic approach for all the literature reviews is described here. Unique features of individual literature reviews are presented in a methods section in each specialty chapter.

Because the objective was to define the current knowledge base, the focus was on recent literature. The general plan was to conduct an English-language search, limited to the human, using MEDLINE (through PubMed or DIALOG). All searches included the terms *65 or older* or *aged* or *geriatric*, followed by a list of content topics of importance in each specialty. The earliest year searched varied, from 1980 to 1994. Searches ended in the first half of 2001, although more recent papers of special significance were often selected and added. The full list of titles of papers resulting from the initial search was sent to the content expert, who selected titles meeting relevance criteria and then obtained abstracts of them. Following this, the content experts chose the papers to examine in full. In general, case reports and letters were excluded at this stage.

In addition, the research consultant maintained a full list of titles from each literature search in an EndNote database. The project director and the research consultant reviewed theses titles (and abstracts, where necessary) for relevance to cross-cutting issue categories. The research consultant obtained full-text copies of the papers selected either from content experts or her local medical library and forwarded these papers to the teams from the Senior Writing Group assigned to each cross-cutting issue category. In some cases, abstracts were substituted for full-text papers. As each chapter was completed, the research consultant added new references to the EndNote database and verified the accuracy of the final list of citations before producing each chapter's citations and references list.

AGENDA ITEMS

The number of agenda items for individual topics varies. Each agenda item is tagged with an abbreviation that indicates the specialty field (eg, "Ophth" for ophthalmology, "GenSurg" for general surgery) and a number, starting with the Arabic 1 in each chapter. The number is *not* meant to indicate importance or priority; it is provided simply to allow for easy cross-reference and citation.

Immediately following its identifying tag, each agenda item is also labeled with a letter from A to D, designating the type of research design and the clinical priority or importance of the proposed study. The word *level* is decidedly not intended to imply degrees of quality. The definitions for A-level through D-level studies are as follows:

- **Level A** identifies important studies with hypothesis-testing intent, using such designs as randomized controlled trials, certain nonrandomized controlled trials, or those cohort studies that focus on a single hypothesis.

- **Level B** identifies important studies with hypothesis-generating intent. Designs would include exploratory, multi-targeted cohort and case-control studies; retrospective or prospective analysis of large databases; cross-sectional observational studies; time series; outcome studies; retrospective case series; or post hoc analyses of randomized controlled trials.

- **Level C** identifies hypothesis-testing studies judged by the content experts to be of lesser importance and priority than those labeled A.

- **Level D** identifies hypothesis-generating studies judged to be of lesser importance than studies labeled B.

Proposed A (or C) studies generally must be preceded by B (or D) studies since research literature on geriatrics aspects of the specialties is today generally deficient in information that would allow for construction of the most efficient and cost-effective controlled trials. Thus, although A studies rank higher in terms of the quality of the evidence they would provide, B studies often have sequence priority over A studies. Therefore, in the chapters that follow, we generally list B studies before the resultant A studies.

The research agenda items are almost entirely focused on clinical research. Where basic science investigations are critically needed to precede any clinical investigation, we have indicated that, classifying such research as level B studies, but we have not suggested details regarding the design and execution of such studies.

The key questions at the end of each chapter are numbered separately from the series of agenda items within the chapter. The hypothesis-generating studies described with each key question are equivalent to level-B designations used elsewhere in the text, and the hypothesis-testing studies are equivalent to level A.

A listing of all research agenda items will be available at the following Web site: <http://www.americangeriatrics.org>.

SPECIALTY DATABASES

Many of the research items call for examination or use of databases maintained by the U.S. Department of Health and Human Services and by various specialty societies. To assist the reader, we have therefore included links to health-related databases used by the authors in their own research, which may be found at <http://www.americangeriatrics.org>. This list does not contain all the relevant databases that are available, but it does include those used most often by the authors. We are not responsible for errors that may exist in the list of links, but we will try to keep it correct and current.

INDEX

All elements in the book are thoroughly indexed by topic: discussions of the literature in all the specialty fields and for each cross-cutting issue, specific studies by name, tables and figures, the agenda items and key questions, descriptions of research design, project history and methods, and more. Wherever the reference in the index is to an agenda item, the page number is bolded, which allows readers to look up a specific topic of particular interest (eg, postoperative delirium) and find all the agenda items in the book that relate to that topic. Index references to tables are signaled by the letter *t* after the page number; figures are likewise referenced with the letter *f* after the page number. When a topic might be referred to by any one of several synonyms, we index it under all the various terms.

REFERENCES

1.   Jones RS, Richards K. Office of Evidence-Based Surgery charts course for improved system of care. Bull Am Coll Surg 2003;88(4):11-21.

2

GERIATRIC ANESTHESIA

David J. Cook, MD*

An aging population carries profound implications for the practice of anesthesiology. Geriatric issues impact every aspect of anesthesiology. First, the preoperative evaluation of the geriatric patient is typically more complex than that of the younger patient because of the heterogeneity of this patient group and the greater number and complexity of comorbid conditions that usually accumulate with age. Perioperative functional status can be difficult to predict because many elderly patients have reduced preoperative function as a consequence of deconditioning, age-related disease, or cognitive impairment. This makes it difficult to adequately assess the patient's ability to respond to the specific stresses associated with surgery. A common example is trying to determine cardiopulmonary reserve in a patient very limited by osteoarthritis. Physiologic heterogeneity and decreased functional reserve are also manifested perioperatively. Normal aging results in changes in cardiac, respiratory, and renal physiology, and the response of the elderly patient to surgical stress is often unpredictable. The pharmacokinetics and pharmacodynamics of elderly and younger patients also differ; moreover, the elderly patient's use of multiple medications may alter homeostatic mechanisms.

This review of research on anesthesia for elderly patients first summarizes the normal physiologic changes that occur with aging, an overview that is essential to frame the discussion of research in the three sections that follow, on preoperative assessment, intraoperative management, and postoperative management of the older surgical patient. Postoperative respiratory complications and delirium are emphasized, and issues of acute and chronic pain management for elderly surgical patients are also highlighted. The goal throughout is to identify needed research in geriatric anesthesiology.

METHODS

The literature search was conducted on the National Library of Medicine's PubMed database. The time period covered was from 1980 to April 2001. The search strategy combined various terms for anesthesia, sedation, analgesics, and opiates with terms for surgical procedures (general or specific commonly performed operations), the terms *elective* and *emergency*, and various terms for the many elements of surgical care: preoperative assessment and management, intraoperative care, perioperative care, postoperative care, complications, and outcomes. Additional requirements were either that the publication be a review, clinical trial, randomized controlled trial, or meta-analysis, or that terms for risk or age factors be present as title words or MeSH headings. Terms denoting age were *age factors, age, aging , elderly, geriatric, gerontologic, older,* or *octogenarian, nonagenarian,* or *centenarian.* Finally, the term *aspirin* was excluded, as it had generated a large number of irrelevant titles in early iterations of this search.

---

* Associate Professor of Anesthesiology, Mayo Clinic and Foundation, Rochester, MN.

AGE-RELATED PHYSIOLOGIC CHANGES AND PERIOPERATIVE CARE

The physiology of aging bears on preoperative assessment, intraoperative and postoperative management, and the types and likelihood of major adverse events. Age-related changes in cardiac, respiratory, neurologic, and renal function as well as in pharmacokinetics have been well defined. The most important generalization from physiologic studies of aging is that the basal function of the various organ systems is relatively uncompromised by the aging process. However, functional reserve, and specifically the ability to compensate for physiologic stress, is greatly reduced (see Figure 2.1). This fact has profound implications for the preoperative assessment and the perioperative care of geriatric patients.

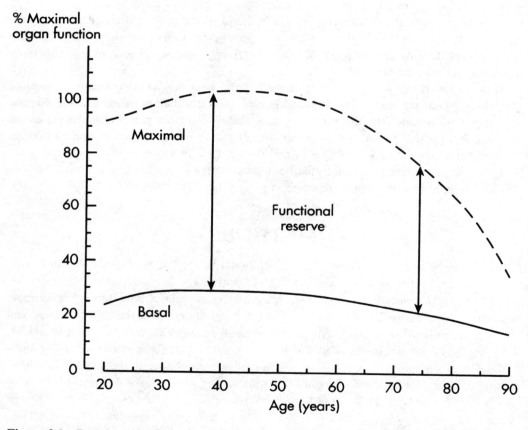

Figure 2.1—Functional reserve is the difference between maximal (*broken line*) and basal (*solid line*) function. Aging inevitably reduces functional reserve even in individuals who are physiologically "young." The configuration of the curve for "basal" function is adapted from longitudinal measurements of total (not weight-specific) basal metabolic rate. (Reprinted with permission with Craven L, ed. *Geroanesthesia: Principles for Management of the Elderly Patient.* St. Louis: Mosby-Year Book, Inc., 1997: figure 1–3.)

CARDIOVASCULAR CHANGES

Numerous changes in cardiovascular function with aging have implications for anesthetic care. With aging, the progressive decrease in the elasticity of the arterial vasculature leads to an increase in systolic blood pressure. Diastolic blood pressure increases through middle age and typically declines after age 60. [1] The cross-sectional area of the peripheral vascular bed also decreases, resulting in a higher peripheral vascular resistance. [2] A decrease in the peripheral vasodilatory response to β-adrenergic stimulation may also contribute to the hypertension of aging. [3]

Progressive ventricular hypertrophy develops in response to increased afterload, resulting in both cellular hypertrophy and deposition of fibrotic tissue. Ventricular hypertrophy increases both wall stress and myocardial oxygen demand and makes the ventricle more prone to ischemia.

Although intrinsic contractility and resting cardiac output are unaltered with aging, the practical effect of ventricular hypertrophy and stiffening is that they limit the ability of the heart to adjust stroke volume. [4] Ventricular hypertrophy impairs the passive filling phase of diastole, making ventricular preload more dependent on the contribution of atrial contraction. At the same time, fatty infiltration and fibrosis of the heart increases the incidence of sinus, atrioventricular, and ventricular conduction defects. [5,6] Myocardial responsiveness to catecholamines also decreases with age; maximal heart rate response is correspondingly decreased. [4,7,8] The reduction in ventricular compliance and the attenuated response to catecholamines compromise the heart's ability to buffer increases in circulatory volume, which results in a predisposition to congestive heart failure. Similarly, even modest decreases in circulatory volume produce hypotension.

From the standpoint of perioperative hemodynamic stability, age-related changes in the autonomic control of heart rate, cardiac output, peripheral vascular resistance, and the baroreceptor response [9–13] are as important as the chronic changes in the myocardium and vasculature. It is evident that age-related changes in the cardiovascular system involve alterations in both mechanics and control mechanisms.

PULMONARY CHANGES

The pulmonary system also undergoes age-related changes in both mechanics and control mechanisms independently of comorbid disease processes. Functionally, there are remarkable parallels with changes in the heart. With aging, the thorax becomes stiffer. [14,15] This may not be evident in the sedentary patient, but reduced chest wall compliance increases the work of breathing and reduces maximal minute ventilation. [14–16] Loss of thoracic skeletal muscle mass aggravates this process. [17] Because of a decrease in elastic lung recoil, the closing volume increases such that by age 65 it exceeds functional residual capacity. [18] Inspiratory and expiratory functional reserve decrease with aging, and the normal matching of ventilation and perfusion decreases. [19,20] The latter process increases the alveolar–arterial O_2 gradient and decreases the resting Pao_2. [18,21] The respiratory response to hypoxia also diminishes in the aged patient. [22] (See Figure 2.2.) In addition, ciliary function is decreased and cough is reduced. [15] Finally, pharyngeal sensation and the motor function required for swallowing are diminished. [23,24]

These changes have important implications in the perioperative period. First, it is difficult to predict from a preoperative interview how an inactive, elderly patient will respond

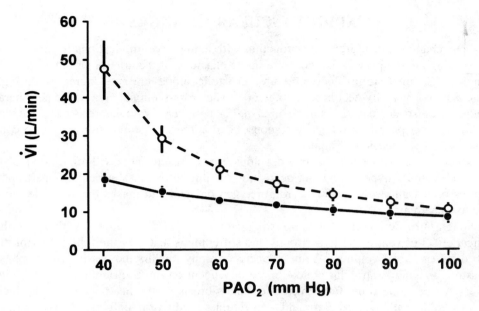

Figure 2.2—Ventilatory response (V_I) to isocapnic progressive hypoxia in eight young normal men (*broken line*) and eight elderly normal men aged 64 to 73 (*solid line*). Values are means ± SEM. BTPS = body temperature, ambient pressure, saturated with water vapor. (Reprinted with permission from Kronenberg RS, Drage CW. Attenuation of the ventilatory and heart rate responses to hypoxia and hypercapnia with aging in normal men. *J. Clin Invest* 1973;52:1812–1819, figure 1.)

to the perioperative respiratory challenges. Anesthetics, postoperative pain, the supine position, narcotics, as well as thoracic and upper abdominal operations impair pulmonary function and further depress respiratory drive. [15,25,26] Although blood gas analysis or spirometric tests may offer some value prior to thoracic operations, the alterations in pulmonary function following surgery are complex and typically not predictable from preoperative pulmonary function testing. [14,20,27] Other implications of age-related changes in pulmonary mechanics and respiratory control are that postoperative hypoxia is likely to occur [28,29] and that the risk of aspiration is significantly increased in the elderly patient. [24,30]

NEUROLOGIC CHANGES

Pulmonary and cardiac complications, respectively, account for most morbidity and mortality in older surgical patients. However, neurologic morbidity affects a large number of patients, and age-related degenerative changes in the central and peripheral nervous systems contribute to a variety of other morbidities. In themselves, neurologic complications have a dramatic impact on length of stay and discharge disposition, translating directly into altered functional status and quality of life.

Independently of any comorbid process, both the central and peripheral nervous systems are affected by aging. [31] There is a loss of cortical gray matter beginning in middle age, resulting in cerebral atrophy, [32] although how much of this is attributable to aging itself or to degenerative diseases is a subject of ongoing investigation. [33] At the level of the neuron, the complexity of neuronal connections decreases, the synthesis of neurotransmitters decreases, and the enzymes responsible for their postsynaptic degradation increase. [32,34,35] While cerebral metabolism, blood flow, and autoregulation generally remain intact, [32] neuronal loss and the deficiency of neurotransmitters limit the ability of the older brain to integrate multiple neural inputs. This has been described as a loss of "fluid" intelligence. Neuronal loss and demyelinization also occur in the spinal cord. [36] Functionally, spinal cord reflexes change and proprioception is reduced. There are also important decreases in hypoxic and hypercarbic drive. [22,37] Declines in visual and auditory function further complicate the ability of the nervous system to acquire and process information. This combination of changes can limit the ability of the older patient to understand and process information in the perioperative period. These changes are probably important contributors to postoperative delirium, drug toxicity, and falls.

Aging is also associated with neuronal loss in the autonomic nervous system. Both sympathetic and parasympathetic ganglia lose neurons, and fibrosis of peripheral sympathetic neurons occurs. This peripheral neuronal adrenergic loss is associated with impairment of cardiovascular reflexes. At the same time, decreases in adrenoceptor responsiveness result in increased adrenomedullary output and plasma catecholamine concentrations. [11,13,36]

Skeletal muscle innervation decreases, translating into loss of motor units and a decrease in strength, coordination, and fine motor control. [38] Joint position and vibration sense may be compromised, and the literature suggests some diminution in the processing of painful stimuli. [39–42] However, this effect, if it exists, appears to be modest at best, and not affecting all nerve types equally. [42–45] Furthermore, given huge inter-patient variability in nervous system function and in the experience of pain, alterations in subtypes of pain perception do not translate into a decreased need for analgesia in the elderly patient. [44–48]

RENAL CHANGES

Aging is accompanied by a progressive decrease in renal blood flow and loss of renal parenchyma. [49,50] By age 80, half of all older persons may have reduced renal blood flow. This is accompanied by renal cortical atrophy, resulting in a 30% decrease in nephrons by the end of middle age. [49,51] Furthermore, aging is associated with sclerosis of remaining nephrons so that some of those remaining are dysfunctional. [50,52] Together, these processes result in a progressive decrease in glomerular capillary surface area and glomerular filtration rate. [50,52–54] However, because of loss of muscle mass, aging is not associated with an increase in serum creatinine. This physiologic, and often occult, aspect of senescence has practical implications in the perioperative period.

The old kidney has difficulty in maintaining circulating blood volume and sodium homeostasis in the perioperative period. [11,53–55] Sodium conservation and excretion are both impaired by aging. Fluid homeostasis is further complicated by alterations in thirst mechanisms and antidiuretic hormone release that frequently result in dehydration. [53–56] In the perioperative period, metabolic acidosis is also relatively common, particularly in elderly patients who are less efficient in the renal excretion of acid. [57]

Reductions in basal renal blood flow render the elderly kidney particularly susceptible to the deleterious effects of low cardiac output, hypotension, hypovolemia, and hemor-

rhage. Anesthetics, surgical stress, pain, sympathetic stimulation, and renal vasoconstric-
tive drugs may all compound subclinical renal insufficiency. The likelihood of acute renal
insufficiency is especially great in intra-abdominal operations and following aortic surgery
and is increased further by many drugs used in the perioperative period. Finally, age-
related decreases in glomerular filtration rate reduce the clearance of a number of drugs
given in the perioperative period.

PHARMACOKINETIC AND PHARMACODYNAMIC CHANGES

Aging is associated with multiple physiologic changes that may affect drug pharmacokinetics.[58] Decreased lean body mass and total body water and an increased proportion of
body fat alter the volume of distribution of drugs, their redistribution among body compartments, and subsequently their rates of clearance and elimination.[59–61] The effect of
changes in body composition on drug distribution and action varies, depending on the
lipid or aqueous solubility of the drug. Water-soluble drugs can have higher serum concentration and lower redistribution, whereas fat-soluble drugs tend to undergo wider distribution and accumulation, followed by delayed release.

Although age-related changes in the proportions of different plasma proteins make predictions about pharmacokinetics complex in the elderly person, for many drugs, decreased
protein binding and increased free fraction have the potential to increase the
pharmacologic effect of drugs administered in the perioperative period.[58] Furthermore,
potential alterations in cardiac output and renal or hepatic clearance may change effective
plasma concentrations and duration of action.[62] Neuronal loss and decreased levels of
neurotransmitters in the central nervous system may increase sensitivity to anesthetic
agents. The changes in pharmacokinetics that occur with aging make it difficult to identify
an independent effect of aging on pharmacodynamics.[59,60] However, age-related changes
in the central nervous system appear to increase the older person's sensitivity to a variety
of anesthetic agents.[63–65] (See Figure 2.3.)

It has been known for decades that pharmacokinetic changes, particularly decreased
metabolism, plus drug interactions coupled with polypharmacy conspire to make the elderly person prone to adverse drug effects.[66–68] There is an almost linear increase in
adverse drug reactions with age, from below 10% at age 25 to above 20% at age 80.[69,70]
The likelihood of adverse drug reactions increases with the number of drugs administered.[66,67] As many elderly patients come to surgery on multiple medications, the addition
of several, even short-acting drugs in the perioperative period makes adverse reactions
likely.[68]

IMPLICATIONS FOR ELDERLY SURGICAL PATIENTS

What is clear from a review of normal changes in physiologic function with aging is that
even the fit elderly patient's ability to compensate for perioperative stress is compromised.
The cardiac, pulmonary, neurologic, and neuroendocrine changes that occur with aging
make hypotension, low cardiac output, hypoxia, hypercarbia, and disordered fluid regulation more likely in the perioperative period. Furthermore, because baseline cardiac, pulmonary, renal, and neurologic function is typically adequate in the absence of acute
challenges, it can be very difficult to predict the effect of perioperative stress on the older
patient.

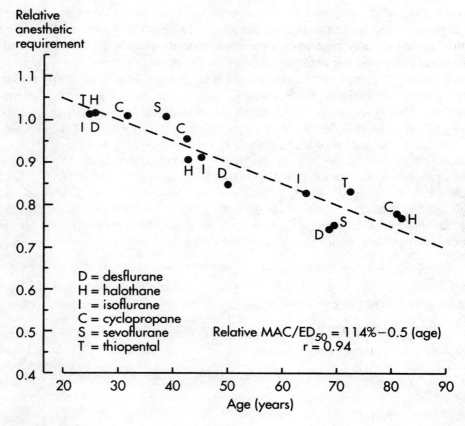

Figure 2.3—With advancing age, anesthetic requirement for unsedated human subjects expressed as relative median effective dose (ED_{50}) or its inhalational equivalent, minimum alveolar concentration (MAC), is progressively and consistently reduced. Anesthetic requirement declines both for inhalational (C, D, H, I, S) and for intravenous (T) anesthetics. (Reprinted with permission from Craven L, ed. *Geroanesthesia: Principles for Management of the Elderly Patient.* St. Louis: Mosby-Year Book, Inc., 1997: figure 3–8.)

PREOPERATIVE ASSESSMENT OF THE ELDERLY PATIENT

The preoperative assessment of the elderly surgical patient is determined by the underlying health of the patient and influenced by the urgency of the procedure. That said, preoperative evaluation could serve several purposes in most patients. Historically, it has served two primary functions: One is to alert the surgical care providers to physiologic conditions that may alter perioperative management, and the other is to determine if medical intervention is indicated before proceeding. Two more contemporary uses of the preoperative assessment are to provide an index of risk and therefore contribute to decisions about the most appropriate intervention, and to provide baseline data on which the success of a surgical intervention might be judged.

Physiologic studies of aging and clinical experience with the elderly population yield three important conclusions that bear on preoperative assessment. First, the geriatric population is tremendously heterogeneous. This concept was superbly expressed by Muravchick, who noted that humans are never so similar as at birth, and never so dissimilar as in old age. [71] The second conclusion is that basal function in most elderly patients is sufficient to meet daily needs, but that under conditions of physiologic stress, impairment in functional reserve becomes evident. Third, it is evident that most older surgical patients have significant comorbidities. Up to 80% of elderly surgical patients have at least one comorbid condition, and one third have three or more pre-existing conditions. [72,73]

In spite of these limitations, even extreme age is not a contraindication to surgery. Acceptable outcomes are reported for operations even in very old patients. [74–78] What is less clear is how to identify which patients will do well and which will do poorly. Even though this has been the subject of considerable research, no area of perioperative anesthetic care and management requires more investigation. The preoperative assessment of the individual patient is composed of four interrelated functions:

■ risk assessment that is based on a stratification of risk derived from population-based studies,

■ the history and physical examination to determine health and functional status,

■ preoperative testing, and

■ in some cases, preoperative optimization.

Each of these functions requires development and better definition for the geriatric surgical population.

RISK ASSESSMENT

Because age itself adds very little additional risk in the absence of comorbid disease, [79] most risk-factor identification and risk-predictive indices have been disease oriented. [80–84] Typically, these investigations have studied a broad age range of patients and in multivariate analyses identified the relative contribution of age and comorbid conditions to surgical morbidity and mortality. [81,82,85–88] Others have looked at the predictive value of the number of comorbid diseases independently of the operative condition or have evaluated the impact of ASA (American Society of Anesthesiologists) status, specific surgical factors, and intra-operative management. [82,88–93]

The applicability of many existing risk indices to the geriatric population is unclear. Because of the prevalence of comorbid conditions, it becomes hard to stratify the older patient population into smaller subsets of more clearly defined risk. The scarcity of population studies of perioperative risk and outcomes specifically in geriatric populations can make choosing the most suitable course of care and providing good information more difficult. Furthermore, elderly patients have some unique risks. In addition to death, myocardial infarction, or congestive heart failure, older patients are particularly more prone than their younger counterparts to postoperative delirium, aspiration, urosepsis, adverse drug interactions, pressure ulcers, malnutrition, falls, and failure to return to ambulation or to home. Therefore, preoperative assessment tools and the variables evaluated in outcomes trials require expansion for application to the geriatric surgical population.

Population studies need to examine not only mortality and major cardiopulmonary morbidity but also outcomes specific to the geriatric population. Once completed, epidemiologic studies that better stratify older patients would help define the preoperative assessment appropriate to older patients.

FUNCTIONAL ASSESSMENT

The efficacy of preoperative functional evaluation in elderly surgical patients requires investigation. This is important for several reasons. The evaluation of the "resting" patient does not indicate how the patient will respond to the cardiac, pulmonary, and metabolic demands of the perioperative period. This approach is emphasized in the guidelines of the American College of Cardiology and the American Heart Association for preoperative cardiac evaluation, in which the patient's activity level, expressed in metabolic units, is a primary determinant of the need for subsequent evaluation. [80] However, this concept must be expanded because the geriatric population has a unique need for functional evaluation in more areas than just cardiopulmonary capacity. Because of patient heterogeneity, functional assessments may be indicated to better characterize patient differences, whether it is for activities of daily living (ADLs), instrumental activities of daily living (IADLs), cognitive and emotional status, or urologic function. [94,95] Scales like the Medical Outcomes Study Short Form–36 (SF-36) [96] have multiple domains that are particularly useful in assessing older patients. Although these metrics have been applied successfully in orthopedic and thoracic surgery [97–99] and can have predictive value for longer term outcomes, [100–104] multidimensional assessment and perioperative functional assessment are largely absent from the surgical literature. [98,105,106]

An example of their application is provided in the study of hip fracture patients by Keene and Anderson, who scored patients preoperatively on the basis of physical condition, ambulation, ADLs, preoperative living situation, and pre-existing disabilities. [102] The scoring system was then used to predict which patients would be discharged to nursing homes following surgery. The actual outcome following surgery was observed for 1 year and compared with the models' predictions (see Table 2.1). Though the study is small, it serves as an example of the type of research needed in geriatric surgery.

Table 2.1—Predicted and Actual Outcomes 1 Year After Hip Fracture Surgery in 39 Elderly Patients

Patients (N)	Residence Before Fracture	Predicted Nursing Home Placement	Actual Nursing Home Placement	Functional Rating* (avg)
10	Home	Temporary	Temporary	72
8	Home	Temporary	Permanent	52
6	Home	Permanent	Permanent	51
15	Nursing Home	Permanent	Permanent	30

* Functional rating was the composite score of five scales: physical condition (maximum 35 points), ambulation (maximum 30 points), activities of daily living (maximum 25 points), prefracture living situation (maximum 10 points), and prefracture disabilities (maximum points 0, maximum deduction for disabilities −40).

SOURCE: Keene JS, Anderson CA. Hip fractures in the elderly: discharge predictions with a functional rating scale. *JAMA* 1982;248:564–567, table 1. Modified with permission.

With regard to preoperative functional assessment, cognitive and psychologic evaluation of the elderly surgical patient deserve special comment. Although frank delirium or dementia at admission clearly predicts poorer acute and long-term outcome, [107,108] subtle forms of cognitive impairment are infrequently diagnosed prior to surgery even though they are more common in elderly patients. In the absence of careful screening, preoperative cognitive deficits may not become evident until the postoperative period. Subtle forms of cognitive impairment can predict subsequent delirium in hospitalized medical patients [109] and worsened cognitive outcome in cardiac, orthopedic, and gastrointestinal surgery patients. [110–114] Preoperative mental status examination [115,116] should be considered for all geriatric surgical patients. Preoperative depression and alcohol abuse are also relatively common and can affect postoperative outcomes in similar ways; [107,117–119] a variety of assessment tools for depression are available. [120,121] The impact of screening for mental status, depression, and alcohol abuse on perioperative management of elderly patients is a huge potential area of investigation.

Preoperative functional assessment is important because the goal should be to return the patient to at least his or her preoperative activity level. The success of surgery must be questioned if the procedure is technically adequate but the patient suffers loss of independence. Multidimensional assessment may help redefine standards for success of surgery and thus reset therapeutic priorities. [97,98,122–124] Application of this type of assessment is exemplified by the work of Mangione et al, who longitudinally measured quality-of-life indicators in patients undergoing hip, thoracic, and aortic surgery. [98] A variety of metrics, including the SF-36, were used to measure physical, psychologic, and social functions and health perceptions preoperatively as well as 1, 6 and 12 months after surgery. (See Figure 2.4 for examples.) Major morbidity and mortality aside, these types of measures address what is fundamentally most important in the medical management of older patients: whether the surgical intervention improves functional status and well-being. These measures are of particular importance to the elderly patient because, unlike the younger patient, the older one is at far greater risk for long-term functional compromise following the stress of surgery.

PREOPERATIVE TESTING

The third dimension of the preoperative evaluation of the elderly surgical patient is preoperative testing. Work in this area has been done for large populations of mixed-age groups. However, it is not clear whether selected preoperative screening tests have a different yield in the elderly age group or, more likely, if specific testing is indicated for elderly patient populations undergoing certain types of surgical procedures.

In the general population there is agreement that most routine tests are not indicated. [125–128] In an evaluation of preoperative screening in 1010 persons undergoing cholecystectomy, abnormal results were found in only 4.5% of tests. [125] In another investigation of 3131 patients aged 0 to 98 years who underwent 38,286 tests, unexpected abnormal results were found in 15% of patients. [126] However, only 3% had a change in their anesthetic or surgical plan that was based on those results. Unfortunately, in neither report was age-specific data provided, so it is unclear if the results can be applied to an elderly surgical population.

Smaller studies of elderly populations suggest that there is a higher yield for specific tests. Seymour et al examined the value of routine chest x-ray (CXR) in 223 patients aged

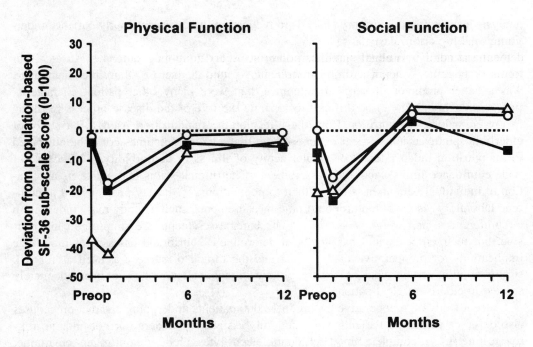

Figure 2.4—Deviation from age- and gender-adjusted population-based SF-36 subgroup scores by surgical procedure. Triangles indicate thoracic surgery for lung cancer; filled squares, total hip arthroplasty; open circles, abdominal aortic aneurysm; dotted line, age- and gender-adjusted population-based value. (Modified with permission from Mangione CM, Goldman L, Orav EJ, et al. Health-related quality of life after elective surgery: measurement of longitudinal changes. *J Gen Intern Med* 1997;12:686–697, figure 2.)

65 years and older undergoing general surgery. [129] Of these, 40% had an abnormality regarded as clinically significant, although in only 5% of the patients did the CXR affect the course of treatment. Seymour et al also examined the value of an electrocardiogram (ECG) in routine screening in 222 patients aged 65 years and older, finding that only 21% of patients had a normal ECG and that 53% had a major abnormality. [130] They reported that although only 1% of patients had abnormalities that delayed surgery, 30% developed new ECG abnormalities postoperatively. The authors concluded that the screening ECG has little or no value for predicting cardiac complications but recommended preoperative ECG for all elderly patients to provide a basis for comparison and as a means of detecting patients for whom surgery should be deferred.

In a small study of acutely ill elderly (mean age 81 years) medical patients (50 admissions), Sewell et al examined the value of full blood cell count, sedimentation rate, urinalysis, electrolyte, liver, thyroid tests, and CXR. [131] Six of 28 patients had abnormalities on CXR (21%), although management was influenced only in one. The most important finding in the screening battery was the frequency of unknown urinary tract infections (16 of 50 patients, 32%). A different retrospective analysis of 86 patients undergoing hip arthroplasty studied the impact of 24 laboratory tests on postoperative course. [132] In four patients (4.6%) care was altered, three of whom had urinary tract infections. A cost-benefit analysis justified routine urinary analysis to reduce hip infections in elderly patients undergoing total hip arthroplasty.

Assessment of nutritional status can also be useful in subpopulations of surgical patients. A 44-center Veterans Administration study found that serum albumin concentration was a better predictor of surgical outcomes than were many other patient characteristics. [133,134] Though it can be difficult to separate the role of the disease process resulting in protein-calorie malnutrition from the effect of the malnutrition itself, [135] a study of elderly hospitalized nonsurgical patients found that adverse outcomes could be attributed to malnutrition independently of greater acuity of illness or comorbidity. [136] Because of wide confidence limits, laboratory assessment of nutritional status may make its application to individual patients less useful than to populations. [135] It may prove useful to combine laboratory tests with anthropomorphic measurements, such as body mass index, limb circumferences, and weight loss. [137–140] The latter assessments are simple and inexpensive, but their clinical yield has not been determined. Nutritional assessment may have implications for preoperative management and the timing of surgery as well as for risk stratification in certain types of surgery, but nutritional evaluation has not been adequately studied in elderly surgical patients.

A recent study on preoperative testing in 18,000 patients undergoing cataract procedures also deserves comment. Patients were randomly assigned to undergo or not undergo routine testing (ECG, complete blood cell count, electrolytes, blood urea nitrogen, creatinine, and glucose). [141] The analysis was stratified by age and showed no benefit to routine testing for any group of patients. Similar conclusions were drawn in a study of 544 elderly noncardiac surgical patients by Dzankic et al. [142]

From these investigations and a body of work in younger subjects, three themes become evident. First, routine screening in a general population of elderly patients does not add significantly to information obtained in the clinical history. Second, in a general population, the positive predictive value of abnormal findings on routine screening is limited. Third, positive results on screening tests have relatively little impact on the course of patient care. In spite of those observations, further research is required.

Even though the yield for routine screening is very low, it can be clinically valuable and cost-effective to develop guidelines for preoperative testing that are based on the type of surgery. It is evident that different types of surgery impose different types and degrees of physiologic stress. The results of the cataract trial will not be applicable to patients undergoing vascular surgery. Preoperative tests such as echocardiography and thallium scanning can have predictive value and potentially alter the course of care and outcomes if applied to specific populations at higher risk. [80,143,144] Similarly, nutritional assessment [134,145] might be very useful prior to abdominal or major orthopedic surgery but would have a much lower impact for carotid endarterectomy. Screening for urinary tract infection prior to orthopedic surgery or pulmonary function testing prior to thoracic surgery are other examples. Because it is the interaction of the patient and the surgical stress that determines outcome, specific testing might be equally indicated in a very physiologically challenged older patient undergoing minimally stressful surgery (hernia repair), and in the mildly compromised older patient undergoing surgery that imposes severe physiologic stress (eg, aortic aneurysm surgery). Future studies of older patients will need to stratify patients according to the severity of their pre-existing risk factors (low, intermediate, or high) and specifically examine the interaction of these factors with the specific surgical challenges most common in the elderly age group.

PREOPERATIVE OPTIMIZATION

The fourth dimension of preoperative evaluation determines whether medical intervention is indicated before proceeding with surgery. To some extent, this dimension has been lost with the foreshortening of the preoperative period, the "AM admit," and a progressive elimination of preoperative testing.

If we are going to define research agendas for the care of elderly surgery patients, preoperative optimization of medical status must be revisited. This is an area where relatively little work has been done. Again, in specific populations undergoing high-risk surgery, the value of preoperative optimization, particularly of cardiac and pulmonary status, can be demonstrated. Examples where the data are compelling include intervention for coronary disease before vascular surgery; pulmonary toilet, antibiotics, and corticosteroid therapy for some types of thoracic surgery; and preoperative β-blockade. [143,144,146–150] Nevertheless, many areas have not been evaluated, particularly in the elderly population. Improving nutritional status before major elective surgery, preoperative hydration, and optimization of renal function in those with chronic or acute insufficiency could have broad impact. Preoperative management of antibiotic therapy, anticoagulation, antiplatelet therapy, and anemia are other obvious areas to examine. There are also suggestions that preoperative education, psychologic support, and physical therapy might facilitate pain management and rehabilitation following some types of surgery, [151,152] but these have not been adequately assessed.

In today's environment it will be difficult to conduct studies on preoperative optimization. It will be difficult to justify randomizing a patient to a control group when he or she is clearly malnourished and surgery can be delayed. Moreover, intervention and delay will add costs. However, limited studies in orthopedic and cardiac surgical patients suggest that appropriately applied preoperative care can be cost-effective in shortening hospital stays or improving functional status following discharge. [152,153] Preoperative optimization will not be practical or necessary in many instances; however, much geriatric surgery is elective, so these studies can be conducted and, if positive, could affect large numbers of patients.

THE PREOPERATIVE RESEARCH AGENDA

The most pressing need for preoperative assessment is to develop better tools to predict which patients will do well and which will do poorly (see also Key Research Questions in Geriatric Anesthesia, end of chapter).

> **Anes 1 (Level B)**: **Prospective epidemiologic studies are needed to describe the relative frequency of various outcomes characteristic of older surgical patients for the most common types of surgery.**

> **Anes 2 (Level B)**: **Once better understanding of characteristic outcomes of specific types of surgery for older patients is attained, patient- and surgery-specific risk factors for geriatric complications should be identified by multivariate analysis that would stratify surgical risk as low, intermediate, or high, depending on type of surgery.**

Anes 3 (Level B): **The positive predictive value of preoperative assessment instruments should be determined in prospective nonrandomized or prospective cohort trials.**

Anes 4 (Level A): **Following evaluation of preoperative assessment instruments (Anes 3), prospective randomized trials should be performed to determine whether the application of these metrics could improve outcomes for elderly surgical patients by altering perioperative intervention, surgical timing, the type or extent of surgery, or postoperative management.**

Anes 5 (Level B): **Prospective cohort studies are needed to determine whether assessment of the older surgical patient's preoperative functional status affects surgical decision making or perioperative care.**

Anes 6 (Level A): **Depending on findings of prospective cohort studies (Anes 5), randomized trials should be performed to determine whether preoperative functional status assessment of elderly patients changes decisions about type or timing of surgery, or pre- or postoperative care strategies and outcomes.**

Anes 7 (Level B): **Cross-sectional or prospective cohort studies are needed to determine by multivariate analysis whether there is an association between pre-existing cognitive impairment, depression, or alcohol abuse and adverse outcomes in geriatric patients.**

Anes 8 (Level A): **For any association that is established by cross-sectional cohort studies between cognitive impairment, depression, or alcohol abuse and adverse outcomes in elderly surgical patients (Anes 7), prospective randomized trials should be performed to determine the effect of pre- or postoperative interventions on these adverse outcomes.**

INTRAOPERATIVE MANAGEMENT

Anesthetic care is episodic, so most of the criteria to judge the success of anesthetic interventions are short-term. Studies of anesthetic drugs and techniques typically address hemodynamic stability, time to awakening, extubation time, postoperative nausea and vomiting, recovery room time, and length of stay. Awareness of the physiologic and pharmacokinetic changes characteristic of the elderly patient have led investigators to examine the effects of a host of anesthetic agents and adjuncts in this population. The effects on elderly patients of intravenous induction agents, narcotics, benzodiazepines, volatile anesthetics, neuromuscular blocking agents, and various types of local anesthetics have all been evaluated. Studies have included the use of these agents for inpatient surgical procedures, outpatient procedures, premedication, sedation, and their administration by bolus and infusion techniques. Because there is a theoretical advantage to shortening recovery time in patients for whom awakening, ambulation, and discharge might otherwise be delayed (ie, elderly patients), much of the more recent work focusing on elderly patients has been devoted to the ultra–short-acting agents.

Some of these studies have identified age-related alterations in the pharmacokinetics, induction, awakening, or recovery room stay. However, perspective is needed. Even though a drug may shorten extubation time by 10 minutes, recovery room time by 45 minutes, or total hospitalization for an outpatient procedure by 90 minutes, the clinical impact of these changes on patient outcomes is probably minimal. There is a role for this type of research in geriatric anesthesia, but in an era of limited time and research dollars, research efforts should probably be directed elsewhere.

REGIONAL VERSUS GENERAL ANESTHESIA

Most general anesthetic agents depress cardiovascular and pulmonary function as well as alter consciousness, which is why it is often advocated that regional anesthesia be used for geriatric patients whenever possible. A major area of research has been to compare the risks and benefits of regional versus general anesthesia in elderly surgical patients. Elderly patients undergoing orthopedic procedures have been the focus of such research. These comparative studies have examined intraoperative cardiovascular stability; cardiac, pulmonary, and thrombotic complications; pain control; and cognitive outcomes. This subject was reviewed recently by Roy. [154]

A few early studies reported that regional anesthesia for hip surgery was associated with better outcomes. Reduced mortality, higher postoperative Pao_2, and fewer mental changes have been reported in patients receiving regional anesthesia. [155,156] However, these studies were very small, and their assessment of cognitive function would not meet current standards for reliability or validity. [157]

Subsequent investigations of elderly patients undergoing hip surgery found that intraoperative hypotension is more common with regional anesthesia, and although the incidence of deep-vein thrombosis (DVT) and blood loss were typically lower with regional techniques, no difference in major morbidity or mortality could be identified. [85,158–163] Because most of these studies are underpowered for rare events, meta-analysis has been used to help address statistical limitations.

The respective benefits of regional and general anesthesia were addressed in a 1992 meta-analysis. [164] Sorenson and Pace examined 13 randomized controlled trials conducted between 1966 and 1991 that reported follow-up to at least 1 month. Meta-analysis endpoints were mortality, DVT, and blood loss. Other complications or adverse events were not evaluated because of inconsistencies in definitions or "the absence of systematic and unbiased application of diagnostic tests to record these events." Sorenson and Pace were unable to identify any statistically significant difference in mortality or blood loss by anesthetic technique, although the study found a clearly reduced incidence of DVT in regional anesthesia groups. Most of the data in the study were recently reanalyzed in another meta-analysis, along with some additional trials. [165] Like Sorenson and Pace's, the analysis by Urwin et al identified reduced DVT and 1-month mortality in 2162 hip-fracture patients receiving regional anesthesia, although no other outcome measure reached statistical significance. [165] (See Figure 2.5.) The reduction in mortality, when that information was available, was not evident at 3, 6, or 12 months. Subsequent large, single-center observational studies involving 741, [166] 1333, [167] and 9425 [168] patients have also not identified meaningful differences in cardiopulmonary morbidity or mortality between regional and general anesthesia in hip-surgery patients.

Outcome Differences in Patients Undergoing Surgery with Regional or General Anesthesia

Outcome	T/P	Incidence (regional)		Incidence (general)		PETO OR (95% CI)	PETO OR (95% CI)
		No.	%	No.	%		
Mortality (1 mo)	7/1,578	49/766	6.4	76/812	9.4		0.66 (0.47-0.96)
Mortality (3 mo)	6/1,491	88/726	12.1	98/765	12.8		0.91 (0.67-1.24)
Mortality (6 mo)	3/1,264	103/613	16.8	105/651	16.1		1.05 (0.78-1.41)
Mortality (12 mo)	2/726	80/354	22.5	78/372	21.0		1.10 (0.77-1.57)
Operative hypotension	7/873	146/426	34.3	116/447	26.0		1.51 (1.12-2.02)+ 1.21 (0.65-2.25)*
Patients receiving transfusion	3/228	63/108	58.3	68/120	56.7		1.02 (0.58-1.80)
Postoperative hypoxia	1/57	10/28	35.7	14/29	48.3		0.60 (0.21-1.71)
Pneumonia	8/1,096	27/529	5.1	31/567	5.5		0.92 (0.53-1.59)
Myocardial infarction	4/888	4/431	0.9	8/457	1.8		0.51 (0.16-1.63)
Cerebrovascular accident	7/1,085	10/529	1.9	6/556	1.1		1.72 (0.64-4.63)
Congestive cardiac failure	6/902	11/439	2.5	12/463	2.6		0.97 (0.42-2.23)
Renal failure	4/796	2/382	0.5	3/414	0.7		0.77 (0.13-4.50)
Acute confusional state	3/167	10/83	12.0	19/84	22.6		0.47 (0.21-1.06)
Urine retention	2/97	10/48	20.8	10/49	20.4		1.02 (0.39-2.71)
Nausea and vomiting	2/95	2/46	4.3	3/49	6.1		0.69 (0.12-4.13)
Deep vein thrombosis	4/259	39/129	30.2	61/130	46.9		0.41 (0.23-0.72)
Pulmonary embolism	9/1,184	8/575	1.4	10/609	1.6		0.84 (0.33-2.13)

B J Anaesth 84:450, 2000

0.1 0.2 0 5 10

CP1044166B-1

Figure 2.5—Comparison of outcome between regional and general anesthesia for dichotomous variables. All results were derived by the use of fixed-effects analysis except for those marked *, which were derived by the use of random-effects analysis. Statistically significant results are indicated by +. Results to the left of the vertical line indicate an advantage for regional anesthesia over general anesthesia. Results show the incidence of each outcome measure. T = number of trials; P = number of patients; OR = odds ratio; CI = confidence intervals. (Reprinted with permission from Urwin SC, Parker MJ, Griffiths R. General versus regional anesthesia for hip fracture surgery: a meta-analysis of randomized trials. *Br J Anaesth* 2000;84:450–455, table 2.)

Another meta-analysis was conducted by Rodgers et al. [169] The authors examined the effects of regional anesthesia in 141 randomized trials involving 9559 patients. As in the report by Urwin et al, these researchers found a reduction in 30-day mortality and DVT in the regional group; the effect on mortality was not evident beyond 1 month. They also describe reductions in pulmonary embolism, transfusion, respiratory depression, myocardial infarction, and renal failure. Although the results are enticing, the reporting of many outcomes was incomplete across studies, so the analysis was based on smaller subsets of patients. Additionally, studies were not rated for quality, and data were used that were not reported in the published trial. Studies for general, obstetrical and gynecologic, urologic, orthopedic, and "other" surgeries were combined, and no information about age is provided. Finally, it is impossible to base practice on the results of this meta-analysis because all of the following groups of patients were combined in the regional anesthesia group: those receiving spinal anesthesia alone, those receiving epidural anesthesia alone, those receiving general anesthesia followed by postoperative regional anesthesia, those receiving general anesthesia combined with intraoperative spinal anesthesia, and those receiving general anesthesia combined with intraoperative epidural anesthesia. Additionally, in 22 studies where general anesthesia was combined with regional anesthesia, the general anesthesia in the regional group differed from that in the general anesthesia alone group. From this, it is difficult to determine if the effects described in the meta-analysis are real and, if so, what their origin is, or which patients they would apply to. It is certainly not possible to recommend any practice on the basis of the results.

In addition to the more typical outcomes measures, several of the studies of orthopedic surgery patients have examined the effect of anesthetic technique on cognitive or functional outcome, often following patients for 3 months or longer. Each of the prospective studies is small, and only the study by Hole et al [156] showed regional anesthesia to be associated with better cognitive outcome in elderly patients undergoing hip or knee surgery. The bulk of investigations could identify no difference. [117,157,170–172]

Even though not all the studies are in agreement, [173,174] similar conclusions must be drawn for patients undergoing regional or general anesthesia for transurethral prostatectomy and peripheral vascular surgery. [172,175–178] In carotid surgery there is a suggestion of a better outcome with a regional technique; however, most investigations are retrospective or nonrandomized, so the effect of patient selection cannot be eliminated. [179–182] Additionally, in the multicenter North American Symptomatic Carotid Endarterectomy Trial, an independent effect of anesthetic technique (or intraoperative monitoring) on carotid surgical outcome could not be found. [183]

The difficulty in identifying clear and meaningful differences between regional and general anesthesia has tremendous implications for the conduct of research in geriatric anesthesia. Probably the most substantive difference in the choice of anesthetic is whether the patient undergoes a regional or a general anesthetic. The pharmacologic difference with that choice is far greater than the difference between different induction agents, narcotics, local anesthetics, or muscle relaxants, or between different doses of those medications. If little or no difference in outcome can be identified for elderly patients undergoing major procedures with general or regional anesthesia, then the yield for similar outcome studies on differing anesthetic agents is likely to be low.

PHYSIOLOGIC MANAGEMENT

In addition to establishing a surgical plane of anesthesia, the anesthesiologist maintains physiologic stability. Although numerous studies have examined the relationship between intraoperative physiologic management and outcome, outside of relatively rare catastrophic events, such as loss of the airway or uncontrolled hemorrhage, it appears that physiologic management plays a modulatory rather than a primary role in outcomes. The best example is in cardiac surgery, where the acute changes in blood pressure, hematocrit, and temperature typically exceed those seen with any other type of surgery. Additionally, most of the patients are older. In spite of that, it has been difficult to demonstrate a direct relationship between physiologic management and outcome. [184–186] Rather, it appears that technical issues during surgery and the comorbidities that the patient brings to the operating room primarily determine outcome. [187,188]

There is a role for specific studies of physiologic or pharmacologic management in elderly surgical patients, but those investigations are likely to have a smaller yield than risk stratification based on population studies and tailoring the surgical procedure to the patient on the basis of preoperative assessment.

It is important to note that these conclusions are not an indictment of anesthetic practice or the role of the anesthesiologist in the operating room. Just the opposite is true. Over the past three decades, anesthesiology has made tremendous strides in patient safety, monitoring, drugs, and education that have made the intraoperative period extraordinarily safe. Those advances will continue to expand what is possible surgically. At the same time, it is because the advances in intraoperative care have been so great that the greatest needs for research lie in the preoperative assessment and the postoperative management of patients.

There are also broad areas related to intraoperative management (rather than the specifics of anesthetic choice) where research focused on the elderly patient would be productive. It is clear that anesthetics and alterations in autonomic function make it more difficult for older patients to maintain their body temperature, and postoperative hypothermia increases the risk of adverse outcomes. [189-193] Studies of temperature control in older patients could be expanded. The appropriate place for prophylactic β-blockade, antiplatelet agents, and H_2 blockers in elderly surgical patients needs to be examined. Given that the immune response may be attenuated in elderly persons and that infectious complications are very common, the appropriate dosage and scheduling for perioperative antibiotics may be a useful area of research. Furthermore, elderly patients receive most of blood given in the perioperative period, so investigation of the immunosuppressive effects of homologous blood transfusion would be instructive. Elderly patients are also at increased risk for musculoskeletal and nerve injury, as well as thrombotic complications. Therefore, documenting the relationship between patient positioning, nerve and skin injury, and thrombotic complications is indicated. Similarly, the appropriateness of nothing-by-mouth (NPO) status, its relationship to hypovolemia, and aspiration risk in the elderly patient would be an area of research with a large potential impact on practice and patient satisfaction.

The fact that anesthetic choice or physiologic management has little independent effect on outcome is not surprising. Very large studies of perioperative morbidity and mortality have found that, apart from catastrophic events, the anesthetic episode per se appears to have little or no impact on 30-day outcomes. [89,92,194] Although certain pathophysiologic processes may be initiated during the intraoperative period, with few exceptions, major morbidity and mortality in the operating room are rare.

THE INTRAOPERATIVE RESEARCH AGENDA

Anes 9 (Level B): **Cross-sectional or retrospective case-control studies are needed to identify the incidence of adverse cardiac or thrombotic-embolic complications in elderly patients undergoing surgery with and without preoperative β-blockade, antithrombotic or antiplatelet therapy, or with a hematocrit above a target value. These studies should be in surgeries identified as having an intermediate or high risk for related complications.**

Anes 10 (Level A): **For any association in elderly patients of cardiac thrombotic-embolic complications with a specific preoperative therapy or hematocrit level, prospective cohort or randomized** studies are needed to determine if pre- or intraoperative therapies would reduce the complications.

Anes 11 (Level D): Prospective nonrandomized investigation of the effect of perioperative temperature management on surgical morbidity in the geriatric population is needed. These investigations should be conducted under conditions where either the surgery is physiologically very challenging or the older patient carries a high burden of comorbidity. Cardiac, respiratory, bleeding, and renal outcomes would be the primary focus of these investigations.

Anes 12 (Level D): Retrospective or cross-sectional research studies should be conducted to identify any relationship between the use or timing of perioperative antibiotic therapy and postoperative pneumonia or wound infection. Differences, if any, between younger and older patients undergoing the same type of surgery should also be examined.

Anes 13 (Level C): Depending on the findings in Anes 12, prospective randomized studies should be used to determine whether preoperative or postoperative antibiotic therapies reduce complications related to infections in elderly surgical patients.

Anes 14 (Level D): Multicenter case-control or prospective cohort studies should be performed to determine whether receiving or not receiving blood in the perioperative period affects the incidence of perioperative infection and immunosuppression in elderly patients. Multivariate analysis would be required to separate the effect of homologous blood transfusion from the comorbid conditions making transfusion more likely.

Anes 15 (Level C): If perioperative infection and immunosuppression in older surgical patients are shown to be associated with receiving blood in the preoperative period (Anes 14), alternative strategies such as delaying surgery or erythropoietin therapy should then be compared with blood transfusion in prospective cohort studies, because a randomized trial could not be justified.

Anes 16 (Level D): Cohort or case-control studies are needed to determine the relationship in older surgical patients between perioperative termination of anticoagulation and thromboembolic or bleeding risk.

Anes 17 (Level C): The effect of timing of termination and resumption as well as the temporizing use of antiplatelet agents in older surgical patients should be compared in case-control or prospective cohort studies.

Anes 18 (Level B): In prospective cohort studies the incidence of perioperative hypotension, aspiration, and renal insufficiency should be compared in elderly patients undergoing standard nothing-by-mouth orders before surgery and in elderly patients

who would be allowed clear liquids closer to the time of surgery. This study would need to be conducted in:

- **patients undergoing specific types of procedures where liberalization of fluid intake is not contraindicated for surgical reasons,**

- **patients undergoing procedures that place them at greater risk for developing hypovolemia (bowel prep), and**

- **instances where preoperative hypovolemia may contribute to complications (angiographic procedures).**

POSTOPERATIVE MANAGEMENT

Most surgical morbidity and mortality occurs in the postoperative period. Pedersen et al examined perioperative mortality in 7306 adult patients undergoing lower-risk surgery (no cardiac, thoracic, or neurosurgical procedures) and found that mortality during anesthesia was 0.05% (1:1800). [85] In the first 24 hours the mortality was twice as high, 0.1%, and it rose fivefold over the next 6 days to 0.56%. Morbidity, including myocardial ischemia and infarction, stroke, renal insufficiency, pneumonia, and delirium, is also most common postoperatively. [183,195,196]

POSTOPERATIVE RESPIRATORY INSUFFICIENCY

The most common morbidity following noncardiac surgery is respiratory. A Veterans Administration study of 84,000 patients (97% male, mean age of 60) found that 17% of patients experienced complications, with pneumonia in 3.6%, ventilatory failure in 3.2%, and unplanned intubation in 2.4%. [88] In a study of 288 general surgical patients aged 65 and over, Seymour and Vaz reported that 17% of patients had atelectasis, 12% had acute bronchitis, and 10% developed pneumonia. [197]

For many reasons, postoperative hypoxia may occur in 20% to 60% of elderly surgical patients. [28,29] As highlighted previously, elderly patients have an increased alveolar-arterial gradient, reduced respiratory muscle strength, and hypoxic and hypercarbic drives at baseline. [14,20,27] Additionally, there is a progressive loss of airway reflexes with age, and apnea and periodic breathing following administration of narcotics are more common. [18,25,198] Postoperative pain, atelectasis, and fluid shifts further increase the likelihood of respiratory complications, as do reductions in cardiac output, hemoglobin concentration, and shivering. [19,191] The supine position during recovery increases the transpulmonary shunt and makes hypoxia more likely. [18] Finally, orthopedic and upper abdominal surgeries, which are common in elderly persons, have an independent effect in increasing postoperative hypoxia and respiratory complications. [26,197,199]

In spite of the frequency of postoperative hypoxia and hypercarbia in elderly surgical patients, clear guidelines for oxygen therapy, pulse oximetry, and capnography in older patients have been poorly defined. [200,201] This issue is of pressing importance, as "day surgery" has increased and continued efforts are made to abbreviate the time to discharge. Further, more and more patients, most of them elderly, undergo conscious sedation outside the operating room environment. Even though the study by Bailey et al is more than 10 years old, its implications are unchanged.[202] In a study of hypoxemia and apnea after sedation with fentanyl and midazolam, they describe deaths associated with the use of these drugs. Of 86 reported U.S. deaths, "All but three . . . occurred outside the operating room . . . where patients are typically unattended by anesthesia personnel." Determination of the requirements for oxygen therapy, pulse oximetry, and capnography in elderly patients undergoing inpatient and outpatient surgery, including procedures with conscious sedation, is indicated.

The risk of postoperative aspiration for the elderly surgical patient also requires attention. Because of alterations in pharyngeal function, diminished cough, and an increased incidence of gastroesophageal reflux, elderly patients are at increased risk of aspiration.[23,24] This risk is accentuated by the effect of anesthesia, sedatives, and narcotics as well as by endotracheal intubation, nasogastric tube placement, and upper abdominal or neck surgery.[30,203,204] Even though the incidence of aspiration in the operative period is low and is uncommonly associated with clinically important pneumonitis or pneumonia,[205] the risk for aspiration extends well beyond the acute operative period.

It is likely that instrumentation of the pharynx, whether from an endotracheal tube,[30] nasogastric tube,[204] or a transesophageal echocardiography probe,[203] alters sensation, motor function, and the protective reflexes preventing aspiration. For patients with prolonged endotracheal intubation ($>$ 24 hours), this effect is persistent for at least 48 hours following extubation.[30] Nasogastric tubes may also contribute to aspiration by increasing the incompetence of the gastroesophageal junction. Pharyngeal dysfunction and aspiration may be related to a greater acuity of illness, but sufficient evidence suggests pharyngeal trespass itself has independent effects.

Given perioperative risk factors, the frequency of aspiration in the elderly population, and the incidence of postoperative respiratory morbidity, insufficient research has been directed to this issue in elderly surgical patients. Pharmacologic interventions to reduce gastric volume or increase pH have received attention in the anesthesia literature, but the investigation by Warner et al of aspiration occurring within 2 hours of surgery[205] implies that research on aspiration and postoperative pneumonia must look beyond the immediate operative period.[206] Additional important research will focus on establishing the appropriate use of nasogastric tubes, the restoration of pharyngeal and tracheal reflexes and gastrointestinal motility, and the advancement of feeding following surgery in the elderly patient. General studies as well as surgery-specific studies are needed.

ACUTE PAIN MANAGEMENT

The same questions that dominate research in pain management in the general population apply to the elderly age group. However, in many ways the questions for elderly persons are more pressing because they might receive the most potential harm as well as the greatest potential benefit from improved treatment of postoperative pain. Because of ischemic heart disease, diminished pulmonary capacity, altered drug clearance, or increased drug sensitivity, the elderly patient is probably more vulnerable to the physiologic consequences of inadequate analgesia, as well as to the side effects of analgesic use. Additionally, there is evidence in the literature indicating that in certain circumstances the older person's pain may be less adequately treated.[48]

PAIN AND ADVERSE OUTCOMES

The perioperative period results in stress and inflammatory responses that peak postoperatively when cardiopulmonary and neurologic complications occur. Therefore, efforts have been made to link the adequacy of analgesia with the magnitude of the stress response. In particular, it has been proposed that inadequate postoperative analgesia may be associated with myocardial ischemia and pulmonary failure. Researchers have examined the effect of the intraoperative anesthetic [207–210] and postoperative epidural analgesia on plasma levels of cortisol, epinephrine, norepinephrine, leucocyte counts, and acute phase proteins and have tried to relate these to cardiopulmonary outcomes. [173,207,211–215] Both negative and positive conclusions have been reached.

When this subject was reviewed by Liu, Carpenter, and Neal, [216] they concluded that intensive analgesia using regional techniques has a limited impact on cardiopulmonary outcomes or the stress response in a general population of surgical patients. They also concluded that pain and the stress response are not directly coupled because the neuroendocrine response is still demonstrated (although blunted) in the presence of intense surgical analgesia with local anesthetics or opioids. However, studies in the groups with highest risk suggest a possible improvement in outcome with intense analgesia that uses regional techniques. [173,217] Intensive pain management strategies may be indicated in high-risk elderly patients or in low-risk elderly patients undergoing high-risk surgery. Defining the circumstances under which epidural analgesia or any other pain management strategy can improve outcomes is an important area for future research.

In addition to the stress response typically associated with the sympathetic-adrenal axis, most types of surgery initiate a significant catabolic state. An inhibitory effect of analgesia on protein wasting has been suggested, [218–220] but a more pressing area for research is to understand postsurgical catabolism in elderly patients. The relationship between preoperative nutritional status and postoperative catabolism must be better understood. Experience with some critically ill patients suggests that catabolism may become dissociated from the initial surgical stress. Because elderly patients have decreased nutritional and metabolic reserve, they are most challenged by the postoperative catabolic state. Basic investigation into postoperative catabolism in the elderly person is important, as are investigations of interventions that might attenuate catabolism or facilitate the transition back to an anabolism.

The adequacy of postoperative analgesia does not appear to be an independent determinant of outcomes in the general population of surgical patients; however, a variety of other issues related to postoperative analgesia require attention. The relative benefit of patient-controlled analgesia (PCA) [221] versus an as-needed or scheduled analgesic administration is of special importance for the elderly surgical patient. Because of the physiologic and psychologic heterogeneity in the geriatric population, it is unlikely that fixed formulae for age-appropriate drug dosing can be identified. Thus, the administration of narcotics on a set schedule in the elderly person is fraught with the potential for both over- and underdosing. These considerations potentially make PCA analgesia an ideal choice. Nevertheless, the issue is complicated. The side-effect profile for PCA analgesics in elderly patients has not been established. [222,223] It has also been suggested that many elderly patients may struggle with the technology. Similarly, the application of PCA for patients with altered mental status is troubling. Outcomes with PCA in the elderly patient must be compared with fixed and as-needed dosing techniques, as well as with postoperative pain control by regional blockade.

The same is true regarding route of administration for analgesic agents. Is there a clear advantage or disadvantage to the use of the intravenous, epidural, or intrathecal routes for analgesic administration in the elderly patient? The elderly person is unusually susceptible to drug interactions and has an increased incidence of respiratory depression, urinary retention, ileus, constipation, and postoperative falls. These are influenced by choices in postoperative analgesia and may differ by route of administration. [222–225] Investigations of analgesic strategies for elderly surgical patients will need to determine not only the quality of analgesia but also the risks and benefits specific to that population. Additionally, because narcotics are commonly associated with side effects in the elderly population, the use of analgesic adjuncts in postoperative pain management requires further investigation. Drugs like ketorolac, clonidine, dexmedetomidine, and COX-2 inhibitors have the potential to achieve adequate analgesia with lower doses of opioids, potentially reducing side effects. [226–230]

A final reason why studies of acute pain management in the elderly person are required is that acute pain management may bear on rehabilitation and subsequently on functional status on discharge. [231] This has been shown with analgesic programs for continuous passive motion machines used following knee replacement. [231–233] Research is required following other types of surgical procedures to determine whether facilitating rehabilitation by effectively managing acute pain can improve other functional outcomes.

Another opportunity for research in the postoperative care of hospitalized elderly patients is related to polypharmacy and adverse drug events. Elderly patients tend to accumulate drug prescriptions over time, and there is a clear relationship between the number of drugs taken and the incidence of adverse drug-related events. [66–70] This problem will be compounded during the surgical period when even more medications are added.

A study by Cullen et al prospectively compared adverse drug events among surgical and medical hospitalized patients in intensive care (ICU) and in general units. [234] The researchers found that the rate of preventable and potential adverse drug events is related to the number of drugs administered rather than to the type of care delivered (ICU or non-ICU, surgical or medical). The earlier report of the same data on 4031 adult hospital admissions identified, among other things, the incidence of adverse drug events, their preventability, and the classes of drugs that caused most events. Those results have particular bearing on the perioperative care of the elderly person. [68]

In the investigation by Bates et al, analgesics were found to be the class of drug that is associated with the highest number of adverse drug events. [68] Antibiotics were found to cause the second greatest number of adverse reactions. Analgesics are also the leading class of drug associated with preventable adverse drug events, followed by sedatives and then antibiotics (see Table 2.2). In the 20 preventable adverse events related to analgesics, 40% were found to be caused by overmedication.

There is a pressing need for research in pain management of the elderly surgical patient. There is also a compelling need for research into the prevention of adverse drug events in elderly hospitalized patients. The intersection of pain management and preventable adverse events associated with analgesics and sedatives places anesthesiologists squarely in a leadership role for research into appropriate analgesic and sedative strategies for the elderly age group.

Table 2.2—Adverse Drug Events and Preventability by Drug Class

Drug Class	Adverse Drug Events N (%) N = 247	Preventable Adverse Drug Events N (%) N = 70
Analgesics	73 (30)	20 (29)
Antibiotics	59 (24)	6 (9)
Sedatives	20 (8)	7 (10)
Antineoplastics	18 (7)	3 (4)
Cardiovascular	9 (4)	3 (4)
Anticoagulants	8 (3)	3 (4)
Antipsychotics	6 (2)	5 (7)
Diabetes	5 (2)	4 (6)
Electrolytes	3 (1)	3 (4)
Other	46 (19)	16 (23)

SOURCE: Bates DW, Cullen DJ, Laird N, et al. Incidence of adverse drug events and potential adverse drug events: implications for prevention. ADE Prevention Study Group. *JAMA* 1995;274:29–34. Used with permission.

In patients who are hospitalized, there is also a window of opportunity to review patient medications, in particular to examine redundancy in therapeutic profile and to look for combinations that may make complications like respiratory depression, aspiration, confusion, postural hypotension, urinary retention, and falls more likely. The development of pharmacy and electronic drug databases for this work would be appropriate; hospitals are more likely than community practitioners to have the resources to support such database development. It would not be practical or appropriate to modify most patients' chronic drug regimens in the postoperative period, but surgical hospitalization nonetheless provides an opportunity for a thorough drug review and recommendations to reduce iatrogenic complications in elderly patients.

DELIRIUM AND COGNITIVE DECLINE

Postoperative delirium or cognitive decline affect 5% to 50% of elderly patients; both disorders have similar predisposing factors, but the syndromes are not equivalent. [111,196,235–237] Disordered thinking and confusion that waxes and wanes characterize postoperative delirium. The onset is typically on the first to third postoperative day, may be sustained for more than a week, and is associated with other medical complications, prolonged hospitalization, and decreased functional status on discharge. [114,121,196,236,238–240] To date, much of the research has centered on the impact of regional versus general anesthesia in orthopedic surgery. [117,118,157,170–172,241] Cognitive dysfunction, a deterioration of such capacities as memory, central processing time, and acquisition of new information, has been well described in both cardiac and noncardiac surgical patients. [242–245]

In anesthesia, the effect of differing anesthetics on postoperative delirium has been studied, [118,157,172,246–249] and a leading hypothesis has been that offending agents aggravate an age-associated central cholinergic insufficiency. [117,250,251] However, from review of the literature it becomes evident that delirium is a syndrome that can be triggered by many different perioperative events, so no single cause is identifiable and no single intervention is likely to be successful.

In addition to being linked to narcotics, sedatives, and anticholinergics, delirium has been associated with urinary tract infection, pneumonia, hypoxia or hypercarbia, fever, blood loss, and electrolyte disturbances. [196,235,236,252–254] Chronic patient factors such as pre-existing frank or subclinical dementia, other organic brain disease, and vision and hearing loss are also predictors of postoperative delirium and cognitive decline. [103,111,114,196,235,255,256] Finally, in the elderly patient it has been suggested that pain, sleep deprivation, sensory deprivation, and an unfamiliar environment may contribute to delirium. [113,196,235,257,258]

Most of the research in the anesthesia literature has focused on the effect of anesthetic and analgesic agents, but the literature in medical patients suggests that the yield for those studies will be low. Studies of the type conducted by Inouye might serve as a model for research in anesthesia. [104,109,254–256,259–261] Inouye describes a multifactorial model for delirium involving the interrelationship between a vulnerable patient and acute insults. [254,259] In a study of elderly medical patients, multivariate modeling identified four risk factors for developing hospitalization delirium: vision impairment, severe illness, pre-existing cognitive impairment, and a blood urea nitrogen–creatinine ratio ≥ 18. [259,262] Patients were then divided into low-, intermediate-, and high-risk groups, depending on the number of risk factors. In a subsequent validation cohort, the rates of delirium in the low-, intermediate-, and high-risk groups were 3%, 16%, and 32%, respectively. [259] In those patients the rate of death or nursing-home placement was 3%, 14%, and 26%, respectively, an eightfold increase from the lowest to highest risk group. [262]

Precipitating factors for delirium in hospitalized medical patients have also been described by Inouye and Charpentier [254] Twenty-five factors occurring at least 24 hours before the onset of delirium were considered. Of those, a multivariate model identified five as predictive: use of physical restraints, malnutrition, more than three medications added, use of a bladder catheter, and any iatrogenic event (eg, volume overload, urinary tract infection, pressure ulcer). Even though the precipitating factors were independent of each other, the authors note that "baseline and precipitating factors are highly interrelated and contribute to delirium in a cumulative fashion."

In a subsequent publication, Inouye et al [260] determined the effect of interventions that were based on their predictive model. Four hundred and twenty-six elderly medical patients in an intervention group were matched to an equal number in a usual care group. In the intervention group, six risk factors for delirium were targeted for intervention: cognitive impairment, sleep deprivation, immobility, visual and hearing impairment, and dehydration. The group receiving intervention by an interdisciplinary team had a 9.9% incidence of delirium versus 15% in the usual care group (a 34% difference). Subdivision of patients into intermediate- or high-risk groups demonstrated that intervention reduced delirium diagnosed by the Confusion Assessment Method (CAM) [263] in intermediate-risk patients, but the tendency to reduce delirium in the high-risk group was not found to be statistically significant.

These studies indicate that presence and severity of cognitive deficit is a strong predictor of the likelihood of delirium during the hospitalization. [259] The same effect has been identified in surgical patients. [111–114] This brings us back to the recurring theme: Subclinical decrements in functional status may become evident during the perioperative period. These findings are extended by the observation that postoperative delirium or cognitive decline may be a harbinger of a potentially permanent decrease in mental status. [242,264]

Together, the data on the predictive value of preoperative cognitive status [259] and the effect of that assessment on the success of intervention [260] provide a compelling rationale to conduct a simple, short mental status examination as part of the preoperative interview. Short functional scales have been designed that might be applicable in the preoperative interview. [116,265,266] The practicality of using such metrics in elderly surgical patients must be established. Following that, the incidence of preoperative cognitive impairment, and its severity, could be identified in populations of elderly patients undergoing different types of procedures. Research into the effectiveness of differing prevention strategies could follow. Those investigations could also examine whether reductions in delirium translate into reduced medical complications or improved functional status on discharge.

For further discussion of the problems of delirium and cognitive decline in the older surgical patient, see Chapter 13, Cross-Cutting Issues.

THE POSTOPERATIVE RESEARCH AGENDA

Anes 19 (Level B): **Prospective studies that better identify patient and procedural risk factors for respiratory failure, aspiration, and pneumonia in elderly surgical patients are needed.**

Anes 20 (Level A): **Randomized trials are needed to determine if respiratory monitoring or O_2 therapy can reduce the incidence of respiratory failure in elderly surgical patients.**

Anes 21 (Level A): **Randomized studies of prophylactic antibiotics, changes in pharyngeal instrumentation, or the way feeding is advanced are needed to determine whether practice changes reduce aspiration and postoperative pneumonia in elderly surgical patients. (See also Key Research Questions in Geriatric Anesthesia, end of chapter.)**

Anes 22 (Level B): **Cross-sectional studies capable of identifying any relationship in elderly surgical patients between intensive nutritional support in high-risk surgery and functional status on discharge (eg, chronic respiratory failure, ambulation, independent living) are needed.**

Anes 23 (Level A): **Data from studies of associations between nutritional support and postoperative functional status after high-risk surgery in elderly patients (Anes 22) should be used to design prospective cohort or randomized controlled trials comparing feeding strategies in elderly patients at risk for malnutrition and muscle wasting following major surgery.**

Anes 24 (Level C): **Randomized trials of interventions that might attenuate postoperative catabolism or facilitate the transition to anabolism in the elderly patient are needed.**

Anes 25 (Level D): Large cross-sectional studies describing analgesic practice and its complications in the elderly surgical patient are needed.

Anes 26 (Level B): Depending in part on findings of large, descriptive studies of analgesia in elderly patients (Anes 25), prospective cohort studies are needed to determine the effect of analgesic modes (patient-controlled versus as-needed versus scheduled dosing), route of administration, the role of nonopioid adjunctive drugs, and nonpharmacologic interventions. These investigations must define a balance between adequate analgesia and reduction of the incidence of adverse drug events in the elderly patient.

Anes 27 (Level A): Prospective randomized controlled trials comparing outcomes with analgesic programs specific to types of surgery are needed to determine whether analgesic regimes designed for the elderly patient reduce in-hospital morbidity or improve functional status on discharge. (See also Key Research Questions in Geriatric Anesthesia, end of chapter.)

Anes 28 (Level D): Improved tools for the assessment of pain in the cognitively impaired elderly patient should be developed.

Anes 29 (Level C): Improved tools for assessing pain in cognitively impaired elderly patients (Anes 28) should be used to determine the adequacy of pain management strategies in this group of patients.

Anes 30 (Level D): A retrospective review is needed to determine the incidence of polypharmacy with combinations of drugs that might contribute to complications (hypotension, bradycardia, falls, confusion, bleeding diathesis, constipation, and urinary retention) in geriatric surgical patients.

Anes 31 (Level A): The effect on outcomes for elderly surgical patients of simplifying drug regimens in hospital or of communicating that information to primary care physicians should be examined in a randomized controlled trial.

Anes 32 (Level B): Cross-sectional studies, with multivariate analysis, are needed to determine whether the risk factors for delirium in elderly surgical patients are the same as those for elderly medical patients.

Anes 33 (Level B): Studies are needed on the utility of the Confusion Assessment Method (CAM) for serial testing of elderly patients before and after surgery to facilitate the diagnosis of postoperative delirium. The CAM should be compared with other tests of cognitive function and with the clinical diagnosis for delirium. At the same time, since dementia is the leading predisposing factor for delirium, the utility of short mental status tests to make the preoperative diagnosis of early dementia should be tested, using a full psychiatric examination as the gold standard.

Anes 34 (Level A): **Prospective controlled (nonrandomized; ie, by ward or unit) trials in patients at moderate to high risk for delirium should be performed to determine the effect of preoperative or postoperative interventions on the incidence of delirium.**

CHRONIC PAIN

A significant proportion of the geriatric population suffers from chronic pain conditions.[46,47] Much of this is related to osteoarthritis; other neuropathic pain disorders that afflict older patients include postherpetic neuralgia (PHN), diabetic neuropathies, and causalgias.[267] Care of these patients is complex, and for many of these painful conditions, therapy is inadequate.

A number of factors limit success in treating chronic pain in elderly persons. First, unlike acute postoperative pain, chronic pain is caused by conditions that typically are not reversible. Second, pain conditions in the elderly person may have a central nervous system component. Third, effective treatment of chronic pain is hampered by the side effects of medications and complications from polypharmacy. Fourth, depression and behavioral changes commonly complicate therapy.[268] Fifth, assessment of pain in older patients can be difficult,[46] and, finally, chronic pain in the elderly person is often associated with unrelated comorbid conditions that may alter treatment plans.[43,269] In spite of these limitations, geriatric patients benefit, as do younger patients, from chronic pain therapy.[43,270,271]

As described by the American Geriatric Society Panel on Persistent Pain in Older Persons, most pain syndromes can be classified into one of four types: nociceptive, neuropathic, mixed or unspecified, and psychogenic.[47] The usefulness of different classes of analgesic agents in these types of syndromes is reasonably well described. Nociceptive pain includes the pain typically associated with arthropathies, myalgias, and ischemic disorders; the mainstays of analgesia are initially acetaminophen and nonsteroidal anti-inflammatory drugs, followed later by narcotics.[46,47,267] In contrast, narcotics are thought to have a lesser place in the treatment of neuropathies such as diabetic neuropathy, PHN, and complex regional pain syndromes.[267,272,273] Instead, the primary pharmacologic therapies are tricyclic antidepressants and anticonvulsant agents.[46,267,274–276] Antiarrhythmic drugs are second-tier agents for neuropathic conditions. Treatment of mixed or unspecified pain syndromes is challenging, as the mechanisms are unknown and treatment may require trials of differing analgesic approaches.[47] For patients whose pain has been classified as psychogenic, psychiatric intervention rather than analgesic agents is indicated.[47]

In addition to familiar analgesics and adjuncts, there is a need for a multidimensional approach to chronic pain in elderly persons. Neuraxial opioids, local anesthetics, and corticosteroids have a role for some patients, as do peripheral or central neuromodulatory techniques and a host of physical, physiatric, and cognitive-behavioral strategies.[43,46,47]

Defining research priorities for anesthesiologists in such a broad and complex area is difficult. The first priority is that chronic pain trials must have sufficient control groups and statistical power. As pointed out by Stanton-Hicks et al regarding neuropathic pain conditions, studies are typically small and anecdotal with few experimental findings, and "without adequate predictors for the choice of therapy, current practice is chaotic, and continues to use the trial-and-error approach."[275]

After design issues are addressed, probably the most basic research recommendation for any of these types of pain conditions is that outcomes should emphasize functional status [271,277] rather than a change in a pain score per se. This is superbly outlined in the consensus report on complex regional pain syndromes. [275] Though quantifying pain is relevant, ultimately the determination of which interventions facilitate rehabilitation, maintain or increase mobility, and support ADLs is a priority. [271,277]

The second broad area requiring further investigation relates to prevention. One of the best examples is in PHN. The rash of acute herpes zoster is very common in elderly persons; a lesser but significant percentage of those affected develop the chronic debilitating pain condition of PHN. [278] Because zoster is chronic and recurring, the percentage of the population affected with PHN increases with age. [278] Although PHN may develop in less than 5% of younger patients with zoster, it may develop in half of patients aged 60 and over. [279] Once established, PHN is difficult to treat. Further research is indicated to determine whether antiviral, analgesic, or anti-inflammatory therapies during acute zoster can prevent the development of chronic PHN. [280–283] A better understanding of precipitating events for other chronic pain conditions, as in PHN, [284] might allow the introduction of preventive measures.

In addition to directing research efforts toward functional effects and trying to define opportunities for prevention of chronic pain conditions, for any strategy it is important to examine the risk-benefit ratio, emphasizing adverse outcomes that are more likely to occur in a geriatric population. As in acute pain management, the effect of chronic therapy on the incidence of complications like confusion, postural hypotension, falls, urinary retention, and constipation must be reported.

Finally, cognitive impairment is a continuum and in milder forms is very common. There is a two-way relationship between pain and cognitive impairment: pain may impair cognition and cognitive impairment can interfere with the communication of pain. [46,285] Therefore, a further area of investigation relevant to the care of patients with chronic pain is its assessment in the cognitively impaired.

THE RESEARCH AGENDA IN CHRONIC PAIN

Anes 35 (Level B): **The first priority in chronic pain trials is large cross-sectional studies that are powered to identify any relationship between pain intervention and functional outcomes.**

Anes 36 (Level A): **With the establishment of any relationship between intervention for chronic pain and functional outcomes in elderly patients (Anes 35), it must be determined prospectively if specific chronic pain therapies can improve functional outcomes in treatment groups relative to a historical or concurrent, nonrandomized control.**

Anes 37 (Level C): **Given the high incidence rate of herpes zoster in the geriatric population, further prospective studies are needed to determine if antiviral, analgesic, or anti-inflammatory therapies during acute zoster can reduce, relative to standard care, the development of chronic post-herpetic neuralgia.**

Anes 38 (Level D): **Cross-sectional studies documenting the association of chronic pain therapy with the incidence of complications like confusion, postural hypotension, falls, urinary retention, and constipation in the elderly population are needed.**

Anes 39 (Level D): **Cross-sectional studies that describe pain management in cognitively impaired patients, relative to a nonimpaired population, are needed.**

Anes 40 (Level D): **Pain assessment tools for chronic pain in the cognitively impaired elderly patient must be compared prospectively with standard assessment methods.**

Anes 41 (Level C): **Prospective trials comparing different analgesic strategies with regard to clinical and functional outcomes are needed.**

SUMMARY

The perioperative care of the geriatric patient is complex. Older patients are at increased risk for a host of complications, and it is probably easier to precipitate these complications than to directly prevent them. This precarious state is a function of decreased functional reserve, variable response to stress, and the number of comorbidities in older patients

Nevertheless, we have learned a great deal that can guide future research. Rather than continuing to focus attention on the choice of anesthetic technique or on short-term outcomes, such as time to extubation or recovery room stay, we should focus attention on better risk stratification of elderly patients in order to better serve the goal of improving patient outcomes. If identified risk factors are amenable to therapy, it should be determined whether improvement in patient status leads to improved outcome. An essential element of both types of investigations will be a focus on preoperative functional status and outcomes appropriate to the geriatric population, rather than just major cardiopulmonary morbidity and mortality.

Outcome is determined by the interaction of patient factors and the challenges introduced by surgery. Surgical impact varies widely by type, so the development of comprehensive care strategies for specific types of surgery common in the elderly age group is indicated. Such an approach is more likely to generate positive results and practical guidelines than pooling elderly patients undergoing differing types of surgery. Developing comprehensive clinical pathways specific to the care of the elderly patient undergoing specific types of surgeries is indicated because these would bring together preoperative, intraoperative, and postoperative management. This approach could improve outcomes and would serve as a foundation for assessing alternative strategies. These might have particular value in postoperative care, particularly with regard to the prevention of delirium, respiratory monitoring, and pain management. In these investigations the anesthesiologist has a unique role, as the clinician responsible for preoperative assessment as well as intraoperative and postoperative management for every elderly patient undergoing every type of surgery.

KEY RESEARCH QUESTIONS IN GERIATRIC ANESTHESIA

Anes KQ1: **What preoperative assessments are useful in developing patient management plans for surgeries common in the elderly population?**

Hypothesis-generating: Large observational studies are needed to identify preoperative risk factors for adverse geriatric outcomes following common surgeries. These will identify both patient- and surgery-dependent factors. Assessment tools for mental status, nutrition, hydration, thrombotic risk, and ADLs must be applied or developed when necessary. It then should be determined which risk factors are potentially modifiable.

Hypothesis-testing: Randomized controlled trials are needed to determine if preoperative or postoperative intervention against modifiable risk factors will decrease perioperative geriatric complications. The adverse effects of such interventions, such as delay of surgery or postoperative bleeding, must be examined along with the potential benefits of interventions.

Examples of interventions that could reasonably be attempted include intensive nourishment for malnutrition and precise management of hydration, multifactorial interventions to prevent postoperative delirium, pre- or postoperative rehabilitation programs to maintain or improve functional status (ADLs, exercise capacity), and antiplatelet therapy for thrombotic and embolic complications.

Anes KQ2: **Can proper choice of postoperative analgesic techniques reduce postoperative morbidity or improve functional status at discharge?**

Hypothesis-generating: Large prospective studies describing analgesic practice and its complications in the elderly patient are needed. The efficacy and complications of regional analgesic techniques, nonopioid adjunctive drugs, and physiatric interventions must be investigated. These investigations must emphasize the type and incidence of adverse drug events in the elderly population.

Hypothesis-testing: Prospective randomized trials are needed to determine if perioperative intensive analgesic techniques (including traditional narcotic, regional, nonopioid adjunctive drugs and physiatric interventions) designed for the elderly patient reduce in-hospital morbidity or improve functional status on discharge.

Anes KQ3: **How can postoperative pulmonary complications in the elderly patient be reduced?**

Hypothesis-generating: Cross-sectional or cohort studies that better identify high-risk procedures or perioperative periods of vulnerability for postoperative hypoxia, respiratory failure, and pneumonia in the elderly surgical patient are needed. These investigations should identify both patient and procedure risk factors, as well as their interaction, for these complications.

Hypothesis-testing: Randomized trials are needed to determine if respiratory monitoring, prophylactic antibiotics, changes in pharyngeal instrumentation, or the way feeding is advanced will reduce respiratory failure, aspiration, and postoperative pneumonia among elderly patients.

REFERENCES

1.   Franklin SS, Gustin WT, Wong ND, et al. Hemodynamic patterns of age-related changes in blood pressure. The Framingham Heart Study. Circulation 1997;96:308-315.
2.   Landahl S, Bengtsson C, Sigurdsson JA, et al. Age-related changes in blood pressure. Hypertension 1986;8:1044-1049.
3.   Pan HY, Hoffman BB, Pershe RA, Blaschke TF. Decline in beta adrenergic receptor-mediated vascular relaxation with aging in man. J Pharmacol Exp Ther 1986;239:802-807.
4.   Folkow B, Svanborg A. Physiology of cardiovascular aging. Physiol Rev 1993;73:725-764.
5.   Falk RH. Etiology and complications of atrial fibrillation: insights from pathology studies. Am J Cardiol 1998;82:10N-17N.
6.   Mackstaller LL, Alpert JS. Atrial fibrillation: a review of mechanism, etiology, and therapy. Clin Cardiol 1997;20:640-650.
7.   Lakatta EG. Age-related alterations in the cardiovascular response to adrenergic mediated stress. Fed Proc 1980;39:3173-3177.
8.   Rodeheffer RJ, Gerstenblith G, Becker LC, et al. Exercise cardiac output is maintained with advancing age in healthy human subjects: cardiac dilatation and increased stroke volume compensate for a diminished heart rate. Circulation 1984;69:203-213.
9.   Collins KJ, Exton-Smith AN, James MH, Oliver DJ. Functional changes in autonomic nervous responses with ageing. Age Ageing 1980;9:17-24.
10. McGarry K, Laher M, Fitzgerald D, et al. Baroreflex function in elderly hypertensives. Hypertension 1983;5:763-766.
11. Phillips PA, Hodsman GP, Johnston CI. Neuroendocrine mechanisms and cardiovascular homeostasis in the elderly. Cardiovasc Drugs Ther 1991;4 Suppl 6:1209-1213.
12. Cleroux J, Giannattasio C, Bolla G, et al. Decreased cardiopulmonary reflexes with aging in normotensive humans. Am J Physiol 1989;257:H961-H968.
13. Rowe JW, Troen BR. Sympathetic nervous system and aging in man. Endocr Rev 1980;1:167-179.
14. Wahba WM. Influence of aging on lung function–clinical significance of changes from age twenty. Anesth Analg 1983;62:764-776.
15. Zaugg M, Lucchinetti E. Respiratory function in the elderly. Anesthesiol Clin North America 2000;18:47-58, vi.
16. Fowler RW. Ageing and lung function. Age Ageing 1985;14:209-215.
17. Tolep K, Kelsen SG. Effect of aging on respiratory skeletal muscles. Clin Chest Med 1993;14:363-378.
18. Pontoppidan H, Geffin B, Lowenstein E. Acute respiratory failure in the adult. 1. N Engl J Med 1972;287:690-698.
19. Kitamura H, Sawa T, Ikezono E. Postoperative hypoxemia: The contribution of age to the maldistribution of ventilation. Anesthesiology 1972;36:244-252.
20. Lynne-Davies P. Influence of age on the respiratory system. Geriatrics 1977;32:57-60.
21. Cerveri I, Zoia MC, Fanfulla F, et al. Reference values of arterial oxygen tension in the middle-aged and elderly. Am J Respir Crit Care Med 1995;152:934-941.
22. Kronenberg RS, Drage CW. Attenuation of the ventilatory and heart rate responses to hypoxia and hypercapnia with aging in normal men. J Clin Invest 1973;52:1812-1819.

23. Aviv JE. Effects of aging on sensitivity of the pharyngeal and supraglottic areas. Am J Med 1997;103:74S-76S.

24. Marik PE. Aspiration pneumonitis and aspiration pneumonia. N Engl J Med 2001;344:665-671.

25. Arunasalam K, Davenport HT, Painter S, Jones JG. Ventilatory response to morphine in young and old subjects. Anaesthesia 1983;38:529-533.

26. Sari A, Miyauchi Y, Yamashita S, et al. The magnitude of hypoxemia in elderly patients with fractures of the femoral neck. Anesth Analg 1986;65:892-894.

27. Kronenberg RS, Drage CW, Ponto RA, Williams LE. The effect of age on the distribution of ventilation and perfusion in the lung. Am Rev Respir Dis 1973;108:576-586.

28. Clayer M, Bruckner J. Occult hypoxia after femoral neck fracture and elective hip surgery. Clin Orthop 2000:265-271.

29. Moller JT, Wittrup M, Johansen SH. Hypoxemia in the postanesthesia care unit: an observer study. Anesthesiology 1990;73:890-895.

30. de Larminat V, Montravers P, Dureuil B, Desmonts JM. Alteration in swallowing reflex after extubation in intensive care unit patients. Crit Care Med 1995;23:486-490.

31. Morris JC, McManus DQ. The neurology of aging: normal versus pathologic change. Geriatrics 1991;46:47-48, 51-44.

32. Creasey H, Rapoport SI. The aging human brain. Ann Neurol 1985;17:2-10.

33. Morrison JH, Hof PR. Life and death of neurons in the aging brain. Science 1997;278:412-419.

34. Severson JA. Neurotransmitter receptors and aging. J Am Geriatr Soc 1984;32:24-27.

35. Wong DF, Wagner HN, Jr., Dannals RF, et al. Effects of age on dopamine and serotonin receptors measured by positron tomography in the living human brain. Science 1984;226:1393-1396.

36. Muravchick S. Central nervous system. In Craven L (ed): Geroanesthesia: Principles for Management of the Elderly Patient. St. Louis: Mosby-Year Book, Inc., 1997:78-113.

37. Peterson DD, Pack AI, Silage DA, Fishman AP. Effects of aging on ventilatory and occlusion pressure responses to hypoxia and hypercapnia. Am Rev Respir Dis 1981;124:387-391.

38. Muravchick S. Peripheral and autonomic nervous system. In Craven L (ed): Geroanesthesia: Principles for Management of the Elderly Patient. St. Louis: Mosby-Year Book, Inc., 1997:114-148.

39. Gibson SJ, Helme RD. Age differences in pain perception and report: a review of physiological, psychological, laboratory and clinical studies. Pain Rev 1995;2:111-137.

40. Tucker MA, Andrew MF, Ogle SJ, Davison JG. Age-associated change in pain threshold measured by transcutaneous neuronal electrical stimulation. Age Ageing 1989;18:241-246.

41. Potvin AR, Syndulko K, Tourtellotte WW, et al. Human neurologic function and the aging process. J Am Geriatr Soc 1980;28:1-9.

42. Chakour MC, Gibson SJ, Bradbeer M, Helme RD. The effect of age on A delta- and C-fibre thermal pain perception. Pain 1996;64:143-152.

43. Helme RD, Gibson SJ. Pain in the elderly. In Jensen TS, Turner JA, Wiesenfeld-Hallin Z (eds): 8th World Congress on Pain. Parkville, Australia: IASP Press, 1997:919-944.

44. Harkins SW. Geriatric pain. Pain perceptions in the old. Clin Geriatr Med 1996;12:435-459.

45. Harkins SW, Davis MD, Bush FM, Kasberger J. Suppression of first pain and slow temporal summation of second pain in relation to age. J Gerontol A Biol Sci Med Sci 1996;51:M260-M265.

46. Ferrell BA. Pain management in elderly people. J Am Geriatr Soc 1991;39:64-73.

47. American Geriatrics Society Panel on Persistent Pain in Older Persons. The management of persistent pain in older persons. J Am Geriatr Soc 2002;50:S205-S224.

48. Jones JS, Johnson K, McNinch M. Age as a risk factor for inadequate emergency department analgesia. Am J Emerg Med 1996;14:157-160.
49. McLachlan MS. The ageing kidney. Lancet 1978;2:143-145.
50. Anderson S, Brenner BM. The aging kidney: structure, function, mechanisms, and therapeutic implications. J Am Geriatr Soc 1987;35:590-593.
51. Epstein M. Aging and the kidney. J Am Soc Nephrol 1996;7:1106-1122.
52. Anderson S, Brenner BM. Effects of aging on the renal glomerulus. Am J Med 1986;80:435-442.
53. Shannon RP, Minaker KL, Rowe JW. Aging and water balance in humans. Semin Nephrol 1984;4:346-353.
54. Miller M. Fluid and electrolyte balance in the elderly. Geriatrics 1987;42:65-68, 71, 75-66.
55. Phillips PA, Rolls BJ, Ledingham JG, et al. Reduced thirst after water deprivation in healthy elderly men. N Engl J Med 1984;311:753-759.
56. Rowe JW, Minaker KL, Sparrow D, Robertson GL. Age-related failure of volume-pressure-mediated vasopressin release. J Clin Endocrinol Metab 1982;54:661-664.
57. Kliger AS. The role of the kidney in fluid, electrolyte, and acid-base disorders. Int Anesthesiol Clin 1984;22:65-82.
58. Lamy PP, Wiser TH. Geriatric anesthesia. In Katlic MR (ed): Pharmacotherapeutic considerations in the elderly surgical patient. Baltimore: Urban & Schwarzenberg, Inc., 1990:209-239.
59. Greenblatt DJ, Sellers EM, Shader RI. Drug therapy: drug disposition in old age. N Engl J Med 1982;306:1081-1088.
60. Shafer SL. The pharmacology of anesthetic drugs in elderly patients. Anesthesiol Clin North America 2000;18:1-29, v.
61. Matteo RS, Ornstein E. Pharmacokinetics and pharmacodynamics of injected drugs in the elderly. Adv Anesthesia 1988;5:25-52.
62. Silverstein JH, Bloom HG, Cassel CK. New challenges in anesthesia: new practice opportunities. Anesthesiol Clin North America 1999;17:453-465.
63. Dundee JW, Robinson FP, McCollum JS, Patterson CC. Sensitivity to propofol in the elderly. Anaesthesia 1986;41:482-485.
64. Jacobs JR, Reves JG, Marty J, et al. Aging increases pharmacodynamic sensitivity to the hypnotic effects of midazolam. Anesth Analg 1995;80:143-148.
65. Homer TD, Stanski DR. The effect of increasing age on thiopental disposition and anesthetic requirement. Anesthesiology 1985;62:714-724.
66. Hurwitz N. Predisposing factors in adverse reactions to drugs. Br Med J 1969;1:536-539.
67. Hurwitz N, Wade OL. Intensive hospital monitoring of adverse reactions to drugs. Br Med J 1969;1:531-536.
68. Bates DW, Cullen DJ, Laird N, et al. Incidence of adverse drug events and potential adverse drug events. Implications for prevention. ADE Prevention Study Group. JAMA 1995;274:29-34.
69. Patterson C. Iatrogenic disease in late life. Clin Geriatr Med 1986;2:121-136.
70. Williamson J, Chopin JM. Adverse reactions to prescribed drugs in the elderly: a multicentre investigation. Age Ageing 1980;9:73-80.
71. Muravchick S. The biology of aging and preoperative evaluation. In Craven L (ed): Geroanesthesia: Principles for Management of the Elderly Patient. St. Louis: Mosby-Year Book, Inc., 1997:1-34.
72. Thomas DR, Ritchie CS. Preoperative assessment of older adults. J Am Geriatr Soc 1995;43:811-821.
73. Vaz FG, Seymour DG. A prospective study of elderly general surgical patients: I. Pre-operative medical problems. Age Ageing 1989;18:309-315.

74. Schneider JR, Droste JS, Schindler N, Golan JF. Carotid endarterectomy in octogenarians: comparison with patient characteristics and outcomes in younger patients. J Vasc Surg 2000;31:927-935.

75. Hoballah JJ, Nazzal MM, Jacobovicz C, et al. Entering the ninth decade is not a contraindication for carotid endarterectomy. Angiology 1998;49:275-278.

76. Hosking MP, Warner MA, Lobdell CM, et al. Outcomes of surgery in patients 90 years of age and older [see comments]. JAMA 1989;261:1909-1915.

77. Warner MA, Saletel RA, Schroeder DR, et al. Outcomes of anesthesia and surgery in people 100 years of age and older. J Am Geriatr Soc 1998;46:988-993.

78. Laskin RS. Total knee replacement in patients older than 85 years. Clin Orthop 1999:43-49.

79. Tiret L, Desmonts JM, Hatton F, Vourc'h G. Complications associated with anaesthesia–a prospective survey in France. Can Anaesth Soc J 1986;33:336-344.

80. Eagle KA, Brundage BH, Chaitman BR, et al. Guidelines for perioperative cardiovascular evaluation for noncardiac surgery. Report of the American College of Cardiology/American Heart Association Task Force on Practice Guidelines. Committee on Perioperative Cardiovascular Evaluation for Noncardiac Surgery. Circulation 1996;93:1278-1317.

81. Goldman L. Cardiac risks and complications of noncardiac surgery. Ann Intern Med 1983;98:504-513.

82. Liu LL, Leung JM. Predicting adverse postoperative outcomes in patients aged 80 years or older. J Am Geriatr Soc 2000;48:405-412.

83. Arvidsson S, Ouchterlony J, Sjostedt L, Svardsudd K. Predicting postoperative adverse events. Clinical efficiency of four general classification systems. The project perioperative risk. Acta Anaesthesiol Scand 1996;40:783-791.

84. Detsky AS, Abrams HB, Forbath N, et al. Cardiac assessment for patients undergoing noncardiac surgery. A multifactorial clinical risk index. Arch Intern Med 1986;146:2131-2134.

85. Pedersen T, Eliasen K, Henriksen E. A prospective study of risk factors and cardiopulmonary complications associated with anaesthesia and surgery: risk indicators of cardiopulmonary morbidity. Acta Anaesthesiol Scand 1990;34:144-155.

86. Pedersen T, Eliasen K, Henriksen E. A prospective study of mortality associated with anaesthesia and surgery: risk indicators of mortality in hospital. Acta Anaesthesiol Scand 1990;34:176-182.

87. Browner WS, Li J, Mangano DT. In-hospital and long-term mortality in male veterans following noncardiac surgery. The Study of Perioperative Ischemia Research Group. JAMA 1992;268:228-232.

88. Khuri SF, Daley J, Henderson W, et al. The National Veterans Administration Surgical Risk Study: risk adjustment for the comparative assessment of the quality of surgical care. J Am Coll Surg 1995;180:519-531.

89. Arvidsson S, Ouchterlony J, Nilsson S, et al. The Gothenburg study of perioperative risk. I. Preoperative findings, postoperative complications. Acta Anaesthesiol Scand 1994;38:679-690.

90. Mohr DN. Estimation of surgical risk in the elderly: a correlative review. J Am Geriatr Soc 1983;31:99-102.

91. Cheng KW, Wang CH, Ho RT, et al. Outcome of surgery and anesthesia in patients 80 years of age and older. Acta Anaesthesiol Sin 1994;32:37-43.

92. Cohen MM, Duncan PG, Tate RB. Does anesthesia contribute to operative mortality? JAMA 1988;260:2859-2863.

93. Cohen MM, Duncan PG. Physical status score and trends in anesthetic complications. J Clin Epidemiol 1988;41:83-90.

94. Goldman L, Hashimoto B, Cook EF, Loscalzo A. Comparative reproducibility and validity of systems for assessing cardiovascular functional class: advantages of a new specific activity scale. Circulation 1981;64:1227-1234.

95. Lawton MP, Brody EM. Assessment of older people: self-maintaining and instrumental activities of daily living. Gerontologist 1969;9:179-186.

96. Ware JE, Jr., Sherbourne CD. The MOS 36-item short-form health survey (SF-36). I. Conceptual framework and item selection. Med Care 1992;30:473-483.

97. Moy ML, Ingenito EP, Mentzer SJ, et al. Health-related quality of life improves following pulmonary rehabilitation and lung volume reduction surgery. Chest 1999;115:383-389.

98. Mangione CM, Goldman L, Orav EJ, et al. Health-related quality of life after elective surgery: measurement of longitudinal changes. J Gen Intern Med 1997;12:686-697.

99. Hannan EL, Magaziner J, Wang JJ, et al. Mortality and locomotion 6 months after hospitalization for hip fracture: risk factors and risk-adjusted hospital outcomes. JAMA 2001;285:2736-2742.

100. Tammela T, Kontturi M, Lukkarinen O. Postoperative urinary retention. I. Incidence and predisposing factors. Scand J Urol Nephrol 1986;20:197-201.

101. Duits AA, Boeke S, Taams MA, et al. Prediction of quality of life after coronary artery bypass graft surgery: a review and evaluation of multiple, recent studies. Psychosom Med 1997;59:257-268.

102. Keene JS, Anderson CA. Hip fractures in the elderly. Discharge predictions with a functional rating scale. JAMA 1982;248:564-567.

103. McCartney JR, Palmateer LM. Assessment of cognitive deficit in geriatric patients. A study of physician behavior. J Am Geriatr Soc 1985;33:467-471.

104. Inouye SK, Peduzzi PN, Robison JT, et al. Importance of functional measures in predicting mortality among older hospitalized patients. JAMA 1998;279:1187-1193.

105. Raja SN, Haythornthwaite JA. Anesthetic management of the elderly: measuring function beyond the immediate perioperative horizon. Anesthesiology 1999;91:909-911.

106. Heyland DK, Guyatt G, Cook DJ, et al. Frequency and methodologic rigor of quality-of-life assessments in the critical care literature. Crit Care Med 1998;26:591-598.

107. Holmes J, House A. Psychiatric illness predicts poor outcome after surgery for hip fracture: a prospective cohort study. Psychol Med 2000;30:921-929.

108. Dolan MM, Hawkes WG, Zimmerman SI, et al. Delirium on hospital admission in aged hip fracture patients: prediction of mortality and 2-year functional outcomes. J Gerontol A Biol Sci Med Sci 2000;55:M527-M534.

109. Inouye SK, Schlesinger MJ, Lydon TJ. Delirium: a symptom of how hospital care is failing older persons and a window to improve quality of hospital care. Am J Med 1999;106:565-573.

110. Millar K, Asbury AJ, Murray GD. Pre-existing cognitive impairment as a factor influencing outcome after cardiac surgery. Br J Anaesth 2001;86:63-67.

111. Dyer CB, Ashton CM, Teasdale TA. Postoperative delirium. A review of 80 primary data-collection studies. Arch Intern Med 1995;155:461-465.

112. Ni Chonchubhair A, Valacio R, Kelly J, O'Keefe S. Use of the abbreviated mental test to detect postoperative delirium in elderly people. Br J Anaesth 1995;75:481-482.

113. Kaneko T, Takahashi S, Naka T, et al. Postoperative delirium following gastrointestinal surgery in elderly patients. Surg Today 1997;27:107-111.

114. Gustafson Y, Berggren D, Brannstrom B, et al. Acute confusional states in elderly patients treated for femoral neck fracture. J Am Geriatr Soc 1988;36:525-530.

115. McDowell I, Kristjansson B, Hill GB, Hebert R. Community screening for dementia: the Mini Mental State Exam (MMSE) and Modified Mini-Mental State Exam (3MS) compared. J Clin Epidemiol 1997;50:377-383.

116. Folstein MF, Folstein SE, McHugh PR. "Mini-mental state". A practical method for grading the cognitive state of patients for the clinician. J Psychiatr Res 1975;12:189-198.

117. Berggren D, Gustafson Y, Eriksson B, et al. Postoperative confusion after anesthesia in elderly patients with femoral neck fractures. Anesth Analg 1987;66:497-504.

118. Williams-Russo P, Urquhart BL, Sharrock NE, Charlson ME. Post-operative delirium: predictors and prognosis in elderly orthopedic patients [see comments]. J Am Geriatr Soc 1992;40:759-767.
119. de Graeff A, de Leeuw JR, Ros WJ, et al. Pretreatment factors predicting quality of life after treatment for head and neck cancer. Head Neck 2000;22:398-407.
120. Lyness JM, Noel TK, Cox C, et al. Screening for depression in elderly primary care patients. A comparison of the Center for Epidemiologic Studies-Depression Scale and the Geriatric Depression Scale. Arch Intern Med 1997;157:449-454.
121. Roca R. Psychosocial aspects of surgical care in the elderly patient. Surg Clin North Am 1994;74:223-243.
122. Bradley EH, Bogardus ST, Jr., van Doorn C, et al. Goals in geriatric assessment: are we measuring the right outcomes? Gerontologist 2000;40:191-196.
123. Heijmeriks JA, Pourrier S, Dassen P, et al. Comparison of quality of life after coronary and/or valvular cardiac surgery in patients > or = 75 years of age with younger patients. Am J Cardiol 1999;83:1129-1132, A1129.
124. Katz S. Assessing self-maintenance: activities of daily living, mobility, and instrumental activities of daily living. J Am Geriatr Soc 1983;31:721-727.
125. Turnbull JM, Buck C. The value of preoperative screening investigations in otherwise healthy individuals. Arch Intern Med 1987;147:1101-1105.
126. Perez A, Planell J, Bacardaz C, et al. Value of routine preoperative tests: a multicentre study in four general hospitals. Br J Anaesth 1995;74:250-256.
127. Kaplan EB, Sheiner LB, Boeckmann AJ, et al. The usefulness of preoperative laboratory screening. JAMA 1985;253:3576-3581.
128. Narr BJ, Warner ME, Schroeder DR, Warner MA. Outcomes of patients with no laboratory assessment before anesthesia and a surgical procedure. Mayo Clin Proc 1997;72:505-509.
129. Seymour DG, Pringle R, Shaw JW. The role of the routine pre-operative chest X-ray in the elderly general surgical patient. Postgrad Med J 1982;58:741-745.
130. Seymour DG, Pringle R, MacLennan WJ. The role of the routine pre-operative electrocardiogram in the elderly surgical patient. Age Ageing 1983;12:97-104.
131. Sewell JM, Spooner LL, Dixon AK, Rubenstein D. Screening investigations in the elderly. Age Ageing 1981;10:165-168.
132. Sanders DP, McKinney FW, Harris WH. Clinical evaluation and cost effectiveness of preoperative laboratory assessment on patients undergoing total hip arthroplasty. Orthopedics 1989;12:1449-1453.
133. Grimes CJ, Younathan MT, Lee WC. The effect of preoperative total parenteral nutrition on surgery outcomes. J Am Diet Assoc 1987;87:1202-1206.
134. Gibbs J, Cull W, Henderson W, et al. Preoperative serum albumin level as a predictor of operative mortality and morbidity: results from the National VA Surgical Risk Study. Arch Surg 1999;134:36-42.
135. Baker JP, Detsky AS, Wesson DE, et al. Nutritional assessment: a comparison of clinical judgement and objective measurements. N Engl J Med 1982;306:969-972.
136. Covinsky KE, Martin GE, Beyth RJ, et al. The relationship between clinical assessments of nutritional status and adverse outcomes in older hospitalized medical patients. J Am Geriatr Soc 1999;47:532-538.
137. Mazolewski P, Turner JF, Baker M, et al. The impact of nutritional status on the outcome of lung volume reduction surgery: a prospective study. Chest 1999;116:693-696.
138. Cohendy R, Gros T, Arnaud-Battandier F, et al. Preoperative nutritional evaluation of elderly patients: the Mini Nutritional Assessment as a practical tool. Clin Nutr 1999;18:345-348.
139. McClave SA, Snider HL, Spain DA. Preoperative issues in clinical nutrition. Chest 1999;115:64S-70S.

140. Moore AA, Siu AL. Screening for common problems in ambulatory elderly: clinical confirmation of a screening instrument. Am J Med 1996;100:438-443.

141. Schein OD, Katz J, Bass EB, et al. The value of routine preoperative medical testing before cataract surgery. Study of Medical Testing for Cataract Surgery. N Engl J Med 2000;342:168-175.

142. Dzankic S, Pastor D, Gonzalez C, Leung JM. The prevalence and predictive value of abnormal preoperative laboratory tests in elderly surgical patients. Anesth Analg 2001;93:301-308.

143. Berlauk JF, Abrams JH, Gilmour IJ, et al. Preoperative optimization of cardiovascular hemodynamics improves outcome in peripheral vascular surgery. A prospective, randomized clinical trial. Ann Surg 1991;214:289-297; discussion 298-289.

144. Leppo JA. Preoperative cardiac risk assessment for noncardiac surgery. Am J Cardiol 1995;75:42D-51D.

145. Roubenoff R, Roubenoff RA, Preto J, Balke CW. Malnutrition among hospitalized patients. A problem of physician awareness. Arch Intern Med 1987;147:1462-1465.

146. Del Guercio LR, Cohn JD. Monitoring operative risk in the elderly. JAMA 1980;243:1350-1355.

147. Smith MS, Muir H, Hall R. Perioperative management of drug therapy, clinical considerations. Drugs 1996;51:238-259.

148. Zaugg M, Tagliente T, Lucchinetti E, et al. Beneficial effects from beta-adrenergic blockade in elderly patients undergoing noncardiac surgery. Anesthesiology 1999;91:1674-1686.

149. Yeager RA, Moneta GL, Edwards JM, et al. Reducing perioperative myocardial infarction following vascular surgery. The potential role of beta-blockade. Arch Surg 1995;130:869-872; discussion 872-863.

150. Bisson A, Stern M, Caubarrere I. Preparation of high-risk patients for major thoracic surgery. Chest Surg Clin N Am 1998;8:541-555, viii.

151. Debigare R, Maltais F, Whittom F, et al. Feasibility and efficacy of home exercise training before lung volume reduction. J Cardiopulm Rehabil 1999;19:235-241.

152. Arthur HM, Daniels C, McKelvie R, et al. Effect of a preoperative intervention on preoperative and postoperative outcomes in low-risk patients awaiting elective coronary artery bypass graft surgery. A randomized, controlled trial. Ann Intern Med 2000;133:253-262.

153. Fisher DA, Trimble S, Clapp B, Dorsett K. Effect of a patient management system on outcomes of total hip and knee arthroplasty. Clin Orthop 1997:155-160.

154. Roy RC. Choosing general versus regional anesthesia for the elderly. Anesthesiol Clin North America 2000;18:91-104, vii.

155. McLaren AD, Stockwell MC, Reid VT. Anaesthetic techniques for surgical correction of fractured neck of femur. A comparative study of spinal and general anaesthesia in the elderly. Anaesthesia 1978;33:10-14.

156. Hole A, Terjesen T, Breivik H. Epidural versus general anaesthesia for total hip arthroplasty in elderly patients. Acta Anaesthesiol Scand 1980;24:279-287.

157. Nielson WR, Gelb AW, Casey JE, et al. Long-term cognitive and social sequelae of general versus regional anesthesia during arthroplasty in the elderly. Anesthesiology 1990;73:1103-1109.

158. Davis FM, Woolner DF, Frampton C, et al. Prospective, multi-centre trial of mortality following general or spinal anaesthesia for hip fracture surgery in the elderly. Br J Anaesth 1987;59:1080-1088.

159. McKenzie PJ, Wishart HY, Dewar KM, et al. Comparison of the effects of spinal anaesthesia and general anaesthesia on postoperative oxygenation and perioperative mortality. Br J Anaesth 1980;52:49-54.

160. McKenzie PJ, Wishart HY, Gray I, Smith G. Effects of anaesthetic technique on deep vein thrombosis. A comparison of subarachnoid and general anaesthesia. Br J Anaesth 1985;57:853-857.

161. Hendolin H, Mattila MA, Poikolainen E. The effect of lumbar epidural analgesia on the development of deep vein thrombosis of the legs after open prostatectomy. Acta Chir Scand 1981;147:425-429.

162. White IW, Chappell WA. Anaesthesia for surgical correction of fractured femoral neck. A comparison of three techniques. Anaesthesia 1980;35:1107-1110.

163. Valentin N, Lomholt B, Jensen JS, et al. Spinal or general anaesthesia for surgery of the fractured hip? A prospective study of mortality in 578 patients. Br J Anaesth 1986;58:284-291.

164. Sorenson RM, Pace NL. Anesthetic techniques during surgical repair of femoral neck fractures. A meta-analysis. Anesthesiology 1992;77:1095-1104.

165. Urwin SC, Parker MJ, Griffiths R. General versus regional anaesthesia for hip fracture surgery: a meta-analysis of randomized trials. Br J Anaesth 2000;84:450-455.

166. Gilbert TB, Hawkes WG, Hebel JR, et al. Spinal anesthesia versus general anesthesia for hip fracture repair: a longitudinal observation of 741 elderly patients during 2-year follow-up. Am J Orthop 2000;29:25-35.

167. Sutcliffe AJ, Parker M. Mortality after spinal and general anaesthesia for surgical fixation of hip fractures. Anaesthesia 1994;49:237-240.

168. O'Hara DA, Duff A, Berlin JA, et al. The effect of anesthetic technique on postoperative outcomes in hip fracture repair. Anesthesiology 2000;92:947-957.

169. Rodgers A, Walker N, Schug S, et al. Reduction of postoperative mortality and morbidity with epidural or spinal anaesthesia: results from overview of randomised trials. BMJ 2000;321:1493.

170. Riis J, Lomholt B, Haxholdt O, et al. Immediate and long-term mental recovery from general versus epidural anesthesia in elderly patients. Acta Anaesthesiol Scand 1983;27:44-49.

171. Bigler D, Adelhoj B, Petring OU, et al. Mental function and morbidity after acute hip surgery during spinal and general anaesthesia. Anaesthesia 1985;40:672-676.

172. Ghoneim MM, Hinrichs JV, O'Hara MW, et al. Comparison of psychologic and cognitive functions after general or regional anesthesia. Anesthesiology 1988;69:507-515.

173. Yeager MP, Glass DD, Neff RK, Brinck-Johnsen T. Epidural anesthesia and analgesia in high-risk surgical patients. Anesthesiology 1987;66:729-736.

174. Chung F, Meier R, Lautenschlager E, et al. General or spinal anesthesia: which is better in the elderly? Anesthesiology 1987;67:422-427.

175. Asbjorn J, Jakobsen BW, Pilegaard HK, et al. Mental function in elderly men after surgery during epidural analgesia. Acta Anaesthesiol Scand 1989;33:369-373.

176. Edwards ND, Callaghan LC, White T, Reilly CS. Perioperative myocardial ischaemia in patients undergoing transurethral surgery: a pilot study comparing general with spinal anaesthesia. Br J Anaesth 1995;74:368-372.

177. Bode RH, Lewis KP, Zarich SW, et al. Cardiac outcome after peripheral vascular surgery. Comparison of general and regional anesthesia. Anesthesiology 1996;84:3-13.

178. Christopherson R, Beattie C, Frank SM, et al. Perioperative morbidity in patients randomized to epidural or general anesthesia for lower extremity vascular surgery. Perioperative Ischemia Randomized Anesthesia Trial Study Group. Anesthesiology 1993;79:422-434.

179. Corson JD, Chang BB, Shah DM, et al. The influence of anesthetic choice on carotid endarterectomy outcome. Arch Surg 1987;122:807-812.

180. Papavasiliou AK, Magnadottir HB, Gonda T, et al. Clinical outcomes after carotid endarterectomy: comparison of the use of regional and general anesthetics. J Neurosurg 2000;92:291-296.

181. Fiorani P, Sbarigia E, Speziale F, et al. General anaesthesia versus cervical block and perioperative complications in carotid artery surgery. Eur J Vasc Endovasc Surg 1997;13:37-42.

182. Bowyer MW, Zierold D, Loftus JP, et al. Carotid endarterectomy: a comparison of regional versus general anesthesia in 500 operations. Ann Vasc Surg 2000;14:145-151.

183. Ferguson GG, Eliasziw M, Barr HW, et al. The North American Symptomatic Carotid Endarterectomy Trial: surgical results in 1415 patients. Stroke 1999;30:1751-1758.

184. Slogoff S, Reul GJ, Keats AS, et al. Role of perfusion pressure and flow in major organ dysfunction after cardiopulmonary bypass. Ann Thorac Surg 1990;50:911-918.

185. Wong BI, McLean RF, Naylor CD, et al. Central-nervous-system dysfunction after warm or hypothermic cardiopulmonary bypass. Lancet 1992;339:1383-1384.

186. Gold JP, Charlson ME, Williams-Russo P, et al. Improvement of outcomes after coronary artery bypass. A randomized trial comparing intraoperative high versus low mean arterial pressure. J Thorac Cardiovasc Surg 1995;110:1302-1311; discussion 1311-1304.

187. Roach GW, Kanchuger M, Mangano CM, et al. Adverse cerebral outcomes after coronary bypass surgery. Multicenter Study of Perioperative Ischemia Research Group and the Ischemia Research and Education Foundation Investigators. N Engl J Med 1996;335:1857-1863.

188. Cook DJ. Neurologic effects. In Gravlee GP, Davis RF, Kurusz M, Utley JR (eds): Cardiopulmonary Bypass: Principles and Practice, 2nd ed. Philadelphia: Lippincott Williams & Wilkins, 2000:403-431.

189. Frank SM, Beattie C, Christopherson R, et al. Unintentional hypothermia is associated with postoperative myocardial ischemia. The Perioperative Ischemia Randomized Anesthesia Trial Study Group. Anesthesiology 1993;78:468-476.

190. Frank SM, El-Rahmany HK, Cattaneo CG, Barnes RA. Predictors of hypothermia during spinal anesthesia. Anesthesiology 2000;92:1330-1334.

191. Frank SM, Fleisher LA, Breslow MJ, et al. Perioperative maintenance of normothermia reduces the incidence of morbid cardiac events. A randomized clinical trial. JAMA 1997;277:1127-1134.

192. Frank SM, Fleisher LA, Olson KF, et al. Multivariate determinants of early postoperative oxygen consumption in elderly patients. Effects of shivering, body temperature, and gender. Anesthesiology 1995;83:241-249.

193. Frank SM, Higgins MS, Breslow MJ, et al. The catecholamine, cortisol, and hemodynamic responses to mild perioperative hypothermia. A randomized clinical trial. Anesthesiology 1995;82:83-93.

194. Cohen MM, Duncan PG, Pope WD, et al. The Canadian four-centre study of anaesthetic outcomes: II. Can outcomes be used to assess the quality of anaesthesia care? Can J Anaesth 1992;39:430-439.

195. Rao TL, Jacobs KH, El-Etr AA. Reinfarction following anesthesia in patients with myocardial infarction. Anesthesiology 1983;59:499-505.

196. O'Keeffe ST, Ni Chonchubhair A. Postoperative delirium in the elderly. Br J Anaesth 1994;73:673-687.

197. Seymour DG, Vaz FG. A prospective study of elderly general surgical patients: II. Post-operative complications. Age Ageing 1989;18:316-326.

198. Pontoppidan H, Beecher HK. Progressive loss of protective reflexes in the airway with the advance of age. JAMA 1960;174:2209-2213.

199. Pedersen T, Viby-Mogensen J, Ringsted C. Anaesthetic practice and postoperative pulmonary complications. Acta Anaesthesiol Scand 1992;36:812-818.

200. Moller JT, Johannessen NW, Espersen K, et al. Randomized evaluation of pulse oximetry in 20,802 patients: II. Perioperative events and postoperative complications. Anesthesiology 1993;78:445-453.

201. Moller JT, Svennild I, Johannessen NW, et al. Perioperative monitoring with pulse oximetry and late postoperative cognitive dysfunction. Br J Anaesth 1993;71:340-347.

202. Bailey PL, Pace NL, Ashburn MA, et al. Frequent hypoxemia and apnea after sedation with midazolam and fentanyl. Anesthesiology 1990;73:826-830.

203. Hogue CW, Jr., Lappas GD, Creswell LL, et al. Swallowing dysfunction after cardiac operations. Associated adverse outcomes and risk factors including intraoperative transesophageal echocardiography. J Thorac Cardiovasc Surg 1995;110:517-522.

204. Mitchell CK, Smoger SH, Pfeifer MP, et al. Multivariate analysis of factors associated with postoperative pulmonary complications following general elective surgery. Arch Surg 1998;133:194-198.

205. Warner MA, Warner ME, Weber JG. Clinical significance of pulmonary aspiration during the perioperative period. Anesthesiology 1993;78:56-62.

206. Roberts JR, Shyr Y, Christian KR, et al. Preemptive gastrointestinal tract management reduces aspiration and respiratory failure after thoracic operations. J Thorac Cardiovasc Surg 2000;119:449-452.

207. Breslow MJ, Parker SD, Frank SM, et al. Determinants of catecholamine and cortisol responses to lower extremity revascularization. The PIRAT Study Group. Anesthesiology 1993;79:1202-1209.

208. Rem J, Nielsen OS, Brandt MR, Kehlet H. Release mechanisms of postoperative changes in various acute phase proteins and immunoglobulins. Acta Chir Scand Suppl 1980;502:51-56.

209. Kilickan L, Toker K. The effects of preemptive intravenous versus preemptive epidural morphine on postoperative analgesia and surgical stress response after orthopaedic procedures. Minerva Anestesiol 2000;66:649-655.

210. Schulze S, Schierbeck J, Sparso BH, et al. Influence of neural blockade and indomethacin on leucocyte, temperature, and acute-phase protein response to surgery. Acta Chir Scand 1987;153:255-259.

211. Klasen JA, Opitz SA, Melzer C, et al. Intraarticular, epidural, and intravenous analgesia after total knee arthroplasty. Acta Anaesthesiol Scand 1999;43:1021-1026.

212. Schulze S, Sommer P, Bigler D, et al. Effect of combined prednisolone, epidural analgesia, and indomethacin on the systemic response after colonic surgery. Arch Surg 1992;127:325-331.

213. Rem J, Brandt MR, Kehlet H. Prevention of postoperative lymphopenia and granulocytosis by epidural analgesia. Lancet 1980;1:283-284.

214. Hjortso NC, Andersen T, Frosig F, et al. Failure of epidural analgesia to modify postoperative depression of delayed hypersensitivity. Acta Anaesthesiol Scand 1984;28:128-131.

215. Rutberg H, Hakanson E, Anderberg B, et al. Effects of the extradural administration of morphine, or bupivacaine, on the endocrine response to upper abdominal surgery. Br J Anaesth 1984;56:233-238.

216. Liu S, Carpenter RL, Neal JM. Epidural anesthesia and analgesia. Their role in postoperative outcome. Anesthesiology 1995;82:1474-1506.

217. Tuman KJ, McCarthy RJ, March RJ, et al. Effects of epidural anesthesia and analgesia on coagulation and outcome after major vascular surgery. Anesth Analg 1991;73:696-704.

218. Giesecke K, Klingstedt C, Ljungqvist O, Hagenfeldt L. The modifying influence of anaesthesia on postoperative protein catabolism. Br J Anaesth 1994;72:697-699.

219. Heindorff H, Schulze S, Mogensen T, et al. Hormonal and neural blockade prevents the postoperative increase in amino acid clearance and urea synthesis. Surgery 1992;111:543-550.

220. Carli F, Halliday D. Continuous epidural blockade arrests the postoperative decrease in muscle protein fractional synthetic rate in surgical patients. Anesthesiology 1997;86:1033-1040.

221. Wasylak TJ, Abbott FV, English MJ, Jeans ME. Reduction of postoperative morbidity following patient-controlled morphine. Can J Anaesth 1990;37:726-731.

222. Petros JG, Alameddine F, Testa E, et al. Patient-controlled analgesia and postoperative urinary retention after hysterectomy for benign disease. J Am Coll Surg 1994;179:663-667.

223. Petros JG, Mallen JK, Howe K, et al. Patient-controlled analgesia and postoperative urinary retention after open appendectomy. Surg Gynecol Obstet 1993;177:172-175.

224. Carpenter RL, Abram SE, Bromage PR, Rauck RL. Consensus statement on acute pain management. Reg Anesth 1996;21:152-156.

225. Carpenter RL. Gastrointestinal benefits of regional anesthesia/analgesia. Reg Anesth 1996;21:13-17.

226. Kumar A, Bose S, Bhattacharya A, et al. Oral clonidine premedication for elderly patients undergoing intraocular surgery. Acta Anaesthesiol Scand 1992;36:159-164.

227. Singelyn FJ, Gouverneur JM. Extended "three-in-one" block after total knee arthroplasty: continuous versus patient-controlled techniques. Anesth Analg 2000;91:176-180.

228. De Kock MF, Pichon G, Scholtes JL. Intraoperative clonidine enhances postoperative morphine patient-controlled analgesia. Can J Anaesth 1992;39:537-544.

229. Wong HY, Carpenter RL, Kopacz DJ, et al. A randomized, double-blind evaluation of ketorolac tromethamine for postoperative analgesia in ambulatory surgery patients. Anesthesiology 1993;78:6-14.

230. Milligan KR, Convery PN, Weir P, et al. The efficacy and safety of epidural infusions of levobupivacaine with and without clonidine for postoperative pain relief in patients undergoing total hip replacement. Anesth Analg 2000;91:393-397.

231. Capdevila X, Barthelet Y, Biboulet P, et al. Effects of perioperative analgesic technique on the surgical outcome and duration of rehabilitation after major knee surgery. Anesthesiology 1999;91:8-15.

232. Mahoney OM, Noble PC, Davidson J, Tullos HS. The effect of continuous epidural analgesia on postoperative pain, rehabilitation, and duration of hospitalization in total knee arthroplasty. Clin Orthop 1990:30-37.

233. Williams-Russo P, Sharrock NE, Haas SB, et al. Randomized trial of epidural versus general anesthesia: outcomes after primary total knee replacement. Clin Orthop 1996:199-208.

234. Cullen DJ, Sweitzer BJ, Bates DW, et al. Preventable adverse drug events in hospitalized patients: a comparative study of intensive care and general care units. Crit Care Med 1997;25:1289-1297.

235. Parikh SS, Chung F. Postoperative delirium in the elderly. Anesth Analg 1995;80:1223-1232.

236. Ritchie K, Polge C, de Roquefeuil G, et al. Impact of anesthesia on the cognitive functioning of the elderly. Int Psychogeriatr 1997;9:309-326.

237. Grichnik KP, Ijsselmuiden AJ, D'Amico TA, et al. Cognitive decline after major noncardiac operations: a preliminary prospective study. Ann Thorac Surg 1999;68:1786-1791.

238. Billig N, Stockton P, Cohen-Mansfield J. Cognitive and affective changes after cataract surgery in an elderly population. Am J Geriatr Psychiatry 1995;4:29-38.

239. Goldstein MZ, Young BL, Fogel BS, Benedict RH. Occurrence and predictors of short-term mental and functional changes in older adults undergoing elective surgery under general anesthesia. Am J Geriatr Psychiatry 1998;6:42-52.

240. Rogers MP, Liang MH, Daltroy LH, et al. Delirium after elective orthopedic surgery: risk factors and natural history. Int J Psychiatry Med 1989;19:109-121.

241. Williams-Russo P, Sharrock NE, Mattis S, et al. Cognitive effects after epidural vs general anesthesia in older adults. A randomized trial. JAMA 1995;274:44-50.

242. Moller JT, Cluitmans P, Rasmussen LS, et al. Long-term postoperative cognitive dysfunction in the elderly ISPOCD1 study. ISPOCD investigators. International Study of Post-Operative Cognitive Dysfunction. Lancet 1998;351:857-861.

243. McKhann GM, Goldsborough MA, Borowicz LM, Jr., et al. Cognitive outcome after coronary artery bypass: a one-year prospective study. Ann Thorac Surg 1997;63:510-515.

244. Newman MF, Kramer D, Croughwell ND, et al. Differential age effects of mean arterial pressure and rewarming on cognitive dysfunction after cardiac surgery. Anesth Analg 1995;81:236-242.

245. Selnes OA, Goldsborough MA, Borowicz LM, et al. Determinants of cognitive change after coronary artery bypass surgery: a multifactorial problem. Ann Thorac Surg 1999;67:1669-1676.

246. Chung FF, Chung A, Meier RH, et al. Comparison of perioperative mental function after general anaesthesia and spinal anaesthesia with intravenous sedation. Can J Anaesth 1989;36:382-387.

247. Marcantonio ER, Juarez G, Goldman L, et al. The relationship of postoperative delirium with psychoactive medications. JAMA 1994;272:1518-1522.

248. Herrick IA, Ganapathy S, Komar W, et al. Postoperative cognitive impairment in the elderly. Choice of patient-controlled analgesia opioid. Anaesthesia 1996;51:356-360.

249. Crul BJ, Hulstijn W, Burger IC. Influence of the type of anaesthesia on post-operative subjective physical well-being and mental function in elderly patients. Acta Anaesthesiol Scand 1992;36:615-620.

250. Tune LE, Damlouji NF, Holland A, et al. Association of postoperative delirium with raised serum levels of anticholinergic drugs. Lancet 1981;2:651-653.

251. Brebner J, Hadley L. Experiences with physostigmine in the reversal of adverse post-anaesthetic effects. Can Anaesth Soc J 1976;23:574-581.

252. Marcantonio ER, Goldman L, Orav EJ, et al. The association of intraoperative factors with the development of postoperative delirium. Am J Med 1998;105:380-384.

253. Dodds C, Allison J. Postoperative cognitive deficit in the elderly surgical patient. Br J Anaesth 1998;81:449-462.

254. Inouye SK, Charpentier PA. Precipitating factors for delirium in hospitalized elderly persons. Predictive model and interrelationship with baseline vulnerability. JAMA 1996;275:852-857.

255. Inouye SK. Delirium in hospitalized older patients: recognition and risk factors. J Geriatr Psychiatry Neurol 1998;11:118-125; discussion 157-118.

256. Inouye SK. Delirium in hospitalized older patients. Clin Geriatr Med 1998;14:745-764.

257. Lynch EP, Lazor MA, Gellis JE, et al. The impact of postoperative pain on the development of postoperative delirium. Anesth Analg 1998;86:781-785.

258. Koenig HG, George LK, Stangl D, Tweed DL. Hospital stressors experienced by elderly medical inpatients: developing a Hospital Stress Index. Int J Psychiatry Med 1995;25:103-122.

259. Inouye SK. Predisposing and precipitating factors for delirium in hospitalized older patients. Dement Geriatr Cogn Disord 1999;10:393-400.

260. Inouye SK, Bogardus ST, Jr., Charpentier PA, et al. A multicomponent intervention to prevent delirium in hospitalized older patients [see comments]. N Engl J Med 1999;340:669-676.

261. Inouye SK, Rushing JT, Foreman MD, et al. Does delirium contribute to poor hospital outcomes? A three-site epidemiologic study. J Gen Intern Med 1998;13:234-242.

262. Inouye SK, Viscoli CM, Horwitz RI, et al. A predictive model for delirium in hospitalized elderly medical patients based on admission characteristics. Ann Intern Med 1993;119:474-481.

263. Inouye SK, van Dyck CH, Alessi CA, et al. Clarifying confusion: the confusion assessment method. A new method for detection of delirium. Ann Intern Med 1990;113:941-948.

264. Goldstein MZ. Cognitive change after elective surgery in nondemented older adults. Am J Geriatr Psychiatry 1993;1:118-125.

265. McDowell I, Newell C. Measuring Health: A Guide to Rating Scales and Questionnaires, 2nd ed. New York: Oxford University Press, Inc., 1996.

266. Froehlich TE, Robison JT, Inouye SK. Screening for dementia in the outpatient setting: the time and change test [see comments]. J Am Geriatr Soc 1998;46:1506-1511.

267. Freedman GM, Peruvemba R. Geriatric pain management. The anesthesiologist's perspective. Anesthesiol Clin North America 2000;18:123-141, vii.
268. Parmelee PA, Katz IR, Lawton MP. The relation of pain to depression among institutionalized aged. J Gerontol 1991;46:15-21.
269. Farrell MJ, Gerontol M, Gibson SJ, Helme RD. The effect of medical status on the activity level of older pain clinic patients. J Am Geriatr Soc 1995;43:102-107.
270. Sorkin BA, Rudy TE, Hanlon RB, et al. Chronic pain in old and young patients: differences appear less important than similarities. J Gerontol 1990;45:64-68.
271. Cutler RB, Fishbain DA, Rosomoff RS, Rosomoff HL. Outcomes in treatment of pain in geriatric and younger age groups. Arch Phys Med Rehabil 1994;75:457-464.
272. Lipman AG. Analgesic drugs for neuropathic and sympathetically maintained pain. Clin Geriatr Med 1996;12:501-515.
273. Arner S, Meyerson BA. Lack of analgesic effect of opioids on neuropathic and idiopathic forms of pain. Pain 1988;33:11-23.
274. Swerdlow M. Anticonvulsants in the therapy of neuralgic pain. In The Pain Clinic. Utrecht: VNU Science Press, 1986:9-19.
275. Stanton-Hicks M, Baron R, Boas R, et al. Complex Regional Pain Syndromes: guidelines for therapy. Clin J Pain 1998;14:155-166.
276. Max MB, Kishore-Kumar R, Schafer SC, et al. Efficacy of desipramine in painful diabetic neuropathy: a placebo-controlled trial. Pain 1991;45:3-9; discussion 1-2.
277. Cutler RB, Fishbain DA, Lu Y, et al. Prediction of pain center treatment outcome for geriatric chronic pain patients. Clin J Pain 1994;10:10-17.
278. Carmichael JK. Treatment of herpes zoster and postherpetic neuralgia. Am Fam Physician 1991;44:203-210.
279. Watson CP, Evans RJ, Watt VR. Post-herpetic neuralgia and topical capsaicin. Pain 1988;33:333-340.
280. Hwang SM, Kang YC, Lee YB, et al. The effects of epidural blockade on the acute pain in herpes zoster. Arch Dermatol 1999;135:1359-1364.
281. Chiarello SE. Tumescent infiltration of corticosteroids, lidocaine, and epinephrine into dermatomes of acute herpetic pain or postherpetic neuralgia. Arch Dermatol 1998;134:279-281.
282. Alper BS, Lewis PR. Does treatment of acute herpes zoster prevent or shorten postherpetic neuralgia? J Fam Pract 2000;49:255-264.
283. Kost RG, Straus SE. Postherpetic neuralgia. Predicting and preventing risk. Arch Intern Med 1997;157:1166-1167.
284. Byrd JC, McGrail LH, Hospenthal DR, et al. Herpes virus infections occur frequently following treatment with fludarabine: results of a prospective natural history study. Br J Haematol 1999;105:445-447.
285. Sengstaken EA, King SA. The problems of pain and its detection among geriatric nursing home residents. J Am Geriatr Soc 1993;41:541-544.

3

GERIATRIC EMERGENCY MEDICINE

*Scott T. Wilber, MD, FACEP**

The emergency department (ED) is commonly the point of entry to the medical system for older adults, who present with a wide variety of problems. Although the ED is generally thought of as a location for the diagnosis and treatment of acute medical and surgical emergencies, it may also be the access point for older adults with chronic conditions or social and psychiatric problems. For younger adults with single, acute problems, an emergency care model that incorporates history, physical examination, diagnostic testing, diagnosis, treatment, and disposition may be appropriate. However, there may be pitfalls when this approach is applied in the ED to older patients. [1]

Older patients may present with vague symptoms or with atypical symptoms of serious disease, which could consequently go undetected. Cognitive impairment, common in older patients, may also go undetected. Comorbidities and polypharmacy are also common and may directly or indirectly affect the older patient's care. The ED may be a presenting location for an elderly patient with functional decline, or the acute illness or injury that provoked the ED visit may result in a decrease in his or her functional abilities. Additionally, treatment may affect the ability of the older patient to live independently; for example, immobilization of an extremity may impact the patient's ability to perform basic activities of daily living (ADLs).

These factors have led to the development of a geriatric emergency care model that differs from the standard emergency care model. The geriatric model emphasizes the consideration of older ED patients as a special population, analogous to pediatric patients. Emergency physicians should include biologic, psychologic, and social factors in the evaluation of the older ED patient. [2]

This chapter reviews the emergency medicine literature to characterize its state of development and to identify important research questions. The goal of research in the emergency care of older patients is to improve patient care through optimum medical management. Other goals include the prevention of disease and injury and the maintenance of physical, social, and emotional functioning. The standard sequence of research leading to these outcomes is descriptive studies, followed by analytic studies and finally by interventional studies. The latter include studies of diagnostic testing, treatments, and outcomes. This scheme is used to classify the stage of existing research in geriatric emergency care and identify areas for future research. This review focuses on ED conditions that practicing physicians and leaders in the field have identified as leading problems.

METHODS

For emergency medicine, the MEDLINE search included the following MeSH headings: "Emergency Medicine," "Emergency Service, Hospital," or "Emergency Treatment." For trauma, the following MeSH headings were used: "Wounds, Penetrating," "Wounds, Non-penetrating," or "Multiple Trauma." This was combined using the Boolean search

* Assistant Professor of Emergency Medicine, Northeastern Ohio Universities College of Medicine, Rootstown, OH; Associate Director, Emergency Medicine Research Center, Summa Health System, Akron, OH.

operator "AND" with articles with the following geriatric identifiers: "Geriatrics" or "Geriatric Assessment" as MeSH headings, or *geriatric*, *geriatrics*, *old*, *older*, or *aged* as title words. Limits placed on the search included English language, human, aged (> 65), and years 1980 to 2001. Articles from outside of the United States or Canada were included only if they provided unique information. They were not used if they presented demographic or observational information only.

The MEDLINE search for emergency medicine resulted in a list of 3348 articles. Following review of titles and abstracts, 299 articles were obtained for inspection. The search for trauma resulted in a list of 1838 articles, of which 133 articles were obtained for inspection.

GENERAL GERIATRIC EMERGENCY CARE

PATTERNS OF ED USE

The patterns of ED use among older patients have been well described. Reports of single-hospital studies, multicenter studies, and analyses of large multihospital databases reveal consistent patterns across all these settings.

A recent population-based cross-sectional study of noninstitutionalized Medicare beneficiaries aged 66 years and older used a Medicare database from 1993. [3] It found that 18% of persons made at least one ED visit per year, including 17% among those aged 66 to 84 and 26% among those 85 years and older. The population-based visit rates were 30 per 100 persons for the group overall, and 28 per 100 in patients in the 66 to 84 age group, and 43 per 100 in the 85 and older age group, which is higher than the percentage of patients making at least one visit because some persons made more than one visit. Logistic regression identified the following as predictors of one or more ED visits over 1 year: age 85 and older (OR [odds ratio] = 1.23), less than 12 years education (OR = 1.22), living alone (OR = 1.15), worsening self-reported health, ADL deficiencies, and comorbidity. Odds ratios for the latter three vary by level of severity.

A similar study using Medicare data from Washington State found identical visit rates but also showed that persons with physicians had fewer visits (185 per 1000 patient years) than did those without physicians (457 visits per 1000 patient years). [4] Older rural patients may also be less likely than their urban counterparts to visit the ED. [5,6]

Analysis of the 1992 National Hospital Ambulatory Medical Care Survey (NHAMCS) database, a national probability sample of ED use performed by the National Center for Health Statistics, found that patients aged 65 and older accounted for 12.6 million ED visits in 1992, or 13% of all ED visits (20% of adult ED visits). [7] The hospitalization rate was 42%, which was four times that of adults aged 18 to 64 years. Cardiopulmonary complaints were most common, with chest pain and dyspnea each constituting 11% of chief complaints. Abdominal pain, vertigo, and generalized weakness each constituted approximately 3% of visits.

Other multicenter studies have shown that ED patients aged 65 and over are more likely to be admitted to the intensive care unit, to arrive by ambulance, to have comorbid illness, to have comprehensive visits, and to have higher rates of test utilization. [8–10]

Descriptive data on ED use by older adults exist, with data from large databases confirming findings of smaller studies. Analytical data are beginning to be published regarding the predictors of visits.

EmergMed 1 (Level D): **Observational and analytic studies on emergency department use by elderly patients should continue to come from large databases or national samples (such as the National Hospital Ambulatory Medical Care Survey database) so that the results can be generalized.**

PHYSICIAN TRAINING AND COMFORT

The Society for Academic Emergency Medicine with the support of the John A. Hartford Foundation formed the Geriatric Emergency Medicine Task Force to evaluate the state of the care of older patients in the ED. The task force did an extensive review of the literature and carried out a series of integrated studies. These included surveys of physicians and patients, prospective and retrospective descriptions of differences between older and younger ED patients, and an analysis of existing data sets. [11]

The task force found that emergency physicians commonly identify the management of older patients as more time-consuming, more difficult, and requiring more resources than that of younger adults. [12] Descriptive studies of physicians' and older patients' comfort with the ED encounter were conducted by the Geriatric Emergency Medicine Task Force in 1991. A survey asked practicing emergency physicians to compare the time required, resources required, and difficulty in managing younger and older patients for seven high-volume complaints (abdominal pain, altered mental status, chest pain, dizziness, fever, headache, trauma); 433 of 971 physicians responded. Two thirds of respondents reported more time and resource use for six of the seven complaints in the older patients. For the seventh, chest pain, more than half reported more time and resource use. The respondents also reported more difficulty in managing abdominal pain, altered mental status, dizziness, and trauma in older than in younger patients. Fifty-three percent of practicing emergency physicians felt that insufficient time had been spent on geriatric issues in their residencies, and 71% felt that research in geriatric emergency medicine was inadequate. [12] This descriptive information is based upon narrowly focused, limited research conducted more than 10 years ago. Only seven complaints were assessed in the former study; therefore, the results may reflect a general sense that resource and time utilization are greater for older patients, rather than a specific concern with these complaints.

EmergMed 2 (Level A): **Randomized controlled trials are needed to assess the effectiveness of interventions (eg, educational models, standardized protocols) for improving quality of care of older emergency department patients.**

ENVIRONMENT

Patient perceptions of ED care have been described through focus-group interviews and small surveys. Issues revealed by these studies include environmental issues, long wait times, anxiety, and poor communication. [13,14]

EmergMed 3 (Level B): **Large studies are needed to confirm the results of patient surveys and focus group interviews. Studies to identify characteristics of the micro-environment that affect outcomes in elderly patients (communication, emergency department environment) are needed to identify target areas for improvement.**

EmergMed 4 (Level A): **Following evidence-based identification of target areas for improvement, controlled studies of the effect of alterations in the micro-environment on outcomes for older emergency department patients should be performed. Such studies likely cannot be based on random assignments of individuals to interventions; rather, whole micro-environments will have to be compared.**

PREHOSPITAL CARE

Descriptive information regarding emergency medical service (EMS) use among older adults comes from single-city retrospective studies. One third of patients aged 65 and older in the ED arrive by ambulance. [8,10] Older patients are responsible for 22% to 39% of EMS runs, which is out of proportion to their representation in the population. [15,16] Population-based estimates of the rate of paramedic runs for older patients show a rate of approximately 100 per 1000 population per year. [15,17] This rate is nearly twice that of patients under age 65, and the rate in patients 65 and older increases with increasing age, to a rate of 291 per 1000 patients aged 85 years and older. [15,17] Given that patients aged 80 and older are the most rapidly increasing demographic group in this country and that nearly one third of patients aged 85 or older require EMS transport per year, one can see that in the years to come an increasing proportion of EMS runs will involve older patients.

Common reasons for EMS transport include respiratory distress (13.1%), unspecified pain (12.3%), and chest pain (12.0%). [17] Older patients are 2.6 times more likely than their younger counterparts to have a cardiopulmonary complaint, 1.8 times more likely to have a fall, and 1.7 times more likely to have a minor medical complaint. Additionally, they are more likely to require advanced cardiac life support care and have longer on-scene times. [16]

Providers of prehospital care have a unique opportunity to assess patients in their home situations. One trial of the feasibility of having paramedics screen older patients for medical, psychiatric, social, and environmental problems has been published. [18] This prospective study involved training paramedics to identify potential problems in older patients, referral of at-risk patients to the Area Agency on Aging for assessment by a trained geriatric assessor, and linkage of the patient to community services. The primary finding of the study was the usefulness of the program to individual patients. The program was defined as useful if a problem was identified, an assessment was done, and the problem was confirmed by the assessor. Additionally, the problem had to have the potential for improvement, and help had to be received. Paramedics identified 197 patients with potential problems out of 6000 evaluated; 124 received assessment. The assessor confirmed problems identified by paramedics in 121 cases (98%). The project was useful for 48% of patients identified as having potential problems.

EmergMed 5 (Level B): **Cohort studies should be performed to describe the ability of prehospital care providers to assess older patients in their home environments. Areas where this may be particularly beneficial include the assessment of the home environment in patients with falls and functional decline, and the assessment of potential abuse. This research should focus on whether information about home environment provided by prehospital care providers affects patient outcomes.**

COGNITIVE IMPAIRMENT

Older patients who present to the ED commonly have cognitive impairment. This may impact the patient's care in many ways, from limiting the reliability of the medical history to reducing his or her understanding of and compliance with discharge instructions. Although recognized or unrecognized dementia is a likely cause of cognitive impairment, delirium is another common cause. Delirium is considered a medical emergency because of its multiple serious medical causes (eg, sepsis, myocardial infarction, drug toxicity, occult fracture, subdural hematoma).[19] For these reasons, the assessment of cognitive impairment is considered an integral part of the evaluation of elderly persons presenting to the ED.

In a retrospective analysis of EMS transports in one county in 1990, Wofford et al reviewed patients aged 60 years and older to identify those transported for altered mental status.[20] Five percent of 4688 transports during this time were for altered mental status, and 74% of these patients were hospitalized, with a mean length of stay of 28 ± 5 days. The diagnoses included infection (26%), toxic-metabolic causes (23%), and cerebrovascular disease (20%).

In a prospective cross-sectional study, Gerson et al used the Orientation Memory Concentration Test, a validated screening instrument for cognitive impairment, to screen ED patients aged 65 years and older.[21] Patients were excluded if they had a prior diagnosis of dementia. The instrument took 1.9 ± 0.91 minutes to perform. Of 547 patients evaluated, 34% had at least moderate impairment of cognition, and an additional 26% had minimal impairment. Only 40% of patients had no impairment of cognition. Using logistic regression, the researchers determined that age 80 and above (OR = 3.68) and nursing-home residence (OR = 13.8) were independent predictors of cognitive impairment. Delirium and dementia were not differentiated.

Naughton et al conducted a prospective cross-sectional study on 188 patients in their ED who were aged 70 or older.[22] Using a combination of the Glasgow Coma Scale, the Folstein Mini–Mental Status Examination (MMSE), and the Confusion Assessment Method (a validated screening tool for delirium), they found that 8.5% of patients had impaired consciousness (patients who did not open their eyes spontaneously or in response to speech, respond to questions, or obey commands), 9.6% had delirium, 22% had cognitive impairment without delirium, and 60% were cognitively intact. Seventeen percent of patients with delirium were not admitted to the hospital. Patients with delirium had ED diagnoses of "congestive heart failure," "rule out MI," "mental status change," "sepsis," "hypertension," "seizure disorder," and "vomiting." Patients with impaired consciousness and delirium had a nonsignificant trend toward higher rates of admission and longer lengths of stay than patients who were cognitively intact. Naughton et al performed a second study to evaluate the use of computed tomography scanning in patients with delirium.[23] Methods for determining cognitive impairment were similar to those of the prior study. In the second study, 4.8% were found to have impaired consciousness, 17% delirium, and 38% cognitive impairment without delirium. Scans were most often ordered for patients with delirium. The authors believe that the differences in the prevalence of cognitive impairment between the two studies may be due to the higher proportion of nursing-home patients in the second study.

Lewis et al performed a similar prospective cross-sectional study of patients aged 65 years or older presenting to their ED.[24] Using the Confusion Assessment Method, they found that 10% of 385 patients had delirium or probable delirium. Using a score of 3 or 4 as the standard, they determined that physician sensitivity for the diagnosis of delirium was 17%. Sixty-two percent of patients with delirium were admitted. The 3-month mortality was higher for those patients with delirium than for those without, but this did not reach statistical significance (14% versus 8%, $P = .20$). For patients discharged from the ED, the increased 3-month mortality in patients with delirium was significant ($P = .048$). The most common diagnoses for admitted patients with delirium was "rule out sepsis," "delirium," and "cerebrovascular accident." "Status post fall" was the most common diagnosis for delirious patients who were discharged from the ED.

Similar results were also found by Elie et al in a prospective cross-sectional study in Montreal of ED patients aged 65 years and older. [25] In this study, research psychiatrists used the MMSE and the Confusion Assessment Method to evaluate patients for delirium. Ten percent of the 447 patients screened had delirium; the sensitivity of ED physicians' diagnosis was 35%, and the specificity was 99%. Diagnoses in patients with delirium included neurologic problems in 65%, pulmonary problems (41%), cardiovascular problems (17%), endocrine problems (11%), infectious disease (7%), and metabolic problems (7%).

It is clear from these studies that older adults presenting to the ED commonly have impaired cognition, and this is often unrecognized by the emergency physician. Discharge from the ED of patients with delirium may result in increased mortality. Emergency physicians are limited by time in assessing older patients and must use brief, sensitive tests to assess for cognitive dysfunction. Which instruments should be used for cognitive assessment of older ED patients is controversial. Currently available instruments include the MMSE, the orientation-memory-concentration test, the Short Portable Mental Status Questionnaire, the clock-drawing test, the Confusion Assessment Method, and others. [26]

> *EmergMed 6 (Level B)*: **Screening tests for cognitive dysfunction for use in the emergency department should be validated against gold-standard assessment, and efforts should be made to determine if new, shorter screening approaches would be effective.**

> *EmergMed 7 (Level B)*: **Prospective cohort studies such as larger-scale longitudinal outcome studies of older patients with impaired cognition are necessary to confirm the finding that patients with undiagnosed delirium have worse outcomes than do those without delirium or with diagnosed and treated delirium.**

> *EmergMed 8 (Level A)*: **If research (EmergMed7) confirms that older patients with delirium that is not diagnosed in the emergency department ultimately have worse outcomes than do those either without delirium or with recognized and treated delirium, interventional trials should be designed to determine the effect on outcomes of better screening and management of cognitive impairment in older emergency department patients.**

FUNCTIONAL ASSESSMENT

Functional assessment is important in the ED evaluation of many older patients. Subacute functional decline may precipitate a visit to the ED, or the acute illness or injury that precipitated the ED visit may cause functional impairment. This may result in frustration for the family if the emergency physician does not recognize the importance of these functional limitations. Likewise, the emergency physician may be frustrated if the patient's other physicians do not recognize the importance of these limitations.

There is little information regarding functional assessment or limitation in the emergency medicine literature. One study of minor traumatic injuries in older ED patients found that 75% of patients had been injured by a fall, 7% had a decline in ADL score, and 23% had a decline in instrumental activities of daily living ADL score. [27]

EmergMed 9 (Level B): **Development and testing of measures for functional assessment that are feasible and valid in elderly emergency department patients are needed.**

EmergMed 10 (Level B): **Case-control or cohort studies are needed to determine whether older emergency department patients with functional impairment have worse outcomes than do those without impairment.**

EmergMed 11 (Level A): **Controlled intervention trials are needed to determine whether the detection and management of functional impairment in older emergency department patients have an effect on these outcomes.**

MEDICATION USE

Explicit criteria for potentially inappropriate medication use in older patients have been defined. [28] These include inappropriate medications as well as drug-disease interactions. In a prospective ED study, Chin et al found that 11% of patients presenting to the ED were already on potentially inappropriate medications, 3.6% were given one in the ED, and 5.6% were prescribed one on discharge from the ED. [29] Drug-disease interactions were less common at presentation (5.2%), in the ED (0.6%), and on discharge (1.2%). The most common inappropriate medications on discharge were indomethacin, diphenhydramine, cyclobenzaprine, and propoxyphene. In the ED, meperidine was also a commonly used inappropriate medication. The study did not find any significant association between potentially inappropriate medications or adverse drug-disease interactions in revisit to the ED, hospitalization, or death over the 3-month follow-up period.

Adverse drug interactions may also be important in the elderly age group. Older patients are more likely to be on multiple medications on presentation to the ED, and medications are commonly added in the ED (one half to two thirds of visits). [30,31] One study showed that 42% of patients presenting to the ED had a drug interaction, but that only 10% were clinically significant. [31] Twenty-six percent of patients had a drug interaction due to medications initiated in the ED, but only 3% were clinically relevant. Multiple regression showed that age 60 and older was the only predictor of clinically significant drug interactions.

Another study showed that 10% of patients who had a drug added in the ED had a potential drug interaction. [30] The rate was significantly different in the two age groups examined by the authors, patients younger than 60 (4%) and patients over age 65 (18%). However, using multiple regression, the researchers found that age was not an independent predictor; rather, the number of medications at presentation and the number of ED medications prescribed were the only significant independent predictors. Eighty-nine percent of all interactions were found to have occurred with prescriptions for narcotics, nonsteroidal anti-inflammatory drugs, benzodiazepines, antacids, and diuretics. Adding medications in the ED may also increase medication complexity and decrease older patients' knowledge of their medications. [32]

Balanced against this negative view of adding medications in the ED is the possibility of oligoanalgesia in older patients. Among patients with long-bone fractures, the older are less likely to receive ED pain medications, wait longer to receive medications, and receive the medications at lower doses than do their younger counterparts. One retrospective review did not correlate this finding with the severity of pain, satisfaction, pain relief, or other outcome measures. [33] Interestingly, in this study, both meperidine and propoxyphene were found to be prescribed more frequently for older than for younger patients, though both are potentially inappropriate for older patients. [28] However, the study was done several years prior to Beers' 1997 update that defined explicit criteria for potentially inappropriate medications for older patients.

> *EmergMed 12 (Level B)*: **Large, long-term studies of the outcomes when older patients are prescribed potentially inappropriate medications are needed.**

> *EmergMed 13 (Level A)*: **Interventional trials (randomized or by comparison of micro-environments) are needed of methods to reduce prescription of potentially inappropriate medications for older patients, such as educational sessions or computer-assisted decision support systems integrated into emergency department discharge instructions.**

SCREENING AND COMPREHENSIVE GERIATRIC ASSESSMENT IN THE ED

The ED is generally considered a location for the treatment of acute medical emergencies rather than for screening. However, for older patients, screening for problems outside of the patient's chief complaint may be beneficial.

COMPREHENSIVE GERIATRIC ASSESSMENT

ED-based comprehensive geriatric screening has been evaluated in two studies. Miller et al performed a nonrandomized controlled trial of a 30-minute comprehensive geriatric assessment in the ED. [34] Patients were enrolled over 11 months and were seen between noon and 8 pm on alternating days. Control patients were obtained by using the ED census to identify patients seen the prior day, matching by gender and age within 5 years. Control patients were not contacted initially and received standard ED care. The intervention group received evaluations by a geriatric nurse clinician who identified medical, dental, and social problems and made recommendations to the patient, family, and physicians. For the intervention group, 434 patients were approached and 385 patients consented to participate. Intervention and control groups were similar in demographic characteristics. Sixty-seven percent of intervention patients were found to be dependent in at least one ADL. Eighty-two percent had at least one geriatric problem identified, and 77% reported at least one unmet dental or social need. The cost of the intervention was low ($5 to identify each geriatric issue and $1 to identify each dental or social issue), but physicians complied with only 62% of suggestions and families with only 37% of suggestions. Mortality and nursing-home residence did not differ between groups at 3 months; however, there were trends toward fewer subsequent ED visits and more advance directives in the intervention group.

Gerson et al conducted a multicenter, prospective, uncontrolled trial of case findings in adults aged 60 and older in five hospital EDs. [35] Medical students were trained in the administration of a 17-item protocol that took a mean time of 17.7 ± 10.2 minutes to complete per patient. Three quarters of 338 eligible patients participated, and 96% of patients had at least one condition detected (281 conditions detected). Most commonly detected conditions were impaired ADLs (79%), decreased vision (55%), lack of influenza vaccination (54%), unhealthy home environment (49%), impaired mental status (46%), falls (40%), and depression (36%). Seventy-six patients were evaluated at follow-up, 47 (17%) conditions were confirmed, and treatment plans were initiated for 25 conditions (9%).

Sinoff et al in a retrospective review of geriatric consults in the ED found that 64% of patients who had consults were admitted, 34% died within 2 years, and 52% were admitted to long-term-care facilities. [36] They found high rates of classic geriatric problems, including falls, incontinence, iatrogenic events, and confusional states. This was an observational study, and only patients for whom a geriatric consultation was obtained in the ED were included. Consultation was not mandatory and was generally initiated by the ED staff.

Jones et al performed a prospective observational study by telephone call-back of adults aged 60 years and older who had been discharged from the ED. [37] They were able to contact 79% of patients and found that 13% of these had moderate deterioration in their ability to care for themselves, and 40% required further clarification of discharge instructions. Four percent were advised to return to the ED, and 3% were referred to a medical social worker.

IDENTIFICATION OF SENIORS AT RISK TOOL

McCusker et al have published multiple studies on screening of ED patients. [38–43] In a prospective, observational study of ED patients aged 75 years and older, they determined predictors of repeat ED visits within 90 days by using multivariate logistic regression. [43] Twenty-four percent of patients made a repeat visit within 90 days. Predictors included male gender (OR = 7.06), living alone (OR = 10.48), and the number of self-reported problems (depression, confusion, incontinence, falls, mobility, and balance) (OR = 2.68).

The Identification of Seniors at Risk (ISAR) screening tool was developed to improve the recognition of older ED patients who are at risk for adverse outcomes. [42] A screening questionnaire was developed from a literature review of predictors of functional decline and by adapting other questionnaires. The initial questionnaire had 27 questions on social, physical, and mental risk factors, on medical history, and on the use of medical services, medications, and alcohol. These questions were compared with validated tools, including the Geriatric Depression Scale and the CAGE questionnaire (Cut down, Annoyed by criticism, Guilty about drinking, Eye-opener). The screening questionnaire itself had good test-retest reliability; however, individual questions were more specific than sensitive and had only modest concurrent validity. The questions with the highest level of sensitivity and specificity were those on visual and hearing impairment, medications, and depression.

A second study looked at the ability of the questionnaire, or a subset of questions from it, to identify patients at risk of adverse health outcome over 6 months (adverse health outcome was defined as death, institutionalization, or a clinically significant decline in physical function). [38] This prospective observational study found that 30% of patients in the development phase had an adverse health outcome, including 10% who died, 3% who were institutionalized, and 16% who had increased functional dependence. The best subset of 6 questions (see Table 3.1) was based upon statistical analysis, as well as input from the ISAR Steering Committee. The area under the curve (AUC) for detection of an adverse outcome was 0.71 in the validation set. Two positive responses had a sensitivity of 75% and a specificity of 58%. Three positive responses had a sensitivity of 27% and a specificity of 81%, and four positive responses a sensitivity of 10% and a specificity of 93%.

The ISAR screening tool and the complete 27-item screening questionnaire have also been found to be predictors of return visits to the ED over 30 days (AUC = 0.63), three or more visits over 6 months (AUC = 0.68), [40] and hospital utilization over 6 months (AUC = 0.68). [39]

Feeling depressed and certain diagnoses also predicted both early and frequent return. [40] A history of heart disease, having ever been married, and not drinking alcohol predicted early return, and a history of diabetes mellitus, a recent ED visit, and lack of support predicted frequent return. [40] Other predictors of high hospital utilization included age 85 or older, living alone, and poor self-reported health. [39]

> **EmergMed 14 (Level B)**: **Comprehensive emergency department screening of older patients is feasible and inexpensive; however, outcomes have not been affected, possibly because of low compliance with recommendations and follow-up. Potential interventions to improve compliance with recommendations and follow-up, including direct referral to geriatric teams, should be prospectively evaluated.**

> **EmergMed 15 (Level B)**: **The Identification of Seniors at Risk tool should be employed at independent sites to determine its value in selecting high-risk elderly patients for interventional trials of geriatric assessment.**

Table 3.1—The Best Subset of Questions from the ISAR Screening Tool

1. *Before* the illness or injury that brought you to Emergency, did you need someone to help you on a regular basis?

2. *Since* the illness or injury that brought you to Emergency, have you needed more help than usual to take care of yourself?

3. Have you been hospitalized for one or more nights during the past 6 months?

4. In general, do you see well?

5. In general, do you have serious problems with your memory?

6. Do you take more than three different medications every day?

Source: Data from McCusker J, Bellavance F, Cardin S, et al. Detection of older people at increased risk of adverse health outcomes after an emergency visit: the ISAR screening tool. J Am Geriatr Soc 1999;47:1229-1237.

SCREENING FOR SPECIFIC CONDITIONS

Visual Deficit

A British study evaluated screening for correctable undetected visual acuity deficit in ED patients aged 65 years or older and found that 36% of patients had a correctable visual acuity deficit of 2 lines or more in one or both eyes. [44] Self-reported problems with vision are associated with adverse health outcomes in older patients discharged from the ED. [38] In a guideline for the ED management of falls in older adults, it was recommended to simply ask the patient whether he or she had had an eye examination in the prior year. [45] No interventional trials of vision screening in the ED have been performed.

Depression

Depression in older adults is common and may be an unrecognized component in a patient's ED presentation. McCusker et al found a prevalence of depression of 26% in ED patients aged 65 and older, using a score of 11 on the Geriatric Depression Scale as a cut-off. [42] The single screening question "In general, do you feel sad and depressed?" had a sensitivity of 56% and a specificity of 88% for detecting depression. Meldon et al found a prevalence of depression in their older ED patients (aged 65 and older) of 27% using the Koenig Scale, a validated 10-question scale for depression screening. [46] Nursing-home patients were found to have a prevalence of depression of 47% versus 24% for those who were living independently. Patients with poor self-reported health were also more likely to be depressed (51% prevalence). Physician sensitivity for the detection of depression was 0%. Clinical characteristics were unable to predict depression in these older patients. [47] In a second study by Meldon et al, 30% of patients were found to meet the criteria for depression, and physician sensitivity was 27% and specificity was 75%. Thirteen percent of depressed patients were referred for mental health evaluation. [48]

Alcohol Abuse

Alcoholism may also go unrecognized in older adults. In a prospective cross-sectional study, Adams et al found 24% of ED patients aged 65 years and over to have a current or prior drinking problem and 14% to be current alcohol abusers (defined as a CAGE score of $\geq$ 2, or a self-reported past or current drinking problem and use of alcohol over the past year). The patients who were current alcohol abusers presented with abdominal pain in 22% of cases and trauma in 7% of cases. ED physicians detected only 17% of current alcohol abusers. [49] McCusker et al reported a prevalence of current alcohol abuse (CAGE score $\geq$ 2) of 2.9%. [42] The question "Do you drink alcohol every day, not counting with meals?" was 33% sensitive and 94% specific for the diagnosis. An analysis of the 1995 NHAMCS database found that the annual rate of alcohol-related ED visits in patients aged 65 and older was 2.6 per 1000 population per year, and this was 0.6% of older persons' ED visits; both were the lowest among all age groups except the below-15 age group. [50] A review of trauma registry data found that 14% of 180 drivers aged 60 or over in motor vehicle crashes had blood alcohol counts of > 100 mg/dL. [51] In men aged 60 and over,

21% had a positive blood alcohol counts. Only one patient was found to have a toxicology screen positive for another drug of abuse.

Elder Abuse

Elder abuse is more widespread than many clinicians realize. Although child abuse is commonly evaluated and screened for in EDs, elder abuse is less so. In fact, surveys of practicing emergency physicians found that elder abuse protocols were available to 27% of respondents, whereas child abuse protocols were available to 75%. [12] In teaching institutions, 93% had protocols for child abuse, but only 42% had protocols for elder abuse. [52] Estimates of the prevalence of elder abuse are that 10% of patients aged 65 and over are subject to some type of abuse. [53] In a stratified random sample of community-dwelling older adults in Boston, Pillemer and Finkelhor found a prevalence of elder abuse of 32 per 1000 population. [54] This included a prevalence of 20 per 1000 for physical abuse, 11 per 1000 for verbal abuse, and 4 per 1000 for neglect. In contrast to other studies and popular thought, 58% of perpetrators were spouses and only 24% were children. The proportion of abused older patients was nearly evenly split between men and women, but the risk among men was more than two times that for women, owing to their smaller representation in the population.

Lachs et al identified 182 older victims of abuse reported to the regional Elder Protection Service. [55] Of these patients, 114 had been seen in the ED over the preceding 5 years, with a median of 3 visits (range 1 to 46 visits). Thirty-eight percent had at least one visit with a high probability of abuse, and 66% had at least one injury visit. Only 9.1% of these visits resulted in a referral to the Elder Protection Service.

Fulmer et al reported on a prospective pilot study of a screening instrument for elder abuse. [56] They screened 484 patients and found a 7% rate of abuse, including physical abuse in 1%, psychologic abuse in 4.1%, and material deprivation in 2.2%. An additional 6% had suspected abuse.

In a retrospective analysis of risk factors, elder abuse was found to be more common among nonwhites (OR = 2.55 for abuse, 3.02 for neglect) and the nonmarried (OR = 2.29 for abuse, 2.49 for neglect). [57] Neglect, but not abuse, was found to be more common among patients with delirium (OR = 4.23) and dementia (OR = 4.07). Two studies present protocols for the evaluation of patients with elder abuse. [56,58]

> ***EmergMed 16 (Level B)***: **Studies are needed to develop brief screening instruments for specific conditions for use with older patients in the emergency department.**

> ***EmergMed 17 (Level A)***: **Screening for asymptomatic conditions in older patients in the emergency department should be done only if detection of the abnormality results in treatment of the disorder and this treatment results in improvement in outcomes. Randomized interventional trials are needed to assess short- and long-term outcomes of patients who have screening and treatment for these conditions.**

SPECIFIC CLINICAL SYNDROMES

ABDOMINAL PAIN

Abdominal pain is the presenting complaint of 3% to 6% of older patients presenting to the ED. Surveys of emergency physicians and emergency medicine residency directors in the early 1990s found that abdominal pain was one of several complaints that physicians found more difficult to manage in the older patient. The mortality in older patients presenting with abdominal pain is 5%. Twenty-two percent will require surgery, and over half (52%) will be admitted to the hospital. Risk factors for death in older patients with abdominal pain include free air on radiograph (RR [relative risk] = 23), age over 84 (RR = 22), other significant radiographic findings (RR = 5.9), and bandemia (RR = 23). [59] If free air is present on abdominal radiographs, the mortality is 75%. Risk factors for surgery include hypotension (RR = 4.7), abnormal bowel sounds (RR = 4.2), other radiographic abnormalities (RR = 4.1), dilated loops on radiographs (RR = 3.2), and leukocytosis (RR = 2.3). Diagnoses in older patients with abdominal pain include infection (19%), mechanical problems (16%), ulcers (8%), genitourinary disease (8%), malignancy (7%), biliary tract disease (6%), cardiac disease (4%), pulmonary disease (2%), other (29%).

In one retrospective review, it was found that emergency physicians correctly classified 67% of patients with abdominal pain who were younger than 65 years but 44% of those who were 65 or older. [60]

Older patients with cholecystitis commonly do not have classic symptoms. In a retrospective review, it was found that 84% had neither epigastric nor right upper quadrant pain, and 5% had no pain at all. [61] Fifty-six percent of patients were afebrile and 41% had a normal white blood cell count. No difference in the presence or absence of these findings was found for the young-old (65 to 74), the old-old (75 to 84), or the oldest-old (85 and older). This mirrors results from another retrospective review, which showed that elevated temperature and abnormal laboratory studies do not differentiate patients who were admitted and underwent surgery from those who did not undergo surgery. [62] Thirteen percent of patients who had normal values for all laboratory studies and normal temperatures required surgery.

Only 20% of older patients with appendicitis present classically. Elevated temperatures are present in less than half (47%), and 23% have tenderness that is diffuse or localized to an area other than the right lower quadrant. [63]

A final retrospective review found that 43% of patients aged 65 and over with abdominal pain were admitted; 20% had immediate surgery, 17% were admitted and had subsequent surgery (41% of admitted patients), and 4% were discharged and had subsequent surgery. [64] Common diagnoses included indeterminate (23%), biliary tract disease (12%), small bowel obstruction (12%), gastritis (8%), perforated viscus (7%), diverticulitis (6%), and appendicitis, incarcerated hernia, and renal colic (4% each). A common limitation of all of these studies is their retrospective nature.

EmergMed 18 (Level B): **Prospective, longitudinal cohort or case-control studies of elderly emergency department patients with abdominal pain are necessary to adequately define which patients with abdominal pain have serious disease and which have benign disease.**

EmergMed 19 (Level B): **The value of history and physical examination findings, laboratory examination, and imaging studies in older emergency department patients should be prospectively evaluated.**

FALLS

Falls are both a common and serious event for older patients. Falls are the most common reason for injury visits in patients aged 65 years and older (52% of such visits). [65] In one study 15% of EMS transports for patients aged 65 years or older were for falls. [17] The risk of falls in older patients increases with increasing age, and women fall more often than men. [17,45] In older patients, fractures occur in 5% of falls, and other serious injuries occur in 5% to 10%. Twelve percent of deaths in the older population are directly or indirectly related to falls. [45]

A practice guideline for the ED management of falls in older patients was published in 1997. [45] This guideline recommended a comprehensive evaluation of ED patients who fall, including an expanded history (eg, ADLs, environmental hazards, last eye examination), physical examination (Timed Get Up and Go test, mental status examination), diagnostic studies and referral (geriatric assessment, social services, optometry, podiatry, physical therapy, occupational therapy). This guideline was implemented in three EDs that were part of a large health maintenance organization in southern California. The guideline was presented to emergency physicians at a 1-hour lecture and to ED nurses at a 30-minute in-service lecture. A pre-post intervention comparison over 2 years found that, following the education, more patients were diagnosed as having fallen as a result of loss of consciousness, stroke, or seizures. There was improved documentation of certain historical elements, visual acuity testing, and the Timed Get Up and Go test. However, there was still low compliance with many of these elements (visual acuity testing in 3.2%, Timed Get Up and Go test in 11.2%). Although there were small improvements in these aspects of the history, there was no difference in the rate of recurrent falls, hospitalization for falls, or hip fractures before and after the implementation of the guideline. [66,67]

Older black Americans may be at high risk of poor outcomes after falls. [68] Older patients may also be at increased risk for occupational injuries due to falls. [69,70]

EmergMed 20 (Level A): **Randomized controlled trials are necessary to assess the value of a falls prevention program in reducing subsequent falls by elderly patients presenting to the emergency department with a fall.**

INFECTIOUS DISEASE

Fever is a common presenting complaint of older ED patients. Morbidity and mortality are high. In one study of ED patients with oral temperatures $\geq$ 100°F, 18% were found to have positive blood cultures, 10% died within a month, and 7% required surgery. [71] Three fourths of patients had signs of serious illness (the above and hospitalization $\geq$ 4 days, intravenous antibiotics $\geq$ 3 days, or repeat ED visit within 72 hours). Predicting serious illness in ED patients with infectious symptoms is difficult. In this study, oral temperature > 103°F, respiratory rate $\geq$ 30, leukocytosis of 11,000 or more, presence of an infiltrate on chest x-ray, and pulse > 120 were found to be independent predictors of serious illness. However, 50% of patients with serious illness had none of these features.

Although the specificity for bacterial infection of such findings as elevated temperature, leukocytosis, and bandemia is relatively high (85% to 97%, varying by cut-off used), the sensitivity is low (24% to 65%). Therefore, the absence of these findings cannot be used to exclude significant bacterial infections in older adults. [72]

Another study found that the only predictive factors for bacteremia in older patients were altered mental status (OR = 2.88), vomiting (OR = 2.63), and bandemia > 6% (OR = 3.5). [73] The sensitivity of $\geq$ 1 factor was 85%, specificity was 46%.

Common infections in older patients with fever are pneumonia or bronchitis (31%), urinary tract infection (22%), sepsis (18%), and cellulitis (5%). [71] Age itself is a risk factor for more serious illness in patients with pneumonia and influenza. [74,75] Patients aged 65 years or older with urinary tract infections are more likely to have multidrug-resistant pathogens (OR = 3.0). [76]

Immunizations have become a routine part of ED practice, especially tetanus immunization. Approximately 50% of older ED patients do not have protective antibodies to tetanus. [77-79] Half of these patients will not seroconvert in 14 days after immunization. [77] One third of patients also have inadequate immunity to diphtheria. [80]

ED immunization for older patients for pneumococcus and influenza has also been evaluated. Sixty-five percent of older adults are immunized for influenza, and 45% are immunized for pneumococcus; persons aged 65 to 74 years are less likely to be immunized than older persons, as are nonwhites and persons with lower socioeconomic status. [81] Studies in urban EDs suggest that only 3% to 18% of high-risk patients (a group that includes patients aged 65 and over) report immunization for pneumococcus, and 28% to 38% report immunization for influenza. [82,83] Feasibility studies of ED-based immunizations for influenza and pneumococcus found that the median time for immunization-related activities was only 4 minutes, and patient length of ED stay is not affected. [82,84]

> *EmergMed 21 (Level B)*: **Up to now, studies of fever and infectious disease in older emergency department patients have been observational and analytic retrospective studies. Prospective observational cohort studies, including longitudinal studies of outcomes and predictors of outcomes, are needed.**

> *EmergMed 22 (Level A)*: **Descriptive studies of emergency-department-based immunization programs have found them to be feasible. Intervention trials for older persons are necessary to determine if such programs are beneficial (because they access an underserved population) and whether they provide more cost-effective care and reduce adverse outcomes in comparison with usual care.**

ACUTE CORONARY SYNDROMES

Chest pain in the older patient has been identified as an area of concern for emergency physicians, who rate this complaint as more time-consuming and requiring more resources to evaluate in older than in younger patients. [12] Increasing age is an independent risk factor for the development of coronary artery disease. [85,86] Of more concern to emergency physicians, though, age is an independent risk factor for acute coronary syndromes (ACS) in patients presenting with symptoms of possible ACS. [86,87] Age is also a risk factor for mortality in patients with ACS. [88,89]

Complicating the evaluation of older patients with possible ACS is the fact that they less commonly present with chest pain and other classic symptoms of ACS. Small, single-center studies and larger, multicenter databases have documented that increasing age increases the likelihood of myocardial infarction (MI) without pain. Bayer et al performed a retrospective study of patients aged 65 to 100 years and found chest pain to be present in the majority of patients up to age 85. [90] After that, shortness of breath was the most common symptom. Approximately 20% to 30% of patients aged 65 to 79, 50% of those aged 80 to 84, and 62% of those 85 and older presented without chest pain. Other presenting complaints in this group included syncope, confusion, weakness, and stroke. Another single-hospital study showed a much higher rate of MI without chest pain, 75%, in patients aged 85 and older. [91] Perhaps the most generalizable study to assess this phenomenon is an analysis of the National Registry of Myocardial Infarction 2, a national registry of patients with confirmed MIs at 1674 hospitals. [92] In this study, one third of all patients did not have chest pain. This included 25% of patients under age 65, 33% of patients aged 65 to 74 years, 42% of patients aged 75 to 84, and 51% of patients 85 and older. Patients without chest pain had longer delays and were less likely to receive thrombolysis, primary angioplasty, aspirin, heparin, and β-blockers. The in-hospital mortality of these patients was 2.21 times greater than that for patients with chest pain.

Although a comprehensive review of the treatment of ACS is beyond the scope of this paper, several points of concern to emergency physicians must be mentioned. Although improvements in care have been documented, there is considerable room for improvement in the acute care of the older patient with ACS. A review of changes in the management of MI between 1987 and 1990 in patients aged 65 and over using Medicare databases found significant improvements in both 30-day mortality (26% to 23%) and 1-year mortality (40% to 36%). [93] During the same period, increases in angiography (13% to 21%), revascularization (13% to 21%), angioplasty (5% to 10%), and bypass (8% to 11%) were noted. However, older patients commonly do not receive as aggressive treatment as their younger counterparts, even though there is evidence to suggest that older patients have greater absolute benefits from such therapy. [94,95] Part of the reason for this may be that older patients are less likely to have indications for and are more likely to have contraindications for thrombolytics. In the Multicenter Chest Pain Study, only 18% of patients aged 75 and older presented with ST elevation or new Q waves on electrocardiogram in less than 6 hours from the onset of their pain, whereas 34% of younger patients did so; 12% of patients aged 65 and over who were eligible by electrocardiogram and time criteria had other contraindications to thrombolysis. [96] However, in a retrospective analysis of Medicare patients in Connecticut, Krumholz et al found that 56% of patients 65 and older who were eligible for thrombolytic therapy and not referred for direct angioplasty or bypass did not receive thrombolytics. [97] Predictors of not using thrombolytics include increasing age, lack of chest pain, altered mental status, presentation after more than 6 hours of symptoms, left bundle branch block, Q waves, ST elevation of less than 6 mm total, and ST elevation in only two leads. Even in "ideal" patients for thrombolytic therapy, ie, those presenting with chest pain, ST elevation, and within 6 hours of the onset of symptoms, 25% of patients did not receive thrombolytic therapy. Although this rate of thrombolytic administration seems low, other studies have shown that only 5% of MI patients aged 75 and older received thrombolytics, and patients in this age group had an 18% mortality. [98] In a prospective study of 4223 patients, Fleming et al found that patients aged 75 years and older were 2.5 times more likely not to be admitted to the coronary care unit, even if the diagnosis was myocardial infarction (RR = 7.1) or exclude MI (RR = 1.5). [99]

Given this information, several things are clear. Older patients, especially the oldest old (age 85 and older), present atypically with ACS. Given the symptoms with which older patients present to the ED, this diagnosis may need to be considered in one third of patients aged 65 or over who present to the ED. Although older patients are less likely to be eligible for thrombolytics, they receive a greater benefit from this treatment. Thus, in patients with ACS, "age is, therefore, best considered as an impetus to pursue prompt therapy rather than a reason to avoid it." [94]

> *EmergMed 23 (Level B)*: **Studies of techniques to improve recognition and appropriate treatment of acute coronary syndromes in older emergency department patients should be performed.**

> *EmergMed 24 (Level A)*: **Older patients should be included in intervention trials of acute coronary syndromes treatment.**

CARDIOPULMONARY ARREST

There have been multiple prospective and retrospective studies on the outcome of out-of-hospital cardiac arrest in older patients. [100–119] Although the results vary, overall, several points become apparent. Some studies have found that age is an independent predictor of mortality from cardiac arrest, [100–102,120] but other studies refute this. [105,109–111] Older patients, including octogenarians and nonagenarians, have acceptable rates of survival to hospital discharge (5% to 10%), [100,102,105,107,109,113,118] especially when the presenting rhythm is ventricular tachycardia or ventricular fibrillation (14% to 24% survival to hospital discharge). [100,107,113] In one prospective cohort, patients aged 90 or over were found to have only a 1% survival rate. [102] However, another retrospective cohort study found patients aged 90 or over to have a 4.4% rate of survival; if the presenting rhythm was ventricular tachycardia or fibrillation, the survival to hospital discharge was 17%. [100] Cerebral outcomes and quality of life are acceptable in both younger and older survivors of out-of-hospital cardiac arrest. [121] In an analysis of the Brain Resuscitation Clinical Trials data, Rogove et al found no difference in neurologic recovery by age. [106] Long-term survival rates appear similar in older and younger patients who survive to hospital discharge (65% in each group in one study). [117]

Data on resuscitation of nursing-home patients with cardiac arrest is mixed. Benkendorf et al performed a prospective cohort study comparing nursing-home with community-dwelling patients with cardiac arrest and found that no nursing-home patient survived, but that 5.6% of community-dwelling patients did. [103] Seventy-five percent of nursing-home patients had an asystolic rhythm. Appelbaum et al found similar poor outcomes in their retrospective study, with 2% of nursing-home patients and 11% of community-dwelling patients surviving to hospital discharge. [114] However, another retrospective study found similar rates of survival to hospital discharge in nursing-home (10.5%) and community-dwelling (9.2%) patients. [66] Tresch et al found a 5% survival to hospital discharge rate in nursing-home patients with cardiac arrest, but a 27% survival when the arrest was witnessed and the rhythm was ventricular tachycardia or fibrillation. [108] Eighty percent of survivors had a functional status similar to their pre-arrest status, and 40% lived for more than 1 year.

Presenting cardiac rhythm and whether the arrest was witnessed are more important than age in predicting the outcome of out-of-hospital cardiac arrest. Given this information, there is no reason to withhold cardiopulmonary resuscitation and advanced cardiac life support on the basis of age alone. Patients with unwitnessed arrests and those with asystole have poorer outcomes at any age. In one large study from Sweden, none of 211 patients aged 70 or over who have unwitnessed, asystolic, out-of-hospital arrests survived to hospital discharge. [101]

> **EmergMed 25 (Level B):** **Cohort or case-control studies are necessary to determine in which patients resuscitation for out-of-hospital arrest is futile. However, it appears that age alone should not be used to make this decision.**

> **EmergMed 26 (Level B):** **Prospective, multicenter, longitudinal studies on the clinical course of older emergency department patients with important conditions (abdominal pain, fever, acute coronary syndromes) are needed (see also Key Research Questions in Emergency Medicine, end of chapter).**

TRAUMA

Injuries in patients aged 65 and over caused 37,560 deaths in 1998, a rate of 109 per 100,000 population. Injuries are therefore the seventh leading cause of death in this age group. Both the crude number of deaths and the death rate increase with age in those aged 65 and over; by age 75, the rate per 100,000 population exceeds all other age groups. [122] In addition to its high mortality, trauma in the older patient can result in significant morbidity, including functional decline and loss of independence.

There are some common limitations in much of the older trauma research. Many reports define "older" to start as young as 55 years of age, rather than the more standard 65 years. However, trauma patients aged 55 and over are a heterogeneous group, and advanced age is associated with increased trauma mortality. Nonstandardized definitions of the "older" age group limit comparisons between studies. Additionally, many of the studies are single-center retrospective analyses of trauma registries at trauma centers. This allows for potential spectrum bias (weighting toward more severe injuries) and makes the results of these studies difficult to generalize to the older trauma patient treated elsewhere. There is often no description of the data quality in these trauma registries. Each study uses different inclusion and exclusion criteria, with some studies including burn patients, patients with penetrating injuries, and patients with isolated orthopedic injuries, and other studies excluding these patients in favor of those with blunt trauma. These factors make comparison difficult and thus lead to confusion about conflicting results. Most of the research is descriptive; very little analytic research and no interventional trials were identified.

Demographics of Trauma in Older Patients

The Northeastern Ohio Trauma Study was a time-stratified random sample of visits to EDs in 1977. [123,124] This large epidemiologic study showed falls to be the leading cause of injury in patients aged 65 and over, followed by motor vehicle crashes. The injury rate for falls was 40 per 1000 population for patients 65 to 74 years, and 69 per 1000 population for patients 75 and older. The injury rate for motor vehicle crashes was 11 and 9 per 1000 for these age groups, respectively. The study also found that the hospital admission rate for injuries rises markedly after age 65 (21% for patients 65 to 74, 34% for patients 75 and older). Population-based mortality rates also increase in older patients, but more striking are case fatality rates, which show sharp increases in patients aged 65 and over (case fatality rate is the death per 1000 injuries). The rate of fractures also increase sharply after age 65; falls were found to cause 87% of all fractures in those aged 65 and over.

Covington et al analyzed the North Carolina Trauma Registry, a statewide registry of all trauma patients admitted for at least 24 hours or dead on arrival in that state's eight level 1 and 2 trauma centers. [125] The researchers found that patients 65 and older have longer stays in the hospital and intensive care unit, higher hospital charges, and higher mortality at all levels of injury severity. Sixty-eight percent of the injuries were caused by falls, and 22% were transportation related.

In an analysis of the National Hospital Discharge Survey, MacKenzie et al found patients aged 65 and older to represent 12% of the population but 23% of the hospitalizations for trauma, and to be responsible for 28% of charges. [126] Patients 75 and older accounted for two thirds of hospitalizations and charges in the older group.

Mortality

In studies of older trauma patients, in-hospital mortality varies from 15% to 45%. [127–135] Finelli et al provided a secondary analysis of data from the Major Trauma Outcome Study of the American College of Surgeons. [135] This was a study of 46,613 major trauma patients admitted to 120 trauma centers between 1982 and 1986; it included 3669 patients aged 65 and over. The elderly group had an 18% case fatality rate; the most common mechanism of injury was fall (46%, 12% mortality), followed by motor vehicle crash (28%, 21% mortality) and pedestrian hit (10%, 33% mortality).

Mortality in trauma patients is related to several factors, including injury severity, host factors, timeliness of care, and quality of care. [136] Several studies have attempted to identify factors that are associated with mortality in older trauma patients, focusing on host factors and injury severity.

One early study of 100 patients aged 70 and over admitted to a single trauma center found that age, sex, Injury Severity Score (ISS), pre-injury ADL dependence, and pre-existing disease do not differ between survivors and nonsurvivors. [127] Central nervous system injury and the presence of shock (blood pressure < 80 systolic) were found to be significantly different between groups. A second study of 39 severely injured patients aged 60 and over also found that ISS is not predictive of mortality, nor is the Trauma Score (TS). [128] These studies are limited by low power to detect an association between predictive variables and mortality. They also had varying inclusion criteria (the former included patients with burns, penetrating injuries, and same-level falls; the latter included only severely injured surgical patients in intensive care who required a pulmonary artery catheter and arterial line). Older patients with isolated hip fractures have been found to have a mortality rate higher than that predicted by anatomic injury scales; [137] thus, the inclusion of this patient subgroup in the former study may have made it more difficult to detect an association between ISS and age.

DeMaria et al retrospectively analyzed 82 patients aged 65 and over admitted to a single center's trauma service between 1982 and 1984. [138] Patients with thermal, penetrating, or isolated orthopedic injuries were excluded. The mortality rate was 21%; factors associated with mortality by univariate analysis included age, ISS, and the Anatomic Injury Severity score for head and neck. Discriminant analysis showed that four variables were associated with survival—ISS, age, and the presence of cardiac or septic complications. A "geriatric trauma survival score" was developed and prospectively tested on 61 additional patients, with 92% accuracy in prediction of mortality. However, one recent study of 326 patients found no difference in this score between survivors and nonsurvivors. [134] Additionally, this score requires knowledge of complications, which limits its use in the early evaluation of trauma patients.

Knudson et al conducted a retrospective study of 852 patients aged 65 and older with blunt trauma identified by trauma registries of three trauma centers and found the ISS to be the single variable that correlates most closely with mortality. [133] In this study, overall mortality was 18.4%. Other risk factors for death were TS < 7 (RR = 6.62), Glasgow Coma Scale score of 3 (RR = 6.11), respiratory rate < 10 (RR = 4.83), blood pressure < 90 (RR = 4.77), abdominal injury (RR = 3.21), chest injury (RR = 2.27), head injury (RR = 2.17), and male sex (RR = 2.07). The authors developed a model for the probability of death using TS, age, and sex, and found this to have similar discriminating ability to the ISS in predicting mortality (sensitivity 37%, specificity 98%, and total correct classification 88% for the model, corresponding percentages of 41%, 97%, and 86% for the ISS).

Morris et al performed a case-control study of the effect of pre-existing conditions on trauma mortality. [136] They evaluated 3074 trauma deaths and 9868 matched controls (injury survivors) identified by the use of computerized hospital discharge data from California. They studied patients of all ages and found the presence of pre-existing conditions to increase with age. Pre-existing conditions associated with mortality included cirrhosis (OR = 4.6), congenital coagulopathy (OR = 3.2), chronic obstructive pulmonary disease (OR = 1.8), ischemic heart disease (OR = 1.8), and diabetes mellitus (OR = 1.2).

Other factors associated with mortality in studies include early intubation, [139] hypotension, [127,132,133] TS, [133,140,141] ISS, [140,141] closed head injury, [127,132,139] base deficit ≤ -6, [142] sepsis, [132] cardiopulmonary complications, [138] bradycardia, prior MI, and history of chronic renal insufficiency. [132]

Accurate prediction of mortality is important for a number of reasons. First, it may provide information to help patients and surrogate decision makers decide on their desired level of care. Second, it allows for comparison between sites for quality-assurance purposes. Third, it may help tailor patient care, by predicting patients who require more aggressive trauma care. Currently, there is no validated, accurate way of predicting mortality in older patients. This is likely due to the multifactorial nature of mortality in older trauma patients.

Several factors must be taken into account when evaluating mortality prediction in older trauma patients. First, what is the intent of the predictive model? A model intended to be used for quality assurance and comparison of mortality between sites may include complications as a predictor; however, this would not be appropriate in a model intended to identify patients for early, aggressive care. Similarly, a model developed in a trauma center may not be accurate when applied to patients in other settings. Therefore, models used to decide on the necessity of specialized trauma care should include patients from settings other than trauma centers. Sensitive models are necessary when determining who requires aggressive care; sensitivity is not as important as correct classification for quality assurance. Also, in developing models for prediction of mortality, investigators should include all potentially relevant predictors in order to improve accuracy. This requires larger data sets; the need for quality data suggests that prospective studies would result in better models than retrospective data could produce. Finally, predicting mortality in heterogeneous groups is difficult. Patients with isolated hip fractures from same-level falls, for instance, have a higher-than-predicted mortality on the basis of anatomic injury scales. Inclusion of these patients in studies with patients with multiple injuries diminishes the predictive value of the equations if this is not taken into account as an independent risk factor.

Functional Outcome

Long-term loss of functional abilities and independence are serious morbidities in older trauma patients. Multiple studies have evaluated the long-term functional outcome of these patients and found better-than-anticipated results. [130,131,143] DeMaria et al performed a follow-up survey of 63 survivors of blunt trauma. [130] These patients were moderately injured (mean ISS 15 $\pm$ 1.1) and had high rates of cardiopulmonary comorbidity (71%), multiple injuries (62%), head injuries (25%), and surgeries (50%, two thirds of these emergent). Prior to their injury, 97% of survivors were independent. At discharge, 33% were independent, with 37% dependent at home and 30% in nursing homes. At follow-up (mean 19.6 $\pm$ 1.2 months), the best functional status obtained was 57% independent, 32% dependent at home, and 11% in nursing homes. Risk factors for permanent nursing-home placement were found to be increased age, longer hospital stay, more complications, and more severe abdominal injuries. van Aalst et al conducted a similar study of long-term outcomes of blunt trauma victims aged 65 and older. [131] They identified 98 such patients over a 5-year period and performed a follow-up survey at a mean of 2.82 years (range 1 to 6 years). Thirty-two patients were independent at follow-up; these were defined as "acceptable outcomes." Fifty patients had died, including 44 patients who died in the hospital. An additional 16 patients were dependent at follow-up. These 66 patients were considered "unacceptable outcomes." Factors associated with unacceptable outcomes included age > 75, Glasgow Coma Scale score $\leq$ 7, shock on admission, closed head injury with Anatomic Injury Severity score $\geq$ 3, and sepsis. Mean values for age, ISS, Revised Trauma Score, probability of survival on Trauma and Injury Severity Score, and Glasgow Coma Scale score differed between the groups. Similar findings for comparisons between survivors and nonsurvivors were found.

Penetrating Trauma

Most published studies of trauma in older patients focus on blunt trauma; penetrating trauma is less common and less well studied. One retrospective analysis of the trauma registry at a level 1 trauma center identified 85 patients aged 65 and over with penetrating trauma who were admitted over a 5-year period and compared them with 85 control persons under age 65 and matched for mechanism of injury and ISS. [144] Older patients were found to have significantly more pre-existing conditions, longer hospital stays (2.6 days longer), and longer stays in intensive care. Complication rates were higher in the older patients (22.3% versus 17.6%), but this was not statistically significant. Mortality was 8.2% in the older group but 3.5% in the younger group. Ninety-one percent of the older patients were discharged home. As the population continues to age, we may begin to see larger numbers of older patients with penetrating trauma, who differ not only from the younger patients but also from older blunt trauma patients.

Aggressive Resuscitation

Scalea et al retrospectively analyzed older blunt multiple trauma patients treated at their level 1 trauma center. [145] The authors describe their experience with 60 patients in 1985 aged 65 and over with diffuse multiple trauma who were stable after initial resuscitation. The overall mortality was 44%; factors that were found to predict mortality were pedestrian-motor vehicle accident, diffuse trauma, initial systolic blood pressure less than 130 mm Hg, systemic acidosis, multiple fractures, and head injuries. The authors did not describe the method used to determine these risk factors or indicate whether they were found to be statistically significant predictors of mortality. The mortality was 85% in the group with any risk factor, and 63% of deaths were in the late post-injury period, commonly from multiple-organ failure.

In 1986 the authors performed invasive monitoring on any patient who had any of the risk factors noted above. Fifteen patients were treated with invasive monitoring; the mortality rate was 93%. The average time to invasive monitoring was 5.5 hours from arrival in the intensive care unit. Because of the low survival rate, after 1986 the authors began a protocol that involved early invasive monitoring. The mortality after this was initiated was 47% ($P < .001$ compared with 1986). The average time to invasive monitoring was 2.2 hours. The groups did not differ in number of injuries, percentage requiring operation, or percentage of patients who died without significant injuries.

The authors suggest that early invasive monitoring of older patients at risk of mortality from multiple-organ failure may improve survival. Given the use of historical controls and the limited comparative information between the groups, it cannot be determined whether the improved survival was due to early invasive monitoring or some other factor.

McKinley et al developed a standardized protocol for resuscitation of trauma patients at risk for post-injury multiple-organ failure. [146] They performed an inception cohort study of patients resuscitated by this protocol, comparing patients aged 65 and older with those under age 65. Patients who had (1) specific injuries (flail chest, two or more abdominal organ injuries, major vascular injury, complex pelvic fracture, or two or more long-bone fractures), (2) base deficit of 6 mEq/L or more, and (3) need for transfusion of six units or more of packed red blood cells, or patients aged 65 and older who have any two of the above criteria, were resuscitated by this protocol; patients with severe brain injury were excluded. The protocol involved resuscitation guided by pulmonary artery catheter using a combination of fluids, blood, inotropics, and vasopressors, with a goal of an oxygen delivery index (DO_2I) of at least 600 mL/min*m2.

Over 19 months, 54 patients under age 65 and 12 patients aged 65 or over were resuscitated by this protocol. Older patients' cardiac index and DO_2I were significantly lower in the older group than in the younger group at the start of resuscitation. Eighty-three percent of older patients required inotropic support with dobutamine, versus 31% of younger patients ($P < .05$); 25% of older patients and 19% of younger patients required vasopressors ($P = NS$). Fifty percent of older patients and 19% of younger patients developed multiple-organ failure. Survival at 7 days was similar between groups (92% older and 94% younger), but 30-day survival was significantly less in the older group (42%) than in the younger group (89%) ($P < .05$ for both comparisons).

Although the authors conclude that aggressive management of older blunt trauma patients is not futile, they provide no comparison with patients who are not managed using this protocol. Thus, it remains unknown whether this protocol results in improved survival over standard care.

> *EmergMed 27 (Level B)*: **Research on older trauma patients would benefit from standardization of outcomes, including short- and long-term survival and also functional outcome.**

> *EmergMed 28 (Level B)*: **Valid and accurate ways to predict outcomes in older trauma patients must be developed on the basis of cohort or case-control studies that can identify risk factors for bad outcomes.**

Early invasive monitoring and aggressive resuscitation of high-risk patients may be beneficial in reducing multiple-organ failure and death in older patients with blunt multiple trauma. A number of research questions are generated on the basis of this hypothesis:

> *EmergMed 29 (Level B)*: **Cohort or case-control studies are needed to determine which older patients are at risk for multiple-organ failure and death after blunt trauma and to construct a predictive model.**

> *EmergMed 30 (Level B)*: **Exploratory studies are needed to identify new noninvasive ways of determining which older trauma patients might benefit from invasive monitoring and aggressive resuscitation.**

> *EmergMed 31 (Level A)*: **To determine whether early invasive monitoring and aggressive resuscitation of high-risk older trauma patients result in improved outcomes, large-scale, randomized controlled trials should be performed, and outcomes that include not only short-term mortality but also long-term mortality and function should be used (see also Key Research Questions in Geriatric Emergency Medicine, next).**

KEY RESEARCH QUESTIONS IN GERIATRIC EMERGENCY MEDICINE

> *EmergMed KQ1*: **Can alterations in the process of emergency department care, such as those found to be beneficial elsewhere (ie, geriatric specialty inpatient units), improve the outcomes of older emergency department patients?**

> Hypothesis-generating studies include the following: evaluation of the micro-environment of the ED to determine the characteristics (eg, communication, physical environment) that affect outcomes in elderly patients, development of brief instruments to detect cognitive and functional impairment in older ED patients, and generation of interventions (educational

models, protocols, computer support systems) to improve physician documentation and medication prescribing.

Hypothesis-testing studies include the study of specific elements of care (ie, improved environment, communication, recognition of delirium, linkage with geriatric teams) on outcomes in older ED patients. This should lead to a controlled study of the effects of a multifaceted approach to geriatric ED care on patient outcomes.

EmergMed KQ2: **What diagnostic and therapeutic interventions can improve outcomes in older emergency department patients with high-risk common complaints, such as abdominal pain and acute coronary syndromes?**

Hypothesis-generating studies include prospective, longitudinal studies of outcomes, evaluation of predictors of adverse outcomes, and evaluation of varied diagnostic approaches to older ED patients with the high-risk common conditions.

Hypothesis-testing studies would be based on the results of the hypothesis-generating studies and would include controlled trials of methods for improving outcomes for older ED patients with the high-risk common conditions.

EmergMed KQ3: **In older blunt multiple trauma patients, does early invasive monitoring and aggressive resuscitation result in improved outcomes?**

Hypothesis-generating studies include the development and validation of sensitive and accurate methods to predict which patients are at risk for multiple-organ failure and death after blunt trauma, and the study of noninvasive methods of determining who may benefit from invasive monitoring and aggressive resuscitation.

Hypothesis-testing studies involve evaluating whether early invasive monitoring and aggressive resuscitation of high-risk older trauma patients results in improved outcomes and comparing the effect of different techniques of aggressive resuscitation on outcomes. These studies should consist of large-scale randomized controlled trials, using outcomes that include not only short-term mortality but also long-term mortality and function.

REFERENCES

1. Sanders AB. Care of the elderly in emergency departments: conclusions and recommendations. Ann Emerg Med 1992;21:830-834.
2. Sanders AB, Witzke DB, Jones JS, et al. Principles of care and application of the geriatric emergency care model. In Sanders AB (ed): Emergency Care of the Elder Person. Geriatric Emergency Medicine Task Force. St. Louis, MO: Beverly Cracom Publications, 1996:59-93.
3. Shah MN, Rathouz PJ, Chin MH. Emergency department utilization by noninstitutionalized elders. Acad Emerg Med 2001;8:267-273.
4. Rosenblatt RA, Wright GE, Baldwin LM, et al. The effect of the doctor-patient relationship on emergency department use among the elderly. Am J Public Health 2000;90:97-102.
5. Lishner DM, Rosenblatt RA, Baldwin LM, Hart LG. Emergency department use by the rural elderly. J Emerg Med 2000;18:289-297.

6. Hamdy RC, Forrest LJ, Moore SW, Cancellaro L. Use of emergency departments by the elderly in rural areas. South Med J 1997;90:616-620.
7. Wofford JL, Schwartz E, Timerding BL, et al. Emergency department utilization by the elderly: analysis of the National Hospital Ambulatory Medical Care Survey. Acad Emerg Med 1996;3:694-699.
8. Strange GR, Chen EH, Sanders AB. Use of emergency departments by elderly patients: projections from a multicenter data base. Ann Emerg Med 1992;21:819-824.
9. Strange GR, Chen EH. Use of emergency departments by elder patients: a five-year follow-up study. Acad Emerg Med 1998;5:1157-1162.
10. Singal BM, Hedges JR, Rousseau EW, et al. Geriatric patient emergency visits. Part I: Comparison of visits by geriatric and younger patients. Ann Emerg Med 1992;21:802-807.
11. Sanders AB. Care of the elderly in emergency departments: where do we stand? Ann Emerg Med 1992;21:792-795.
12. McNamara RM, Rousseau E, Sanders AB. Geriatric emergency medicine: a survey of practicing emergency physicians. Ann Emerg Med 1992;21:796-801.
13. Baraff LJ, Bernstein E, Bradley K, et al. Perceptions of emergency care by the elderly: results of multicenter focus group interviews. Ann Emerg Med 1992;21:814-818.
14. Hedges JR, Singal BM, Rousseau EW, et al. Geriatric patient emergency visits. Part II: Perceptions of visits by geriatric and younger patients. Ann Emerg Med 1992;21:808-813.
15. Gerson LW, Shvarch L. Emergency medical service utilization by the elderly. Ann Emerg Med 1982;11:610-612.
16. Dickinson ET, Verdile VP, Kostyun CT, Salluzzo RF. Geriatric use of emergency medical services. Ann Emerg Med 1996;27:199-203.
17. Wofford JL, Moran WP, Heuser MD, et al. Emergency medical transport of the elderly: a population-based study. Am J Emerg Med 1995;13:297-300.
18. Gerson LW, Schelble DT, Wilson JE. Using paramedics to identify at-risk elderly. Ann Emerg Med 1992;21:688-691.
19. Sanders AB. Recognition of cognitive problems in older adults by emergency medicine personnel. Ann Emerg Med 1995;25:831-833.
20. Wofford JL, Loehr LR, Schwartz E. Acute cognitive impairment in elderly ED patients: etiologies and outcomes. Am J Emerg Med 1996;14:649-653.
21. Gerson LW, Counsell SR, Fontanarosa PB, Smucker WD. Case finding for cognitive impairment in elderly emergency department patients. Ann Emerg Med 1994;23:813-817.
22. Naughton BJ, Moran MB, Kadah H, et al. Delirium and other cognitive impairment in older adults in an emergency department. Ann Emerg Med 1995;25:751-755.
23. Naughton BJ, Moran M, Ghaly Y, Michalakes C. Computed tomography scanning and delirium in elder patients. Acad Emerg Med 1997;4:1107-1110.
24. Lewis LM, Miller DK, Morley JE, et al. Unrecognized delirium in ED geriatric patients. Am J Emerg Med 1995;13:142-145.
25. Elie M, Rousseau F, Cole M, et al. Prevalence and detection of delirium in elderly emergency department patients. CMAJ 2000;163:977-981.
26. Maddens ME. Should elderly emergency department patients be screened for dementia? Ann Emerg Med 1994;23:873-874.
27. Shapiro MJ, Partridge RA, Jenouri I, et al. Functional decline in independent elders after minor traumatic injury. Acad Emerg Med 2001;8:78-81.
28. Beers MH. Explicit criteria for determining potentially inappropriate medication use by the elderly. An update. Arch Intern Med 1997;157:1531-1536.
29. Chin MH, Wang LC, Jin L, et al. Appropriateness of medication selection for older persons in an urban academic emergency department. Acad Emerg Med 1999;6:1232-1242.

30. Beers MH, Storrie M, Lee G. Potential adverse drug interactions in the emergency room. An issue in the quality of care. Ann Intern Med 1990;112:61-64.

31. Herr RD, Caravati EM, Tyler LS, et al. Prospective evaluation of adverse drug interactions in the emergency department. Ann Emerg Med 1992;21:1331-1336.

32. Hayes KS. Adding medications in the emergency department: effect on knowledge of medications in older adults. J Emerg Nurs 1999;25:178-182.

33. Jones JS, Johnson K, McNinch M. Age as a risk factor for inadequate emergency department analgesia. Am J Emerg Med 1996;14:157-160.

34. Miller DK, Lewis LM, Nork MJ, Morley JE. Controlled trial of a geriatric case-finding and liaison service in an emergency department. J Am Geriatr Soc 1996;44:513-520.

35. Gerson LW, Rousseau EW, Hogan TM, et al. Multicenter study of case finding in elderly emergency department patients. Acad Emerg Med 1995;2:729-734.

36. Sinoff G, Clarfield AM, Bergman H, Beaudet M. A two-year follow-up of geriatric consults in the emergency department. J Am Geriatr Soc 1998;46:716-720.

37. Jones JS, Young MS, LaFleur RA, Brown MD. Effectiveness of an organized follow-up system for elder patients released from the emergency department. Acad Emerg Med 1997;4:1147-1152.

38. McCusker J, Bellavance F, Cardin S, et al. Detection of older people at increased risk of adverse health outcomes after an emergency visit: the ISAR screening tool. J Am Geriatr Soc 1999;47:1229-1237.

39. McCusker J, Bellavance F, Cardin S, et al. Prediction of hospital utilization among elderly patients during the 6 months after an emergency department visit. Ann Emerg Med 2000;36:438-445.

40. McCusker J, Cardin S, Bellavance F, Belzile E. Return to the emergency department among elders: patterns and predictors. Acad Emerg Med 2000;7:249-259.

41. McCusker J, Bellavance F, Cardin S, Belzile E. Validity of an activities of daily living questionnaire among older patients in the emergency department. J Clin Epidemiol 1999;52:1023-1030.

42. McCusker J, Bellavance F, Cardin S, Trepanier S. Screening for geriatric problems in the emergency department: reliability and validity. Identification of Seniors at Risk (ISAR) Steering Committee. Acad Emerg Med 1998;5:883-893.

43. McCusker J, Healey E, Bellavance F, Connolly B. Predictors of repeat emergency department visits by elders. Acad Emerg Med 1997;4:581-588.

44. Reinstein DZ, Dorward NL, Wormald RP, et al. 'Correctable undetected visual acuity deficit' in patients aged 65 and over attending an accident and emergency department. Br J Ophthalmol 1993;77:293-296.

45. Baraff LJ, Della Penna R, Williams N, Sanders A. Practice guideline for the ED management of falls in community-dwelling elderly persons. Kaiser Permanente Medical Group. Ann Emerg Med 1997;30:480-492.

46. Meldon SW, Emerman CL, Schubert DS, et al. Depression in geriatric ED patients: prevalence and recognition. Ann Emerg Med 1997;30:141-145.

47. Meldon SW, Emerman CL, Moffa DA, Schubert DS. Utility of clinical characteristics in identifying depression in geriatric ED patients. Am J Emerg Med 1999;17:522-525.

48. Meldon SW, Emerman CL, Schubert DS. Recognition of depression in geriatric ED patients by emergency physicians. Ann Emerg Med 1997;30:442-447.

49. Adams WL, Magruder-Habib K, Trued S, Broome HL. Alcohol abuse in elderly emergency department patients. J Am Geriatr Soc 1992;40:1236-1240.

50. Li G, Keyl PM, Rothman R, et al. Epidemiology of alcohol-related emergency department visits. Acad Emerg Med 1998;5:788-795.

51. Higgins JP, Wright SW, Wrenn KD. Alcohol, the elderly, and motor vehicle crashes. Am J Emerg Med 1996;14:265-267.

52. Jones JS, Rousseau EW, Schropp MA, Sanders AB. Geriatric training in emergency medicine residency programs. Ann Emerg Med 1992;21:825-829.

53. Council on Scientific Affairs, American Medical Association. Elder abuse and neglect. JAMA 1987;257:966-971.

54. Pillemer K, Finkelhor D. The prevalence of elder abuse: a random sample survey. Gerontologist 1988;28:51-57.

55. Lachs MS, Williams CS, O'Brien S, et al. ED use by older victims of family violence. Ann Emerg Med 1997;30:448-454.

56. Fulmer T, Street S, Carr K. Abuse of the elderly: screening and detection. J Emerg Nurs 1984;10:131-140.

57. Fulmer T, McMahon DJ, Baer-Hines M, Forget B. Abuse, neglect, abandonment, violence, and exploitation: an analysis of all elderly patients seen in one emergency department during a six-month period. J Emerg Nurs 1992;18:505-510.

58. Jones J, Dougherty J, Schelble D, Cunningham W. Emergency department protocol for the diagnosis and evaluation of geriatric abuse. Ann Emerg Med 1988;17:1006-1015.

59. Marco CA, Schoenfeld CN, Keyl PM, et al. Abdominal pain in geriatric emergency patients: variables associated with adverse outcomes. Acad Emerg Med 1998;5:1163-1168.

60. Kizer KW, Vassar MJ. Emergency department diagnosis of abdominal disorders in the elderly. Am J Emerg Med 1998;16:357-362.

61. Parker LJ, Vukov LF, Wollan PC. Emergency department evaluation of geriatric patients with acute cholecystitis. Acad Emerg Med 1997;4:51-55.

62. Parker JS, Vukov LF, Wollan PC. Abdominal pain in the elderly: use of temperature and laboratory testing to screen for surgical disease. Fam Med 1996;28:193-197.

63. Horattas MC, Guyton DP, Wu D. A reappraisal of appendicitis in the elderly. Am J Surg 1990;160:291-293.

64. Bugliosi TF, Meloy TD, Vukov LF. Acute abdominal pain in the elderly. Ann Emerg Med 1990;19:1383-1386.

65. Burt CW, Fingerhut LA. Injury visits to hospital emergency departments: United States, 1992-95. Vital Health Stat 13 1998:1-76.

66. Baraff LJ, Lee TJ, Kader S, Della Penna R. Effect of a practice guideline for emergency department care of falls in elder patients on subsequent falls and hospitalizations for injuries. Acad Emerg Med 1999;6:1224-1231.

67. Baraff LJ, Lee TJ, Kader S, Della Penna R. Effect of a practice guideline on the process of emergency department care of falls in elder patients. Acad Emerg Med 1999;6:1216-1223.

68. Grisso JA, Schwarz DF, Wolfson V, et al. The impact of falls in an inner-city elderly African-American population. J Am Geriatr Soc 1992;40:673-678.

69. Layne LA, Landen DD. A descriptive analysis of nonfatal occupational injuries to older workers, using a national probability sample of hospital emergency departments. J Occup Environ Med 1997;39:855-865.

70. Sanders AB. Changing clinical practice in geriatric emergency medicine. Acad Emerg Med 1999;6:1189-1193.

71. Marco CA, Schoenfeld CN, Hansen KN, et al. Fever in geriatric emergency patients: clinical features associated with serious illness. Ann Emerg Med 1995;26:18-24.

72. Wasserman M, Levinstein M, Keller E, et al. Utility of fever, white blood cells, and differential count in predicting bacterial infections in the elderly. J Am Geriatr Soc 1989;37:537-543.

73. Fontanarosa PB, Kaeberlein FJ, Gerson LW, Thomson RB. Difficulty in predicting bacteremia in elderly emergency patients. Ann Emerg Med 1992;21:842-848.

74. Fine MJ, Auble TE, Yealy DM, et al. A prediction rule to identify low-risk patients with community-acquired pneumonia. N Engl J Med 1997;336:243-250.

75. Cox FM, Cobb MM, Chua WQ, et al. Cost of treating influenza in emergency department and hospital settings. Am J Manag Care 2000;6:205-214.

76. Wright SW, Wrenn KD, Haynes M, Haas DW. Prevalence and risk factors for multidrug resistant uropathogens in ED patients. Am J Emerg Med 2000;18:143-146.

77. Gareau AB, Eby RJ, McLellan BA, Williams DR. Tetanus immunization status and immunologic response to a booster in an emergency department geriatric population. Ann Emerg Med 1990;19:1377-1382.

78. Stair TO, Lippe MA, Russell H, Feeley JC. Tetanus immunity in emergency department patients. Am J Emerg Med 1989;7:563-566.

79. Alagappan K, Rennie W, Kwiatkowski T, et al. Seroprevalence of tetanus antibodies among adults older than 65 years. Ann Emerg Med 1996;28:18-21.

80. Alagappan K, Rennie W, Kwiatkowski T, Narang V. Antibody protection to diphtheria in geriatric patients: need for ED compliance with immunization guidelines. Ann Emerg Med 1997;30:455-458.

81. Influenza and pneumococcal vaccination levels among adults aged > or = 65 years–United States, 1997. MMWR Morb Mortal Wkly Rep 1998;47:797-802.

82. Slobodkin D, Zielske PG, Kitlas JL, et al. Demonstration of the feasibility of emergency department immunization against influenza and pneumococcus. Ann Emerg Med 1998;32:537-543.

83. Rodriguez RM, Baraff LJ. Emergency department immunization of the elderly with pneumococcal and influenza vaccines. Ann Emerg Med 1993;22:1729-1732.

84. Slobodkin D, Kitlas JL, Zielske PG. A test of the feasibility of pneumococcal vaccination in the emergency department. Acad Emerg Med 1999;6:724-727.

85. Hoeg JM. Evaluating coronary heart disease risk. Tiles in the mosaic. JAMA 1997;277:1387-1390.

86. Diamond GA, Forrester JS. Analysis of probability as an aid in the clinical diagnosis of coronary-artery disease. N Engl J Med 1979;300:1350-1358.

87. Braunwald E, Mark DB, Jones RH, et al. Unstable angina: diagnosis and management. Clinical Practice Guideline No.10. Rockville MD: Agency for Health Care Policy and Research. National Heart, Lung and Blood Institute, 1994. AHCPR publication no. 94-0602.

88. Lee TH, Ting HH, Shammash JB, et al. Long-term survival of emergency department patients with acute chest pain. Am J Cardiol 1992;69:145-151.

89. Karlson BW, Herlitz J, Strombom U, et al. Improvement of ED prediction of cardiac mortality among patients with symptoms suggestive of acute myocardial infarction. Am J Emerg Med 1997;15:1-7.

90. Bayer AJ, Chadha JS, Farag RR, Pathy MS. Changing presentation of myocardial infarction with increasing old age. J Am Geriatr Soc 1986;34:263-266.

91. Muller RT, Gould LA, Betzu R, et al. Painless myocardial infarction in the elderly. Am Heart J 1990;119:202-204.

92. Canto JG, Shlipak MG, Rogers WJ, et al. Prevalence, clinical characteristics, and mortality among patients with myocardial infarction presenting without chest pain. JAMA 2000;283:3223-3229.

93. Pashos CL, Newhouse JP, McNeil BJ. Temporal changes in the care and outcomes of elderly patients with acute myocardial infarction, 1987 through 1990. JAMA 1993;270:1832-1836.

94. Forman DE, Bernal JL, Wei JY. Management of acute myocardial infarction in the very elderly. Am J Med 1992;93:315-326.

95. Topol EJ, Califf RM. Thrombolytic therapy for elderly patients. N Engl J Med 1992;327:45-47.

96. Krumholz HM, Friesinger GC, Cook EF, et al. Relationship of age with eligibility for thrombolytic therapy and mortality among patients with suspected acute myocardial infarction. J Am Geriatr Soc 1994;42:127-131.

97. Krumholz HM, Murillo JE, Chen J, et al. Thrombolytic therapy for eligible elderly patients with acute myocardial infarction. JAMA 1997;277:1683-1688.

98. Weaver WD, Litwin PE, Martin JS, et al. Effect of age on use of thrombolytic therapy and mortality in acute myocardial infarction. The MITI Project Group. J Am Coll Cardiol 1991;18:657-662.

99. Fleming C, D'Agostino RB, Selker HP. Is coronary-care-unit admission restricted for elderly patients? A multicenter study. Am J Public Health 1991;81:1121-1126.

100. Kim C, Becker L, Eisenberg MS. Out-of-hospital cardiac arrest in octogenarians and nonagenarians. Arch Intern Med 2000;160:3439-3443.

101. Engdahl J, Bang A, Lindqvist J, Herlitz J. Can we define patients with no and those with some chance of survival when found in asystole out of hospital? Am J Cardiol 2000;86:610-614.

102. Swor RA, Jackson RE, Tintinalli JE, Pirrallo RG. Does advanced age matter in outcomes after out-of-hospital cardiac arrest in community-dwelling adults? Acad Emerg Med 2000;7:762-768.

103. Benkendorf R, Swor RA, Jackson R, et al. Outcomes of cardiac arrest in the nursing home: destiny or futility? [see comment]. Prehosp Emerg Care 1997;1:68-72.

104. Ghusn HF, Teasdale TA, Pepe PE, Ginger VF. Older nursing home residents have a cardiac arrest survival rate similar to that of older persons living in the community. J Am Geriatr Soc 1995;43:520-527.

105. Wuerz RC, Holliman CJ, Meador SA, et al. Effect of age on prehospital cardiac resuscitation outcome. Am J Emerg Med 1995;13:389-391.

106. Rogove HJ, Safar P, Sutton-Tyrrell K, Abramson NS. Old age does not negate good cerebral outcome after cardiopulmonary resuscitation: analyses from the brain resuscitation clinical trials. The Brain Resuscitation Clinical Trial I and II Study Groups. Crit Care Med 1995;23:18-25.

107. Bonnin MJ, Pepe PE, Clark PS. Survival in the elderly after out-of-hospital cardiac arrest. Crit Care Med 1993;21:1645-1651.

108. Tresch DD, Neahring JM, Duthie EH, et al. Outcomes of cardiopulmonary resuscitation in nursing homes: can we predict who will benefit? Am J Med 1993;95:123-130.

109. Juchems R, Wahlig G, Frese W. Influence of age on the survival rate of out-of-hospital and in-hospital resuscitation. Resuscitation 1993;26:23-29.

110. Joslyn SA, Pomrehn PR, Brown DD. Survival from out-of-hospital cardiac arrest: effects of patient age and presence of 911 Emergency Medical Services phone access. Am J Emerg Med 1993;11:200-206.

111. Van Hoeyweghen RJ, Bossaert LL, Mullie A, et al. Survival after out-of-hospital cardiac arrest in elderly patients. Belgian Cerebral Resuscitation Study Group. Ann Emerg Med 1992;21:1179-1184.

112. Awoke S, Mouton CP, Parrott M. Outcomes of skilled cardiopulmonary resuscitation in a long-term-care facility: futile therapy? J Am Geriatr Soc 1992;40:593-595.

113. Longstreth WT, Cobb LA, Fahrenbruch CE, Copass MK. Does age affect outcomes of out-of-hospital cardiopulmonary resuscitation? JAMA 1990;264:2109-2110.

114. Applebaum GE, King JE, Finucane TE. The outcome of CPR initiated in nursing homes. J Am Geriatr Soc 1990;38:197-200.

115. Tresch DD, Thakur RK, Hoffmann RG, et al. Comparison of outcome of paramedic-witnessed cardiac arrest in patients younger and older than 70 years. Am J Cardiol 1990;65:453-457.

116. Murphy DJ, Murray AM, Robinson BE, Campion EW. Outcomes of cardiopulmonary resuscitation in the elderly. Ann Intern Med 1989;111:199-205.

117. Tresch DD, Thakur RK, Hoffmann RG, et al. Should the elderly be resuscitated following out-of-hospital cardiac arrest? Am J Med 1989;86:145-150.

118. Tresch DD, Thakur R, Hoffmann RG, Brooks HL. Comparison of outcome of resuscitation of out-of-hospital cardiac arrest in persons younger and older than 70 years of age. Am J Cardiol 1988;61:1120-1122.

119. Gulati RS, Bhan GL, Horan MA. Cardiopulmonary resuscitation of old people. Lancet 1983;2:267-269.

120. Herlitz J, Ekstrom L, Wennerblom B, et al. Prognosis among survivors of prehospital cardiac arrest. Ann Emerg Med 1995;25:58-63.

121. Nichol G, Stiell IG, Hebert P, et al. What is the quality of life for survivors of cardiac arrest? A prospective study. Acad Emerg Med 1999;6:95-102.

122. Murphy SL. Deaths: Final Data for 1998. National Vital Statistics Reports, Vol. 48, No. 11. Hyattsville, MD: National Center for Health Statistics, 2000.

123. Fife D, Barancik JI, Chatterjee BF. Northeastern Ohio Trauma Study: II. Injury rates by age, sex, and cause. Am J Public Health 1984;74:473-478.

124. Fife D, Barancik JI. Northeastern Ohio Trauma Study III: incidence of fractures. Ann Emerg Med 1985;14:244-248.

125. Covington DL, Maxwell JG, Clancy TV. Hospital resources used to treat the injured elderly at North Carolina trauma centers. J Am Geriatr Soc 1993;41:847-852.

126. MacKenzie EJ, Morris JA, Jr., Smith GS, Fahey M. Acute hospital costs of trauma in the United States: implications for regionalized systems of care. J Trauma 1990;30:1096-1101; discussion 1101-1093.

127. Oreskovich MR, Howard JD, Copass MK, Carrico CJ. Geriatric trauma: injury patterns and outcome. J Trauma 1984;24:565-572.

128. Horst HM, Obeid FN, Sorensen VJ, Bivins BA. Factors influencing survival of elderly trauma patients. Crit Care Med 1986;14:681-684.

129. Carrillo EH, Richardson JD, Malias MA, et al. Long term outcome of blunt trauma care in the elderly. Surg Gynecol Obstet 1993;176:559-564.

130. DeMaria EJ, Kenney PR, Merriam MA, et al. Aggressive trauma care benefits the elderly. J Trauma 1987;27:1200-1206.

131. van Aalst JA, Morris JA, Jr., Yates HK, et al. Severely injured geriatric patients return to independent living: a study of factors influencing function and independence. J Trauma 1991;31:1096-1101; discussion 1101-1092.

132. Zietlow SP, Capizzi PJ, Bannon MP, Farnell MB. Multisystem geriatric trauma. J Trauma 1994;37:985-988.

133. Knudson MM, Lieberman J, Morris JA, Jr., et al. Mortality factors in geriatric blunt trauma patients. Arch Surg 1994;129:448-453.

134. Tornetta P, 3rd, Mostafavi H, Riina J, et al. Morbidity and mortality in elderly trauma patients. J Trauma 1999;46:702-706.

135. Finelli FC, Jonsson J, Champion HR, et al. A case control study for major trauma in geriatric patients. J Trauma 1989;29:541-548.

136. Morris JA, Jr., MacKenzie EJ, Edelstein SL. The effect of preexisting conditions on mortality in trauma patients. JAMA 1990;263:1942-1946.

137. Wardrope J, Cross SF, Fothergill DJ. One year's experience of major trauma outcome study methodology. BMJ 1990;301:156-159.

138. DeMaria EJ, Kenney PR, Merriam MA, et al. Survival after trauma in geriatric patients. Ann Surg 1987;206:738-743.

139. Broos PL, D'Hoore A, Vanderschot P, et al. Multiple trauma in elderly patients. Factors influencing outcome: importance of aggressive care. Injury 1993;24:365-368.

140. Pellicane JV, Byrne K, DeMaria EJ. Preventable complications and death from multiple organ failure among geriatric trauma victims. J Trauma 1992;33:440-444.
141. Jones JM, Maryosh J, Johnstone S, Templeton J. A multivariate analysis of factors related to the mortality of blunt trauma admissions to the North Staffordshire Hospital Centre. J Trauma 1995;38:118-122.
142. Davis JW, Kaups KL. Base deficit in the elderly: a marker of severe injury and death. J Trauma 1998;45:873-877.
143. Battistella FD, Din AM, Perez L. Trauma patients 75 years and older: long-term follow-up results justify aggressive management. J Trauma 1998;44:618-623; discussion 623.
144. Nagy KK, Smith RF, Roberts RR, et al. Prognosis of penetrating trauma in elderly patients: a comparison with younger patients. J Trauma 2000;49:190-193; discussion 193-194.
145. Scalea TM, Simon HM, Duncan AO, et al. Geriatric blunt multiple trauma: improved survival with early invasive monitoring. J Trauma 1990;30:129-134; discussion 134-126.
146. McKinley BA, Marvin RG, Cocanour CS, et al. Blunt trauma resuscitation: the old can respond. Arch Surg 2000;135:688-693; discussion 694-685.

4

GERIATRIC GENERAL SURGERY

*Walter E. Pofahl II, MD, FACS**

General surgery encompasses many organ systems. This chapter, organized broadly by organ systems, highlights issues concerning the surgical care of elderly patients and reviews current understanding of specific disease states, covering recent research on such topics as the epidemiology, evaluation, management, and outcomes for each condition. Disorders of several organ systems that are also often treated by general surgeons are discussed separately (see Chapter 5 on noncardiac thoracic surgery and Chapter 3 on emergency medicine).

METHODS

The MEDLINE database was searched via the DIALOG Information Service. The time period covered was from 1980 to December 2000. The search strategy combined the MeSH terms for specific surgical procedures with terms denoting old age and also with the various terms for risk factors, postoperative care, postoperative complications, comorbidity, mortality, quality of life, prognosis, recovery, outcome, length of stay, and functional status. An additional requirement was that the term *age* or *aged* be present in the title or that the term *age factors* be present in the MeSH heading. Finally, terms that were excluded were those for specific surgical procedures relating to the specialties that are covered in other chapters and those terms for procedures in the realm of surgical specialties not included in this project, as well as those for liver transplantation, esophagoscopy, gastroscopy, and colonoscopy. The search resulted in 582 references. A final selection from these was made on the basis of a review of titles and abstracts.

OVERVIEW: PROCEDURES AND OUTCOMES

Emergency procedures account for a significant proportion of the operations on older people. A retrospective review of general surgery procedures performed in patients aged 70 and over at a large urban hospital found that 15% of the cases were emergencies.[1] Infection, intestinal obstruction, incarcerated hernia, and hemorrhage were the leading indications for operation. The review found postoperative morbidity and mortality rates to be significantly higher for emergency procedures (31% and 20%, respectively) than for elective procedures (6.8% and 1.9%, respectively) in the same age group. A companion study from the same group found that inguinal herniorrhaphy, colectomy, and cholecystectomy were the most common elective procedures.[2] In another study, of patients aged 90 years and over, operations on the digestive system were found to be the most common.[3] In this population, the observed 5-year survival rate was not significantly different from the expected survival rate for persons aged 90 years and over not undergoing an operation. A prospective audit of 1111 general surgical procedures in 1040 patients aged 65 and older revealed an overall mortality of 5.4%.[4] Patients aged 75 and older had

* Associate Professor, Chief, Division of General Surgery, Brody School of Medicine, East Carolina University, Greenville, NC.

a significantly higher postoperative mortality rate. Among patients aged 65 to 74 years, 14.5% required emergency operations, with a mortality rate of 12.9%. For patients aged 75 and older, 27.9% underwent emergency operations, with a mortality rate of 22.5%.

Two studies from Scandinavian countries have included data on the discharge disposition of elderly patients after general surgical and urologic operations. Schoon and Arvidsson found that in 1981, 78% of patients aged 80 years and older were admitted from home and 58% were discharged directly home. [5] In 1987, 85% were admitted from home and 73% were discharged directly home. Other researchers found that 74% of patients aged 80 and older undergoing general surgical procedures were admitted from home and 70% were discharged home. [6] Seventeen percent were admitted from a nursing home and 16% were discharged back to a nursing home.

In a prospective longitudinal study of 900 general surgical patients, 5-year survival was found to be lower in patients aged 65 years and over undergoing a general surgical procedure than in an aged-matched population. [7] Following an initially higher mortality in the 6 months after surgery, the survival rates in older patients undergoing operations matched that of controls. Specific factors associated with higher early mortality included nonelective admission, age over 75 years, American Society of Anesthesiologists (ASA) class 4 or 5, and major surgery. Although survival rates for specific diseases were not analyzed, survival rates for patients undergoing operation for malignant disease were calculated. Patients without malignancy had survival curves resembling those of an age-matched population. Although the postoperative mortality was similar in patients with and without malignancy, patients with malignant disease had a higher mortality rate for the first year after operation.

A cost analysis of resource utilization by older surgical patients found that this age group consumes a disproportionate share of resources. [8] Beginning at age 55, elderly patients were found to begin using a greater share of resources, and patients aged 65 and over, to account for 30% of all surgical admissions. The mean cost per patient stabilizes at 75 years of age. Because reimbursement per patient plateaus at about 55 years of age, the surgical care of patients aged 75 and older leads to significant financial losses. The proportion of emergency admissions and of intensive care unit use, and the need for blood transfusions progressively increases in the elderly patients. Only intensive care unit use was found to stabilize (at 25% to 30% of admissions) after age 65 years.

A 2-year study of 8899 patients aged 65 years and older undergoing surgery found that severity of illness is a better predictor than age of morbidity, mortality, and length of stay. [9] Outcomes for a given disease severity were found to be stable in patients from age 65 to 85 years and older.

To summarize the findings of recent research:

- Emergency operations, especially on the gastrointestinal system, account for a significant fraction of the general surgery procedures performed on older people.

- The survival rates of elderly patients undergoing elective general surgery operations are similar to those of age-matched groups.

- Costs associated with surgical care are significantly higher in older people.

- Severity of illness, rather than chronologic age, predicts postoperative morbidity, mortality, and length of stay.

GenSurg 1 (Level B): **Prospective cohort studies of specific surgical procedures are needed to identify the risk factors in the geriatric population for specific negative and positive outcomes.**

GenSurg 2 (Level B): **Prospective studies are needed to compare outcomes in younger and older patients for specific surgical procedures in outpatient settings or with short hospital stays. For example, is it possible to safely perform laparoscopic antireflux surgery in older patients with a 23-hour hospital stay?**

GenSurg 3 (Level B): **Case-control studies are needed to identify factors that place elderly patients at high risk for requiring emergency surgical procedures.**

GenSurg 4 (Level B): **Basic studies are needed to elucidate the differences in pathophysiology of the diseases and disorders in the elderly patient that lead to a high risk of requiring emergency surgical procedures.**

GenSurg 5 (Level B): **Guidelines for educating physicians to recognize diseases and risk factors that might predict an older patient's need for emergency surgical procedure should be developed; the guidelines would be based on findings of the research recommended in GenSurg 3 and GenSurg 4.**

ENDOCRINE DISEASE

The incidence of primary hyperparathyroidism is higher in older than in younger people, with estimates ranging as high as 1.5 per 100 patients. A comparison of preoperative symptoms, signs, and laboratory assessment has revealed more severe hyperparathyroidism in elderly (aged 70 years and older) than in younger patients.[10] Despite these differences, the cure rates and postoperative complication and death rates are similar in younger and elderly patients.

Similarly, thyroid disease is common among older people. In a study of 1631 patients aged 50 or older undergoing thyroid surgery, the most common indications for operation were found to be compression symptoms and risk of malignancy.[11] On analysis of resected specimens, the most common diagnosis was found to be multinodular goiter. A significantly higher prevalence of malignancy was found in patients aged 75 years and over. Postoperative complication rates were similar in patients aged 50–60, 61–74, and 75 and older.

To summarize the findings of recent research:

■ Hyperparathyroidism and diseases of the thyroid are common in older people.

■ Treatment outcomes for hyperparathyroidism are equivalent in older and younger patients.

■ The results of surgical treatment of thyroid diseases are similar in older and younger patients.

> *GenSurg 6 (Level B)*: **Research is needed to determine the effect of hyperparathyroidism on quality of life, longevity, functional status, and cognitive status of older patients.**

> *GenSurg 7 (Level B)*: **Observational comparison of older and younger patients is needed to suggest whether hyperparathyroidism is recognized and treated surgically in the same percentage of older and younger patients.**

BREAST CANCER

Although breast cancer is not unique to older people, this age group is at the greatest risk for this malignancy. The incidence of invasive breast cancer in women aged 65 and older is almost six times greater than in younger women, and approximately two thirds of new breast cancers occur in women aged 50 and over. [12] The majority of patients present with stage I and II disease. [13] However, despite this stage distribution, most elderly patients undergo modified radical mastectomy instead of breast conservation surgery. [12–14] One analysis of treatment found that, adjusted for stage, patients aged 70 and older were less likely to receive therapy that is in agreement with National Institutes of Health treatment recommendations. [13] In a series of 184 patients aged 70 and older treated at the M. D. Anderson Cancer Center, [14] the postoperative mortality rate was found to be 1.6%, with all three deaths due to myocardial infarction. With a median follow-up of 80 months, 40% of deaths were due to breast cancer and 60% to other causes. The survival rate specific to breast cancer was 79% at 7 years. Data from the Surveillance, Epidemiology, and End Results Program (SEER) reveal 5-year relative survival rates of 85.2% and 86.5% for patients aged under 65 years and 65 years and older, respectively. [12] During a 30-month follow-up of 1800 postmenopausal women aged 55 years and older with breast cancer, 15% died. [13] Breast cancer was the cause of death in 51% of these cases. However, among patients aged 75 and older, only 38% of deaths were due to breast cancer; cardiovascular disease was the cause of death in 34% of these patients. Multivariate analysis revealed that age above 74 years was a significant determinant of decreased survival in patients with unknown stage or stage I or II breast cancer. Renal failure, liver disease, and stroke or transient ischemic attack were associated with a greater than twofold mortality risk.

Several randomized prospective European trials have investigated tamoxifen as primary therapy for patients aged 70 and over with operable breast cancer. In an early study by Gazet et al, [15] 116 patients aged 70 and over with surgically resectable breast cancer were randomized to tamoxifen (20 mg per day) or surgical resection (mastectomy or wide local excision) as primary therapy. Of the 56 patients in the surgical arm, 43 underwent wide local excision and 13 underwent mastectomy. Local recurrences, development of distant metastases, and death rates (overall and cancer-specific) were equivalent in the two groups, with a median follow-up of 3 years. A subsequent study by Robertson et al [16] evaluated tamoxifen (20 mg b.i.d.) versus wedge mastectomy as primary treatment of resectable breast cancer in 135 patients aged 70 and over. At 5 years, there were no significant differences between the two treatment arms in overall survival or metastasis-free survival. However, there was a significant difference in locoregional recurrence. In the tamoxifen group, 59% of patients experienced locoregional disease progression. In contrast, only 30% of patients in the surgical arm had a locoregional recurrence.

Several additional randomized trials compared tamoxifen alone and surgery with adjuvant tamoxifen in the treatment of resectable breast cancer in patients older than 70 years. A multicenter trial with 171 patients in the surgery-plus-tamoxifen arm (40 mg per day) and 183 in the tamoxifen-alone arm (40 mg per day) found no difference in survival or quality of life between the two groups at a median follow-up of 34 months. [17] Surgical treatment in the surgery-plus-tamoxifen arm consisted of local excision in the majority of patients, mastectomy in 23%, and quadrantectomy in 2%. However, there was a significant rate of local failure necessitating surgical intervention in the tamoxifen-only arm. These findings were confirmed in a larger study of 237 patients in the surgery-plus-tamoxifen arm (20 mg per day) and 236 patients in the tamoxifen-alone arm (160 mg loading dose, then 20 mg per day). [18] Although overall survival was unchanged, the surgery-plus-tamoxifen arm had a significantly greater disease-free survival, with a median follow-up of 3 years. A prospective randomized trial compared tamoxifen (20 mg per day) and placebo in elderly women (older than 65 years) with node-positive breast cancer after modified radical mastectomy. [19] The time to treatment failure was prolonged in the tamoxifen group (7.4 versus 4.4 years). Overall survival was improved in the tamoxifen group (P = .063).

Much of the research in breast cancer in older patients has dealt with the role of axillary lymph node dissection (ALND) because of the potential morbidity associated with this aspect of breast surgery. The data on complications after ALND are mixed. An early prospective study of arm lymphedema in patients undergoing ALND found a prevalence of 25% in patients aged 60 or older. [20] In contrast, this complication occurred in only 7% of younger patients, all of whom had a postoperative wound infection. Radiotherapy, including axillary radiation, had no effect on the rate of lymphedema. Lymphedema was also associated with division of the insertion of the pectoralis minor muscle in elderly patients undergoing ALND, 55% compared with 10% when the muscle was not divided. A subsequent randomized clinical trial of lumpectomy and axillary dissection with and without radiation therapy evaluated upper-extremity morbidity. [21] In contrast to the previous study, this trial found a higher frequency of upper-extremity symptoms in patients younger than 65 at up to 36 months after therapy. On multivariate analysis, only the number of lymph nodes removed and younger age were found to have a significant impact on arm morbidity at 3 to 12 months post-treatment.

A comparison of 63 older (aged 65 or older) and younger women receiving breast irradiation following partial mastectomy found no increase in complications among the older women. [22] Although radiography is safe in older women, a retrospective study found that only approximately 40% of women aged 60 and older were referred for postoperative irradiation after segmental mastectomy. [23] In contrast, 82% of similar patients younger than 60 received postoperative radiotherapy. Among older women receiving postoperative radiation therapy, the local recurrence rate was significantly lower than in older women treated by segmental mastectomy alone (4.0% versus 39.1%). However, this improvement in locoregional control did not translate into improved survival in elderly patients receiving postoperative radiotherapy. Comparison of responses to radiation therapy found no differences in overall survival, disease-free survival, or local recurrence rates between patients aged 70 or older and a younger cohort undergoing lumpectomy and breast irradiation for stage I and II breast cancers. [24]

Several studies have examined the possibility of omitting axillary dissection in elderly patients. A study of 73 patients aged 65 years and older with stage I and II breast cancers and clinically negative axillary nodes assessed the outcomes for tumor excision followed by breast and regional lymph node irradiation. [25] Sixty-six of these patients were also treated with tamoxifen because of positive estrogen receptors or tumor size greater than 2 cm. With a median follow-up of 54 months, the 8-year probabilities of disease-free, metastasis-free, and overall survival were 84%, 86%, and 53%, respectively. A retrospective study of 78 patients aged 70 and older undergoing resection of T1 lesions followed 14 patients who did not undergo axillary dissection. [26] These patients were older (79 years versus 74 years) than patients undergoing ALND. Among patients having ALND, lymph nodes were positive in only 17%. Adjuvant therapy consisted of tamoxifen alone or in conjunction with radiation in 9 of the 14 patients not undergoing ALND and radiation alone in 1 of the 14 patients. The mean follow-up was 48, 43, and 31 months in node-positive, node-negative, and patients not having ALND, respectively. There were no significant differences in disease-free survival, recurrences, or death rates among the three groups. A randomized prospective trial comparing modified radical mastectomy to lumpectomy and tamoxifen (20 mg per day) found a significantly improved overall survival in the tamoxifen group at 6 years. [27] There was no difference in disease-free survival rates.

Following mastectomy, immediate or delayed breast reconstruction is an option. A retrospective review of 242 patients undergoing postmastectomy breast reconstruction found that only 18 were aged 60 or older. [28] Although 34% of the patients undergoing mastectomy were in the elderly age group, only 7% underwent reconstruction. In contrast, 38% of patients younger than 60 had postmastectomy reconstruction. Older patients undergoing reconstruction were more likely than younger patients to have a prosthetic implant. Overall, the elderly patients had a lower rate of postoperative complications than did younger patients, except among patients undergoing reconstruction with autogenous tissue flaps, where there were no significant differences between the postoperative complication rates in older or younger patients.

The role of screening mammography for older women remains uncertain. A retrospective cohort study of over 690,000 California women aged 66 to 79 years found a screening rate of 46%. [29] This rate declined with age to 40% in women aged 75 to 79. Screening was associated with a significantly lower rate of metastatic disease. However, no determination of impact on mortality could be made.

To summarize the findings of recent research:

- Breast cancer is more common in elderly than in younger women.

- The stage distribution of breast cancer is similar in younger and older patients.

- Survival appears to be diminished in older breast cancer patients; however, as breast cancer patients age, they are more likely to die from comorbidities than from breast cancer.

- Tamoxifen can be used as sole therapy in early-stage breast cancer in older patients; however, it has a significantly higher rate of local and regional recurrence than is found with surgery or surgery plus adjuvant tamoxifen.

- Tamoxifen is beneficial in older patients with node-positive breast cancer.

GenSurg 8 (Level A): **Randomized controlled trials should be performed to determine the effect of screening mammography on survival, treatment morbidity, functional outcomes, and costs as a function of age.**

GenSurg 9 (Level A): **Randomized controlled trials of breast cancer therapy in older women should be performed to compare the use of tamoxifen alone with tamoxifen plus surgery, in subgroups of ages ranging from 50 to 90 years. Outcomes measured would include survival, treatment morbidity, function, and cost. Subgroup analyses would identify which patients are likely to respond well to tamoxifen alone.**

GenSurg 10 (Level A): **Randomized controlled trials are needed to determine the minimum duration of tamoxifen therapy that is required for optimal effect in older breast cancer patients.**

GenSurg 11 (Level A): **Randomized controlled trials are needed to compare rates of recurrence and survival in groups of older breast cancer patients who are treated with and without axillary dissection.**

STOMACH DISORDERS

Disorders of the stomach requiring surgery can be a source of significant morbidity and mortality in older patients. Many reports regarding gastric disease in the older population focus on the management of gastric cancer, and most are from Asian and European centers because of the higher incidence of gastric malignancy in these locations than in the United States.

GASTROESOPHAGEAL REFLUX

Gastroesophageal reflux disease (GERD) is common among both younger and older people, with similar reported prevalence rates of approximately 20%.[30] However, the frequency of complications of GERD is higher in elderly patients. This may be due to differences in symptom thresholds for younger patients. A study of symptoms in 195 elderly patients with foregut symptoms found that 30% of patients with severe esophagitis had no symptoms of GERD.[31] A more recent study compared symptoms and response to esophageal acid perfusion in veterans younger than age 60 and in those aged 60 and older.[32] The younger patients reported more severe reflux symptoms than the older cohort, despite similarities in degrees of esophagitis and pH studies. In addition, the younger patients reported a shorter time to symptom perception and greater sensitivity to acid perfusion than did the elderly patients.

The evaluation and treatment of GERD in older and younger people is similar. The main treatment modality is acid suppression, typically with a proton-pump inhibitor. These medications are well tolerated by older patients. The role of laparoscopic antireflux surgery has not been well defined in elderly patients. A retrospective analysis of data prospectively collected on 36 patients aged 65 or higher found that their outcomes were similar to those of younger patients also undergoing laparoscopic antireflux surgery.[33] The older patients accounted for approximately 11% of the operations over a 6-year period. Minor complications were more common in the elderly patients (13.9%) than in the younger patients (2.6%). The incidence of more severe complications was similar in the two groups. The only death occurred with a younger patient. At a median follow-up of 27 months, elderly and younger patients had similar rates of recurrent GERD symptoms, dysphagia, and fundoplication failure.

ULCER DISEASE

A recent report from the Mayo Clinic outlines the role of a specialized management team for the treatment of acute gastrointestinal bleeding. [34] In this series of patients (average age = 65 years), upper gastrointestinal hemorrhages accounted for 75% to 80% of the cases of gastrointestinal bleeding. Over half of these patients had a history of recent nonsteroidal anti-inflammatory drug (NSAID) use. Although no supporting data are provided, the author contends that early operative intervention should occur in elderly patients because of their limited physiologic reserve.

In a retrospective review of 40 high-risk patients presenting with perforated gastric ulcer, 18 (45%) were aged 70 years or older. [35] The mortality for this group of elderly patients was 44%. For the 12 patients aged 70 and older treated with omental patch closure of the perforated ulcer, the mortality was 58%. The mortality rate was 17% in the 6 patients undergoing partial gastrectomy. Analysis of 136 patients undergoing surgical treatment for complications of peptic ulcers found that perforation accounted for 67% of the cases and bleeding for 31%. [36] The postoperative complication rate was 66%, and the overall mortality was 30%. The death rates were equivalent in patients suffering perforation or bleeding, at 31%. Twenty-five of the 28 deaths in patients with perforation occurred in patients aged 70 or over. Similarly, almost three quarters of the deaths in patients requiring operation for bleeding were in this older age group.

GASTRIC CANCER

A retrospective study attempted to clarify risk factors associated with postoperative complications in elderly patients undergoing total gastrectomy for cancer. [37] The prevalence of preoperative cardiopulmonary disease was found to be significantly higher in patients aged 65 and older than in the younger cohort. Both groups had similar distributions of tumor stage; there were no significant differences in preoperative renal function or nutritional status between the two groups. The rate of postoperative complications was significantly higher in the older patients (44.4%) than in the younger patients (19.2%). Although mortality was also higher in the older group (11.1%) than in the younger group (3.5%), this difference was not statistically significant. A report from Japan of 382 patients undergoing curative resection of early gastric cancer found that increasing age is associated with a lower long-term survival rate. [38] Of the 25 patients dying of recurrent disease, median survival was significantly shorter in patients aged 55 years or over (1.7 years) than in younger patients (5.6 years). In another study of 380 patients undergoing total gastrectomy, 43% were aged 70 or older. [39] Chronic lung disease, hypoalbuminemia, diabetes mellitus, and electrocardiogram changes were found to be more common among the older patients. The postoperative complication rate was higher in the older cohort. However, postoperative mortality was not significantly different in the two groups, nor was there a significant difference in long-term survival.

A study by Wu et al examined the quality of life after gastric resection for cancer in 433 patients aged 65 and older. [40] The two groups compared were patients aged 65 to 74 years and patients aged 74 years and over. The postoperative morbidity and mortality rates were higher in the older group. Multivariate analysis found that age and extent of gastric resection were independent predictors of postoperative mortality. There was no difference in long-term survival between the two age groups. After accounting for 261 deaths (180 due to gastric cancer, 21 due to postoperative mortality) and 22 patients lost to follow-up, researchers assessed quality of life using the Spitzer index in 125 of the patients aged 65 to 74 and 25 of the patients over age 74 and found no significant differences in Spitzer index scores between the two groups. All patients, except one receiving chemotherapy, had normal work and daily activities; 16% had a lack of energy and 14% had experienced a period of anxiety or depression.

To summarize the findings of recent research:

- The prevalence of GERD is similar in younger and older patients; however, the incidence of severe and complicated GERD is higher in elderly patients.

- The morbidity and mortality rates for complications of peptic ulcer disease in older patients are high.

- Emergency operations for gastric disease are associated with high rates of postoperative complications and death.

- The postoperative morbidity rates after gastrectomy for gastric cancer are higher in elderly patients than in younger patients. The postoperative mortality rates are similar for these two groups of patients.

- Long-term survival rates after gastric resection for gastric cancer are similar in younger and older patients.

GenSurg 12 (Level B): **Observational cohort studies are needed to determine if presentation and pathophysiology of peptic ulcer disease are different in older and younger people.**

GenSurg 13 (Level B): **Prospective cohort studies are needed to seek clues as to how complications of peptic ulcer disease in older patients can be prevented.**

GenSurg 14 (Level B): **Cohort studies on older patients are needed to identify risk factors for peptic ulcer disease.**

GenSurg 15 (Level B): **Observational cohort studies tests are needed of putative methods to reduce the morbidity and mortality of emergency operations for peptic ulcer disease in older patients.**

GenSurg 16 (Level A): **Randomized controlled trials of the most promising method for reducing the morbidity and mortality of emergency surgery for peptic ulcer disease in older patients are needed.**

GenSurg 17 (Level B): **Cohort studies are needed to seek alternatives to nonsteroidal anti-inflammatory drugs for use by older patients.**

GenSurg 18 (Level A): **As possibly safer nonsteroidal anti-inflammatory drugs are developed, they should be tested in randomized controlled trials for safe use by older patients.**

GenSurg 19 (Level B): **Outcome studies and prospective cohort studies are needed to build evidence as to optimum treatment for each stage of gastric cancer, including ways to palliate the near-terminal and terminal phases.**

GenSurg 20 (Level B): **Cohort or outcome studies are needed to gain information about the effectiveness of using newer treatment methods, such as photodynamic therapy, for treating elderly patients with stomach disorders.**

COLORECTAL DISEASE

Colorectal disease is a significant concern for older people. Many report abnormalities in bowel function. The incidence of benign and malignant conditions of the large intestine increases with age. For American women between the ages of 60 and 79, the probability of developing colorectal cancer is 3%; for American men in the same age group, the probability is 4%. [41]

DIVERTICULAR DISEASE

Diverticulosis and diverticulitis are more common in older than in younger people. Colon resection to manage these problems is occasionally required and represents the most common indication for colectomy for benign disease in older people. One evaluation of the metabolic responses to elective colon resection found no age-related changes. [42] In a nonrandomized prospective comparison of elective laparoscopic and open colectomy for sigmoid diverticulitis, it was found that laparoscopic surgery was associated with a lower requirement for postoperative parenteral analgesics, lower postoperative morbidity, a shortened length of stay, and a reduced requirement for postoperative inpatient rehabilitation. [43] The main factors associated with the reduction in postoperative morbidity are lower rates of wound infection and pulmonary infection. Another prospective cohort study of elective laparoscopic colorectal surgery in older patients found that 80% of previously independent patients undergoing laparoscopic procedures return home but that only 43% undergoing open procedures were able to do so ($P = .025$). [44] A higher proportion of the patients undergoing open colorectal surgery (46%) were discharged to a rehabilitation facility; only 11% of those undergoing laparoscopic procedures needed such facilities ($P = .016$). Earlier retrospective studies had also demonstrated the safety of laparoscopic colorectal surgery in older patients. One study found that although patients aged 70 years and older had more cardiopulmonary comorbidities than younger patients, there was no difference in major or minor postoperative complication rates for younger and older patients. [45] Another study, in which 38% of the patients aged 60 years and older had medical comorbidities, showed equivalent rates of postoperative complications, conversion to open procedures, length of ileus, and hospital length of stay for older patients and a procedure-matched group younger than 60 years. [46]

In contrast to elective resection for diverticulosis, emergent management of lower gastrointestinal bleeding can have significant death and complication rates. Among 49 patients at a single institution undergoing total abdominal colectomy for bleeding, 71% were found to require an emergency operation, with a mortality rate of 34%. [47] The mortality rate was found to increase with advancing age, from 20% in patients younger than 70 years to 39% in patients aged 70 years and older.

COLORECTAL CANCER

Given the prevalence of colorectal cancer and the fact that the risk of developing the disease increases with age, colorectal malignancy is a common problem in older people. One analysis found that 75% of new colorectal cancers occur in patients aged 65 years or older. [48] The same analysis found 40% of patients to have five or more comorbidities, and 80%, one or more conditions considered to have a high or moderate life impact threat. There was no significant relationship between age and stage at presentation; however, the risk ratio for death was almost twice as high in patients aged 75 or over. An analysis of Medicare claims data found a 5% perioperative mortality for colectomy for colon cancer in patients aged 65 years and older. [49] Furthermore, the risk of mortality was significantly increased in men and with increasing age. The risk of perioperative mortality was found to be 31% higher in men than in women. The relative mortality risk was twice that of patients younger than 85 years and three times that of patients younger than 75 years. Overall, 1- and 2-year survival rates were 76% and 63%, respectively. Even after adjusting for differences in life expectancy, logistic regression analysis demonstrated a detrimental impact of increasing age on survival. Contradictory results were found in a study from Ireland that investigated outcomes for colorectal cancer in patients aged 70 years or more who constituted 44% of the patients treated for colorectal cancer at a single institution over a 6-year period. [50] Although the elderly patients presented more commonly than younger patients with complications of their malignancy requiring emergency intervention (18% versus 11%), there were no differences between younger and older patients in the postoperative mortality rates overall, for elective procedures, or for emergency procedures. Differences in 5-year survival rates for the elderly and younger groups were not statistically significant. Overall 5-year survival was 52% for the elderly patients and 45% for the younger cohort. For those patients undergoing potentially curative resection, the respective rates were 68% and 59%.

A study from Japan found more advanced colorectal cancer among patients aged 80 years and over with a sedentary as opposed to active lifestyle. [51] Furthermore, sedentary patients with stage III colorectal cancer had shorter survival. Postoperative mortality was also highest in the sedentary group undergoing palliative operations, although the mortality rate for sedentary patients undergoing potentially curative resection was the same as for active patients. Unfortunately, the mortality rates were not controlled for pre-existing morbidities. Another study comparing total rectal resection and coloanal anastomosis found no difference in outcomes between young and elderly patients with rectal tumors. [52] Specifically, there were no differences in perioperative morbidity or functional results, quality of life, and performance status. This is counter to the commonly held belief that older patients do not do well with coloanal anastomoses because of debilitating diarrhea. The functional outcome of coloanal anastomosis in elderly patients was subsequently confirmed in a study by Dehni et al. [53] This nonrandomized study found no significant difference in functional results of coloanal anastomosis with colonic J-pouch between patients older than 75 years and younger patients (mean age = 58 years). Similar functional outcomes with ileoanal reservoir have been demonstrated in patients aged 50 years and older [54,55] or 60 years [56] and in younger patients, even though the procedure is performed for benign colonic disease and typically in a younger patient population.

Whether older patients more commonly require colostomy is unknown; however, most surgeons seem to be more likely to perform a colostomy in older patients than to forgo surgery and risk anastomotic leakage. These colostomies are frequently performed as part of an emergency procedure and commonly are never closed. A study by Wong et al [57] confirms the morbidity associated with colostomy closure in older patients. This retrospective review of 84 patients aged 70 years and older showed a higher incidence (13% versus 5%) of postoperative complications in older than in younger patients.

To summarize the findings of recent research:

- Benign and malignant colorectal diseases are more common in older people.

- Postoperative complication rates for elective laparoscopic colectomy are lower than for elective open colectomy in older patients.

- Emergency procedures are associated with significantly higher complication and death rates.

   GenSurg 21 (Levels B and A): **Nonrandomized or randomized trials comparing appropriate management options for complications of diverticular disease in older patients are needed.**

   GenSurg 22 (Level A): **Randomized controlled trials are needed to compare the various colorectal cancer screening methods now in use for their efficacy in elderly patients.**

   GenSurg 23 (Level B): **Exploratory studies are needed to elucidate the roles of emerging technologies in the management of colorectal cancer in elderly patients.**

LIVER RESECTION

Few general surgery procedures are as strongly associated with the potential for physiologic disruption, morbidity, and mortality as are major liver resections. One would anticipate that, given older patients' limited physiologic reserve, they would tolerate this procedure poorly. Because of the increased incidence of colorectal cancer and other gastrointestinal cancers causing liver metastases with advancing age, the need for liver-directed therapy will continue to increase in this patient population. Because colorectal liver metastases represent the most common indication for liver resection in this country and the incidence of hepatocellular carcinoma is significantly lower, only liver resection for metastatic disease will be reviewed herein.

A retrospective review of 41 patients undergoing liver resection showed a similar rate of postoperative morbidity and mortality in patients aged 70 years and older when they were compared with a group with a mean age of 57 years. [58] An earlier study demonstrated similar morbidity and mortality rates following major liver resection in older patients (mean age = 74 years) and a younger cohort (mean age = 46 years). [59] In addition, postoperative liver function was similar in the elderly and the younger patients. Fong et al analyzed outcomes from liver resection for colorectal cancer metastases in a group of 128 patients aged 70 years and older, constituting 22% of the liver resections performed at a single institution over an 11-year period. [60] The perioperative mortality and complication rates of 4% and 41%, respectively, were comparable to the rates in younger patients. Additionally, long-term survival rates were not found to be significantly different in elderly and younger patients following resection.

Overall, it seems that liver resection can be performed safely in older people. However, most reports are from high-volume specialty centers whose results may be better than those of lower-volume centers.

> **GenSurg 24 (Level B)**: **Cohort studies are needed to determine the role, safety, and efficacy of newer liver-directed therapies in older patients, for example, cryoablation, radiofrequency ablation, and hepatic artery infusion.**

BILIARY DISEASE

Cholecystectomy is one of the most commonly performed general surgery procedures. In an analysis of more than 42,000 cholecystectomies performed in 1989, the overall mortality was found to be less than 1%. [61] Postoperative mortality was highest in patients aged 65 years and older (0.5% versus 0.03% for those younger than 65 years). Complication rates, length of stay, and charges were also higher in these older patients. Subsequent studies have evaluated laparoscopic cholecystectomy in older patients. Pessaux et al prospectively evaluated laparoscopic cholecystectomy in 102 patients aged 75 years or older. [62] Over one third of these patients were ASA class III or IV, and one third had acute cholecystitis, whereas only 14% of younger patients did. Older patients had higher rates of postoperative complications (13.7% versus 6.6%) and higher rates of conversion to an open procedure (21.6% versus 12.9%). An earlier study had similar findings: an overall complication rate of 14.5% in patients aged 60 years and older. [63] No significant difference between the complication rates of patients aged 60 to 69 (11%) and of those aged 70 or greater (20%) was found. An analysis of 18,500 patients aged 80 to 105 years undergoing cholecystectomy found that significantly more patients undergoing laparoscopic cholecystectomy were discharged home (75% versus 68% for open cholecystectomy), and fewer were discharged to a skilled nursing facility (8% versus 11%). [64] The postoperative mortality rate was significantly lower for patients undergoing laparoscopic cholecystectomy (1.8%) than for patients undergoing open cholecystectomy (4.4%). In a study of 144 patients aged 65 and older undergoing laparoscopic cholecystectomy, no episodes of hypercarbia or hypotension were found despite the presence of cardiopulmonary disease in 64% of these patients. [65]

Laparoscopic cholecystectomy also has a significant role in the management of biliary pancreatitis in elderly patients. A retrospective analysis of the management of gallstone pancreatitis found similar morbidity and mortality rates for laparoscopic cholecystectomy in patients aged 65 or older and in younger patients. [66] In each age group, slightly over 20% of patients were initially treated without cholecystectomy or endoscopic retrograde cholangiography, usually because the patient refused treatment. Among those managed without cholecystectomy or endoscopic retrograde cholangiography, 20% were readmitted with recurrent pancreatitis and subsequently underwent surgery.

To summarize the findings of recent research:

- Cholecystectomy is one of the most frequently performed operations in older patients.

- Elderly patients present with a greater proportion of complicated biliary disease.

- The morbidity and mortality rates for cholecystectomy are higher in elderly than in younger patients.

- In elderly patients laparoscopic cholecystectomy has a lower mortality rate than does open cholecystectomy.

> ***GenSurg 25 (Level A)***: **Randomized controlled trials are needed to compare the safety and effectiveness for older patients of outpatient or short-stay cholecystectomy with the safety and effectiveness of longer hospital stays.**

> ***GenSurg 26 (Level B)***: **Basic physiologic and biochemical studies are needed to learn why older patients are more likely than younger patients to present with complicated biliary disease.**

PANCREATIC DISEASE

Pancreatic cancer remains a significant source of cancer deaths. As with most malignancies, the risk increases with age. Although the perioperative morbidity and mortality associated with pancreatic resection has historically been high, these rates have markedly improved over the past decade. A study of 42 patients with a mean age of 75 years found perioperative morbidity and mortality rates of 31% and 9%, respectively, for radical pancreatic resection. [67] Another early report by Hannoun et al of 44 patients aged 70 and older undergoing pancreaticoduodenectomy (Whipple procedure) between 1970 and 1990 showed a mortality rate of 4.5%. [68] The postoperative morbidity rate was 36% in this group. The mortality and morbidity rates in patients undergoing operations after 1985 were 3.7% and 33.0%, respectively. The death and complication rates in a younger cohort of 179 patients (mean age = 57 ± 10 years) were 10% and 35%, respectively. The mortality and morbidity rates in younger patients undergoing operations after 1985 were 1.8% and 32%, respectively. Five-year survival rates were equivalent in the two groups. Subsequent studies have confirmed low postoperative mortality following pancreatic resection in older patients, [60,69–72] with several having no mortality in elderly patients undergoing resection. In these reports, long-term survival after pancreatic resection was equivalent in the elderly and younger patients.

Research has made it clear that pancreatic resection can be performed safely in older people. However, as with liver resection, most reports are from high-volume specialty centers whose results may be better than those at lower-volume centers.

> ***GenSurg 27 (Level B)***: **Cohort or case-control studies are needed to determine what are the most appropriate selection criteria for pancreatic resection in older patients.**

> ***GenSurg 28 (Level A)*:** **Exploratory prospective cohort studies are needed to suggest how elderly patients with pancreatic cancer are best palliated.**

CEREBROVASCULAR DISEASE

The incidence of atherosclerotic vascular disease increases with age. The mean age of patients in most reports approaches or exceeds 65 years. An analysis of the economic impact of vascular surgery in older people showed that elderly patients undergoing peripheral vascular surgery accounted for almost half of the hospital admissions and generated a disproportionately higher percentage (58%) of total hospital costs. [73] Older people have a significantly higher mortality associated with emergency vascular procedures (38.2%) than with elective procedures (2.3%). [74] Assessment of functional outcome after vascular procedures showed that 65% of patients were living at home and 35% in a nursing facility; 58% were fully ambulatory and 15% were confined to a wheelchair or bedridden. [74]

As the third leading cause of death in the United States, cerebrovascular disease is a significant source of morbidity and mortality in older people. Carotid endarterectomy is an accepted therapy in selected patients for the prevention of stroke in the presence of extracranial atherosclerotic vascular disease. On the basis of the Asymptomatic Carotid Atherosclerosis Study (ACAS), carotid endarterectomy is indicated in patients with asymptomatic carotid lesions causing at least 60% stenosis and whose surgical risk is less than 3% and life expectancy is at least 5 years. [75,76] On the basis of the European Carotid Surgery and the North American Symptomatic Carotid Endarterectomy (NASCET) trials, carotid endarterectomy is recommended in patients with symptomatic lesions causing 70% to 99% stenosis. [77,78] For symptomatic patients with 50% to 69% stenosis, carotid endarterectomy was found to yield a moderate reduction in stroke risk in the NASCET [79] but not in the European trial. [78] Unfortunately, both ACAS and NASCET excluded patients over the age 79 years.

A comparison of carotid endarterectomy in patients older and younger than 75 years found equivalent stroke and death rates in the two groups. [80] The combined stroke and death rates were 4% and 6% for patients younger than 75 years and 75 years and older, respectively. Perioperative strokes were the most common cause of death in the younger age group. In contrast, the most common cause of death in the older age group was cardiac. Additional studies have confirmed the safety of carotid endarterectomy. This is especially important given the fact that patients older than 79 years were excluded from the original NASCET [77] and from the ACAS. [76] In the follow-up NASCET report on symptomatic patients with moderate stenosis (50% to 69%), patients aged 80 years and over were included. [79] Sixty-four percent of the patients in the surgical arm and 59% of the patients in the medical arm were aged 65 or older. Seventeen percent of the patients randomized to carotid endarterectomy were aged 75 or older, and 14% of patients randomized to medical therapy were in this age group. Although older patients were eligible for enrollment, no age-specific results were provided. Patients with moderate carotid stenosis had only a moderate reduction in stroke risk with endarterectomy, and patients with less than 50% stenosis had no benefit from operation.

The incidence of perioperative stroke in elderly patients has been reported to vary, from approximately 1% to 19%. [81-86] The highest stroke rate reported was 19.2% in 26 patients older than 80 years, as compared with 2.2% in younger patients. [84] These strokes accounted for half of the strokes in the entire cohort of 254 patients. Other single-institution studies have reported postoperative combined stroke and death rates of 1.1% [85] and 2.9% [82] for patients aged 80 years and older. These studies reported stroke-free survival rates greater than 95%. A single-institution report on carotid endarterectomy in 58 patients 75 years and older showed a combined stroke and death rate of 6.4% and a rate of 3.2% in 115 younger patients, but this difference was not statistically significant. [81] There was no significant difference in cardiac morbidity between the two groups (7.9% for the older group and 7.2% for the younger patients).

In a statewide analysis of almost 10,000 patients undergoing carotid endarterectomy over a 5-year period, over half of the patients were aged 70 or older and 10% were aged 80 or older. [83] As patient age increased, so did medical complexity. There were no significant differences in stroke and mortality rates for patients younger than 65 (1.7%, 0.8%), aged 65 to 69 (1.6%, 0.9%), aged 70 to 79 (1.8%, 0.9%), or aged 80 and older (1.3%, 1.4%). However, lengths of stay and hospital charges were significantly higher in patients aged 70 and older. Examination of a sample of Medicare beneficiaries undergoing carotid endarterectomy found no increased stroke risk in patients over 80 years old; [86] however, the mortality risk was doubled.

To summarize the findings of recent research:

■ Stroke is a significant source of morbidity and mortality in older people.

■ Stroke can be prevented with appropriate performance of carotid endarterectomy.

■ The results of carotid endarterectomy are similar across the age spectrum.

GenSurg 29 (Level B, then A): **Cohort studies followed possibly by randomized controlled trials are needed to determine beyond what age carotid endarterectomy is minimally or not beneficial.**

GenSurg 30 (Level B): **Prospective studies are needed to determine the incidence and prevalence of cerebrovascular disease in older patients. As with screening for other conditions, prospective studies are needed to evaluate the impact of screening for carotid disease on longevity, quality of life, stroke rate, and financial implications. Cohort studies are needed to determine if there is a subset of older patients (eg, smokers, those with hypertension) who benefit from screening for carotid disease.**

PERIPHERAL OCCLUSIVE DISEASE

As with cerebrovascular disease, elderly patients have an increased incidence of atherosclerotic disease of the lower extremities. In one study of patients undergoing lower-extremity bypass, patients aged 75 years and over represented 28% of all reconstructions during a 9-year period. [87] Among the group of 166 elderly patients undergoing lower-extremity revascularization, 26% had incapacitating claudication and 74% had critical limb ischemia as manifested by rest pain (20%) or ulceration or gangrene (54%). The perioperative mortality rate was 5.4%, and the early and late limb salvage rates were 93%

and 83%, respectively, in the elderly patients. One report of 108 patients aged 80 and over with more severe limb ischemia—all had rest pain and 40% presented with acute ischemia—found much worse results, with a limb salvage rate of only 51% and an overall mortality rate of 25%. [88] The limb salvage, amputation, and mortality rates were best for patients with chronic ischemia who underwent active treatment consisting of angioplasty, thrombolytic therapy, vascular reconstruction, or embolectomy. In contrast, limb salvage and amputation rates were the worst for patients with chronic ischemia who received only supportive care. The mortality rate was higher for patients with acute ischemia undergoing active treatment than for patients with chronic ischemia.

Choi et al analyzed data prospectively collected over a 10-year period on 629 consecutive patients aged 80 or older who underwent infrainguinal vascular reconstruction. [89] These elderly patients constituted 16% of the 3886 procedures performed. There were significantly lower proportions of males, patients with diabetes, and active smokers in the elderly age group than in the younger group. Sixty-eight percent of the older patients underwent reconstruction for tissue loss, as compared with 55% of patients younger than age 80. Only 4.5% of elderly patients underwent surgery for claudication, whereas in 14.6% of the younger patients this was the indication for surgery. Postoperative mortality was higher among the older patients, 4.6% versus 2.8%. Long-term patency and limb salvage rates were higher in the elderly patients; however, cumulative survival was significantly less.

A review of distal bypasses (below the tibioperoneal trunk) in 125 patients aged 75 and older found a limb salvage rate of 81.7% at 5 years and a cumulative graft patency rate of 81.6%. [90] The proportion of patients aged 85 and older progressively increased such that they accounted for 22% of all distal bypasses in the 75 and older group during the last 6 years of the study. The perioperative mortality was 8% in patients aged 75 and older. The primary cause of death was perioperative myocardial infarction. Of the 10 patients suffering myocardial infarction, 7 died.

Tretinyak et al administered the Medical Outcomes Study 36-item Short Form (SF-36) to 46 male veterans (mean age = 67 years) prior to and after lower-extremity bypass. [91] These patients had lower health-related quality-of-life scores than did age-matched controls, and following revascularization only physical function scores improved significantly. Using a different assessment tool, Gibbons et al administered a health status questionnaire to 276 patients undergoing infrainguinal bypass. [92] Among the 156 patients completing questionnaires before and 6 months after infrainguinal revascularization, significant improvements in the mean vitality, instrumental activities of daily living, mental well-being, and lower-extremity discomfort scores were reported after bypass surgery. There was no significant improvement in the mean general health rating.

To summarize the findings of recent research:

■ The likelihood of critical limb ischemia increases with age.

■ Good patency and limb salvage rates can be obtained.

■ The primary cause of postoperative mortality is cardiac disease.

GenSurg 31 (Level B): **Cohort studies comparing the results of endovascular therapy, thrombolytic therapy, and interventional vascular radiology in older patients are needed.**

GenSurg 32 (Level B): **Cohort studies are needed to determine selection criteria for lower-extremity bypass in older patients.**

GenSurg 33 (Level B): **Exploratory studies (eg, case series, cohort studies, outcomes studies) are needed to learn how best to improve limb salvage rates in peripheral vascular disease in older patients.**

ABDOMINAL AORTIC ANEURYSM

Abdominal aortic aneurysm (AAA) repair has traditionally been associated with a high perioperative mortality, to be weighed against the fact that aneurysm rupture has a significant death rate. Recent studies have reported improved complication and death rates following aneurysm repair. In one, patients aged 80 and over undergoing elective repair were found to have a 3% postoperative mortality rate. [93] The perioperative mortality of patients undergoing emergency repair was found to be 20%. Other studies have also documented large differences in mortality and morbidity rates between elective and emergent AAA repair. [74,82,94] A report from Australia found no difference in the mortality rates for elective AAA repair between patients older than 80 years and patients younger than 80 years. [94] However, the mortality rate of emergency AAA repair was 60% for the patients older than 80 years but only 20% for the younger cohort. Comparison of long-term survival at 5 years in elderly patients undergoing elective AAA repair with survival of the general population (United States) matched for aged, sex, and race found no difference. [74]

Recently, endovascular repair of AAA has been proposed as a technique to diminish the morbidity and mortality and enhance recovery from AAA repair. Using a decision analysis model, Finlayson et al evaluated the effect of availability of endovascular repair on the threshold size for performing AAA repair. [95] The threshold aneurysm diameter for recommending endovascular repair was significantly reduced only in men aged 80 and over. However, this reduction of the threshold for repair resulted in only a small increase (0.2 years) in quality-adjusted life expectancy.

The costs of screening for and treating AAA in older people are substantial. When a simulation model incorporating several different screening scenarios is used, costs for screening by palpation and ultrasound for positive physical examination findings are estimated to lead to an estimated gain of 20 life-years (0.2 years per person) at $28,741 per life-year for a model cohort of 10,000 men aged 60 to 80 years followed for 20 years. [96] Screening by a single ultrasound would yield 57 additional life-years at a cost of $41,550 per life-year. A second ultrasound examination after 5 years would gain 1 life-year at an estimated cost of $906,769. This must be counterbalanced by the costs associated with emergent AAA repair. A cost analysis of Australian patients undergoing AAA repair found little difference in the cost of elective repair among patients younger than 80 years and those 80 years and older ($8081 and $10,305 per patient, respectively). [94] In contrast, the costs associated with emergency repair were $28,243 and $24,555 per patient for younger and older patients, respectively. However, the cost per survivor of emergency AAA repair was significantly higher for the older patients ($61,384) than for the younger patients ($35,303).

To summarize the findings of recent research:

■ As with other conditions, emergency repair for AAA is associated with significantly higher rates of complications and death, as well as higher cost.

■ Elective AAA repair in older patients has perioperative morbidity and mortality rates and a survival rate similar to that in younger patients.

> **GenSurg 34 (Level B)**: **Studies are needed to identify criteria for selecting patients who should be screened for abdominal aortic aneurysm and the screening methods to use.**

> **GenSurg 35 (Level A)**: **Randomized controlled trials are needed to compare results using newer endovascular repairs in elderly high-risk patients with results in traditional surgical abdominal aortic aneurysm repair.**

PRESSURE ULCERS

Pressure ulcers are due to prolonged periods of immobility. Elderly patients are at greater risk for this. Furthermore, the incidence of pressure ulcers in surgical patients is significantly higher than in other hospitalized populations. [97] Attempts to identify and prevent pressure ulceration in surgical patients have been difficult owing to the length of operative procedures, operating room bed design, and lack of knowledge about the intrinsic and extrinsic factors responsible for ulceration. A prospective study of a method for predicting pressure-ulcer development found no significant difference in the rate of ulceration between patients aged 65 years and older (22%) and patients younger than 65 (15%). [98] A randomized prospective trial found a 21.5% incidence of pressure ulcers, predominantly on the buttocks and coccyx, within 6 days of surgery. [97] The use of a special mattress overlay had no effect on the incidence of pressure ulceration.

To summarize: because of their general immobility, elderly patients undergoing surgery may be at increased risk for pressure ulceration.

> **GenSurg 36 (Level B)**: **Cohort studies are needed to suggest whether prevention and treatment strategies for pressure ulcers that are applicable to younger patients are also applicable to older patients.**

CHALLENGES IN GENERAL SURGERY FOR ELDERLY PATIENTS

Older people represent the fastest growing segment of the U.S. population. They also represent the segment most likely to require medical and surgical care. As shown in this review, in most instances the outcomes for elective operations in elderly patients are similar to those in younger patients. However, emergency procedures in the older people are associated with especially high rates of complications and death. The challenge is to identify at-risk patients and intervene before the condition necessitates emergency intervention.

In addition to this challenge, the role of emerging technology and techniques in caring for older patients remains poorly defined. In several instances, such as laparoscopic cholecystectomy and laparoscopic colectomy, this patient group appears to have benefited from the development of minimally invasive techniques. However, the place of other therapies, such as endovascular repair of aneurysms and gene therapy, is undefined.

KEY RESEARCH QUESTIONS IN GERIATRIC GENERAL SURGERY

GenSurg KQ1: **How can elderly patients at high risk for emergency procedures be identified?**

Hypothesis-generating studies will require prospective cohort studies that determine the most common general surgical emergencies in older patients, the underlying causes of those emergencies, and whether the emergencies could be avoided. These conditions will probably include peptic ulcer disease, biliary disease, hernias, colonic disease, and trauma. It is essential that outcome measures are not limited to the usual surgical indices, that is, 30-day morbidity and mortality figures. In the older population, the measures must also include long-term outcomes, quality of life, and the effect of these interventions on the families.

Hypothesis-testing studies would be based on relationships delineated in the hypothesis-generating studies. The success of the therapies for preventing or lessening the impact of these conditions would be the basis for clinical trials. For example, elderly patients present with a greater proportion of complicated biliary disease. If specific factors associated with complicated biliary disease were identified, then a trial of intervention to ameliorate those factors could be undertaken. The same would occur for other diseases associated with a significant incidence of emergency presentations and high morbidity and mortality, such as ulcer disease and gastrointestinal hemorrhage. In addition, when high-risk patients are identified, outcomes for different treatment modalities can be compared in prospective trials.

GenSurg KQ2: **What are the differences in pathophysiology of the disease processes in the older patient leading to surgical emergencies?**

Hypothesis-generating studies would require large, prospective databases and cohort studies similar to those for GenSurg KQ1. This priority also requires measurement of physiologic, biochemical, immunologic, and genetic variables to determine the underlying physiologic differences of biliary disease, ulcer disease, and other gastrointestinal abnormalities that commonly require emergent intervention.

Hypothesis-testing studies would be based on the findings generated by the cohort studies. For example, is there a specific protein, hormone, or other factor that accounts for a higher incidence of complicated biliary disease in older people? Once the pathologic "factor" is identified, randomized trials of treatments manipulating the factor could be undertaken. Several areas of research appear promising at this time: the molecular biology of aging, the effects of malnutrition, the impaired immune response in the older patient, and infectious disease, especially viral disease and susceptibility to "normal" pathogens.

GenSurg KQ3: **What factors impact on procedure-specific risk-benefit projections in elderly patients?**

Hypothesis-generating studies will require the use of existing databases, the development of newer prospective databases, and prospective cohort studies. Current databases that could be accessed include the American College of Surgeons Tumor Registry, the National VA Surgical Quality Improvement Program, and the Centers for Medicare and Medicaid Services. Newer databases would need to be developed that incorporate information related to elderly patients. Input variables would include demographics, specific comorbidities, specific procedural data, and outcomes such as morbidity, mortality, discharge destination, quality of life, and functional status. From these studies, specific factors and procedure-related outcomes could be categorized.

Hypothesis-testing studies would be based on factors and outcomes following the above studies. Large, multi-institutional randomized clinical trials would be required to answer such questions as these: At what age (in the absence of other comorbidities) do the risks of carotid endarterectomy outweigh the benefits? When does screening mammography cease to be effective from the standpoint of breast cancer mortality or cost?

REFERENCES

1. Keller SM, Markovitz LJ, Wilder JR, Aufses AH, Jr. Emergency surgery in patients aged over 70 years. Mt Sinai J Med 1987;54:25-28.
2. Keller SM, Markovitz LJ, Wilder JR, Aufses AH, Jr. Emergency and elective surgery in patients over age 70. Am Surg 1987;53:636-640.
3. Warner MA, Hosking MP, Lobdell CM, et al. Surgical procedures among those greater than or equal to 90 years of age. A population-based study in Olmsted County, Minnesota, 1975-1985. Ann Surg 1988;207:380-386.
4. Barlow AP, Zarifa Z, Shillito RG, et al. Surgery in a geriatric population. Ann R Coll Surg Engl 1989;71:110-114.
5. Schoon IM, Arvidsson S. Surgery in patients aged 80 years and over. A retrospective comparative study from 1981 and 1987. Eur J Surg 1991;157:251-255.
6. Rorbaek-Madsen M, Dupont G, Kristensen K, et al. General surgery in patients aged 80 years and older. Br J Surg 1992;79:1216-1218.
7. Edwards AE, Seymour DG, McCarthy JM, Crumplin MK. A 5-year survival study of general surgical patients aged 65 years and over. Anaesthesia 1996;51:3-10.
8. Munoz E, Friedman R, Schroder W, et al. Age, resource consumption, and outcome for surgical patients at an academic medical center. Surgery 1988;103:335-343.
9. Dunlop WE, Rosenblood L, Lawrason L, et al. Effects of age and severity of illness on outcome and length of stay in geriatric surgical patients. Am J Surg 1993;165:577-580.
10. Chen H, Parkerson S, Udelsman R. Parathyroidectomy in the elderly: do the benefits outweigh the risks? World J Surg 1998;22:531-535; discussion 535-536.
11. Bliss R, Patel N, Guinea A, et al. Age is no contraindication to thyroid surgery. Age Ageing 1999;28:363-366.
12. Ries LAG, Eisner MP, Kosary CL, et al. (eds): SEER Cancer Statistics Review, 1973-1998. Bethesda, MD: National Cancer Institute, 2001.
13. Yancik R, Wesley MN, Ries LA, et al. Effect of age and comorbidity in postmenopausal breast cancer patients aged 55 years and older. JAMA 2001;285:885-892.
14. Singletary SE, Shallenberger R, Guinee VF. Breast cancer in the elderly. Ann Surg 1993;218:667-671.
15. Gazet JC, Markopoulos C, Ford HT, et al. Prospective randomised trial of tamoxifen versus surgery in elderly patients with breast cancer. Lancet 1988;1:679-681.

16. Robertson JF, Ellis IO, Elston CW, Blamey RW. Mastectomy or tamoxifen as initial therapy for operable breast cancer in elderly patients: 5-year follow-up. Eur J Cancer 1992;28A:908-910.

17. Bates T, Riley DL, Houghton J, et al. Breast cancer in elderly women: a Cancer Research Campaign trial comparing treatment with tamoxifen and optimal surgery with tamoxifen alone. The Elderly Breast Cancer Working Party. Br J Surg 1991;78:591-594.

18. Mustacchi G, Milani S, Pluchinotta A, et al. Tamoxifen or surgery plus tamoxifen as primary treatment for elderly patients with operable breast cancer: The G.R.E.T.A. Trial. Group for Research on Endocrine Therapy in the Elderly. Anticancer Res 1994;14:2197-2200.

19. Cummings FJ, Gray R, Tormey DC, et al. Adjuvant tamoxifen versus placebo in elderly women with node-positive breast cancer: long-term follow-up and causes of death. J Clin Oncol 1993;11:29-35.

20. Pezner RD, Patterson MP, Hill LR, et al. Arm lymphedema in patients treated conservatively for breast cancer: relationship to patient age and axillary node dissection technique. Int J Radiat Oncol Biol Phys 1986;12:2079-2083.

21. Liljegren G, Holmberg L. Arm morbidity after sector resection and axillary dissection with or without postoperative radiotherapy in breast cancer stage I. Results from a randomised trial. Uppsala-Orebro Breast Cancer Study Group. Eur J Cancer 1997;33:193-199.

22. Wyckoff J, Greenberg H, Sanderson R, et al. Breast irradiation in the older woman: a toxicity study. J Am Geriatr Soc 1994;42:150-152.

23. Kantorowitz DA, Poulter CA, Sischy B, et al. Treatment of breast cancer among elderly women with segmental mastectomy or segmental mastectomy plus postoperative radiotherapy. Int J Radiat Oncol Biol Phys 1988;15:263-270.

24. Peschel RE, Wilson L, Haffty B, et al. The effect of advanced age on the efficacy of radiation therapy for early breast cancer, local prostate cancer and grade III-IV gliomas. Int J Radiat Oncol Biol Phys 1993;26:539-544.

25. Wazer DE, Erban JK, Robert NJ, et al. Breast conservation in elderly women for clinically negative axillary lymph nodes without axillary dissection. Cancer 1994;74:878-883.

26. Feigelson BJ, Acosta JA, Feigelson HS, et al. T1 breast carcinoma in women 70 years of age and older may not require axillary lymph node dissection. Am J Surg 1996;172:487-489; discussion 489-490.

27. van Zyl JA, Muller AG. Tumour excision plus continuous tamoxifen compared with modified radical mastectomy in patients over 70 years of age with operable breast cancer. J Surg Oncol 1995;59:151-154.

28. August DA, Wilkins E, Rea T. Breast reconstruction in older women. Surgery 1994;115:663-668.

29. Smith-Bindman R, Kerlikowske K, Gebretsadik T, Newman J. Is screening mammography effective in elderly women? Am J Med 2000;108:112-119.

30. Linder JD, Wilcox CM. Acid peptic disease in the elderly. Gastroenterol Clin North Am 2001;30:363-376.

31. Raiha I, Hietanen E, Sourander L. Symptoms of gastro-oesophageal reflux disease in elderly people. Age Ageing 1991;20:365-370.

32. Fass R, Pulliam G, Johnson C, et al. Symptom severity and oesophageal chemosensitivity to acid in older and young patients with gastro-oesophageal reflux. Age Ageing 2000;29:125-130.

33. Brunt LM, Quasebarth MA, Dunnegan DL, Soper NJ. Is laparoscopic antireflux surgery for gastroesophageal reflux disease in the elderly safe and effective? Surg Endosc 1999;13:838-842.

34. Gostout CJ. Gastrointestinal bleeding in the elderly patient. Am J Gastroenterol 2000;95:590-595.

35. Di Quinzio C, Phang PT. Surgical management of perforated benign gastric ulcer in high-risk patients. Can J Surg 1992;35:94-97.

36. Bulut OB, Rasmussen C, Fischer A. Acute surgical treatment of complicated peptic ulcers with special reference to the elderly. World J Surg 1996;20:574-577.

37. Pacelli F, Bellantone R, Doglietto GB, et al. Risk factors in relation to postoperative complications and mortality after total gastrectomy in aged patients. Am Surg 1991;57:341-345.

38. Moriguchi S, Odaka T, Hayashi Y, et al. Death due to recurrence following curative resection of early gastric cancer depends on age of the patient. Br J Cancer 1991;64:555-558.

39. Bittner R, Butters M, Ulrich M, et al. Total gastrectomy. Updated operative mortality and long-term survival with particular reference to patients older than 70 years of age. Ann Surg 1996;224:37-42.

40. Wu CW, Lo SS, Shen KH, et al. Surgical mortality, survival, and quality of life after resection for gastric cancer in the elderly. World J Surg 2000;24:465-472.

41. American Cancer Society. Table 3. Probability of developing invasive cancers within selected age intervals by gender, U.S., 1995-1997. CA Cancer J Clin 2001;51:19.

42. Watters JM, Redmond ML, Desai D, March RJ. Effects of age and body composition on the metabolic responses to elective colon resection. Ann Surg 1990;212:213-220.

43. Tuech JJ, Pessaux P, Rouge C, et al. Laparoscopic vs open colectomy for sigmoid diverticulitis: a prospective comparative study in the elderly. Surg Endosc 2000;14:1031-1033.

44. Stewart BT, Stitz RW, Lumley JW. Laparoscopically assisted colorectal surgery in the elderly. Br J Surg 1999;86:938-941.

45. Schwandner O, Schiedeck TH, Bruch HP. Advanced age–indication or contraindication for laparoscopic colorectal surgery? Dis Colon Rectum 1999;42:356-362.

46. Reissman P, Agachan F, Wexner SD. Outcome of laparoscopic colorectal surgery in older patients. Am Surg 1996;62:1060-1063.

47. Bender JS, Wiencek RG, Bouwman DL. Morbidity and mortality following total abdominal colectomy for massive lower gastrointestinal bleeding. Am Surg 1991;57:536-540; discussion 540-531.

48. Yancik R, Wesley MN, Ries LA, et al. Comorbidity and age as predictors of risk for early mortality of male and female colon carcinoma patients: a population-based study. Cancer 1998;82:2123-2134.

49. Whittle J, Steinberg EP, Anderson GF, Herbert R. Results of colectomy in elderly patients with colon cancer, based on Medicare claims data. Am J Surg 1992;163:572-576.

50. Mulcahy HE, Patchett SE, Daly L, O'Donoghue DP. Prognosis of elderly patients with large bowel cancer. Br J Surg 1994;81:736-738.

51. Sunouchi K, Namiki K, Mori M, et al. How should patients 80 years of age or older with colorectal carcinoma be treated? Long-term and short-term outcome and postoperative cytokine levels. Dis Colon Rectum 2000;43:233-241.

52. Leo E, Audisio RA, Belli F, et al. Total rectal resection and colo-anal anastomosis for low rectal tumours: comparative results in a group of young and old patients. Eur J Cancer 1994;30A:1092-1095.

53. Dehni N, Schlegel D, Tiret E, et al. Effects of aging on the functional outcome of coloanal anastomosis with colonic J-pouch. Am J Surg 1998;175:209-212.

54. Jorge JM, Wexner SD, James K, et al. Recovery of anal sphincter function after the ileoanal reservoir procedure in patients over the age of fifty. Dis Colon Rectum 1994;37:1002-1005.

55. Lewis WG, Sagar PM, Holdsworth PJ, et al. Restorative proctocolectomy with end to end pouch-anal anastomosis in patients over the age of fifty. Gut 1993;34:948-952.

56. Reissman P, Teoh TA, Weiss EG, et al. Functional outcome of the double stapled ileoanal reservoir in patients more than 60 years of age. Am Surg 1996;62:178-183.

57. Wong RW, Rappaport WD, Witzke DB, et al. Factors influencing the safety of colostomy closure in the elderly. J Surg Res 1994;57:289-292.

58. Brand MI, Saclarides TJ, Dobson HD, Millikan KW. Liver resection for colorectal cancer: liver metastases in the aged. Am Surg 2000;66:412-415; discussion 415-416.

59. Cosenza CA, Hoffman AL, Podesta LG, et al. Hepatic resection for malignancy in the elderly. Am Surg 1995;61:889-895.

60. Fong Y, Blumgart LH, Fortner JG, Brennan MF. Pancreatic or liver resection for malignancy is safe and effective for the elderly. Ann Surg 1995;222:426-434; discussion 434-427.

61. Roslyn JJ, Binns GS, Hughes EF, et al. Open cholecystectomy. A contemporary analysis of 42,474 patients. Ann Surg 1993;218:129-137.

62. Pessaux P, Tuech JJ, Derouet N, et al. Laparoscopic cholecystectomy in the elderly: a prospective study. Surg Endosc 2000;14:1067-1069.

63. Mayol J, Martinez-Sarmiento J, Tamayo FJ, Fernandez-Represa JA. Complications of laparoscopic cholecystectomy in the ageing patient. Age Ageing 1997;26:77-81.

64. Maxwell JG, Tyler BA, Rutledge R, et al. Cholecystectomy in patients aged 80 and older. Am J Surg 1998;176:627-631.

65. Behrman SW, Melvin WS, Babb ME, et al. Laparoscopic cholecystectomy in the geriatric population. Am Surg 1996;62:386-390.

66. McGrath MF, McGrath JC, Gabbay J, et al. Safe laparoendoscopic approach to biliary pancreatitis in older patients. Arch Surg 1996;131:826-831; discussion 831-823.

67. Spencer MP, Sarr MG, Nagorney DM. Radical pancreatectomy for pancreatic cancer in the elderly. Is it safe and justified? Ann Surg 1990;212:140-143.

68. Hannoun L, Christophe M, Ribeiro J, et al. A report of forty-four instances of pancreaticoduodenal resection in patients more than seventy years of age. Surg Gynecol Obstet 1993;177:556-560.

69. Cameron JL, Pitt HA, Yeo CJ, et al. One hundred and forty-five consecutive pancreaticoduodenectomies without mortality. Ann Surg 1993;217:430-435; discussion 435-438.

70. Chijiiwa K, Yamaguchi K, Yamashita H, et al. ASA physical status and age are not factors predicting morbidity, mortality, and survival after pancreatoduodenectomy. Am Surg 1996;62:701-705.

71. al-Sharaf K, Andren-Sandberg A, Ihse I. Subtotal pancreatectomy for cancer can be safe in the elderly. Eur J Surg 1999;165:230-235.

72. Vickers SM, Kerby JD, Smoot TM, et al. Economics of pancreatoduodenectomy in the elderly. Surgery 1996;120:620-625; discussion 625-626.

73. Munoz E, Cohen J, Chang J, et al. Socioeconomic concerns in vascular surgery: a survey of the role of age, resource consumption, and outcome in treatment cost. J Vasc Surg 1989;9:479-486.

74. Cogbill TH, Landercasper J, Strutt PJ, Gundersen AL. Late results of peripheral vascular surgery in patients 80 years of age and older. Arch Surg 1987;122:581-586.

75. Biller J, Feinberg WM, Castaldo JE, et al. Guidelines for carotid endarterectomy: a statement for healthcare professionals from a Special Writing Group of the Stroke Council, American Heart Association. Circulation 1998;97:501-509.

76. Executive Committee for the Asymptomatic Carotid Atherosclerosis Study (ACAS). Endarterectomy for asymptomatic carotid artery stenosis. JAMA 1995;273:1421-1428.

77. North American Symptomatic Carotid Endarterectomy Trial (NASCET) Collaborators. Beneficial effect of carotid endarterectomy in symptomatic patients with high-grade carotid stenosis. N Engl J Med 1991;325:445-453.

78. Farrell B, Fraser A, Sandercock P, et al. Randomised trial of endarterectomy for recently symptomatic carotid stenosis: final results of the MRC European Carotid Surgery Trial

(ECST). ECST Writing Committee of the European Carotid Surgery Trialists' Collaborative Group. Lancet 1998;351:1379-1387.

79. Barnett HJ, Taylor DW, Eliasziw M, et al. Benefit of carotid endarterectomy in patients with symptomatic moderate or severe stenosis. North American Symptomatic Carotid Endarterectomy Trial Collaborators. N Engl J Med 1998;339:1415-1425.

80. Maxwell JG, Rutherford EJ, Covington DL, et al. Community hospital carotid endarterectomy in patients over age 75. Am J Surg 1990;160:598-603.

81. Perler BA. The impact of advanced age on the results of carotid endarterectomy: an outcome analysis. J Am Coll Surg 1996;183:559-564.

82. Wong DT, Ballard JL, Killeen JD. Carotid endarterectomy and abdominal aoritc aneurysm repair: are these reasonable treatments for patients over age 80? Am Surg 1998;64:998-1001.

83. Perler BA, Dardik A, Burleyson GP, et al. Influence of age and hospital volume on the results of carotid endarterectomy: a statewide analysis of 9918 cases. J Vasc Surg 1998;27:25-31; discussion 31-23.

84. Hallett JW, Pietropaoli JA, Ilstrup DM, et al. Comparison of North American Symptomatic Carotid Endarterectomy Trial and population-based outcomes for carotid endarterectomy. J Vasc Surg 1998;27:845-850; discussion 851.

85. Schneider JR, Droste JS, Schindler N, Golan JF. Carotid endarterectomy in octogenarians: comparison with patient characteristics and outcomes in younger patients. J Vasc Surg 2000;31:927-935.

86. Estes JM, Guadagnoli E, Wolf R, et al. The impact of cardiac comorbidity after carotid endarterectomy. J Vasc Surg 1998;28:577-584.

87. Smith JJ, Toogood GJ, Galland RB. Reconstruction for lower limb occlusive disease in the elderly. Cardiovasc Surg 1999;7:58-61.

88. Davies B, Heather BP, Earnshaw JJ. Poor outcome in patients aged over 80 with limb-threatening ischaemia. Cardiovasc Surg 1999;7:56-57.

89. Choi D, Darling RC, Roddy SP, et al. Infrainguinal reconstruction in octogenarians: should age be a contraindication? Ann Vasc Surg 2000;14:67-72.

90. Nunnelee JD, Kurgan A, Auer AI. Distal bypasses in patients over age 75. With a thorough medical evaluation, patients over 75 in need of distal bypass may not be at greater risk than younger patients. Geriatr Nurs 1993;14:252-254.

91. Tretinyak AS, Lee ES, Kuskowski MM, et al. Revascularization and quality of life for patients with limb-threatening ischemia. Ann Vasc Surg 2001;15:84-88.

92. Gibbons GW, Burgess AM, Guadagnoli E, et al. Return to well-being and function after infrainguinal revascularization. J Vasc Surg 1995;21:35-44; discussion 44-35.

93. Paty PS, Lloyd WE, Chang BB, et al. Aortic replacement for abdominal aortic aneurysm in elderly patients. Am J Surg 1993;166:191-193.

94. Bagia JS, Robinson D, Kennedy M, et al. The cost of elective and emergency repair of AAA in patients under and over the age of 80. Aust N Z J Surg 1999;69:651-654.

95. Finlayson SR, Birkmeyer JD, Fillinger MF, Cronenwett JL. Should endovascular surgery lower the threshold for repair of abdominal aortic aneurysms? J Vasc Surg 1999;29:973-985.

96. Frame PS, Fryback DG, Patterson C. Screening for abdominal aortic aneurysm in men ages 60 to 80 years. A cost-effectiveness analysis. Ann Intern Med 1993;119:411-416.

97. Schultz A, Bien M, Dumond K, et al. Etiology and incidence of pressure ulcers in surgical patients. AORN J 1999;70:434, 437-440, 443-439.

98. Stotts NA. Predicting pressure ulcer development in surgical patients. Heart Lung 1988;17:641-647.

5

GERIATRIC GENERAL
THORACIC SURGERY

Joseph LoCicero III, MD, FACS; John Yee, MD*

Continuing improvements in instrumentation, anesthetic and surgical techniques, and post-operative management allow the thoracic surgeon to operate on the oldest patients with the expectation of successful outcomes. However, when elderly patients require thoracic surgery and scarce resources in support of such specialized care must be allocated, the need to provide care to younger patients may become a factor in the decision whether to operate on the elderly patient. One may argue that age-based criteria for therapy merely reflect the balance that must be struck between the cost of treatment and its potential long-term benefit. The implication is that age, either alone or combined with other factors, may so profoundly decrease the clinical efficacy of certain treatments as to make them either useless or potentially harmful to older people. The potential benefit of treatment must then be weighed against the few remaining years of life to be gained. The countervailing point of view sees age as a very poor predictor of clinical outcome and highlights the possibility that elderly patients may be denied potentially effective care as a consequence of false assumptions that are based on their age alone. Faulty medical information or physician bias are the sources of these assumptions. Medical decision making concerning elderly patients, although anchored in risk-benefit estimates among individuals, is inseparable from broader social issues related to the perceived value of the elderly age group. Resource allocation in health care institutions, priority setting in medical education, and the direction of research initiatives all reflect the way our society views the older person, and they directly affect decision making by physicians. The general tendency of the literature from surgeons on benign and malignant diseases of the lungs and esophagus has been to report what one was able to get away with and not to shed light on mechanisms of injury and repair in the older patients that might affect outcomes and thus attitudes about recommending major operations on elderly patients. This review is intended to bring together the accumulated experience of the past 20 years with the older population and serious lung and esophageal disease, and thus to highlight the areas most in need of further research.

METHODS

The search was conducted on the National Library of Medicine's PubMed database. The time period covered was from January 1982 to October 2002. The search strategy combined various terms for general thoracic surgical procedures (general or specific commonly performed operations, including the esophagus, lung, and mediastinum), the terms *elective* and *emergency*, and various terms for perioperative care, complications, and outcomes. Additional requirements were either that the publication be a review, clinical trial, randomized controlled trial, or meta-analysis, or that terms for risk or age factors be present as title words or MeSH headings. Terms denoting advanced age were *age factors,*

* LoCicero: The Point Clear Charities Professor, Chair of Surgery, Director of the Center for Clinical Oncology, and Director of the Center for Interventional Technologies, The University of South Alabama, Mobile, AL; Yee: Assistant Professor of Surgery, University of Michigan Medical Center, Ann Arbor, MI.

age, aging, elderly, geriatric, gerontologic, older, or *octogenarian, nonagenarian,* or *centenarian.* Finally, animal research was systematically excluded.

LUNG CANCER

Lung cancer accounts for 15% of all cancers. It is responsible for 30% of cancer deaths, more than cancers of the breast, colon, prostate, and ovary combined, and the incidence is growing throughout the world. Currently, it is the leading cause of cancer death among both men and women. The American Cancer Society estimated that there would be 169,500 new cases of lung cancer in the United States in 2001. [1] The number of Americans who would die from this disease was estimated at 157,400. The peak incidence of lung cancer in the life span of Americans occurs in their fifties. The effects of toxic exposures accumulate with age, and lung cancer is increasingly a disease of those aged 65 years and over. The treatment of lung cancer relies predominantly on surgery, chemotherapy, and radiation. All these modalities impose considerable demands on patient physiology. Age-related declines in cardiovascular or respiratory reserve may limit the utility of these treatments.

The majority of lung cancers fall into one of two histologic categories. Small-cell lung cancers are derived from neuroendocrine cells, and non–small-cell lung cancers are epithelial in origin. Surgery is generally limited to the early stages of small-cell lung cancer, where little lung is removed and the physiologic stresses are smaller. In contrast, surgical resection is potentially curative for non–small-cell lung cancer. Adenocarcinoma and squamous cell cancers are the predominant subtypes.

Sociodemographic differences appear in both the incidence and the outcome of lung cancer. The risk of lung cancer for men in the United States is approximately twice that for women. The peak incidence occurs between the ages of 75 and 79, at the rate of 357 per 100,000. [2] This compares with an incidence among persons aged 50 to 54 years of only 58.2 per 100,000. The overall probability of 5-year survival is currently 15.6%. The age at diagnosis affects the probability of survival to a much greater degree than that which can be explained by actuarial factors. A person diagnosed with lung cancer at age 45 has a 22.8% chance at 5-year survival, but those diagnosed past the age of 65 have a 13.7% rate.

Cigarette smoking is the prime risk factor for the development of lung cancer. The current epidemic of lung cancer reflects smoking patterns of the years 1950 to 1980. Recently, there has been a significant decline in the incidence of lung cancer among men. Among women, there has been an increase in both its incidence and mortality. This rise parallels changes in smoking patterns. The percentage of men who smoked fell 19% between 1965 and 1985, while the rate for women decreased by only 6%. Any optimism regarding the end of the current epidemic is dampened by the fact that there is a significant increase in the percentage of teenagers who smoke. Public education regarding the risks of smoking, combined with legislative limits on the sale or promotion of cigarettes, may help reverse this tide. [3]

The majority of lung cancers are diagnosed when the disease is already advanced. This accounts for the very high mortality rate. At presentation, only 15% of patients have disease that is localized within the lung and potentially amenable to surgical removal. [4] Overall, 85% of all patients die within 5 years of their diagnosis. In cases of distant spread, no available therapy is curative. Several clinical trials among elderly patients have demonstrated improvement in overall survival as well as quality of life with chemotherapy for advanced non–small-cell lung cancer. [5] Despite numerous advances in surgery, chemotherapy, and radiation, median survival for most patients after treatment remains only 2 years. Long-term survival is most common among asymptomatic patients with stage I cancers that undergo resection. The proportion of patients who present for treatment at such an early stage is quite small, ranging from 5% to 10%. The diagnosis may be made as a result of chest radiographs done for other indications or screening procedures among high-risk individuals. The percentage of stage I non–small-cell cancers that prove to be resectable is approximately 90%. [6] The few remaining patients are usually unresectable because they have inadequate pulmonary reserve or major contraindications for general anesthesia. In recent published series, operative mortality for stage I lung cancer approaches zero. The 5-year survival rate after operation for stage I cancer ranges from 53% to 100%, with those patients with stage IA having 73% to 100% survival. [7–13] This compares with a 5-year survival rate of only 10% among patients with screen-detected stage I disease that was not operated upon. [14] Cancer progression accounted for the mortality of these nonresected patients in 80% of cases. Patients who are free of disease at 5 years have a 90% chance of surviving 10 or more years after operation. The high rate of resectability and the low operative mortality associated with early lung cancers are compelling arguments for those who are working to introduce screening programs among populations at risk.

The study at Johns Hopkins, the Mayo Clinic, and Memorial Sloan Kettering sponsored by the National Cancer Institute found that mass screening for lung cancer with sputum cytology and standard chest radiography failed to reduce lung cancer mortality. [15,16] This was interpreted as evidence against the utility of screening for lung cancer. There were concerns that screening resulted in the overdiagnosis of lung cancers. It was possible that screening had led to the detection of slowly growing lung cancers that would otherwise not threaten the life of the patient before death occurred from other causes. Screening was also quite expensive, given the small number of cancers detected. The public health issues of cost and accessibility are still pertinent to the implementation of any mass screening program. Governments have developed population health models that may be useful in the economic evaluation of cancer control interventions and in the guidance of policy decision making. [17] Costs are not limited to those of screening itself. The cost of any screening program includes not only the price of the tests but also the burden of any additional testing borne by patients who were initially positive on the screening test but ultimately found not to have cancer. Any increase in the survival rate among patients with screening-detected lung cancer may be offset by the morbidity and mortality of unnecessary surgery on patients who are falsely identified as having cancer. Lead-time bias is an additional confounding factor that may further limit the survival benefit of early detection programs for lung cancer.

Screening programs for lung cancer have focused on improving the diagnostic test. The development of new tools for the early detection of lung cancer has paralleled progress in molecular biology and computerized imaging technology. Standard sputum cytology now uses molecular probing of atypical cells. [18] Immunostaining for heterogeneous nuclear ribonucleoproteins has led to the detection of preclinical lung cancer. [19] The finding that molecular changes in shed epithelial cells may predict bronchial metaplasia and the subsequent development of lung cancer brings up the issues of chemoprevention, limited removal of mucosal cells via photodynamic laser therapy, and the potential use of aerosolized drug delivery systems. The Early Lung Cancer Action Project recently reported on the use of an annual helical computed tomography (CT) scan for the screening of lung cancer among 1000 heavy smokers aged 60 and over. [20] Almost one fourth of all screened individuals had a noncalcified nodule (233 of 1000). The researchers discovered 27 cancers; 87% of them were stage I. The CT detection rate was six times higher than that obtained by chest radiography alone. It would be expected that an increase in the sensitivity of the screening procedure would translate into more patients' being found at an earlier stage of the disease, when there is the greatest potential for resection and cure. Lead-time bias may, however, make any survival benefit more apparent than real. There are currently no prospective data on what impact, if any, that helical CT may have on the long-term outcome of patients with asymptomatic screen-detected lung cancer. A recent economic analysis of lung cancer screening, combining data from the Surveillance, Epidemiology and End Results (SEER) registry public-use database and published results from the Early Lung Cancer Action Project, found annual screening over a period of 5 years to be cost-effective (at approximately $19,000 per life-year saved) when limited to a high-risk cohort of patients between ages 60 and 74 years. [21] The widespread implementation of mass screening programs for lung cancer will likely await the development of less expensive CT scanners and automated forms of sputum cytology analysis. Annual screening among selected groups of high-risk elderly patients already may be economically justifiable and warranted.

Outcome studies in the surgical management of lung cancer have generally not included large cohorts of elderly patients, and little information exists as to age-specific changes in quality of life. Recent clinical trials using radiation and chemotherapy for the treatment of lung cancer have used quality-of-life indices as primary measures of outcome. [22–24] Auchter et al used the Functional Assessment of Cancer Therapy-Lung (FACT-L) patient questionnaire to score the quality of life in patients enrolled in a radiotherapy trial for advanced inoperable lung cancer. This tool, which includes 33 scores for physical, functional, emotional, and social well-being and a 10-item subscale of lung cancer symptoms, was used to generate a trial outcome index. [25] Specific analyses of how chemotherapy may affect the aged patient are now reaching publication stage. The Elderly Lung Cancer Vinorelbine Italian Study (ELVIS) involved a multicenter randomized trial of single-agent chemotherapy versus best supportive care in patients over the age of 70 and used both survival and quality of life as endpoints. [26,27] One-year survival in the vinorelbine group was 32% as compared with 14% in the best supportive-care arm. This trial, the first to examine chemotherapy for advanced lung cancer in elderly patients, found that the survival benefit was not gained at the expense of a poorer quality of life. Dyspnea, pain, and social, cognitive, and physical functioning scores were found to improve with treatment. The clinical efficacy of treatment was therefore measured in terms of patient well-being rather than simply months survived.

The standard surgical treatment for a localized cancer of the lung is surgery via thoracotomy and either lobectomy or pneumonectomy. There is a historical bias toward offering surgery only to younger patients. Many physicians have had grave reservations about proposing surgery to elderly patients, given the risks posed by general anesthesia, thoracotomy, and the loss of pulmonary function. It was also unclear whether lung cancer is inherently different in older patients, more specifically, whether the elderly patient has a significantly more aggressive progression to death. If lung cancer in elderly patients is proven to be slow growing and of low potential for fatal outcome, a more conservative treatment approach can be justified that weighs natural life expectancy against the chronic progression of disease. Conversely, if lung cancer in the elderly person is significantly more aggressive and less amenable to surgery, a rather more conservative approach can be justified, with palliative treatment aimed mainly at preserving the patient's quality of life. The core of this debate has been settled; lung cancer among older patients is not an indolent disease. In a retrospective study of 80 patients aged 70 years and over, Harviel et al reported a mean survival of 3.5 months for untreated patients, 9.8 months for those receiving chemotherapy or radiation, and 30.6 months after resection, with an operative mortality of 18.2%. [28] Berggren et al reported a 5-year survival rate of 32% in a series of 82 patients aged 70 years and older who were operated upon for bronchogenic carcinoma. This contrasted with a 0% survival rate without operation. [29] Shirakusa et al reviewed their experience with resections among patients aged 80 years and over. A cumulative 5-year survival of 79% was noted for patients with stage I carcinoma. [30] A survival advantage has therefore been established among elderly patients undergoing resection for lung cancer.

Long-term survival among elderly patients after surgery for lung cancer must be balanced against the mortality risk of the operation itself. Studies from almost two decades ago had clearly correlated age above 65 years with increased mortality after thoracotomy. In 1973, Evans reported a postoperative mortality of 20% after major pulmonary resection for bronchogenic carcinoma among 114 patients aged 65 years and older. [31] These patients came from 1804 cases of lung cancer, of all age groups, diagnosed between 1950 and 1971. The percentage of patients ultimately found to have resectable disease was 15%. The rate of resectability was not influenced by age. The age at diagnosis did not appear to correlate with the potential for curative resection and, by inference, clinical stage. Postoperative mortality rates were age related. Patients younger than 65 years had a hospital mortality of 10%. Patients aged 65 to 69 years had a 16% rate. Hospital mortality for patients aged 75 to 83 years was 26.6%. A 4-year survival rate of 39% was reported. This was compared with data from 780 patients over the age of 65 who were not candidates for surgery. A 1-year survival rate of less than 7% was documented in this group and was comparable to that seen among inoperable patients younger than 65 years. Surgery was justifiable among older patients since the natural history of lung cancer was not more indolent or slow growing among those who were elderly. Despite a higher rate of peri-operative mortality, the prospect of long-term survival after pulmonary resection in elderly patients was sufficiently high to justify the risk of operation. Ten years later, the Lung Cancer Study Group of North America again demonstrated a clear association between age and operative mortality after thoracotomy. Their 1983 report showed a 30-day postoperative mortality of only 1.3% for patients younger than 50 years. The mortality rate was found to rise with increasing age. Patients aged 60 to 69 years, 70 to 79 years, and over 80 years had mortality rates of 4.1%, 7%, and 8.1%, respectively. [32]

More recent studies have indicated that the operative mortality rate after standard lung resection for patients between the ages of 70 and 80 is starting to approach that obtained among younger patients. In a review of 1079 patients undergoing thoracotomy for lung cancer, de Perrot et al noted a mortality rate of 1.3% for lobectomy or lesser resection among patients younger than 60 years as compared with a 5.5% rate for older patients. [33] Cancer-specific long-term survival was equivalent for all age groups. Pagni et al studied 385 patients aged 70 years and older operated upon for lung cancer with curative intent. The operations consisted of lobectomy (77%), pneumonectomy (6%), bilobectomies (4%), and wedge or segmental resections (13%). The 30-day mortality risk for the elderly patients (aged 70 years and older) was compared with a cohort of 180 patients aged 69 years and younger. The mortality for all resections in the elderly group was higher (4.2% versus 1.6%). Mortality in the octogenarian group was 2.8%. Major morbidity was similar in the two groups (13.2% versus 13%). Pneumonectomy carried a higher risk for death, with 3 of 24 deceased. Mortality rates over time were also evaluated. Mortality among elderly patients in the early period of the study (1971 to 1982) was 11.1%. This declined to a rate of 2.6% over time (1983 to 1994). The authors concluded that functional elderly patients should not be denied curative lung resection on the basis of age alone, but they also cautioned against the use of pneumonectomy. [34] Harvey et al found the risk of operative mortality not to increase until after the age of 80. [35] In their study of 81 patients with surgery for non–small-cell lung cancer, these authors observed a mortality rate of 1.4% for patients under 70, 1.6% for patients between 70 and 79, and 17.6% for patients 80 years or older. The use of heparin prophylaxis against deep-vein thrombosis and pulmonary embolism was emphasized. The authors cautioned against the use of extended pulmonary resection. They also preferred limited wedge resection to lobectomy in patients with preoperative impairment of pulmonary reserve. Hanagiri et al reported no mortality among 18 octogenarians after resection. Half were lobectomies, and the remainder constituted various forms of parenchyma-sparing procedures. A 5-year survival rate of 42.6% was found, comparable to that obtained in younger patients. [36] Other centers have noted overall operative mortality rates of less than 2% for selected patients aged 70 and over, with intermediate-term survival rates comparable to those for younger patients. [37,38]

A correlation between operative mortality and the extent of pulmonary resection was demonstrated in elderly patients. Evans noted a mortality rate of 15% after lobectomy as compared with 27% after pneumonectomy among patients aged 65 years and older. [31] Bates reported on 100 patients over the age of 70 who had 26% mortality after pneumonectomy as compared with 14% after lobectomy. [39] No deaths were noted after segmental resection. Oliaro et al had a 9.1% mortality rate after pneumonectomy as compared with an overall mortality rate of only 3.1% among patients over 70 years of age. [40] Jensik et al advocated limited pulmonary resection for elderly patients with lung cancer and marginal physiologic reserve. [41] More recent reports indicate that mortality may be decreasing even for pneumonectomy and suggest that there are fewer differences in operative mortality between different types of resection in properly selected patients older than 75 years. [42] Tanita et al recorded no operative deaths in a highly selected series of 24 octogenarians undergoing more than single lobectomy. [43]

Age alone is not a contraindication for pulmonary resection. A 1990 review of 185 patients 70 years old or older with non–small-cell lung cancer noted a 5-year survival of 48% after resection and an operative mortality rate of 3%. [44] Mortality and prognosis were similar to those associated with younger patients. No differences based on age were found with regard to histologic type, TNM (tumor. node, and metastasis) classification, and curability. Pulmonary complications occurred in 21% of the elderly patients and were correlated with impaired preoperative pulmonary function and smoking. Nonoperative therapy or limited resection was recommended when postoperative pulmonary function was predicted to be less than 0.8 L/m^2 for vital capacity and 0.6 L/m^2 for forced expiratory volume in 1 second (FEV_1). [45,46] Mane et al similarly found that age was not a predictor of poor long-term survival after resection for lung cancer. [47] Aoki et al analyzed the risks associated with pulmonary resection in 35 patients over the age of 80. [48] The operative mortality rate was 0%, with morbidity in 60%. There were 10 major pulmonary complications, including respiratory insufficiency following bacterial pneumonia and sputum retention. Although they concluded that surgical treatment was not contraindicated for octogenarians with lung cancer, the authors cautioned that preoperative low arterial oxygen, high alveolar-arterial oxygen diffusion gradient, and long operative times may place older patients at risk for serious postoperative pulmonary complications. A gross survey of 7099 patients in Japan evaluated 30-day operative mortality and its relationship to patient age. The mortality was 0.4% for patients younger than 60 years, 1.3% for those 60 to 69, 2.0% for those 70 to 79, and 2.2% for patients aged 80 and over. [49] In 2000, Bernet et al compared 92 patients younger than 50 years of age undergoing surgery for lung cancer with a comparable group of 120 patients older than 70 years. No difference was found in operative mortality between the two groups (2.2% versus 2.5%). Survival was similar in younger and older patients after surgical resection. The survival rate at 5 years, when adjusted for tumor stage, was 56% in patients younger than 50 years as compared with 53% in patients older than 70 years. [46] Oliaro et al assessed postoperative complications, mortality, and long-term survival after surgical therapy for non–small-cell cancer in 258 patients aged 70 years and older. [40] Overall postoperative mortality was 3.1%, with a morbidity rate of 39.1%. The rate of complication was significantly increased among patients with multiple concomitant diseases. Multivariate analysis found that survival was dependent on tumor stage and not on age. Five-year survival for stage I cancers was 73.6% as compared with 23% for stage II. They additionally found that highly selected elderly patients had a significantly higher rate of survival than did those patients who were operated upon when the criteria for surgery were less strict. The proper selection of patients for surgery was found to have as much influence on survival as the stage of the tumor. This finding highlights the importance of functional status, rather than chronologic age, as a determinant for good outcome after resection. The low mortality and acceptable survival data confirmed to the authors that surgery is worthwhile for selected elderly patients.

Advancements in anesthesia and pain management have certainly helped to reduce the mortality of standard pulmonary resections. Mortality rates after lobectomy among elderly patients are therefore now similar to those found among younger patients. Data indicate that although age is not associated with postoperative mortality, advanced age is associated with increased morbidity. A report on 331 patients undergoing major resection for lung cancer prospectively found that age over 60 years, male sex, pneumonectomy, and predicted postoperative FEV_1 are univariate predictors of increased risk for major complications. [50] When the effect of these variables was controlled for in a multivariate analysis, a low predicted postoperative FEV_1 remained the only significant independent predictor of complications. The researchers concluded that pulmonary resection should not be denied on the basis of traditionally cited preoperative pulmonary variables, and that this very simple calculated prediction of postoperative pulmonary function may help identify patients at increased risk for complications. Wang et al found low diffusing capacity for carbon dioxide (Dlco) to predict a high risk for pulmonary complications after surgery and an increased length of hospital stay. [51] Exercise testing, 6-minute walk distances, and stair climbing are used as adjuncts to the standard spirometric testing of high-risk patients. [52]

Relatively small patient numbers and the fact that the patients are already highly selected for good performance status limit most studies dealing with the results of pneumonectomy in elderly patients. Specific inferences with respect to age-associated mortality and morbidity are therefore difficult to draw from retrospective descriptions. Although advanced age alone generally has not been predictive of death after pneumonectomy, retrospective studies have demonstrated higher mortality among elderly patients. Mizushima et al found a significantly higher operative mortality after pneumonectomy among patients over the age of 70 (22.2%) than among younger patients (3.2%). [53] The cancer-related prognosis for the elderly group was, however, comparable to that for younger patients across all stages. Age was not found to predict a poor prognosis for long-term survival. Despite the higher operative mortality, pneumonectomy was thought to be justified for the treatment of lung cancer in carefully selected elderly patients.

Bernard et al reviewed the results of pneumonectomy among 639 patients at the Mayo Clinic. [54] Associated conditions were found in 47.7%. These concurrent illnesses included chronic obstructive pulmonary disease (COPD) (28.6%), coronary artery disease (13.1%), cardiac arrhythmia (9.1%), and diabetes mellitus (8.5%). Complications occurred in 43.2% of patients; the vast majority of these were cardiopulmonary. The mortality rate observed was 7.0%. Advanced age was associated with postoperative cardiopulmonary morbidity in univariate analysis ($P < .0001$). Age was as important in determining morbidity as decreased FEV_1 and the presence of pre-existing cardiovascular disease. In multivariate analysis, advanced age was again found to be strongly associated with cardiopulmonary morbidity. Age alone did not prove to adversely affect postoperative mortality in either univariate or multivariate analysis. Appropriate selection of patients and meticulous peri-operative care were deemed paramount in minimizing the risk of pneumonectomy. These researchers recommended aggressive screening for the presence of occult cardiovascular disease and optimizing the patient's pulmonary function. Reversible conditions, such as smoking, infection, or bronchospasm, also should be addressed prior to surgery. Intra-operative techniques, such as intra-pericardial control of hilar vessels and tissue reinforcement of the bronchial stump, were recommended to minimize technical complications. Similar findings were found for patients undergoing combined pulmonary and chest wall resection for locally invasive lung cancer. An analysis of 201 patients undergoing surgical resection of lung cancers invading the chest wall was performed by the use of both univariate and multivariate methods. Age, nodal involvement, and depth of invasion were found to be the only independent factors predicting survival in completely resected patients. [55]

Efforts have been made to identify factors that may be responsible for the higher operative mortality among elderly patients. Kirsh et al, in a 1976 report from the University of Michigan, reviewed 55 patients who had undergone curative resection for lung cancer. [56] This cohort came from a group of 75 patients, older than 70 years of age, who had been diagnosed with lung cancer between 1959 and 1969. Seventeen patients were deemed inoperable because of comorbidity, and three were found at operation to have unresectable disease. The remaining 55 patients had an operative mortality of 14% after lobectomy and

17% after pneumonectomy. Five-year survival was 30% and was comparable to that seen among younger patients. Overall operative mortality rates, for all age groups, from the same institution were 7% for pneumonectomy, 5.7% for lobectomy, 0% for segmentectomy, and 1.6% for thoracotomy alone. The researchers concluded that age per se does not have an adverse influence on long-term survival after pulmonary resection for bronchogenic carcinoma and that a decision to proceed with surgery should be made on the basis of cardiovascular status and pulmonary reserve. The higher rate of peri-operative mortality among elderly patients was attributed to difficulties in properly identifying poor-risk elderly patients prior to surgery. Accurate and precise guidelines for excluding patients from operation were therefore proposed. The guidelines proposed to indicate inoperability included:

- resting hypercapnia ($Pco_2 > 45$ mm Hg) or hypercapnia with exercise;

- hypoxemia ($PO_2 < 50$ mm Hg);

- $FEV_1 < 2000$ mL, FVC < 2000, or MVV $< 50\%$ of predicted for pneumonectomy;

- $FEV_1 < 1500$ mL for lobectomy;

- calculated $FEV_1 < 800$ mL after surgery.

All these indices related the risk of surgery to physiologic function without any specific reference to age. The researchers concluded that surgery for lung cancer can be safely offered to properly selected elderly patients with acceptable mortality and good potential for long-term survival.

Harpole et al found that age greater than 65 years, right-sided procedures, and the presence of dysrhythmia are associated with increased risk for major complication after pneumonectomy.[57] No identifiable factors were noted to predict mortality. Supraventricular dysrhythmias were found to be the most common complications reported to occur after pneumonectomy (24%), typically presenting 1 to 5 days after surgery. The patients at highest risk for these dysrhythmias were those older than 65 years and patients undergoing right-sided procedures, extrapleural pneumonectomy, or intrapericardial dissection. Joo et al reviewed 105 patients after pneumonectomy and noted a 10% complication rate with atrial fibrillation and respiratory failure predominating.[58] Continuous electrocardiographic monitoring for the early diagnosis of cardiac dysfunction was therefore recommended.

Despite the higher operative mortality documented among older patients, most authors advocated an aggressive surgical approach to lung cancer in elderly patients. Meticulous patient selection and preservation of pulmonary tissue were the hallmarks of studies that showed improved surgical outcome after resection in elderly patients. Breyer et al reported on 150 pulmonary resections for primary lung carcinoma among a highly selected group of patients over the age of 70 years.[59] Parenchyma-sparing procedures were used whenever possible, with segmental resection performed in 52 cases. Multiple logistic regression analysis determined that the amount of lung tissue removed, a history of congestive heart failure, and a history of previous pulmonary resection are all significantly related to an increased risk of major complications or death. The risk of major complication or death was not found to be related to age. Overall 5-year survival was 27%, with a hospital mortality of only 4%. The aggressive use of chest physiotherapy and aspiration bronchoscopy among these elderly patients was credited for the low rates of complication and death after surgery. It was recommended that age alone is not a criterion to reject a patient for pulmonary resection. In 1987, Sherman and Guidot compared two groups of patients, under and over the age of 70, in terms of operative outcome after thoracotomy. [60] Although operative mortality in the elderly group was greater (9.4% versus 4.0%), no statistically significant difference in the postoperative complications, postoperative hospital stay, or actuarial survival was found. The researchers concluded that advanced age does not adversely affect prognosis, and they also urged that elderly patients with reasonable cardiopulmonary function have a potentially curative pulmonary resection. This conclusion was echoed in the geriatric literature of the day, as continued refinements in surgical care gradually lowered the mortality risk for lung cancer surgery among elderly patients to levels that began to approach those obtained in younger patients. [61]

The number of elderly patients who will require treatment for lung cancer is certain to increase. Standard lobectomy is safe and effective for older patients. The mortality and morbidity after either segmental or lobar resection is generally comparable to that achieved in younger patients. Elderly patients do appear to have an increased rate of complication after more extended resections that include either removal of chest wall or pneumonectomy. The majority of complications are either cardiac or respiratory. Mortality after extended resection is not substantially increased among elderly patients in most surgical series, likely because of the rigorous selection process that occurs prior to considering patients for radical surgery. Any consideration of pulmonary resection in elderly patients therefore mandates a rigorous review of preoperative cardiopulmonary reserve. [62,63] Data from standard spirometry may be supplemented by exercise testing, blood gas analysis, measurement of diffusing capacity, and nuclear ventilation-perfusion studies. In multivariate analysis, advanced age and increasing extent of pulmonary resection was found to predispose the patient to cardiac arrhythmias. [64] A comprehensive system of surgical care must be considered for elderly patients undergoing major resection. Preoperative physical conditioning with incentive spirometry, graded exercise, and smoking cessation represents one aspect of this program. Intra-operative technique must be meticulous in order to minimize bleeding and tissue trauma. Effective pain control, early mobilization, chest physiotherapy, prophylaxis for deep-vein thrombosis, and electrocardiographic monitoring are important components of postoperative care. The Society of Thoracic Surgeons has a large database of perioperative outcomes and long-term results for coronary artery bypass grafting. [65] Recently, the society initiated a similar database for patients undergoing major thoracic surgical procedures.

Minimally invasive techniques of pulmonary resection may offer unique advantages to the elderly patient. Because a significant part of the morbidity of lung resection can be attributed to the pain of the incision with its resultant deleterious effects on pulmonary function, any reduction in the extent of the incision used to access the lung may result in decreased postoperative morbidity and mortality. Muscle-sparing thoracotomy was shown to decrease pain, length of hospital stay, and narcotic requirements as compared with standard incisions. [66] Video-assisted thoracic surgery (VATS) has been used for wedge resection and lobectomy in elderly patients. [67–71] Specialized surgical centers have demonstrated that these techniques are feasible and safe. [72] Early results with VATS lobectomy have shown that survival results are comparable to those of open surgery in stage I lung cancer. [73,74] Reductions in surgical complications, mortality, pain, narcotic use, postoperative delirium, hospital cost, and length of stay have been described. [75,76] Long-term survival data comparing VATS lobectomy with standard resection in elderly patients are not currently available.

The optimal care of the elderly patient undergoing pulmonary resection includes meticulous attention to detail before, during, and after operation. A multimodality approach to the surgical management of lung cancer in the elderly patient is therefore needed. Although few centers have a dedicated clinical pathway specifically designed for elderly patients, standard practice guidelines incorporate many of the core elements necessary for optimal care of the aged thoracic surgery patient. Key components of this approach begin with increased educational efforts to overcome potential bias among physicians who may not fully consider elderly patients as candidates for surgery. Additional features are lung cancer screening among older people, optimal preoperative testing of elderly patients, and appropriate referral to centers of specialized care. Cost-effective methods of preoperative conditioning will need to be developed.

ThoracicSurg 1 (Level A): **Randomized controlled trials are needed of the effect on mortality and morbidity of the use of computed tomography screening for elderly patients with high-risk factors for the development of cancer.**

ThoracicSurg 2 (Level B): **An instrument to assess age-specific outcomes, functional status, and quality of life for elderly lung cancer patients that is applicable to both preoperative and postoperative situations needs to be developed and validated.**

ThoracicSurg 3 (Level A): **Ongoing large therapeutic lung cancer trials need to incorporate the age-specific instrument described in ThoracSurg 2.**

ThoracicSurg 4(Level B): **A preoperative tool to assess the general function of the elderly patient having a major pulmonary procedure needs to be developed and validated.**

ThoracicSurg 5 (Level B): **A multivariate analysis using the Society of Thoracic Surgeons Database or other collections of cases and aimed at defining the most important risk factors for adverse surgical outcomes should be performed. The instrument should include measures of the patient's functional capacity as well as pulmonary functions.**

ThoracicSurg 6 (Level B): **A method of preoperative optimization that addresses the most important risk factors for morbidity and mortality from pneumonectomy should be developed and tested.**

ThoracicSurg 7 (Level A): **Randomized controlled trials are needed to compare the efficacy of preoperative optimization methods with current best medical practices.**

ThoracicSurg 8 (Level A): **Randomized controlled trials are needed to evaluate video-assisted thoracic surgery techniques for lobectomy; the trials should compare outcomes, including long-term survival in elderly patients, with those of standard open procedures.**

BENIGN DISEASES OF THE LUNGS

The two most common disease states that impact the lung health of elderly persons are pneumonia and chronic bronchitis. The Centers for Disease Control and Prevention published the discharge statistics for 2000 in advance form in 2002. [77] The data demonstrate that hospitalization for those aged 65 and over continues to rise while all other groups have shown a continued decline. Pneumonia was found to be the third most common reason behind heart disease and fractures for hospitalization in this age group. Pneumonia and chronic bronchitis combined were second only to heart disease as the first diagnosis at the time of discharge from the hospital. In the elderly age group, pneumonia is the fifth most common cause of death.

Chronic bronchitis and emphysema are the subject of intense investigation by the government. The National Emphysema Treatment Trial (NETT), supported by the National Heart, Lung, and Blood Institute (NHLBI), the Health Care Financing Administration (HCFA, now the Center for Medicare and Medicaid Services), and the Agency for Health Care Policy and Research (AHCPR, now the Agency for Healthcare Research and Quality), is the first multicenter clinical trial designed to determine the role, safety, and effectiveness of surgery to reduce lung volume. Patient screening for entry into the study began in the fall of 1997. It is expected to run for a few more years, and multiple reports are anticipated that will help to define the altered physiology, the best diagnostic evaluations, the optimum rehabilitation, and the role of surgery in the long-term management of severe emphysema. This investigation, coupled with the Lung Health Study, [78] will continue to provide a focus on emphysema for years to come. In March of 2002, the NHLBI reported on a workshop on COPD. [79] The report discussed the new results, concepts, and opportunities in COPD research: protease functions, oxidant injury, viral infection, mucous hypersecretion, apoptosis, alveolar regulation, biomarkers, genetics, inflammation, imaging technologies, molecular characterization, and drug development. It recommended research into characterization of the disease process, pathogenesis, and therapy. However, it did not include the effects of trauma or surgery, or the additive effects of aging on patients with COPD.

Pneumonia per se is not a surgical condition, but the consequences and complications of pneumonia such as empyema require intervention. Gavazzi et al investigated empyema in elderly patients [80] and found that many very old patients present with a pleural effusion that is not associated with classic symptoms of pneumonia. Prompt attention to pleural drainage and institution of antibiotic therapy are the most important prognostic factors. These researchers recommended that, because of the diversity of clinical presentation in the elderly population and because of the efficiency of rapid treatment, physicians should perform an examination of pleural fluid when the cause of pleural effusion in an older patient is uncertain. Chu et al echoed the same sentiments, emphasizing that failure of early recognition leads to a protracted course. [81]

Although thoracotomy and decortication have been the mainstay of empyema management in all patients for many years, clinicians constantly look for less invasive methods to manage these very ill patients. Tube thoracostomy with the installation of fibrinolytic agents was introduced more than 30 years ago. It has met with some success, particularly for the frail patient or the patient who is too ill to undergo a major surgical procedure. Cameron reviewed the use of fibrinolytics, including several randomized trials. [82] At this time, there is insufficient evidence to support routine use of intrapleural fibrinolytic therapy in the treatment of parapneumonic effusion and empyema. Ongoing trials may shift the balance toward the use of fibrinolytic therapy.

Another technique that has been popularized is the use of VATS for the management of empyema. This technique specifically for empyema was first described in 1985.[83] Since then, there have been a number of reports verifying the usefulness of thoracoscopy.[84,85] Coote reviewed the trials comparing thoracoscopy with tube thoracostomy and with tube thoracostomy plus fibrinolytic therapy.[86] This reviewer concluded that thoracoscopy seems to offer an advantage in terms of chest tube time and length of stay but that there is insufficient level I evidence to conclude that thoracoscopy is clearly superior.

> *ThoracicSurg 9*: (Levels B, A): **The effects of lung volume reduction procedures and their complications on elderly patients with chronic obstructive pulmonary disease need to be investigated in cohort studies that compare younger and older patients. Subsequently, a randomized controlled trial might be needed to compare outcomes in elderly patients who undergo a standard volume-reduction procedure with similar patients who do not.**

> *ThoracicSurg 10 (Level A)*: **Randomized trials are needed to evaluate the efficacy of minimally invasive techniques and compare them with standard thoracotomy for the management of empyema in elderly patients.**

ESOPHAGEAL CANCER

Esophageal cancer is one of the 10 most common solid tumors in humans. There are approximately 12,500 cases per year in the United States.[87] Over 90% of these patients will die of their disease despite therapy.[88] Early symptoms of esophageal cancer may be subtle or entirely lacking. Intermittent dysphagia may be ignored by the patient or under-investigated by treating physicians. More than 60% of patients, at presentation, therefore have metastatic or unresectable disease. Of the patients who proceed on to surgery, 75% have locally advanced disease.[89,90] In a study of the interval between onset of dysphagia and treatment, Rothwell et al found a median delay of 15 weeks for patients with dysphagia and 17 weeks for patients with other symptoms. The most frequent cause of delay was late presentation to the family doctor.[91]

The incidence of squamous cell cancers varies tremendously across the globe. Its incidence in Western countries is approximately 5 to 10 cases per 100,000 persons. Areas in Iran and China report an incidence of up to 500 cases per 100,000. Factors related to the development of squamous cell cancers include age, sex, race, diet, alcohol consumption, and tobacco abuse. The average age at presentation for squamous cell cancer of the esophagus in the United States is 67 years. The overall incidence is 4 to 6 times higher in men than in women.[92] Tobacco and alcohol consumption are strong predisposing factors in the development of squamous cell carcinoma of the esophagus. Case studies have revealed a strong dose-related risk among smokers that is 5 to 10 times the risk among nonsmokers.[93] The same is true of alcohol, with the greatest increased risk among those consuming hard liquor as opposed to wine or beer.[94] The combination of smoking and heavy alcohol consumption appears to have a synergistic effect on the development of esophageal cancer and to cause a 100-fold increase in relative risk.[95] Nutritional deficiencies in vitamins A, B_2, and C also have been implicated in the development of squamous cell cancers of the esophagus, as have mineral deficiencies involving zinc and magnesium. The risk was found to be elevated with high meat intake, and protective effects were found with increased consumption of raw fruits and vegetables.[96] These risk factors are of specific importance to elderly patients and to their family physicians. High cumulative exposure to tobacco and alcohol, combined with nutritional deficiencies that are often seen among seniors, should prompt the physician to specifically ask questions on the quality of patient swallowing. There should be a low threshold for further investigations, such as a contrast esophagram and esophagoscopy.

Adenocarcinomas of the esophagus are generally not associated with any of the risk factors typically found among patients with squamous cell cancer.[97–101] Patients with adenocarcinomas usually are well-nourished middle- to upper-class men with no history of alcohol abuse. Obesity and gastroesophageal reflux have been linked to the subsequent development of esophageal adenocarcinoma.[102–104] Benign columnar metaplasia of the esophagus (Barrett's esophagus) is found in 10% of patients with symptomatic gastroesophageal reflux and is present in 70% of resected adenocarcinomas of the gastric cardia and esophagus.[105,106] Patients with Barrett's esophagus are at risk of developing dysplasia within the areas of columnar metaplasia. The presence of dysplasia in a columnar-lined esophagus represents a premalignant condition that substantially increases the risk for the subsequent development of invasive cancer.[107] The risk of developing adenocarcinoma in the presence of Barrett's esophagus is estimated to be 1/400 to 1/170 patient years. This is 40 times greater than that seen in patients without Barrett's esophagus.[108–110] The histologic progression of Barrett's esophagus to carcinoma may be related to mutations of the p53 tumor suppressor gene.[111] Growth factor mutations involving *erb*-b2 and EGFR may further contribute to malignant transformation.[112] Other studies have suggested that destruction of cyclin kinase inhibitors may promote uninhibited growth of the cancers.[113] The prevalence of gastroesophageal reflux and its influence on the subsequent development of Barrett's esophagus has resulted in a dramatic change in the epidemiology of esophageal cancer over the past 20 years in the United States. Adenocarcinomas of the gastroesophageal junction have become the predominant histologic subtype, now accounting for more than 70% of esophageal cancers. In the United States between 1976 and 1987, the average annual rate of increase in incidence of esophageal adenocarcinoma among white males was 9.4%, exceeding that of any other malignancy.[114] Similar trends were noted in western European countries.[115] This is in marked contrast to worldwide statistics, where squamous cell cancers still account for the majority of cases. Patients with a long history of reflux should be screened for Barrett's changes by esophagoscopy. The presence of dysplasia must be specifically sought, as it represents a premalignant condition. High-grade dysplasia is an indication for esophagectomy because of the prevalence of occult adenocarcinoma.[116] Educational efforts must therefore be aimed toward the general public and health care personnel in order to enhance recognition of the relationship between reflux and esophageal cancer. This knowledge may lead to the early investigation of symptoms and improve patient acceptance of either surveillance or therapeutic procedures.

In the past few years, investigations into the possibility of preventing cancer with simple agents have borne fruit. Moran reviewed the use of anti-inflammatory drugs to decrease the risk of developing cancer in general.[117] The Mayo Clinic group, working with a well-established model of Barrett's cancer, demonstrated a decrease in the rate of cancer development in rats fed COX-2 inhibitors. [118] Kaur et al gave patients with Barrett's esophagus COX-2 inhibitors and demonstrated a decrease in COX-2 and prostaglandin E_2 expression in mucosal biopsies. [119] In a novel approach, Lin et al gave the Chinese herbal medicine zeng sheng ping to patients with high-grade dysplasia and riboflavin with calcium to patients with mild dysplasia. [120] The patients with high-grade dysplasia had a 50% reduction in relative risk, and the patients with mild dysplasia had an 80% reduction in relative risk. Clinical trials with COX-2 inhibitors are now starting in the United States.

Esophageal resection is the standard treatment of both squamous cell cancers and adenocarcinomas of the esophagus. Improvements in patient selection, anesthesia, operative technique, and peri-operative care have dramatically reduced operative mortality over the past 20 years. [121] Surgical resection can provide an 80% 5-year survival in patients with stage I disease. The 5-year survival of patients after surgery for locally advanced disease is approximately 20% to 30%. Unfortunately, the majority of patients are unable to undergo surgery because they have extensive disease at the time of diagnosis. The formidable physiologic stress posed by the operation itself also renders many additional patients inoperable because of their comorbidities. Two surgical approaches are widely used for esophageal resection: trans-hiatal esophagectomy with cervical esophagogastric anastomosis and Ivor Lewis transthoracic esophagectomy. The major difference between the two techniques relates to the location of the anastomosis and the need for thoracotomy. The trans-hiatal esophagectomy involves an upper midline laparotomy and a left cervical neck incision. Mobilization of the esophagus is done through the hiatus, and a thoracotomy is not required. The esophagogastric anastomosis is placed in the left neck at the level of the clavicle. The Ivor Lewis esophagectomy is performed via a laparotomy incision and a right thoracotomy. [122] The anastomosis is located in the chest at the level of the azygous vein. The equivalence of trans-hiatal esophagectomy to transthoracic esophagectomy for long-term survival has been well documented at different centers throughout the world in both retrospective case series and prospective clinical trials. [123–130]

Surgery may have its most important functional impact by changing the mode of recurrence in esophageal cancer. Autopsy findings comparing resected and nonresected patients treated for esophageal cancer found local residual cancer to be much more common among patients who had not undergone surgery as part of their therapy (94.4% versus 21.2%, $P < .0001$). The low incidence of localized disease suggests that esophagectomy, though often palliative in terms of overall survival benefit, may be very effective in minimizing the incidence of local recurrence and its attendant disabling symptoms. [131] Recurrence patterns after trans-hiatal esophagectomy indicate that almost 40% of patients will later develop loco-regional disease, either alone or in combination with systemic metastases. In multivariate analysis, recurrence was found to be related to postoperative lymph node status and the radical nature of the operation. [132] Surgery will result in better long-term control of local symptoms. The choice of operation may have some impact on the risk for local recurrence. The potential benefit of more radical forms of local resection, such as total thoracic esophagectomy with radical lymphadenectomy, must be balanced against the risk for increased peri-operative morbidity and mortality. Among elderly patients, the trans-hiatal esophagectomy is likely to be a less physiologically demanding operation. It obviates the need for thoracotomy and therefore avoids the attendant pain and decline in respiratory performance associated with a second incision into the chest. The location of the anastomosis in the neck, as opposed to the right chest, maximizes the extent of the proximal margin and makes management of any potential leak less complicated. [133] Anastomotic leaks are generally well tolerated, as the cervical esophagogastric anastomosis is easily accessed and drained, and strictures are safely dilated. [134] The use of a side-to-side stapled anastomosis in the neck has resulted in a substantial reduction in frequency of anastomotic leaks and later strictures. It represents the latest in a series of technical refinements of this operation. [135] Orringer et al at the University of Michigan have provided benchmark data regarding the safety and efficacy of trans-hiatal esophagectomy. Data from 1085 patients were reported, with a hospital mortality rate of 4%. [136] Actuarial survival of patients with carcinoma equaled or exceeded that reported for transthoracic esophagectomy. Late functional results were good or excellent in 70% of patients. Greater safety, fewer complications, and comparable long-term survival have led many to consider trans-hiatal esophagectomy to be the approach of choice for patients with limited functional reserve. [137,138]

Age-related declines in cardiopulmonary capacity are important in evaluating patients for esophagectomy. A multivariate analysis of postoperative complications after esophageal resection found age and volume of transfusion to be associated significantly with postoperative hypoxemia and the need for prolonged respiratory support. [139] In a study using the National Medicare claim database for patients aged 65 years and older, the operative mortality of 1.2 million patients who were hospitalized between 1994 and 1999 for major elective surgery was reviewed. Operative mortality was found to vary widely according to the type of procedure. Esophagectomy and pneumonectomy were associated with the highest risk of death, with mortality rates of 13.6% and 13.7 %, respectively. [140] Operative mortality among patients 80 years and older was more than twice that observed for patients 65 to 69 years old. A retrospective analysis for risk factors associated with poor outcome after esophagectomy in a series of 269 patients found age ($P = .001$, relative risk [RR] = 2.6) and performance status ($P = .04$, RR = 1.9) to predict operative mortality. Multivariate analysis determined the optimal predictive model to be defined by age (RR = 3.9), intraoperative blood loss (RR = 1.7), pulmonary complications (RR = 6.6), and the need for inotropic support (RR = 10.2). [141]

Several authors specifically reviewed their experience with esophagectomy among elderly patients. Poon et al studied 167 patients over the age of 70 and compared the results of esophagectomy with that found in 570 younger patients. [142] The resection rate in the elderly population was lower than that in younger patients (48% versus 65%, $P < .001$). No significant differences were observed in the rate of surgical complications. The 30-day mortality was higher in the elderly patients (7.2% versus 3.0%, $P = .02$), but the hospital mortality rate was not significantly different between the elderly and younger age groups (18.0% versus 14.4%, $P = .27$). Survival was similar between the two age groups when deaths from unrelated medical conditions were excluded from analysis. The authors concluded that in the elderly patient, esophagectomy for carcinoma of the esophagus could be carried out with acceptable risk and that intensive peri-operative support would be required. Alexiou et al reviewed 337 patients under the age of 70 and compared them with 150 patients aged 70 to 79 and 36 patients aged 80 to 86 undergoing esophagectomy at a specialty center for thoracic surgery in England. These three groups were analyzed with regard to preoperative medical status, resectability, complications, operative mortality, and long-term survival. Patients over the age of 70 had fewer pre-existing respiratory problems than younger patients. No significant differences in resectability rate were detected among the three groups (80.8%, 77.7%, and 80%, respectively). Elderly patients had a higher incidence of overall (34% and 36.1%), respiratory (24.7% and 19.4%), and cardiovascular (7.3% and 11.1%) complications than did those aged under 70 years (24.6%, 16.3%, and 2.1%, respectively). However, operative mortality (4.7%, 6.7%, and 5.6%) and 5-year survivals inclusive of operative mortality (25.1%, 21.2%, and 19.8%) were similar among the three groups. Esophagectomy in this specialist thoracic unit was safe and associated with acceptable long-term survival in all age groups. [143] Jougon et al noted the same in a study that compared 89 patients over the age of 70 years with 451 younger patients. The older patients had a 24.7% morbidity rate and 7.8% mortality. No significant differences between the two groups were found in terms of morbidity, mortality, mean hospital stay, or long-term survival. [144] Chino et al reported a 60% incidence of postoperative complications in a series of 45 patients over the age of 80 years. Five-year survival after resection was 30.8% and comparable to that for younger patients. [145] Xijiang et al reported on a series of 63 elderly patients operated upon for esophageal cancer between 1978 and 1992. A complication rate of 25.4% was noted, with pulmonary problems being most commonly encountered. The 3-year survival rate among patients undergoing surgery with curative intent was 100%, 35%, and 25% in stages I, II, and III, respectively. [146] Naunheim et al described 38 patients over the age of 70 who underwent transthoracic (71%) or trans-hiatal (29%) esophagectomy. Pneumonia was again the most prevalent postoperative complication, occurring in 29% of patients. [147] Thomas et al reported on 56 patients over the age of 70 and compared them with 330 younger patients undergoing esophagectomy for cancer. Pulmonary function, as assessed by spirometry, was significantly worse among the older patients. Operative mortality was comparable in the two groups (10.7% versus 11.2%). Postoperative morbidity included anastomotic leak (10.7% versus 13.6%) and pulmonary complications (17.9% versus 20.6%) in both groups. Excellent palliation of dysphagia was achieved in 92% of the elderly patients who survived operation. Five-year survival was not different for elderly and younger patients (17% versus 18.9%). [148] Among even older patients, the report by Adam et al on 31 octogenarians undergoing esophagectomy demonstrated an elective operative mortality rate of 10.7%, with the successful palliation of dysphagia in 73%. The 5-year survival rate was 17%. [149] Emergency operation was associated with an increased risk of complications and death. Karl et al noted no significant difference in preoperative risk factors, operative mortality, length of stay, length of procedure, estimated blood loss, rate of major complication, or Kaplan-Meier survival rate between patients older than 70 years and those who were younger. [150]

Minimally invasive esophagectomy holds the potential for further reducing operative morbidity and mortality. [151,152] No prospective trials have directly compared traditional open esophagectomy with minimally invasive surgery among elderly patients. There are also no long-term data to determine whether the minimally invasive approach is equivalent to open procedures in terms of stage-specific long-term survival and patterns of tumor recurrence. [153,154] The same is also true for endoscopic mucosal resection, a minimally invasive technique developed for the treatment of superficial esophageal carcinoma and high-grade dysplasia in Barrett's esophagus. [155,156]

Improvement in pain control is an essential element in promoting early patient mobilization and preventing respiratory complications such as atelectasis or pneumonia. A multimodality approach to control postoperative pain and the physiologic stress response has led to earlier extubation, earlier discharge from intensive care, and improved patient mobilization. [157] A balanced program of preemptive and postoperative analgesia has been proposed for elderly high-risk patients undergoing esophagectomy. [158] A paravertebral block may be combined with general anesthesia, opioids, and nonsteroidal anti-inflammatory drugs prior to incision. Postoperative analgesia can be provided with either continuous extrapleural intercostal nerve block or thoracic epidural infusion. Regional analgesia in elderly patients may help reduce the need for systemic narcotics. The sedative and neuropsychologic side effects of these drugs may be avoided. Pain scores upon mobilization among patients in whom epidural analgesia was continued for 5 days were found to be significantly decreased in comparison with those from patients who were switched over to patient-controlled analgesia with intravenous morphine in the early postoperative period. [159] The increased use of advanced thoracoscopic and laparoscopic techniques for minimally invasive esophagectomy may further reduce the physiologic impact of the operation and resultant risk of complications related to inadequate analgesia. [160,161]

One of the prime questions facing physicians caring for elderly patients relates to whether the proposed treatment will yield an acceptable quality of life for the patient. Esophageal obstruction related to tumor progression leads to multiple problems that are, in aggregate, devastating to the patients' sense of well-being. Oral food intake is severely limited, and many patients are unable to swallow their own saliva. This will lead to the persistent need to regurgitate the contents of an obstructed esophagus during the day and predispose to episodes of aspiration. Persistent pain may also result from stasis and inflammation within the obstructed esophagus. The need for tube feeding further limits patient autonomy. A consideration of esophagectomy in an elderly patient must therefore take into account survival benefit, functional outcome, and quality of life. Among patients of advanced age, for whom the potential for long life is quite limited, functional outcome is of paramount importance. Esophagectomy must be examined in terms of its ability to palliate dysphagia and to restore normal swallowing. The functional results after esophagectomy will have to be compared with results obtained after chemoradiation, stenting, or endoscopic ablation. [162]

Comprehensive strategies have been devised to reduce the complications of esophagectomy. Gillinov and Heitmiller reported on a management program from 1990 to 1995 that was designed to maximize airway protection in the postoperative period and discussed their results with trans-hiatal esophagectomy. The clinical pathway consisted of overnight mechanical ventilation, chest physiotherapy, video pharyngo-esophagram on postoperative day 6 or 7, and graduated postesophagectomy therapeutic diet. Pulmonary complications were classified as major or minor, depending upon whether or not a change in therapy was required. Ten patients (10%) had 11 major pulmonary complications that included pneumonia, pleural effusion, exacerbation of pre-existing COPD, and mucus plug requiring bronchoscopy or mechanical ventilation. Patients with major pulmonary complications were older (69.3 ± 9.8 versus 59.2 ± 12.1 years, $P < .02$) and more likely to have pre-existing lung disease. Pneumonia was the most common cause of death following trans-hiatal esophagectomy. [163] The introduction of clinical care pathways was also associated with a 34% reduction in total hospital costs, with major decreases in pharmacy, laboratory, radiology, and miscellaneous charges. [164] Orringer et al, in their large series of patients undergoing trans-hiatal esophagectomy at the University of Michigan, emphasized smoking cessation, preoperative incentive spirometry, and walking 1 to 2 miles per day prior to surgery as key elements for early postoperative mobilization and minimizing pulmonary complications. [136] Intensive-care monitoring was not routinely used in their series of trans-hiatal esophagectomies, as patients were usually extubated in the operating room, immediately after surgery. These strategies reflect the practices of highly experienced centers and may form the framework of clinical guidelines that will optimize the care of elderly patients.

Most clinical trials have focused on morbidity and mortality as measures of patient outcome. The physician's assessment of the relative harms or benefits of treatment may differ considerably from the patient's. Quality-of-life scores are patient based and more likely to accurately reflect the efficacy of various treatments. Complications such as vocal cord palsy may have marked detrimental effects on speech and comfortable swallowing that are difficult to quantify within the context of a clinical trial unless quality of life is taken into account. [165] Simple questionnaire studies have shown only 22% of patients to have no complaints after esophagectomy. [166] Gross measures, such as the ability to return to work, appear to indicate that the majority of patients can achieve a satisfactory quality of life after esophagectomy. [167] However, return to work may be an inappropriate endpoint for elderly patients. Less reflux, regurgitation, and esophagitis are associated with cervical esophagogastric anastomoses than with intrathoracic anastomoses. [168]

Few studies have prospectively measured quality of life by using validated and appropriate instruments that are sufficiently sensitive to small but clinically important changes in quality of life. Disease-specific modules have been developed for use in conjunction with generic measures. The European Organization for Research and Treatment of Cancer (EORTC) QLQ-OES24 is an adjunct to the EORTC QLQ-C30 core quality-of-life instrument and was specifically designed for patients undergoing potentially curative treatment or palliation of malignant dysphagia. [169] There is evidence to suggest that these quality-of-life indices may help predict survival in patients with esophageal cancer. Blazeby et al reported on 89 consecutive patients with esophageal cancer who completed the EORTC QLQ-C30 questionnaire and the dysphagia scale from the esophageal cancer module. Univariate analysis revealed that better baseline physical and role function scores were significantly associated with increased survival, and that worse fatigue, appetite loss, and constipation scores were significantly associated with shorter survival ($P < .01$). Multivariate analysis, taking account of associations between the quality-of-life scores and adjusting for age, comorbidity, and tumor stage, showed that only physical function at baseline remained significantly associated with survival. [170] In a related study, consecutive patients undergoing potentially curative esophagectomy or purely palliative treatment were studied with the EORTC QLQ-C30 and the dysphagia scale from the QLQ-OES24 before treatment and at regular intervals for 3 years or until death. Six weeks after esophagectomy, patients reported worse functional, symptom, and global scores than before treatment. In patients who survived at least 2 years, quality-of-life scores returned to preoperative levels within 9 months, but patients who died within 2 years of surgery never regained their former quality of life. In both groups, dysphagia improved after surgery, and the improvement was maintained until death or for the duration of the study. Patients undergoing palliative treatment reported gradual deterioration in most aspects until death.

Esophagectomy was thus found to provide lasting palliation of dysphagia at the cost of a transient reduction in global quality-of-life scores among patients surviving more than 2 years. [171]

Studies on the functional outcome of esophageal resection have generally focused on patient symptoms. McLarty et al reported on 359 patients undergoing esophagectomy for stage I or stage II esophageal carcinoma. Long-term function and quality of life were measured in 107 patients who survived 5 or more years. Median age at operation was 62 years, with Ivor Lewis resection performed in 72% and trans-hiatal esophagectomy in 13%. Median survival was 10.2 years. Gastroesophageal reflux was present in 60%, symptoms of dumping in 50%, and dysphagia to solid food in 25%. Factors affecting late functional outcome were analyzed, and it was determined that a cervical anastomosis was associated with significantly fewer reflux symptoms and that dumping syndrome occurred more often in younger patients. Quality of life was assessed separately by the Medical Outcomes Study 36-item Short-Form Health Survey (SF-36) and compared with the national norm. Scores measuring physical functioning were decreased. Scores measuring ability to work, social interaction, daily activities, emotional dysfunction, perception of health, and levels of energy were similar to national norms, and mental health scores were higher. [172]

Johansson and Walther compared 50 patients over the age of 70 with 89 younger patients at 3, 6, and 12 months after esophagectomy in an effort to determine the influence of age on survival and functional outcome after surgery. The overall hospital mortality rate was only 1.4%, with all deaths occurring in the younger age group. Between 71% and 77% of the patients experienced no dysphagia at the three evaluations during the first postoperative year. The 5-year survival rate was 31%. Survival correlated with tumor stage but not with age. Functional outcome, as measured by dysphagia scores, was equivalent in patients over and under 70 years of age. [173]

Information regarding long-term functional outcome and quality of life after esophagectomy has also been collected from patients undergoing surgery for benign disease. These data are particularly relevant because the length of follow-up is not limited by the progression of malignancy. The Mayo Clinic published their results with esophagectomy for benign disease. Eighty-one patients completed a combined two-part questionnaire regarding esophageal function and quality of life (SF-36) a median of 9.8 years (range, 10 months to 18.9 years) after surgery. Median age at time of esophageal reconstruction was 51 years, and alimentary continuity was re-established with stomach in 71.6%. Dysphagia to solids was present in 59.3%, with one third requiring at least one postoperative dilatation. Heartburn was present in 61.7%. The number of bowel movements per day increased in 45.7% and was unchanged in 44.4%. Age, sex, and type of esophageal reconstruction did not affect late functional outcome. Physical functioning, social functioning, and health perception were decreased ($P < .05$). No significant change was observed in role-physical, mental health, bodily pain, energy or fatigue, and role-emotional scores. [174] Another study from the same institution found that 175 of 255 patients had functional improvement after esophagectomy for benign disease, with a median follow-up of 52 months. Functional results were classified as excellent in 31.8%, good in 10.2%, fair in 35.4%, and poor 22.6%. [175] These data indicate that esophagectomy is associated with an acceptable quality of gastrointestinal function and that the results are durable over time.

The effect of hospital volume on hospital mortality after esophagectomy in the Netherlands was studied over the period from 1993 to 1998. Fifty-two percent of the procedures were performed in low-volume centers averaging 1 to 10 resections per year, 6% were performed in medium-volume centers with 11 to 20 resections a year, and 42% were performed in two high-volume centers averaging more than 50 resections a year. Hospital mortality was found to be 12.1% in low-volume centers and 7.5% in medium-volume hospitals; a 4.9% mortality rate was found in high-volume centers, despite the observation that these specialty units appeared to manage slightly more advanced tumors than the low- and medium-volume centers. [176] The increased operative experience among specialty surgeons who perform high numbers of complex procedures at tertiary-care hospitals may be one of the most critical determinants of patient mortality. Familiarity with the technical pitfalls of procedure and their potential consequences in the postoperative period allows the experienced surgeon to either avoid complications or recognize them earlier once they occur. High-volume hospitals are also more likely to have a wider range of advanced diagnostic or therapeutic services that may salvage patients who become gravely ill after operation.

Studies in the United States have indicated that hospitals with a high volume of esophagectomy, and therefore more experienced surgical teams, can perform the procedure with lower costs and patient mortality rates than low-volume centers can achieve. Logistic regression analysis was used to determine the relationship between hospital volume and mortality in 1561 patients who had esophagectomy for cancer in California between 1990 and 1994. [177] An average of two or fewer resections was performed annually in 88% of hospitals. The mortality rate in hospitals performing more than 30 esophagectomies during the 5-year period was 4.8%. This compared with a mortality rate of 16% for hospitals that performed the procedure less frequently. These results strongly support the importance of an experienced surgical team for complex procedures associated with a high risk of complication. Similar conclusions came from a retrospective cohort study using the SEER-Medicare linked database that examined 5013 patients aged 65 years or older at diagnosis who underwent pancreatectomy, esophagectomy, pneumonectomy, liver resection, or pelvic exenteration between 1984 and 1993. [178] Thirty-day mortality in relation to procedure volume was adjusted for comorbidity, patient age, and cancer stage. Higher volume was linked with lower mortality for pancreatectomy ($P = .004$), esophagectomy ($P < .001$), liver resection ($P = .04$), and pelvic exenteration ($P = .04$), but not for pneumonectomy ($P = .32$). The most striking results were for esophagectomy, for which the operative mortality rose to 17.3% in low-volume hospitals, compared with 3.4% in high-volume hospitals. Adjustments for case mix and other patient factors did not change the finding that low volume is strongly associated with excess mortality. As age increases, other factors that are not controllable, such as delirium and other geriatric complications, may erode the advantage of the experienced surgeon. Mortality may be no different for the oldest-old patients.

The relationship between hospital volume and cost was recently evaluated for 1136 patients undergoing esophageal resection in Maryland. High hospital volume was associated with a fivefold reduction in the risk of death, a 6-day reduction in length of stay, and a savings of $11,673 in hospital charges. [179] In a study on the relationship between operative volume, hospital size, and cancer specialization on morbidity, mortality, and hospital use after esophagectomy for cancer, data from the Health Care Utilization Project was used to evaluate all Medicare-reimbursed esophagectomies for treatment of cancer from 1994 to 1996 in 13 national cancer institutions and 88 community hospitals. Complications, length of stay, hospital costs, and mortality were assessed according to hospital size, institutional specialization, and operative volume. Mortality was found to be lower in national cancer institution hospitals than in community hospitals (4.2% versus 13.3%, $P < .05$) or in hospitals performing a large number of esophagectomies (3. 0% versus 12.2%, $P < .05$). Multivariate analysis revealed that the independent risk factor for operative mortality is the volume of esophagectomies performed and not the number of other operations, hospital size, or institutional specialization. Hospitals performing a large number of esophagectomies were found to show a tendency toward fewer complications (55% versus 68%, $P = .06$), decreased length of stay (14.7 days versus 17.7 days, $P = .006$), and lower charges ($39,867 versus $62,094, $P < .005$). The analysis indicated that the increased experience of the surgical team, and not merely hospital size or cancer specialization, can account for improved patient outcome with lower cost. [180] These data were not stratified by age and did not explicitly report on whether the improvement in overall patient mortality reflects a uniform improvement in all age groups or advances limited to patients of a specific age.

ThoracicSurg 11 (Level B): **Screening endoscopic trials should be performed for elderly patients with longstanding reflux or a history of Barrett's esophagus to determine if early detection and treatment of high-grade dysplasia is cost-effective.**

ThoracicSurg 12 (Levels B, A): **Nonrandomized chemoprevention trials targeted specifically toward at-risk elderly patients should be continued, to be followed by a randomized controlled trial of chemoprevention using the most promising agent and comparing it with usual care.**

ThoracicSurg 13 (Level B): **The Society of Thoracic Surgeons database and other similar databases should be used to gather data on the impact of age-related comorbidities and other factors related to operative management on the outcomes of esophagectomy for elderly patients.**

ThoracicSurg 14 (Level B): **A national database for collecting morbidity and long-term survival rates of minimally invasive techniques for esophageal cancer should be established.**

ThoracicSurg 15 (Level B): **Esophagectomy needs to be evaluated for effectiveness as a procedure for improving quality of life and preventing complications of aspiration in elderly patients.**

ThoracicSurg 16 (Level B): **Instruments to measure age-specific outcomes of surgery for esophageal caner need to be developed and validated. Functional status and quality of life should be among the outcomes assessed.**

ThoracicSurg 17 (Level A): **Large clinical esophageal cancer trials should incorporate the age-specific instruments described in ThoracicSurg 16.**

ThoracicSurg 18 (Level B): **Esophagectomy could be used as a model for highly complex surgical procedures in the elderly patient to answer the following questions:**

■ **What makes the high-volume center able to provide better care for elderly esophagectomy patients?**

■ **Do high-volume centers achieve better surgical outcomes with the oldest-old patients?**

■ **In what ways can care be improved for the elderly patient after esophagectomy?**

■ **Once a formula for success is characterized, is it applicable to the care of elderly patients receiving other types of major operations?**

BENIGN ESOPHAGEAL DISEASE

Among elderly persons, disorders of deglutition are quite common.[181,182] With increasing age, patients develop significant dysphagia, along with achalasia, gastroesophageal reflux disease (GERD), and constipation. Neurologic problems that accompany normal aging and the increased incidence of cerebrovascular accidents also add to dysphagia in the older population. Several swallowing clinics around the country have begun to concentrate the necessary interdisciplinary expertise in one location and have met with some success. The chapter on otolaryngology addresses issues surrounding dysphagia (see Chapter 8).

Disorders of digestion commonly require therapy. They are treated by a variety of nonsurgical methods but sometimes require surgical intervention. Some 750 references deal specifically with operations for achalasia and reflux in the geriatric population. Surgeons and gastroenterologists tend to disagree on the right approach to all patients with reflux regardless of age. Sarani et al performed a survey to understand the variation in approach to the patient with GERD.[183] Surveys were sent to 1000 randomly selected members of the American Gastroenterological Association (AGA) and to 1000 randomly selected members of the Society of American Gastrointestinal Endoscopic Surgeons (SAGES). Twenty percent of the AGA surveys and 33% of the SAGES surveys were completed and returned. The AGA group considered patients whose symptoms are not well controlled, those who have complications of disease, and those who require significant lifestyle changes to control their symptoms as the best candidates for surgical evaluation. As a group, gastroenterologists remain somewhat hesitant to refer patients for laparoscopic antireflux surgery. Surgeons considered patients whose symptoms have been well controlled with medical therapy, those who have complications of disease, and those who require significant lifestyle changes to control their symptoms as ideal candidates for fundoplication. As new, less invasive approaches emerge, the therapy for GERD will likely continue to be controversial.

Surgeons agree that the trend is to perform less invasive procedures and that results are equal to or better than open procedures. However, laparoscopic antireflux surgery is commonly denied to older patients with GERD because of a perceived higher operative complication rate, a decreased impact of the intervention on quality of life, and decreased cost-effectiveness. Several series of procedures on elderly patients are now available for evaluation. These are either retrospective reviews or historical prospective studies. One of the first reviews to directly address the issues relating to elderly patients was reported by Trus et al in 1998. [184] They had operated upon 42 patients aged 65 years and over out of a total of 359 patients with GERD. These patients did as well as the younger patients. Brunt et al reported an almost identical study the following year from Washington University. [185] In 2001, Kamolz et al evaluated the quality-of-life issues in elderly patients who had antireflux operations. [186] They followed 72 elderly patients after surgery for 1 to 3 years. Three patients developed significant complications, and two required reoperation. The remaining patients did well, with a significant increase in their perceived quality of life.

In 2002, two prospective cohort studies were reported. Bammer et al examined the safety and long-term outcome of patients aged 80 years and older who were having laparoscopic antireflux surgery. [187] Immediate results were good, with two major complications and no deaths. At follow-up, 96% stated that their surgical outcome was satisfactory. Two patients were suffering from severe symptoms. Overall well-being at a mean follow-up time of 3.1 years was 7.5 (range 3 to 10) on a 10-point scale in comparison with 2.2 (range 1 to 5) before surgery ($P = .03$). Khajanchee et al culled from their database of 1100 patients 30 patients with a mean age of 71 years who had severe symptoms of GERD and compared them with a young cohort of patients from the same database. [188] All patients had at least 6 months of follow-up. Each group demonstrated a significant improvement in the postoperative symptom assessment scores and the esophageal functional studies ($P < .05$). No significant differences were found in postoperative complications, postoperative hospital stay, postoperative symptom scores, Demeester scores, or the quality-of-life data. Even reoperative procedures seem to be safe in experienced hands. Kamolz et al described their series of 11 patients aged 65 years and over who required reoperation. [189] There were no serious postoperative complications, and the 3- and 1-year follow-up demonstrated continued good results.

Newer techniques for even less invasive procedures than those now used are being developed. These will require some refinement before they can be considered to be appropriate for trials in the elderly population.

ThoracicSurg 19 (Level B): **A structured literature review should be performed and a consensus conference between gastroenterologists and surgeons should be organized to establish criteria, based on symptoms and quality of life, for intervention in the management of gastroesophageal reflux disease, particularly in elderly patients.**

ThoracicSurg 20 (Level A): **A prospective trial of laparoscopic antireflux surgery comparing elderly patients with younger matched control patients operated on during the same period should be performed to determine the suitability of this operation for the elderly patient.**

RESEARCH IN SUPPORT OF IMPROVED CARE

Thoracic surgeons have extended the indications for operation into the oldest segment of the population. This coincides with advances in the medical management of comorbidities and improvements in critical care. Operative interventions are an integral part of advanced therapy for the aging population. Technical improvements, including minimally invasive approaches, continue to be investigated. Complex operations such as esophagectomies are performed routinely on older patients, with excellent results.

Accurate data are needed to determine the population at risk for the development of esophageal and chronic lung diseases and those who might benefit from surgical intervention. At the primary care level, surveys must be performed to identify age bias or aberration from evaluation protocols and to determine whether surgical candidates are referred appropriately. Surgeons using evidence-based protocols in conjunction with pulmonologists, gastroenterologists, and oncologists must collaborate to identify appropriate candidates for surgical intervention and to manage them successfully through the perioperative period.

Older patients undergoing operations require more advanced techniques to reduce morbidity. Preoperative preparation through organized care is important in preparing the older person for the stress of a large thoracic procedure. Safer anesthetic techniques and greater use of minimally invasive operations may yield better outcomes. The postoperative phase, which includes intensive care, hospital stay, and rehabilitation periods, require refinement in protocols and procedures to afford the best results. Thoracic surgeons require the latest data and educational support to be able to treat their older patients optimally.

KEY RESEARCH QUESTIONS IN GERIATRIC THORACIC SURGERY

The most important research areas identified in the specialty of geriatric thoracic surgery are the impact of preoperative preparation on improving the perioperative experience, the design and assessment of geriatric clinical management programs to accommodate the increasingly older and sicker patients who may require thoracic operations, and the analysis of short- and long-term quality-of-life outcomes among geriatric thoracic surgical patients. Studies to address these issues include clinical trials, observational studies, subgroup analyses, and expansion of databases to address key questions about the care of elderly thoracic surgical patients.

ThoracicSurg KQ1: **How effective is preoperative preparation in improving the immediate surgical outcome for elderly patients?**

Hypothesis-generating research studies should focus on the technical aspects of specific thoracic operations. Database analyses and observational studies of specific procedures for preoperative evaluation, education, and preparation of elderly patients should elucidate the risk factors and specific preparation necessary for thoracic surgical procedures. Newer methods of assessment may ultimately shape management decisions in thoracic surgery for the elderly patient, as they may alter practices of surgeons, revise risk stratification, and further clarify the expectations for postoperative recovery from thoracic surgery by the geriatric patient. Cohort studies to compare various preoperative preparation strategies for elderly patients are needed. Multivariate analyses of such studies may clarify the minimum functional capacity and the role of treatment techniques to achieve the desired outcome.

Hypothesis-testing research should include randomized trials of elderly patients with and without specific preoperative habilitation.

ThoracicSurg KQ2: **What changes in perioperative care are needed to improve outcomes in the elderly thoracic surgical patient?**

Hypothesis-generating research should include methodologic studies to identify high-risk elderly patients and devise clinical pathways for their care. Database analyses of the pre-hospital, in-hospital, and rehabilitative periods of elderly surgical patients should be performed to identify clinical management strategies that result in decreased morbidity and improved functional recovery. Prospective cohort studies of patients aged 75 and over treated by nonoperative means, standard operation, and minimally invasive modalities are needed to clarify the potential benefits of each therapy.

Hypothesis-testing research studies include randomized trials of perioperative management strategies, with emphasis on reduction in morbidity. Case-control or randomized studies of elder-specific pathways to elucidate the benefit of pathways in obtaining better functional outcomes and reducing in-hospital adverse events are needed. The aim of these studies would be to identify treatment strategies that reduce the incidence of perioperative pulmonary complications, wound-related problems, and end-organ failure, which have been shown to be especially prevalent in elderly thoracic patients.

ThoracicSurg KQ3: **To what extent do thoracic surgical operations improve quality-of-life outcomes in the elderly patient population?**

Hypothesis-generating research should include the expansion of current clinical databases to include short- and long-term quality-of-life outcomes of elderly thoracic surgical patients. The ability to satisfactorily gauge the success of thoracic operations in improving quality of life for elderly patients depends heavily on the accurate measure of preoperative and perioperative functional capabilities. Observational studies and database analysis should focus on the refinement of risk factors for poor outcomes in elderly surgically treated patients.

Hypothesis-testing research studies to address this question would be aimed at comparing surgical and medical therapy for lung and esophageal disease in older patients. Randomized trials of elderly patients treated for specific disease entities, particularly chronic lung disease and thoracic cancers, using age-specific instruments are needed to clarify the role of operative therapy in improving survival and quality of life.

REFERENCES

1. American Cancer Society: Cancer Facts and Figures. American Cancer Society, 2002. p 10.
2. Feinstein MB, Bach PB. Epidemiology of lung cancer. Chest Surg Clin N Am 2000;10:653-661.
3. Cooley ME, Kaiser LR, Abrahm JL, Giarelli E. The silent epidemic: tobacco and the evolution of lung cancer and its treatment. Cancer Invest 2001;19:739-751.
4. Fry WA, Phillips JL, Menck HR. Ten-year survey of lung cancer treatment and survival in hospitals in the United States: a national cancer data base report. Cancer 1999;86:1867-1876.
5. Haura EB. Treatment of advanced non-small-cell lung cancer: a review of current randomized clinical trials and an examination of emerging therapies. Cancer Control 2001;8:326-336.

6. Flehinger BJ, Kimmel M, Melamed MR. The effect of surgical treatment on survival from early lung cancer: implications for screening. Chest 1992;101:1013-1018.

7. Martini N, Beattie EJ, Jr. Results of surgical treatment in Stage I lung cancer. J Thorac Cardiovasc Surg 1977;74:499-505.

8. Williams DE, Pairolero PC, Davis CS, et al. Survival of patients surgically treated for stage I lung cancer. J Thorac Cardiovasc Surg 1981;82:70-76.

9. Pairolero PC, Williams DE, Bergstralh EJ, et al. Postsurgical stage I bronchogenic carcinoma: morbid implications of recurrent disease. Ann Thorac Surg 1984;38:331-338.

10. Harpole DH, Jr., Herndon JE, 2nd, Young WG, Jr., et al. Stage I nonsmall cell lung cancer: a multivariate analysis of treatment methods and patterns of recurrence. Cancer 1995;76:787-796.

11. Wada H, Tanaka F, Yanagihara K, et al. Time trends and survival after operations for primary lung cancer from 1976 through 1990. J Thorac Cardiovasc Surg 1996;112:349-355.

12. Mountain CF. Revisions in the International System for Staging Lung Cancer. Chest 1997;111:1710-1717.

13. Strauss GM. Screening for lung cancer: an evidence-based synthesis. Surg Oncol Clin N Am 1999;8:747-774, viii.

14. Sobue T, Suzuki T, Matsuda M, et al. Survival for clinical stage I lung cancer not surgically treated: comparison between screen-detected and symptom-detected cases. The Japanese Lung Cancer Screening Research Group. Cancer 1992;69:685-692.

15. Eddy DM. Screening for lung cancer. Ann Intern Med 1989;111:232-237.

16. Bailar JC, III. Early lung cancer detection: summary and conclusions. National Cancer Institute Early Lung Cancer Detection Program Cooperative Study Group. Am Rev Respir Dis 1984;130:565-570.

17. Will BP, Berthelot JM, Nobrega KM, et al. Canada's Population Health Model (POHEM): a tool for performing economic evaluations of cancer control interventions. Eur J Cancer 2001;37:1797-1804.

18. Tockman MS, Mulshine JL. The early detection of occult lung cancer. Chest Surg Clin N Am 2000;10:737-749.

19. Tockman MS, Mulshine JL, Piantadosi S, et al. Prospective detection of preclinical lung cancer: results from two studies of heterogeneous nuclear ribonucleoprotein A2/B1 overexpression. Clin Cancer Res 1997;3:2237-2246.

20. Henschke CI, McCauley DI, Yankelevitz DF, et al. Early Lung Cancer Action Project: overall design and findings from baseline screening. Lancet 1999;354:99-105.

21. Marshall D, Simpson KN, Earle CC, Chu CW. Economic decision analysis model of screening for lung cancer. Eur J Cancer 2001;37:1759-1767.

22. Hollen PJ, Gralla RJ, Kris MG, Cox C. Quality of life during clinical trials: conceptual model for the Lung Cancer Symptom Scale (LCSS). Support Care Cancer 1994;2:213-222.

23. Anderson H, Hopwood P, Stephens RJ, et al. Gemcitabine plus best supportive care (BSC) vs BSC in inoperable non-small cell lung cancer–a randomized trial with quality of life as the primary outcome. UK NSCLC Gemcitabine Group. Non-Small Cell Lung Cancer. Br J Cancer 2000;83:447-453.

24. Pater JL, Zee B, Palmer M, et al. Fatigue in patients with cancer: results with National Cancer Institute of Canada Clinical Trials Group studies employing the EORTC QLQ-C30. Support Care Cancer 1997;5:410-413.

25. Auchter RM, Scholtens D, Adak S, et al. Quality of life assessment in advanced non-small-cell lung cancer patients undergoing an accelerated radiotherapy regimen: report of ECOG study 4593. Eastern Cooperative Oncology Group. Int J Radiat Oncol Biol Phys 2001;50:1199-1206.

26. The Elderly Lung Cancer Vinorelbine Italian Study Group. Effects of vinorelbine on quality of life and survival of elderly patients with advanced non-small-cell lung cancer. J Natl Cancer Inst 1999;91:66-72.

27. Gridelli C. The ELVIS trial: a phase III study of single-agent vinorelbine as first-line treatment in elderly patients with advanced non-small cell lung cancer. Elderly Lung Cancer Vinorelbine Italian Study. Oncologist 2001;6 Suppl 1:4-7.

28. Harviel JD, McNamara JJ, Straehley CJ. Surgical treatment of lung cancer in patients over the age of 70 years. J Thorac Cardiovasc Surg 1978;75:802-805.

29. Berggren H, Ekroth R, Malmberg R, et al. Hospital mortality and long-term survival in relation to preoperative function in elderly patients with bronchogenic carcinoma. Ann Thorac Surg 1984;38:633-636.

30. Shirakusa T, Tsutsui M, Iriki N, et al. Results of resection for bronchogenic carcinoma in patients over the age of 80. Thorax 1989;44:189-191.

31. Evans EW. Resection for bronchial carcinoma in the elderly. Thorax 1973;28:86-88.

32. Ginsberg RJ, Hill LD, Eagan RT, et al. Modern thirty-day operative mortality for surgical resections in lung cancer. J Thorac Cardiovasc Surg 1983;86:654-658.

33. de Perrot M, Licker M, Reymond MA, et al. Influence of age on operative mortality and long-term survival after lung resection for bronchogenic carcinoma. Eur Respir J 1999;14:419-422.

34. Pagni S, McKelvey A, Riordan C, et al. Pulmonary resection for malignancy in the elderly: is age still a risk factor? Eur J Cardiothorac Surg 1998;14:40-44; discussion 44-45.

35. Harvey JC, Erdman C, Pisch J, Beattie EJ. Surgical treatment of non-small cell lung cancer in patients older than seventy years. J Surg Oncol 1995;60:247-249.

36. Hanagiri T, Muranaka H, Hashimoto M, et al. Results of surgical treatment of lung cancer in octogenarians. Lung Cancer 1999;23:129-133.

37. Morandi U, Stefani A, Golinelli M, et al. Results of surgical resection in patients over the age of 70 years with non small-cell lung cancer. Eur J Cardiothorac Surg 1997;11:432-439.

38. Ciriaco P, Zannini P, Carretta A, et al. Surgical treatment of non-small cell lung cancer in patients 70 years of age or older. Int Surg 1998;83:4-7.

39. Bates M. Results of surgery for bronchial carcinoma in patients aged 70 and over. Thorax 1970;25:77-78.

40. Oliaro A, Leo F, Filosso PL, et al. Resection for bronchogenic carcinoma in the elderly. J Cardiovasc Surg (Torino) 1999;40:715-719.

41. Jensik RJ, Faber LP, Milloy FJ, Monson DO. Segmental resection for lung cancer: a fifteen-year experience. J Thorac Cardiovasc Surg 1973;66:563-572.

42. Sioris T, Salo J, Perhoniemi V, Mattila S. Surgery for lung cancer in the elderly. Scand Cardiovasc J 1999;33:222-227.

43. Tanita T, Hoshikawa Y, Tabata T, et al. Functional evaluations for pulmonary resection for lung cancer in octogenarians: investigation from postoperative complications. Jpn J Thorac Cardiovasc Surg 1999;47:253-261.

44. Ishida T, Yokoyama H, Kaneko S, et al. Long-term results of operation for non-small cell lung cancer in the elderly. Ann Thorac Surg 1990;50:919-922.

45. Wada H, Nakamura T, Nakamoto K, et al. Thirty-day operative mortality for thoracotomy in lung cancer. J Thorac Cardiovasc Surg 1998;115:70-73.

46. Bernet F, Brodbeck R, Guenin MO, et al. Age does not influence early and late tumor-related outcome for bronchogenic carcinoma. Ann Thorac Surg 2000;69:913-918.

47. Mane JM, Estape J, Sanchez-Lloret J, et al. Age and clinical characteristics of 1433 patients with lung cancer. Age Ageing 1994;23:28-31.

48. Aoki T, Yamato Y, Tsuchida M, et al. Pulmonary complications after surgical treatment of lung cancer in octogenarians. Eur J Cardiothorac Surg 2000;18:662-665.

49. Wada H, Nakamura T, Nakamoto K, et al. Thirty-day operative mortality for thoracotomy in lung cancer. J Thorac Cardiovasc Surg 1998;115:70-73.

50. Kearney DJ, Lee TH, Reilly JJ, et al. Assessment of operative risk in patients undergoing lung resection: importance of predicted pulmonary function. Chest 1994;105:753-759.

51. Wang J, Olak J, Ultmann RE, Ferguson MK. Assessment of pulmonary complications after lung resection. Ann Thorac Surg 1999;67:1444-1447.

52. Holden DA, Rice TW, Stelmach K, Meeker DP. Exercise testing, 6-min walk, and stair climb in the evaluation of patients at high risk for pulmonary resection. Chest 1992;102:1774-1779.

53. Mizushima Y, Noto H, Sugiyama S, et al. Survival and prognosis after pneumonectomy for lung cancer in the elderly. Ann Thorac Surg 1997;64:193-198.

54. Bernard A, Deschamps C, Allen MS, et al. Pneumonectomy for malignant disease: factors affecting early morbidity and mortality. J Thorac Cardiovasc Surg 2001;121:1076-1082.

55. Magdeleinat P, Alifano M, Benbrahem C, et al. Surgical treatment of lung cancer invading the chest wall: results and prognostic factors. Ann Thorac Surg 2001;71:1094-1099.

56. Kirsh MM, Rotman H, Bove E, et al. Major pulmonary resection for bronchogenic carcinoma in the elderly. Ann Thorac Surg 1976;22:369-373.

57. Harpole DH, Liptay MJ, DeCamp MM, Jr., et al. Prospective analysis of pneumonectomy: risk factors for major morbidity and cardiac dysrhythmias. Ann Thorac Surg 1996;61:977-982.

58. Joo JB, DeBord JR, Montgomery CE, et al. Perioperative factors as predictors of operative mortality and morbidity in pneumonectomy. Am Surg 2001;67:318-321; discussion 321-312.

59. Breyer RH, Zippe C, Pharr WF, et al. Thoracotomy in patients over age seventy years: ten-year experience. J Thorac Cardiovasc Surg 1981;81:187-193.

60. Sherman S, Guidot CE. The feasibility of thoracotomy for lung cancer in the elderly. JAMA 1987;258:927-930.

61. O'Rourke MA, Crawford J. Lung cancer in the elderly. Clin Geriatr Med 1987;3:595-623.

62. von Knorring J, Lepantalo M, Lindgren L, Lindfors O. Cardiac arrhythmias and myocardial ischemia after thoracotomy for lung cancer. Ann Thorac Surg 1992;53:642-647.

63. Yano T, Yokoyama H, Fukuyama Y, et al. The current status of postoperative complications and risk factors after a pulmonary resection for primary lung cancer: a multivariate analysis. Eur J Cardiothorac Surg 1997;11:445-449.

64. Asamura H, Naruke T, Tsuchiya R, et al. What are the risk factors for arrhythmias after thoracic operations? A retrospective multivariate analysis of 267 consecutive thoracic operations. J Thorac Cardiovasc Surg 1993;106:1104-1110.

65. Ferguson TB, Jr., Hammill BG, Peterson ED, et al. A decade of change–risk profiles and outcomes for isolated coronary artery bypass grafting procedures, 1990-1999: a report from the STS National Database Committee and the Duke Clinical Research Institute. Society of Thoracic Surgeons. Ann Thorac Surg 2002;73:480-489; discussion 489-490.

66. Tovar EA, Roethe RA, Weissig MD, et al. Muscle-sparing minithoracotomy with intercostal nerve cryoanalgesia: an improved method for major lung resections. Am Surg 1998;64:1109-1115.

67. McKenna RJ, Jr. Thoracoscopic lobectomy with mediastinal sampling in 80-year-old patients. Chest 1994;106:1902-1904.

68. Ishida T, Ishii T, Yamazaki K, et al. Thoracoscopic limited resection of bronchogenic carcinoma in patients over the age of 80. Int Surg 1996;81:237-240.

69. Kaga K, Park J, Nishiumi N, et al. Usefulness of video-assisted thoracic surgery (Two Windows Method) in the treatment of lung cancer for elderly patients. J Cardiovasc Surg (Torino) 1999;40:721-723.

70. Yim AP. Thoracoscopic surgery in the elderly population. Surg Endosc 1996;10:880-882.

71. Asamura H, Nakayama H, Kondo H, et al. Video-assisted lobectomy in the elderly. Chest 1997;111:1101-1105.

72. Shennib HA, Landreneau R, Mulder DS, Mack M. Video-assisted thoracoscopic wedge resection of T1 lung cancer in high-risk patients. Ann Surg 1993;218:555-558; discussion 558-560.

73. McKenna RJ, Jr., Fischel RJ, Wolf R, Wurnig P. Video-assisted thoracic surgery (VATS) lobectomy for bronchogenic carcinoma. Semin Thorac Cardiovasc Surg 1998;10:321-325.

74. Lewis RJ, Caccavale RJ. Video-assisted thoracic surgical non-rib spreading simultaneously stapled lobectomy (VATS(n)SSL). Semin Thorac Cardiovasc Surg 1998;10:332-339.

75. Jaklitsch MT, Bueno R, Swanson SJ, et al. New surgical options for elderly lung cancer patients. Chest 1999;116:480S-485S.

76. Lewis RJ, Caccavale RJ, Bocage JP, Widmann MD. Video-assisted thoracic surgical non-rib spreading simultaneously stapled lobectomy: a more patient-friendly oncologic resection. Chest 1999;116:1119-1124.

77. Kozak LJ, Hall MJ, Owings MF. National Hospital Discharge Survey: 2000 Annual Summary with detailed diagnosis and procedure data. Vital Health Stat 2002;Series 13.

78. Scanlon PD, Connett JE, Waller LA, et al. Smoking cessation and lung function in mild-to-moderate chronic obstructive pulmonary disease. The Lung Health Study. Am J Respir Crit Care Med 2000;161:381-390.

79. Croxton TL, Weinmann GG, Senior RM, Hoidal JR. Future research directions in chronic obstructive pulmonary disease. Am J Respir Crit Care Med 2002;165:838-844.

80. Gavazzi G, Orliaguet O, Coume M, et al. [Thoracic empyema in very old patients: two types of clinical presentation]. Rev Med Interne 2001;22:1124-1127.

81. Chu MW, Dewar LR, Burgess JJ, Busse EG. Empyema thoracis: lack of awareness results in a prolonged clinical course. Can J Surg 2001;44:284-288.

82. Cameron R. Intra-pleural fibrinolytic therapy vs. conservative management in the treatment of parapneumonic effusions and empyema. Cochrane Database Syst Rev 2000;(3):CD002312.

83. Hutter JA, Harari D, Braimbridge MV. The management of empyema thoracis by thoracoscopy and irrigation. Ann Thorac Surg 1985;39:517-520.

84. Landreneau RJ, Keenan RJ, Hazelrigg SR, et al. Thoracoscopy for empyema and hemothorax. Chest 1996;109:18-24.

85. Angelillo-Mackinlay T, Lyons GA, Piedras MB, Angelillo-Mackinlay D. Surgical treatment of postpneumonic empyema. World J Surg 1999;23:1110-1113.

86. Coote N. Surgical versus non-surgical management of pleural empyema. Cochrane Database Syst Rev 2002;(2):CD001956.

87. Greenlee RT, Murray T, Bolden S, Wingo PA. Cancer statistics, 2000. CA Cancer J Clin 2000;50:7-33.

88. Blot WJ, Devesa SS, Kneller RW, Fraumeni JF, Jr. Rising incidence of adenocarcinoma of the esophagus and gastric cardia. JAMA 1991;265:1287-1289.

89. Lund O, Hasenkam JM, Aagaard MT, Kimose HH. Time-related changes in characteristics of prognostic significance in carcinomas of the oesophagus and cardia. Br J Surg 1989;76:1301-1307.

90. Forastiere AA, Heitmiller RF, Kleinberg L. Multimodality therapy for esophageal cancer. Chest 1997;112:195S-200S.

91. Rothwell JF, Feehan E, Reid I, et al. Delay in treatment for oesophageal cancer. Br J Surg 1997;84:690-693.

92. Kirby TJ, Rice TW. The epidemiology of esophageal carcinoma: the changing face of a disease. Chest Surg Clin N Am 1994;4:217-225.

93. Rogot E, Murray JL. Smoking and causes of death among U.S. veterans: 16 years of observation. Public Health Rep 1980;95:213-222.

94. Yu MC, Garabrant DH, Peters JM, Mack TM. Tobacco, alcohol, diet, occupation, and carcinoma of the esophagus. Cancer Res 1988;48:3843-3848.

95. Tuyns AJ. Oesophageal cancer in non-smoking drinkers and in non-drinking smokers. Int J Cancer 1983;32:443-444.
96. Kjaerheim K, Gaard M, Andersen A. The role of alcohol, tobacco, and dietary factors in upper aerogastric tract cancers: a prospective study of 10,900 Norwegian men. Cancer Causes Control 1998;9:99-108.
97. Brown LM, Silverman DT, Pottern LM, et al. Adenocarcinoma of the esophagus and esophagogastric junction in white men in the United States: alcohol, tobacco, and socioeconomic factors. Cancer Causes Control 1994;5:333-340.
98. Gammon MD, Schoenberg JB, Ahsan H, et al. Tobacco, alcohol, and socioeconomic status and adenocarcinomas of the esophagus and gastric cardia. J Natl Cancer Inst 1997;89:1277-1284.
99. Zhang ZF, Kurtz RC, Sun M, et al. Adenocarcinomas of the esophagus and gastric cardia: medical conditions, tobacco, alcohol, and socioeconomic factors. Cancer Epidemiol Biomarkers Prev 1996;5:761-768.
100. Kabat GC, Ng SK, Wynder EL. Tobacco, alcohol intake, and diet in relation to adenocarcinoma of the esophagus and gastric cardia. Cancer Causes Control 1993;4:123-132.
101. Gray JR, Coldman AJ, MacDonald WC. Cigarette and alcohol use in patients with adenocarcinoma of the gastric cardia or lower esophagus. Cancer 1992;69:2227-2231.
102. Brown LM, Swanson CA, Gridley G, et al. Adenocarcinoma of the esophagus: role of obesity and diet. J Natl Cancer Inst 1995;87:104-109.
103. Lagergren J, Bergstrom R, Lindgren A, Nyren O. Symptomatic gastroesophageal reflux as a risk factor for esophageal adenocarcinoma. N Engl J Med 1999;340:825-831.
104. Chow WH, Blot WJ, Vaughan TL, et al. Body mass index and risk of adenocarcinomas of the esophagus and gastric cardia. J Natl Cancer Inst 1998;90:150-155.
105. Cameron AJ, Lomboy CT. Barrett's esophagus: age, prevalence, and extent of columnar epithelium. Gastroenterology 1992;103:1241-1245.
106. Altorki NK, Oliveria S, Schrump DS. Epidemiology and molecular biology of Barrett's adenocarcinoma. Semin Surg Oncol 1997;13:270-280.
107. Spechler SJ, Robbins AH, Rubins HB, et al. Adenocarcinoma and Barrett's esophagus: an overrated risk? Gastroenterology 1984;87:927-933.
108. Skinner DB, Walther BC, Riddell RH, et al. Barrett's esophagus: comparison of benign and malignant cases. Ann Surg 1983;198:554-565.
109. Williamson WA, Ellis FH, Jr., Gibb SP, et al. Barrett's esophagus: prevalence and incidence of adenocarcinoma. Arch Intern Med 1991;151:2212-2216.
110. Cameron AJ, Ott BJ, Payne WS. The incidence of adenocarcinoma in columnar-lined (Barrett's) esophagus. N Engl J Med 1985;313:857-859.
111. Schneider PM, Casson AG, Levin B, et al. Mutations of p53 in Barrett's esophagus and Barrett's cancer: a prospective study of ninety-eight cases. J Thorac Cardiovasc Surg 1996;111:323-331; discussion 331-323.
112. D'Amico TA, Harpole DH, Jr. Molecular biology of esophageal cancer. Chest Surg Clin N Am 2000;10:451-469.
113. Singh SP, Lipman J, Goldman H, et al. Loss or altered subcellular localization of p27 in Barrett's associated adenocarcinoma. Cancer Res 1998;58:1730-1735.
114. Blot WJ, Fraumeni JF, Jr. Trends in esophageal cancer mortality among US blacks and whites. Am J Public Health 1987;77:296-298.
115. Bytzer P, Christensen PB, Damkier P, et al. Adenocarcinoma of the esophagus and Barrett's esophagus: a population-based study. Am J Gastroenterol 1999;94:86-91.
116. Heitmiller RF, Redmond M, Hamilton SR. Barrett's esophagus with high-grade dysplasia: an indication for prophylactic esophagectomy. Ann Surg 1996;224:66-71.
117. Moran EM. Epidemiological and clinical aspects of nonsteroidal anti-inflammatory drugs and cancer risks. J Environ Pathol Toxicol Oncol 2002;21:193-201.

118. Buttar NS, Wang KK, Leontovich O, et al. Chemoprevention of esophageal adenocarcinoma by COX-2 inhibitors in an animal model of Barrett's esophagus. Gastroenterology 2002;122:1101-1112.

119. Kaur BS, Khamnehei N, Iravani M, et al. Rofecoxib inhibits cyclooxygenase 2 expression and activity and reduces cell proliferation in Barrett's esophagus. Gastroenterology 2002;123:60-67.

120. Lin P, Chen Z, Hou J, et al. [Chemoprevention of esophageal cancer]. Zhongguo Yi Xue Ke Xue Yuan Xue Bao 1998;20:413-418.

121. Krasna MJ. Surgical staging and surgical treatment in esophageal cancer. Semin Oncol 1999;26:9-11.

122. Visbal AL, Allen MS, Miller DL, et al. Ivor Lewis esophagogastrectomy for esophageal cancer. Ann Thorac Surg 2001;71:1803-1808.

123. Jauch KW, Bacha EA, Denecke H, et al. Esophageal carcinoma: prognostic features and comparison between blunt transhiatal dissection and transthoracic resection. Eur J Surg Oncol 1992;18:553-562.

124. Bolton JS, Sardi A, Bowen JC, Ellis JK. Transhiatal and transthoracic esophagectomy: a comparative study. J Surg Oncol 1992;51:249-253.

125. Goldminc M, Maddern G, Le Prise E, et al. Oesophagectomy by a transhiatal approach or thoracotomy: a prospective randomized trial. Br J Surg 1993;80:367-370.

126. Horstmann O, Verreet PR, Becker H, et al. Transhiatal oesophagectomy compared with transthoracic resection and systematic lymphadenectomy for the treatment of oesophageal cancer. Eur J Surg 1995;161:557-567.

127. Putnam JB, Jr., Suell DM, McMurtrey MJ, et al. Comparison of three techniques of esophagectomy within a residency training program. Ann Thorac Surg 1994;57:319-325.

128. Jacobi CA, Zieren HU, Muller JM, Pichlmaier H. Surgical therapy of esophageal carcinoma: the influence of surgical approach and esophageal resection on cardiopulmonary function. Eur J Cardiothorac Surg 1997;11:32-37.

129. Millikan KW, Silverstein J, Hart V, et al. A 15-year review of esophagectomy for carcinoma of the esophagus and cardia. Arch Surg 1995;130:617-624.

130. Gluch L, Smith RC, Bambach CP, Brown AR. Comparison of outcomes following transhiatal or Ivor Lewis esophagectomy for esophageal carcinoma. World J Surg 1999;23:271-275; discussion 275-276.

131. Mafune KI, Tanaka Y, Takubo K. Autopsy findings in patients with esophageal carcinoma: comparison between resection and nonresection groups. J Surg Oncol 2000;74:196-200.

132. Hulscher JB, van Sandick JW, Tijssen JG, et al. The recurrence pattern of esophageal carcinoma after transhiatal resection. J Am Coll Surg 2000;191:143-148.

133. Blewett CJ, Miller JD, Young JE, et al. Anastomotic leaks after esophagectomy for esophageal cancer: a comparison of thoracic and cervical anastomoses. Ann Thorac Cardiovasc Surg 2001;7:75-78.

134. Honkoop P, Siersema PD, Tilanus HW, et al. Benign anastomotic strictures after transhiatal esophagectomy and cervical esophagogastrostomy: risk factors and management. J Thorac Cardiovasc Surg 1996;111:1141-1146; discussion 1147-1148.

135. Orringer MB, Marshall B, Iannettoni MD. Eliminating the cervical esophagogastric anastomotic leak with a side-to-side stapled anastomosis. J Thorac Cardiovasc Surg 2000;119:277-288.

136. Orringer MB, Marshall B, Iannettoni MD. Transhiatal esophagectomy: clinical experience and refinements. Ann Surg 1999;230:392-400; discussion 400-393.

137. Tilanus HW, Hop WC, Langenhorst BL, van Lanschot JJ. Esophagectomy with or without thoracotomy: is there any difference? J Thorac Cardiovasc Surg 1993;105:898-903.

138. Bolton JS, Ochsner JL, Abdoh AA. Surgical management of esophageal cancer: a decade of change. Ann Surg 1994;219:475-480.

139. Tsutsui S, Moriguchi S, Morita M, et al. Multivariate analysis of postoperative complications after esophageal resection. Ann Thorac Surg 1992;53:1052-1056.

140. Finlayson EV, Birkmeyer JD. Operative mortality with elective surgery in older adults. Eff Clin Pract 2001;4:172-177.

141. Ferguson MK, Martin TR, Reeder LB, Olak J. Mortality after esophagectomy: risk factor analysis. World J Surg 1997;21:599-603; discussion 603-594.

142. Poon RT, Law SY, Chu KM, et al. Esophagectomy for carcinoma of the esophagus in the elderly: results of current surgical management. Ann Surg 1998;227:357-364.

143. Alexiou C, Beggs D, Salama FD, et al. Surgery for esophageal cancer in elderly patients: the view from Nottingham. J Thorac Cardiovasc Surg 1998;116:545-553.

144. Jougon JB, Ballester M, Duffy J, et al. Esophagectomy for cancer in the patient aged 70 years and older. Ann Thorac Surg 1997;63:1423-1427.

145. Chino O, Makuuchi H, Machimura T, et al. Treatment of esophageal cancer in patients over 80 years old. Surg Today 1997;27:9-16.

146. Xijiang Z, Xizeng Z, Xishan H, Hongjing J. Surgical treatment for carcinoma of the esophagus in the elderly patient. Ann Thorac Cardiovasc Surg 1999;5:182-186.

147. Naunheim KS, Hanosh J, Zwischenberger J, et al. Esophagectomy in the septuagenarian. Ann Thorac Surg 1993;56:880-883; discussion 883-884.

148. Thomas P, Doddoli C, Neville P, et al. Esophageal cancer resection in the elderly. Eur J Cardiothorac Surg 1996;10:941-946.

149. Adam DJ, Craig SR, Sang CT, et al. Esophagectomy for carcinoma in the octogenarian. Ann Thorac Surg 1996;61:190-194.

150. Karl RC, Smith SK, Fabri PJ. Validity of major cancer operations in elderly patients. Ann Surg Oncol 1995;2:107-113.

151. Luketich JD, Nguyen NT, Weigel T, et al. Minimally invasive approach to esophagectomy. JSLS 1998;2:243-247.

152. Watson DI, Davies N, Jamieson GG. Totally endoscopic Ivor Lewis esophagectomy. Surg Endosc 1999;13:293-297.

153. Peracchia A, Rosati R, Fumagalli U, et al. Thoracoscopic esophagectomy: are there benefits? Semin Surg Oncol 1997;13:259-262.

154. Luketich JD, Schauer PR, Christie NA, et al. Minimally invasive esophagectomy. Ann Thorac Surg 2000;70:906-911; discussion 911-902.

155. Noguchi H, Naomoto Y, Kondo H, et al. Evaluation of endoscopic mucosal resection for superficial esophageal carcinoma. Surg Laparosc Endosc Percutan Tech 2000;10:343-350.

156. Ell C, May A, Gossner L, et al. Endoscopic mucosal resection of early cancer and high-grade dysplasia in Barrett's esophagus. Gastroenterology 2000;118:670-677.

157. Brodner G, Pogatzki E, Van Aken H, et al. A multimodal approach to control postoperative pathophysiology and rehabilitation in patients undergoing abdominothoracic esophagectomy. Anesth Analg 1998;86:228-234.

158. Sabanathan S, Shah R, Tsiamis A, Richardson J. Oesophagogastrectomy in the elderly high risk patients: role of effective regional analgesia and early mobilisation. J Cardiovasc Surg (Torino) 1999;40:153-156.

159. Flisberg P, Tornebrandt K, Walther B, Lundberg J. Pain relief after esophagectomy: thoracic epidural analgesia is better than parenteral opioids. J Cardiothorac Vasc Anesth 2001;15:282-287.

160. Nguyen NT, Follette DM, Wolfe BM, et al. Comparison of minimally invasive esophagectomy with transthoracic and transhiatal esophagectomy. Arch Surg 2000;135:920-925.

161. Fernando HC, Christie NA, Luketich JD. Thoracoscopic and laparoscopic esophagectomy. Semin Thorac Cardiovasc Surg 2000;12:195-200.

162. Chan A, Wong A. Is combined chemotherapy and radiation therapy equally effective as surgical resection in localized esophageal carcinoma? Int J Radiat Oncol Biol Phys 1999;45:265-270.

163. Gillinov AM, Heitmiller RF. Strategies to reduce pulmonary complications after transhiatal esophagectomy. Dis Esophagus 1998;11:43-47.

164. Zehr KJ, Dawson PB, Yang SC, Heitmiller RF. Standardized clinical care pathways for major thoracic cases reduce hospital costs. Ann Thorac Surg 1998;66:914-919.

165. Baba M, Aikou T, Natsugoe S, et al. Quality of life following esophagectomy with three-field lymphadenectomy for carcinoma, focusing on its relationship to vocal cord palsy. Dis Esophagus 1998;11:28-34.

166. Suzuki H, Abo S, Kitamura M, et al. An evaluation of symptoms and performance status in patients after esophagectomy for esophageal cancer from the viewpoint of the patient. Am Surg 1994;60:920-923.

167. Collard JM, Otte JB, Reynaert M, Kestens PJ. Quality of life three years or more after esophagectomy for cancer. J Thorac Cardiovasc Surg 1992;104:391-394.

168. De Leyn P, Coosemans W, Lerut T. Early and late functional results in patients with intrathoracic gastric replacement after oesophagectomy for carcinoma. Eur J Cardiothorac Surg 1992;6:79-84; discussion 85.

169. Blazeby JM, Alderson D, Farndon JR. Quality of life in patients with oesophageal cancer. Recent Results Cancer Res 2000;155:193-204.

170. Blazeby JM, Brookes ST, Alderson D. Prognostic value of quality of life scores in patients with oesophageal cancer. Br J Surg 2000;87:362-373.

171. Blazeby JM, Farndon JR, Donovan J, Alderson D. A prospective longitudinal study examining the quality of life of patients with esophageal carcinoma. Cancer 2000;88:1781-1787.

172. McLarty AJ, Deschamps C, Trastek VF, et al. Esophageal resection for cancer of the esophagus: long-term function and quality of life. Ann Thorac Surg 1997;63:1568-1572.

173. Johansson J, Walther B. Clinical outcome and long-term survival rates after esophagectomy are not determined by age over 70 years. J Gastrointest Surg 2000;4:55-62.

174. Young MM, Deschamps C, Allen MS, et al. Esophageal reconstruction for benign disease: self-assessment of functional outcome and quality of life. Ann Thorac Surg 2000;70:1799-1802.

175. Young MM, Deschamps C, Trastek VF, et al. Esophageal reconstruction for benign disease: early morbidity, mortality, and functional results. Ann Thorac Surg 2000;70:1651-1655.

176. van Lanschot JJ, Hulscher JB, Buskens CJ, et al. Hospital volume and hospital mortality for esophagectomy. Cancer 2001;91:1574-1578.

177. Patti MG, Corvera CU, Glasgow RE, Way LW. A hospital's annual rate of esophagectomy influences the operative mortality rate. J Gastrointest Surg 1998;2:186-192.

178. Begg CB, Cramer LD, Hoskins WJ, Brennan MF. Impact of hospital volume on operative mortality for major cancer surgery. JAMA 1998;280:1747-1751.

179. Dimick JB, Cattaneo SM, Lipsett PA, et al. Hospital volume is related to clinical and economic outcomes of esophageal resection in Maryland. Ann Thorac Surg 2001;72:334-339; discussion 339-341.

180. Swisher SG, Deford L, Merriman KW, et al. Effect of operative volume on morbidity, mortality, and hospital use after esophagectomy for cancer. J Thorac Cardiovasc Surg 2000;119:1126-1132.

181. Wade PR. Aging and neural control of the GI tract. I. Age-related changes in the enteric nervous system. Am J Physiol Gastrointest Liver Physiol 2002;283:G489-G495.

182. Schindler JS, Kelly JH. Swallowing disorders in the elderly. Laryngoscope 2002;112:589-602.

183. Sarani B, Scanlon J, Jackson P, Evans SR. Selection criteria among gastroenterologists and surgeons for laparoscopic antireflux surgery. Surg Endosc 2002;16:57-63.
184. Trus TL, Laycock WS, Wo JM, et al. Laparoscopic antireflux surgery in the elderly. Am J Gastroenterol 1998;93:351-353.
185. Brunt LM, Quasebarth MA, Dunnegan DL, Soper NJ. Is laparoscopic antireflux surgery for gastroesophageal reflux disease in the elderly safe and effective? Surg Endosc 1999;13:838-842.
186. Kamolz T, Bammer T, Granderath FA, et al. Quality of life and surgical outcome after laparoscopic antireflux surgery in the elderly gastroesophageal reflux disease patient. Scand J Gastroenterol 2001;36:116-120.
187. Bammer T, Hinder RA, Klaus A, et al. Safety and long-term outcome of laparoscopic antireflux surgery in patients in their eighties and older. Surg Endosc 2002;16:40-42.
188. Khajanchee YS, Urbach DR, Butler N, et al. Laparoscopic antireflux surgery in the elderly. Surg Endosc 2002;16:25-30.
189. Kamolz T, Granderath FA, Bammer T, et al. Failed antireflux surgery: surgical outcome of laparoscopic refundoplication in the elderly. Hepatogastroenterology 2002;49:865-868.

6
GERIATRIC CARDIAC SURGERY

Nicola Francalancia, MD; Joseph LoCicero III, MD, FACS*

Cardiovascular disease is the leading cause of death in the United States; 84% of deaths from cardiovascular disease occur in people aged 65 and older. [1] The health care of the geriatric patient population includes a growing number of cardiothoracic surgical interventions intended to improve the quality of life of older persons, and the challenges of providing surgical therapy for coronary and valvular diseases in older patients are increasing.

METHODS

To identify issues that will affect decisions about the role and potential benefits of surgery for heart disease, we reviewed the current body of knowledge in the field of cardiac surgery for the geriatric patient. We searched the National Library of Medicine's PubMed database for the period from 1994 to April 6, 2001. The time frame was narrower than for many other of the topics covered by this project because examination of initial search results indicated that only the more recent references were relevant. The search strategy combined terms for specified cardiac surgical procedures with terms for complications, and it was further qualified by adding the various terms for risk factors, age factors, outcomes, quality of life, and rehabilitation. The search resulted in 1799 references. From among the relevant papers, we chose those that emphasize the management of such issues as perioperative care, postoperative complications, and quality of life for the elderly cardiac surgical patient. Age as a risk factor for specific cardiac surgical procedures was also examined.

THE CHANGING PATTERN OF PATIENTS UNDERGOING HEART SURGERY

The characteristics of patients undergoing heart surgery have changed over time. The patients undergoing operations for coronary artery disease (CAD) and valve replacement or repair are now older, with more comorbid conditions. Warner et al prospectively studied and compared 23,512 patients undergoing coronary artery bypass grafting (CABG) during three time periods from 1981 to 1995. [2] The mean age and the percentage of patients aged 65 years or older were significantly higher in the later time periods. In a multivariate analysis for predictors of mortality, these researchers found that patients aged 65 and older in the more recent cohort of patients had an odds ratio of 2.7 for mortality. Patients aged 80 and over were found to have a significantly higher risk of any complication with surgery, including neurologic events, pneumonia, arrhythmias, or wound infection. Other researchers reviewed aortic and mitral valve replacements in 2898 patients over two separate 4-year periods. [3] The later group had significantly more patients with preoperative

* Francalancia: Associate Professor of Surgery, Department of Surgery, Division of Cardiothoracic Surgery, University of Massachusetts Medical School, Worcester, MA; LoCicero: The Point Clear Charities Professor, Chair of Surgery, Director of the Center for Clinical Oncology, Director of the Center for Interventional Technologies, The University of South Alabama, Mobile, AL.

risk factors for mortality and low cardiac output syndrome. Patients in the later group were more likely to be aged 70 or older. A prospective analysis of 4839 CABG procedures over three time periods by Abramov et al showed a time-related increase in severity of preoperative risk profile. [4] Age, urgent surgery, chronic renal failure, peripheral vascular disease, and prior CABG were found to be independent predictors of operative morbidity and mortality. These authors suggest the revision and expansion of criteria for CABG referral.

The mortality rate for patients aged 65 and over was shown to be higher than that for younger patients (6.1% versus 3.5%). [5] Risk factors for in-hospital death after heart surgery among elderly patients include diabetes mellitus, hypertension, myocardial infarction, and congestive heart failure. Retrospective multivariate analysis of 436 patients aged 75 or older who underwent cardiac surgery at a single institution showed that emergency operation, renal dysfunction, and cardiomegaly negatively influence hospital survival. [6]

Decisions regarding resource allocation for future health care delivery to older people must acknowledge the impact of heart disease on cost. Patients with multivessel CAD and diabetes mellitus have higher costs of care with greater length of stay. In a retrospective analysis, Culler et al demonstrated this effect, with age being one of eight important factors that contribute to these costs. [7]

A common misconception among clinicians treating elderly patients is that advanced age alone precludes aggressive interventions, including surgical therapies. An older patient with myocardial ischemia may receive either less aggressive or delayed intervention wherever this bias persists. Bearden et al demonstrated this when they observed that when patients enrolled in a multicenter hypertension study developed CAD, the elderly patients, regardless of comorbid conditions, socioeconomic status, and social support, are offered cardiac interventions that are less intensive than those offered to younger patients. [8] Similarly, according to a study by Paul et al, [9] elderly patients who sustain acute myocardial infarctions are often treated less aggressively. These researchers noted that, despite higher rates of mortality among elderly patients (19% versus 5%), younger patients are three times as likely to undergo percutaneous transluminal coronary angioplasty (PTCA) or CABG.

The treatment of cardiovascular diseases in elderly persons consists largely of the management of symptoms and sequelae of atherosclerotic disease. Initial management at the primary care level consists of risk reduction to minimize onset and progression of atheromatous disease. When surgical intervention is required, atheromatous disease of the aorta may be encountered, a condition that may increase the risk of emboli and stroke. Protruding atheromas have a higher incidence in patients aged 60 and over. [10] Trehan et al examined 6138 patients undergoing CABG and formulated specific surgical approaches for patients with evidence of carotid and aortic atheromatous disease to attain low rates of stroke. [11] Detection of atheromatous disease by carotid screening and intraoperative transesophageal echocardiography may contribute to risk adjustment and surgical planning for a growing number of elderly patients with extensive vascular disease.

The medical community has appropriately emphasized the need for improved treatment of congestive heart failure in elderly patients. The best surgical option for end-stage heart failure, however, after correction of ischemic states or repair of valvular dysfunction, consists of cardiac transplantation. The limitations of this therapy, particularly for elderly patients, are well known; older age negatively influences candidacy for transplantation, as demand for suitable organs far outweighs supply. Pennington et al note that older age affects transplant candidacy, noting that only 3.2% of patients listed for cardiac transplantation in 1995 were 65 years or older.[12] An aging population will potentially increase the demand for donor organs if the upper age limit for candidacy for transplantation is increased. Therefore, one additional surgical strategy to be considered is implantation of permanent ventricular assist devices into the growing number of patients who will present with end-stage congestive heart failure with little or no option of undergoing cardiac transplantation. This approach will require further experience in the use of cardiac assist devices in the elderly patient population to identify those who have potential for improvement in quality of life with the ultimate cardiac therapy—permanent cardiac replacement with a mechanical device.

An important component of providing surgical therapy to all elderly patients with cardiac disease is acknowledgment of age-specific changes in cardiac response to ischemia or stress. Clinical studies show that elderly patients with CAD have lower left ventricular pump performance and efficiency than do younger patients.[13] Patients aged 70 and over have also been shown to have a reduction in myocardial perfusion reserve.[14] The presence of angina before an acute myocardial infarction does not appear to confer the protection against in-hospital death in patients aged 65 and over that it has been shown to offer for younger patients, which suggests the possible loss of ischemic preconditioning in the senescent myocardium.[15] Animal studies that demonstrate variance between adult and senescent myocardial response to blood cardioplegia, which is commonly used for clinical heart surgery, suggest that strategies for myocardial protection may need to be reexamined if the less contractile hearts of elderly patients are to be accommodated.[16] The understanding of aging as a physiologic response has profound ramifications in cardiac surgery as it relates to varied clinical presentation of disease, recovery from reperfused states, and maintenance of perioperative hemodynamic stability.

Further research in geriatric cardiac surgery is needed to accurately define the populations at risk for heart disease and the indications for surgical evaluation. This will require institutional and multicenter databases that allow cardiac surgeons to monitor outcomes. Specific areas of investigation include the following:

> *CardiacSurg 1 (Level B)*: **Risk profiles must be revised to accurately reflect current medical and surgical practices with regard to advanced age and heart surgery. Existing databases must be expanded to include functional outcomes in elderly patients and to monitor cardiac care patterns for elderly patients. This will yield important outcome data to guide clinical decision making for the aging population.**

> *CardiacSurg 2 (Level A)*: **Intervention studies (clinical trials) of specific geriatric clinical pathways in cardiac surgery are needed to identify possible beneficial effects on outcomes.**

> *CardiacSurg 3 (Level D)*: **Methods for estimating future total costs of cardiac surgery in elderly patients, including the perioperative and rehabilitative periods, need to be developed.**

> *CardiacSurg 4 (Level A)*: **Multicenter randomized controlled trials comparing catheter-based interventions and coronary artery bypass**

grafting for the treatment of coronary artery disease in geriatric cardiac patients is needed.

CardiacSurg 5 (Level D): Studies are needed to review resources that accommodate potentially longer hospital stays by elderly heart surgery patients who present with greater acuity and complications following surgery.

CardiacSurg 6 (Level B): Predictive models are needed to estimate the numbers of patients with risk factors for heart disease who may ultimately require surgical care (eg, the current diabetic population that will require surgery in their 60s through their 80s).

CardiacSurg 7 (Level B): Prospective cohort studies are needed that investigate the potential role of cardiac assist devices in the treatment of congestive heart failure in elderly patients deemed unlikely to undergo heart transplantation.

CardiacSurg 8 (Level B): Further investigation of the senescent myocardium and age-specific physiologic response to stress is needed to identify reasons for pump failure or for low-output syndrome.

CORONARY ARTERY DISEASE

Advances in the treatment of CAD, including early intervention, prevention, risk modification, and general public awareness, have resulted in improved clinical outcomes in myocardial ischemia. For patients who present with acute coronary syndromes, early reperfusion to myocardium at risk is considered the standard of care. The benefit of reperfusion in elderly patients (aged 75 or older) was shown by Gottlieb et al in a comparison of two cohorts (1981–1983, 1992–1994) of patients who had sustained acute myocardial infarction. [17] The more recent cohort of elderly patients who received thrombolysis, angioplasty, or CABG were found to have fewer in-hospital complications and mortality rates approximately 30% lower than those of the earlier cohort of patients. The treatment of CAD for all patient populations, however, has dramatically changed over time. The availability of new interventional techniques and drug therapies necessitate a re-evaluation of the care of elderly cardiac patients to determine the benefit that is specific to this group at risk.

Stouffer et al noted in a comparison of older and younger patients that age influences the risk factors but not the clinical signs and symptoms of left main CAD. [18] The older CABG patients (N = 798, mean age 59) were found to have significantly greater incidence of hypertension, obesity, and prior myocardial infarction than did the younger CABG patients (N = 112, mean age 40). [19]

Surgical revascularization continues to play an important role in treating older people with CAD. CABG is the operation performed most frequently by most cardiac surgeons. The typical CABG patient, however, may have already exhausted other medical options for symptomatic angina or heart failure. Aldea et al examined patients undergoing CABG or percutaneous intervention and noted that the CABG patients generally are older. [20] Harris et al retrospectively studied 7099 patients at Mayo Clinic treated with CABG and

4937 who underwent coronary angioplasty over a 10-year period (divided into three equal intervals). [21] Operative mortality rates for both procedures changed little over the study period despite the significantly greater number of patients aged 65 and over undergoing both procedures in the later time periods. These researchers noted an increase from 23% to 84% in the use of the internal mammary artery as a bypass conduit in the latest period. They also noted the trend for CABG to be performed more often following acute myocardial infarction or as an emergency operation for unstable angina. In a retrospective analysis, O'Keefe et al compared two concurrent cohorts of patients aged 70 and over who underwent either coronary angioplasty or CABG. [22] The groups were found to have similar rates of survival over 5 years; however, patients undergoing angioplasty were found to have significantly greater numbers of cardiac events, including Q-wave myocardial infarction, repeat revascularization, CABG, or angioplasty than did those treated by CABG initially. This suggests that this older group of patients had greater freedom from repeated revascularization when treated with CABG.

In a retrospective analysis over a 2-year period of 109 patients aged 70 and over who presented with refractory angina, Vassilikos et al showed that the patients who were revascularized by CABG had better long-term outcomes than did those treated by angioplasty. [23] The patients who underwent CABG had fewer events, such as the need for repeat revascularization or the development of myocardial infarctions. The study confirms and strengthens the earlier findings by O'Keefe. In the more recent study, the selection of procedure, however, was determined by the cardiologist; at the time of the study, coronary stents were not routinely used in conjunction with angioplasty.

In the Bypass Angioplasty Revascularization Investigation (BARI) trial where 1829 patients were randomly assigned to either undergo CABG or PTCA, 39% of patients were aged 65 and over at the start of the trial. [24] Cardiac mortality was shown to be greater at 5 years in the patients undergoing PTCA, although there was no difference when nondiabetic patients were excluded from the analysis. For older patients in that trial, stroke was more common after CABG than for younger patients (1.7% versus 0.2%). Older patients in the trial were found to have less recurrent angina and to be less likely to undergo repeat procedures if they initially underwent CABG.

As percutaneous coronary interventional techniques have improved with the development of intracoronary stents, studies to compare CABG and angioplasty with stent placement have become necessary to appropriately compare current treatment modalities for CAD. In a study of 1200 patients randomized to undergo either CABG or stent placement for multivessel CAD, Serruys et al noted no significant difference between the rates of death, stroke, or myocardial infarction between the two treatment groups. [25] At 1 year, however, a second revascularization was required by 16.8% of those in the stenting group but only by 3.5% of those who underwent CABG. The two groups were similar with respect to age (mean age = 61 years in both groups). Patients in the CABG group showed greater freedom from angina at 1 year than the stenting group. In a study of 200 patients with normal left ventricular function, Kim et al showed similar results in CABG and multivessel coronary stenting. [26] Angina returned in 19% of the stenting group but only 8% of the CABG group. Repeat revascularization was required in 19% of the stenting group and 2% of the CABG group at mean follow-up of 21 ± 10 months, despite the fact that ventricular function was normal in all patients upon enrollment.

The use of coronary stents in elderly patients has also been studied. Ritchie et al examined the impact of stents on the management of CAD in the Medicare population over time periods when stent use became more widespread. [27] The study showed that patients who have stents have lower hospital mortality and less same-admission CABG than patients having angioplasty alone. Munoz et al compared coronary stenting in patients older than 75 years to that in a younger cohort of patients. [28] A similar incidence of major adverse cardiac events (27.7% versus 28.2%) was observed in the two groups of patients. Long-term event-free survival rates also showed no differences at 5 years between the two groups. The older group of patients, however, were found to present more often with multivessel coronary disease and lower ejection fractions, and more frequently to have unstable angina. The older patient group showed a significantly higher in-hospital mortality rate (6.6% versus 2.4%) and rate of myocardial infarction (5.3% versus 1.7%) than did the stented patients aged 75 or younger.

In another study, patients undergoing isolated CABG between 1970 and 1989 demonstrated stable perioperative mortality rates. [29] However, temporal trends showed an increased number of patients older than 65 and a greater number of emergency operations. In this study, the leading cause of death was found to be cardiac pump failure and postoperative myocardial infarction, both occurring more commonly in older patients. Elderly patients undergoing CABG present with a higher frequency of hypertension, hyperlipidemia, prior myocardial infarction, and diabetes mellitus. These patients more often present with unstable angina and diffuse coronary artery disease. [30] The operative mortality for CABG among elderly patients has declined, however. Ivanov et al showed in examination of 3330 consecutive patients aged 70 and over that the prevalence of high-risk elderly patients rises over time and that poor ventricular function, diabetes, female sex, prior CABG, and peripheral vascular disease are independent predictors for poor outcome among elderly patients. [31]

Hannan and Burke demonstrated increased in-hospital mortality for elderly patients by reviewing the 30,972 CABG procedures performed in New York State in 1991 and 1992. [32] Patients aged 80 and over had mortality of 8.31%. The group aged 75 to 79 had mortality of 5.28%. These data were compared with the mortality rates of 1.10%, 1.65%, 2.17%, 2.76%, and 3.36% for ages 40–49, 50–59, 60–64, 65–69, and 70–74, respectively. The mortality rates for 33 risk factors were found to be higher in patients aged 75 and over than in younger patients. These factors include emergency surgery (14.08% versus 5.73% mortality), hemodynamic instability (23.45% versus 9.52% mortality), and renal failure (21.34% versus 10.35% mortality).

Peigh et al examined the records of 250 patients undergoing isolated CABG who were divided into five age groups and found that the elderly patients had more complications, a longer length of hospital stay, and a higher mortality rate than did the younger patients. [33] In addition, the older patients had a reduced performance status measured by the Karnofsky scale. However, in a retrospective analysis by Ott et al of patients undergoing CABG, the mortality rates and postoperative complications were not found to be significantly different in a group of patients aged 70 or over and in a younger group. [34] This study emphasized the application of a rapid recovery protocol. Such protocols feature rapid extubation, aggressive fluid management, and early patient mobilization. Using data collected prospectively from 20,614 patients undergoing isolated CABG from 1982 to 1997, Yau et al showed that age, reoperation, ventricular dysfunction, operative urgency, and left main coronary artery disease are predictors of mortality for coronary artery bypass. [35] The prevalence of patients with moderate ventricular dysfunction (left ventricular ejection fraction 20% to 40%) increased from 18.4% in 1982–1986 to 21.7% in 1992–1997. Mortality decreased from the 1982–1986 cohort to the 1987–1991 cohort; the reduction in mortality was most marked in patients with ejection fraction of under 40%.

Other studies have shown some specific increased risk profiles in elderly patients undergoing surgical revascularization. CABG following acute myocardial infarction carries added risk for mortality. Kaul et al observed that age above 70 years is an independent predictor of early mortality for patients who undergo CABG within 30 days of an acute myocardial infarction. [36] In a study of over 4500 patients undergoing CABG at the Toronto Hospital, patients who had low-output syndrome were found to have a greater mortality (16.9% versus 0.9%). Importantly, one of the nine independent predictors of developing low-output syndrome was found to be age above 70 years, resulting in an odds ratio increase of 1.5. [37] This suggests that efforts to reduce myocardial ischemia, a known precipitating factor for low-output syndrome, should be investigated, with particular emphasis on the aging myocardium. In multivariate analysis of 2264 patients undergoing CABG, Del Rizzo et al noted that age above 70, re-do surgery, poor left ventricular function, renal impairment, and the presence of preoperative intra-aortic balloon pump are predictors of mortality. [38]

In a retrospective study of 1127 patients aged 70 years and over who underwent CABG between 1985 and 1996, Busch et al noted that, despite a decreased number of emergent operations, the incidence of respiratory failure and neurologic disorders rose over that period. [39] They also observed that the percentage of septuagenarians operated upon rose from 6.4% in 1985 to 21.5% in 1996.

Technical aspects of the operation have been investigated in an attempt to identify strategies that would improve outcome and long-term survival or minimize morbidity for CABG. The use of bilateral grafting with skeletonized internal thoracic arteries in elderly patients was found to result in low morbidity and mortality. [40] Elderly patients undergoing CABG who received internal mammary artery grafting were found to have fewer postoperative complications. [41] Among elderly patients who receive internal mammary artery grafting, other factors such as smoking, reoperation, or left main coronary artery disease are risk factors for mortality. [42] In a study to improve outcomes in an elderly high-risk CABG patient population, Gutfinger et al showed that liberal use of preoperative intra-aortic balloon pump could be performed safely with no significant increase in complication or mortality rates. [43]

For elderly patients undergoing CABG, time to recovery may determine needs for postoperative resources and rehospitalization. Paone et al studied 146 patients aged 70 and over with the expectation that these patients would progress through the postoperative clinical pathway in much the same way as a younger comparison group. [44] Although age was one significant factor in contributing to increased length of stay, the study suggests that extraordinary modifications of the clinical pathways are not necessary for success with elderly patients. Advanced age was not found to be significantly associated with 30-day hospital readmission following CABG. [45]

Samuels et al identified a group of older patients at particularly high risk for mortality following CABG. [46] In patients aged 75 and older with chronic obstructive pulmonary disease (COPD) who are receiving corticosteroid therapy, mortality was 50%. Older patients with COPD not receiving steroids had a mortality rate of 17%. These data support investigation into nonsurgical therapy for elderly patients with severe COPD.

Recently, cardiac surgeons have used minimally invasive techniques to perform cardiac operations in an effort to reduce morbidity and decrease hospital stay and postoperative recovery period. These novel methods include coronary artery bypass performed on a beating heart and without the use of cardiopulmonary bypass (off-pump coronary artery bypass). The avoidance of cardiopulmonary bypass may reduce morbidity that has been attributed to inflammatory responses and fluid shifts known to occur with extracorporeal circulation.

Two cohorts of elderly CABG patients were compared by Boyd et al. [47] Off-pump patients were found to have significantly shorter hospital stay, intensive care unit stay, and rates of postoperative atrial fibrillation than did conventional CABG patients. Koutlas et al showed that two groups of patients aged 75 or over, those who underwent beating-heart coronary artery bypass surgery and those who underwent conventional CABG, had similar neurologic complications, renal failure, rates of atrial fibrillation, and rates of postoperative myocardial infarction. [48] These researchers noted significantly shorter postoperative length of stay, lower transfusion rates, and a lower mortality rate in the beating-heart surgery group.

Yokoyama et al studied high-risk groups undergoing off-pump and on-pump CABG. [49] They found that off-pump and on-pump CABG have comparable results in the high-risk group consisting of patients 80 years of age or older. They noted that off-pump CABG reduces but does not eliminate neurologic events in elderly patients. Other methods for adapting conventional operations are being performed, including port-access operations where percutaneous cannulation techniques and limited incisions are used in an attempt to limit surgical trauma. Such adaptations do not eliminate the use of cardiopulmonary bypass, but these techniques are rapidly evolving as tools that potentially reduce the morbidity of open cardiac procedures.

Research in coronary artery surgery should continue to focus on technical aspects of the operations that allow safer perioperative management of the elderly CABG patient. Recent studies indicate that coronary revascularization can often be safely performed by novel techniques that may avoid use of cardiopulmonary bypass. Cardiac surgical specialists are also active in the investigation of other therapies intended to ameliorate the symptoms of coronary artery disease. This includes transmyocardial laser revascularization and gene therapy for inoperable CAD. As medical and surgical options for the treatment of coronary artery disease expand, treatments that benefit elderly patients should be investigated to determine suitability on the basis of outcomes in this patient population. Potential areas of investigation for cardiac surgery include the following:

CardiacSurg 9 (Level B): **Prospective studies of young and elderly patients are needed to investigate lung function as a risk for coronary artery bypass grafting by determining the degree of pulmonary compromise that would shift risk from surgical to medical management of coronary artery disease.**

CardiacSurg 10 (Level B): **Cohort studies on various cardiopulmonary bypass techniques are needed, with morbidity in elderly patients as the chief outcome measure.**

CardiacSurg 11 (Level A): Randomized controlled trials are needed that select the most promising cardiopulmonary bypass techniques and compare them, again with morbidity in elderly patients as the chief outcome measure.

CardiacSurg 12 (Level B): Cohort studies are needed to identify risk factors and benefit predictors of myocardial protective techniques for both on- and off-pump coronary artery bypass in elderly patients. This includes myocardial protective strategies aimed specifically at the aged myocardium and mechanical or chemical protective techniques when off-pump procedures are used.

CardiacSurg 13 (Level A): Randomized controlled trials are needed that select the most promising myocardial protective techniques and compare them with each other and with traditional bypass techniques; morbidity, need for reintervention, and relief of symptoms in elderly patients should be the main outcome measures. The best on-pump method could also be compared with the best off-pump method.

CardiacSurg 14 (Level B): Cohort studies are needed of innovative and emerging therapies for coronary artery disease (eg, gene therapy, transmyocardial laser revascularization), as well as of other complementary treatments in the elderly patient population.

CardiacSurg 15 (Level B): Cohort studies are needed to investigate the profiles and clinical course of elderly patients who undergo angioplasty and to establish future risks of reintervention or need for coronary artery bypass grafting.

CardiacSurg 16 (Level B): Outcome studies are needed of conduit use (mammary artery, radial artery, saphenous vein graft) in elderly patients, specifically to analyze a possible selection bias by surgeon in the choice of conduit.

CardiacSurg 17 (Level B): Studies are needed that apply and test minimally invasive techniques that may reduce cost, decrease length of stay, and yield good long-term outcome in elderly coronary artery bypass grafting patients.

VALVE SURGERY

Valvular surgery in the elderly patient is performed as an intervention for stenotic or insufficient native valves. The aortic and mitral valves are most often involved; aortic stenosis is the most common indication for cardiac valve surgery. The aortic valve is typically replaced with either a mechanical or bioprosthetic prosthesis, or, alternatively, a homograft may be used. For mitral valvular disease, reparative procedures including annular supportive operations are preferred, although replacement with mechanical or bioprosthetic valves is also performed. Cardiac valvular procedures become more complex when they need to be combined with procedures such as CABG.

For patients with mild symptoms, Stahle et al noted that postoperative survival rates for those aged 70 and over who were undergoing aortic valve (AVR) or mitral valve replacement are comparable to those for the general population without valvular disease. The study therefore recommends early identification and surgical intervention for valvular heart disease. [50] Hannan et al showed that the number of years in excess of age 55 is a significant multivariate predictor of mortality for patients undergoing cardiac valve replacement. [51] This was found to be consistent across multiple groups when other risk factors are controlled.

For mitral valve surgery, Lee et al compared 190 elderly patients with 424 younger patients and noted that late surgery contributes far more than age to poor outcome, as the elderly group typically presented with advanced heart failure and poor ventricular function. [52] Survival was studied in 2359 patients undergoing AVR, showing excellent relative survival at 15 years of 74.9. [53] In these studies, old age was not consistently shown to be a risk factor for excess mortality after AVR.

In another study on elderly patients (aged 75 years and over) undergoing AVR for aortic stenosis, the independent predictive factors for mortality were found to be left ventricular failure, lack of sinus rhythm, and emergency operation. [54] The presence of severe preoperative symptoms due to advanced aortic stenosis also translates into longer intensive care stay for elderly patients. [55]

Mitral valve repair in the elderly patient may be compatible with acceptable mortality and outcomes. Grossi et al showed that mitral valve reconstruction in 278 patients aged 70 or greater had 6.5% mortality, rising to 17.0% when CABG was added. [56] The 5-year rate of freedom from reoperation in this patient population was 91.2%. However, advanced age was found in another study to be a predictor of long-term mortality in patients with pulmonary hypertension who were undergoing mitral valve surgery for mitral stenosis. [57]

The choice of valve prosthesis in the elderly patient has been investigated extensively. The excellent durability of mechanical prosthetic valves when compared with tissue or bioprosthetic valves is weighed against the need for long-term anticoagulation, which in an elderly population may lead to bleeding complications. In the Veterans Affairs randomized study comparing mechanical and bioprosthetic valves in valve replacement, the rate of primary valve failure after AVR was not found to be significantly different between the valve types in patients aged 65 and over. [58] In long-term follow-up of patients aged 65 and over, Helft et al showed that bioprosthetic valve replacement has low structural deterioration rates and low mortality rates but ultimately has high mortality rates attributable to causes not related to valves. [59] In patients aged 70 and over, a bioprosthetic valve offers lower risk of thromboembolic complications and acceptable rates of structural deterioration. [60] Banbury et al concluded that the Carpentier-Edwards pericardial aortic valve, with low incidence of structural deterioration and acceptable rates of freedom from hemorrhage (91%), endocarditis (93%), and thromboembolism (87%) at 12 years, is an appropriate choice of prosthesis in patients aged 65 and older. [61]

In a prospective randomized study of AVR in patients aged 75 years and over, Santini et al noted that stentless valves (ie, biologic valves with nonrigid sewing rings) carry no advantage over conventional bioprosthetic valves with respect to mortality rates, transvalvular gradients, or regression of left ventricular mass. [62] The stentless valves typically require longer operative times for implantation. Elderly patients were found to have satisfactory survival after AVR with stentless xenografts at 3 years. [63] Schmidtke et al also showed that the Ross procedure (AVR with pulmonary autograft) can be safely performed in selected patients aged 60 and over. [64]

Milano et al showed that elderly patients who receive mechanical valves in the aortic position have significantly increased risk of anticoagulant-related hemorrhages during the next 10 years in comparison with patients who receive bioprosthetic valve replacements. [65] Jamieson et al compared older patients with a younger cohort and noted that older patients undergoing AVR with bileaflet mechanical prosthesis have a significantly greater rate of thromboembolic and hemorrhagic complications than do the younger group of patients. [66] Masters et al, however, found no difference in thromboembolism when comparing mechanical valve replacement in an elderly group (aged 65 and over) and a younger group of patients. [67] These studies indicate that anticoagulation risks in elderly patients are not firmly established. The degree to which thrombotic or hemorrhagic complications occur in elderly patients as a consequence of ineffective monitoring, drug interactions, or noncompliance requires further study. For elderly patients with known coronary artery disease, the shorter survival expectations may justify the use of bioprosthetic valve replacement. [68]

Excellent quality of life after isolated valvular surgery was shown in a study of 147 patients aged 75 and over. The study found that 59.2% of patients are able to perform moderate to vigorous activities and 88.5% are able to climb at least one flight of stairs. [69]

Efforts to intervene early in the course of valvular heart disease in elderly patients have the potential for improving outcomes. Continued research in the technical aspects of valve surgery is warranted. Minimally invasive techniques with their potential for reduced morbidity following valvular surgery are currently being employed with increasing frequency. The minimally invasive procedures include those that limit incisions and surgical trauma. Minimal-access surgery for aortic valvular procedures has focused on parasternal incisions or mini-sternotomy. Mitral valve operations have also been developed to allow endoscopic or robotic manipulations of instruments placed through the right chest via small incisions. Methods to establish cardiopulmonary bypass have been devised to allow percutaneous arterial and venous access coupled with tissue-sparing incisions. These techniques are in rapid developmental stages and will require data collection to demonstrate their efficacy and the durability of repair. Early data suggest reduced hospital stay and good patient tolerance. Data that are specific to the elderly patient undergoing operations with the new techniques are needed. The choice of valvular prosthesis continues to evolve. Thrombotic or hemorrhagic complications in elderly patients need to be examined. Anticoagulant monitoring by newly developing home-based tests have the potential for reducing dosage errors that lead to those complications. An important question to be answered is whether a patient with a mechanical valve device requires any anticoagulation other than antiplatelet therapy. Specific studies that should be performed include the following:

CardiacSurg 18 (Level A): **Prospective randomized trials are needed to compare regimens of anticoagulant therapy for elderly patients with a mechanical prosthesis to minimize valvular complications and thromboembolic complications. Such studies may require cost-benefit analysis of decreasing anticoagulation as a function of age in patients with valvular prostheses.**

CardiacSurg 19 (Level A): **Prospective randomized trials comparing minimally invasive aortic valve replacement with conventional** methods in elderly patients are needed to assess the benefits of improved morbidity and decreased hospitalization.

CardiacSurg 20 (Level A): **Randomized prospective trials comparing minimally invasive with conventional mitral valve operations in elderly patients are needed. These studies should include the efficacy and duration of repair and outcomes with respect to operative and perioperative morbidity when thoracoscopic and robotic techniques are employed.**

REOPERATIVE CARDIAC SURGERY

Reoperative surgery in elderly patients carries a high risk for morbidity and mortality. In a comparison of younger and older (aged 70 and above) patients undergoing reoperative CABG, Christenson et al noted that the older patients had poorer New York Heart Association (NYHA) functional classification and more generalized atherosclerosis. [70] These older patients had a higher occurrence of low cardiac output syndrome, a higher incidence of gastrointestinal and renal complications, and longer cardiopulmonary bypass times. Hospital mortality rates for the older patients were 17.9% and 7.1% for younger patients; however, the 5-year survival rates and cardiac event-free survival rates for the older and younger patients were 76.2% and 69.9%, respectively. In an analysis comparing reoperative CABG and primary CABG, Christenson also noted that age above 80 years, urgent operation, poor ventricular function, and generalized atherosclerosis are among the independent risk factors for postoperative death in both the primary and reoperative CABG patients. [71] Weintraub et al reviewed the course of 2030 patients who underwent reoperative CABG and noted that hospital mortality increases from 5.7% for patients less than age 50 to 10% for patients aged 70 and older. [72] In that study, older age was found to be a marker for increased mortality by multivariate analysis. Neurologic events also were found to be significantly greater for the older patients undergoing reoperative surgery, with an occurrence of 4.1% for those aged 70 and over. Pellegrini et al noted significantly greater mortality, occurrence of low-output syndrome, renal failure, and sepsis in reoperative CABG patients aged 70 to 79 than in those 60 to 69 years of age. [73]

Reoperation carries increased risk for the elderly patient. Technical aspects of re-do procedures must be investigated to identify potential areas of improvement. These include myocardial protective schemes, modifications of cardiopulmonary bypass techniques, and minimally invasive operative strategies where possible. Topics for research include the following:

CardiacSurg 21 (Level B): **Cohort studies are needed that focus on patency and outcomes related to conduit choice in elderly patients who have had prior coronary artery bypass grafting and who require reoperation.**

CardiacSurg 22 (Level A): **Randomized trials of myocardial protective strategies in reoperative heart surgery in the elderly patient are needed to identify the optimal approach in recurrent coronary disease.**

CardiacSurg 23 (Level B): **Feasibility and outcomes analyses of off-pump techniques in elderly patients are needed to define morbidity and mortality in repeat revascularization procedures.**

CardiacSurg 24 (Level B): **Cohort studies are needed of outcomes in elderly patients who have undergone reoperative coronary artery bypass grafting with arterial grafts after venous conduits developed stenosis or other flow-limiting changes occurred.**

CardiacSurg 25 (Level B): **Longitudinal studies are needed to determine outcomes in valvular repair or replacement operations in elderly patients who have had prior coronary revascularization procedures.**

AORTIC DISSECTION

Surgery for aortic dissection often presents as an acute syndrome with hemodynamic compromise, ischemia, and multi-organ dysfunction. This condition is poorly tolerated by elderly patients with poor cardiac reserve and other comorbid conditions. An emergency surgical procedure is commonly required early in the course of ascending aortic dissection for survival benefit. In reviewing the course of 124 consecutive patients who underwent operation for acute ascending aortic dissection, Ehrlich et al showed in multivariate analysis that age above 60, hemodynamic compromise, and the absence of hypertension are predictors for hospital death. [74] In a similar study Ehrlich et al found that older age, hemodynamic instability, preoperative cardiopulmonary resuscitation, and lack of retrograde cerebral perfusion are significant predictors of death from operation for acute ascending aortic dissection. [75]

To improve outcome and reduce perioperative morbidity in elderly patients with acute dissection, it is necessary to identify the problem expediently and attempt to control factors that lead to hemodynamic instability. Intraoperative measures to improve reconstructive techniques include the use of glue-type substances for aortic repair. [76] Further research on methods to preserve cerebral perfusion and prevent accumulation of metabolites during periods of circulatory arrest is also indicated, as elderly patients fare poorly from neurologic complications often associated with major aortic procedures.

The technical aspects of surgery for aortic dissection require ongoing refinement. Techniques that improve cerebral protection and reduce visceral injury are being investigated. Further understanding of circulatory arrest physiology, with particular emphasis on the geriatric patient, may elicit the development of maneuvers and medications that minimize the morbidity and mortality of the operations. Studies comparing medical and surgical treatment for aortic dissection in older patients need to be performed to establish survival benefit and refine indications for either rapid operation or stabilization and medical treatment. Potential topics for investigation include the following:

CardiacSurg 26 (Level B): **Longitudinal studies of elderly patients treated nonoperatively for aortic dissection are needed to determine the profile of patients at greatest risk of early death that is related to initial dissection.**

CardiacSurg 27 (Level B): **Outcome analyses of operative treatment for ascending and descending aortic dissection in elderly patients are** needed to further clarify risk profiles. Emphasis should be on comparison of acute and chronic presentation.

CardiacSurg 28 (Levels B, A): Cohort studies and ultimately randomized clinical trials of cerebral protection techniques in elderly patients are needed to identify surgical techniques that lead to fewer neurologic complications, transfusion requirements, and other perioperative complications.

COMPLICATIONS OF CARDIAC SURGERY

Complications following cardiac surgery result in increased mortality, longer hospital and intensive care unit stays, and greater costs. Stroke, arrhythmias, postoperative bleeding, wound infections, and renal failure are among the most common complications. These complications have been shown to be particularly prevalent in elderly patients, as demonstrated by some of the studies discussed here and in the next section. Stroke is also considered in Chapters 4 (General Surgery) and 12 (Rehabilitation), as it is known to have increased occurrence with worse outcomes in elderly patients as both a disease entity and a surgical complication.

The occurrence of atrial fibrillation following cardiac surgical procedures is approximately 20% to 30%. This arrhythmia has been shown to increase the length of both intensive care unit and hospital stay. In their study of 570 patients undergoing CABG, Aranki et al showed that atrial fibrillation occurs more commonly in older patients, with the median age being 71 years; 66 years was the median age for those patients who did not have postoperative arrhythmias. [77]

Postoperative bleeding following CABG which requires re-exploration may be associated with increased mortality and length of hospital stay. In a multicenter regional cohort study of 8586 patients undergoing CABG, increased age and prolonged cardiopulmonary bypass time were found to be among the factors associated with increased bleeding risk. [78]

Gastrointestinal complications after cardiac surgery may occur in approximately 1% to 3% of patients; mortality from these events may be high. Christenson et al noted a 16.4% overall mortality from gastrointestinal complications following CABG. Cholecystitis and mesenteric ischemia were the most common events noted in that study. [79] In addition to poor ventricular function, cardiac reoperation, urgency of operation, and poor preoperative NYHA functional classification, age greater than 70 years was also found to be independently associated with post-CABG gastrointestinal complications. [80,81] Visser et al concluded that advanced age, valve replacement, emergency procedures, and prolonged bypass or clamp times are risk factors for the development of colorectal complications following cardiac surgery. [82] No independent risk factors for mortality associated with these complications could be established.

In a study of changing patterns among patients undergoing cardiopulmonary bypass between 1990 and 1997–98, Ostermann et al observed not only that the patient population became older and more severely ill, but also that the incidence of patients requiring perioperative continuous veno-venous hemofiltration for acute renal failure actually declined slightly (2.0 versus 2.7%). [83]

Wound complications following any surgical procedure may significantly increase the length of hospital stay, overall costs, and even mortality rates. In a retrospective study of 12,267 consecutive cardiac surgical patients over a 5-year period with 100% follow-up, Borger et al noted that advanced age is an independent risk factor for the development of serious sternal wound infections. [84]

In another study, in multivariate analysis advanced age also proved to be an independent risk factor for mortality after development of postsurgical mediastinitis. [85] For patients who develop sepsis following cardiac surgery, an increased mortality was found to be associated with advanced age or the development of low cardiac output syndrome. [86]

In a case-control retrospective analysis of post-CABG patients, silent aspiration, a severe form of pharyngeal dysfunction where oral contents spill into the tracheobronchial tree without elicitation of gagging or coughing, was studied. Advanced age was identified as a significant predictor of this entity. The study suggested that intraoperative cerebral injury might contribute to its development. [87]

Delirium in elderly patients following heart surgery is often attributable to multiple causes, including acute illness, prolonged pre- and postoperative intensive care unit stay, and drug interactions. [88] The chapter on cross-cutting issues addresses this common geriatric surgical complication (see the section on delirium in Chapter 13).

Complications are an expected part of surgical procedures and have a great impact on the outcomes in an elderly population. Potential areas for research include the following:

CardiacSurg 29 (Levels B, A): **Exploratory cohort studies are needed to seek evidence of success with treatments designed to reduce perioperative arrhythmias associated with a large percentage of cardiac operations. It would be important to establish whether postoperative atrial arrhythmias in elderly patients lead to lessened mobility and subsequent added risk for pneumonia, deep-vein thrombosis, and other complications. Subsequently, randomized controlled trials might be carried out to compare success rates and possible benefits from the treatments that show promise.**

CardiacSurg 30 (Level B): **Outcome studies of specific technical aspects of operations are needed to identify potential means of reducing wound complications in elderly patients. The use of minimally invasive techniques for both cardiac exposure and vein harvest to reduce surgical trauma in elderly patients should be evaluated.**

CardiacSurg 31 (Level B): **Cohort studies are needed to establish the incidence of and risk factors for complications in the geriatric cardiac patient, including delirium, bowel dysfunction, and swallowing difficulties.**

CardiacSurg 32 (Level B): **Studies of the susceptibility to hospital-acquired infections of elderly cardiac patients are needed. This should include efforts to determine if wound complications in the older patient are a result of prolonged hospital stay, lessened mobility, or age-related depression of the immune system.**

STROKE, NEUROLOGIC DEFICITS, AND CARDIAC SURGERY

Stroke is a leading cause of serious, long-term disability in the United States. About 88% of stroke deaths occur in people aged 65 and older. [1] Studies of patients undergoing cardiac surgical procedures have attempted to identify technical and patient-related factors contributing to risk of stroke.

Most strokes after cardiac surgery occur after an initial uneventful recovery, and atrial fibrillation has not been found to impact postoperative stroke rate unless it is accompanied by low cardiac output syndrome. [89] In a multicenter prospective study of 2108 patients undergoing CABG, Roach et al showed that independent predictors of focal-injury stroke, coma, or stupor are proximal aortic atherosclerosis, a history of neurologic disease, age above 70, and history of pulmonary disease. [90] Older age is an important predictor of more subtle neurologic injury, such as deterioration in intellectual function, memory deficit, or seizures. The strongest independent predictor for focal stroke was found to be proximal aortic atherosclerosis (judged by the surgeon's intraoperative palpation), which was associated with a fourfold increase in risk. Janssen et al observed that age greater than 75 years is a risk factor for the development of all neurologic complications (mild or major) after CABG. [91] Notably, the preoperative neurologic deficits, including the presence of mild dementia and delirium with acute illness in the elderly patient with heart disease, may not be recognized or fully documented, resulting in inaccurate risk assessment and misinterpretation of the patient's postoperative neurologic recovery.

In a prospective study of consecutive CABG patients, D'Agostino et al noted that age is a significant predictor of carotid stenosis, with stenosis > 50% resulting in significantly increased risk of postoperative neurologic event. [92] The role of preoperative carotid screening of elderly patients undergoing cardiac procedures should be investigated. In elderly patients (aged 70 and over) undergoing CABG, Morino et al found that calcification of the ascending aorta is associated with cerebral complications. [93]

Five factors were identified by McKhann et al as being correlated with post-CABG stroke: increased age, prior stroke, presence of carotid bruit, hypertension, and diabetes mellitus. [94] The only intraoperative factor showing correlation with stroke was cardiopulmonary bypass time. Mickleborough et al studied 1631 consecutive patients undergoing CABG and noted that age above 60 years has an odds ratio 2.9 for developing stroke of by multivariate analysis of preoperative, intraoperative, and postoperative variables. [95] Carotid scanning to identify high-risk groups was advocated. Another study reported that age above 70 years predisposes patients to stroke after CABG (N = 3910, multivariate odds ratio 3.88). [96] Almassi et al studied stroke in the setting of cardiac surgery. [97] Their database consisted of 4941 patients, 72% of whom were aged 60 and over. Stroke predictors were found to include age, renal insufficiency, use of inotropic agents in the postoperative period, total cardiopulmonary bypass time, and surgical priority. They found that stroke results in increased intensive care unit and hospital stay as well as increased mortality. In a multicenter review of preoperative risk factors for stroke after CABG, the independent factors found to be significantly associated with stroke include increased age, prior stroke, increased duration of cardiopulmonary bypass period, renal dysfunction, and carotid and peripheral vascular disease. [98]

Hammon et al studied neurobehavioral changes after CABG and noted that increasing patient age, multiple emboli detected by cranial Doppler, and palpable aortic plaque are associated with increased neurologic deficits. [99] They suggested that technical maneuvers to reduce embolic production (such as minimal aortic clamping) might result in fewer adverse neurobehavioral events. Such studies to correlate specific aortic manipulations with resultant postoperative neurologic events warrant further investigation. In a retrospective analysis of 2480 younger and older (aged 70 and over) patients undergoing coronary or valvular heart surgery, Ahlgren and Aren showed that the older patients have increased cerebral complication rates (4.1% versus 2.5%). [100] The nature of the complications ranged from coma and hemiparesis to confusion and visual deficits. Nearly one half of the noted cerebral symptoms were recorded in the period beyond immediate anesthetic recovery. Higher incidence rates of cerebral complications were found in patients who had combined valve and coronary procedures.

Reducing the stroke rate among elderly cardiac surgical patients warrants investigation into the technical aspects of cardiac procedures and the refinement of preoperative assessment and risk reduction. Carotid duplex scanning may identify patients at risk. Minimally invasive operative techniques have the potential for decreasing stroke rates, if indeed cardiopulmonary bypass is contributory to higher rates of cerebral complications. Risk modification, including improved diabetic management and control of hypertension, also deserves investigative attention, with emphasis on the elderly patient at risk. Future research should include the following:

> *CardiacSurg 33 (Level A)*: **Randomized clinical trials are needed to compare the neurologic results of coronary artery bypass grafting alone with the results of this procedure preceded by carotid endarterectomy when carotid stenosis > 50% is present.**

> *CardiacSurg 34 (Level A)*: **More randomized clinical trials should be conducted to investigate the occurrence of stroke and neurocognitive behavioral symptoms in elderly patients on whom coronary artery bypass grafting is performed with or without the use of cardiopulmonary bypass. This would include the development of widely acceptable neurobehavioral assessment tools (eg, cognitive tests) to be used as benchmarks in the evaluation of elderly patients before and after cardiac surgery.**

> *CardiacSurg 35 (Level B)*: **To identify possible modifiable risk factors for stroke in elderly patients undergoing cardiac surgery, investigation is needed of available and novel techniques (eg, epi-aortic ultrasound, cerebral oximetry, and transesophageal echocardiography) in elderly patients. Studies of the role of pharmacologic agents as risk factors are also needed.**

THE OCTOGENARIAN AS CARDIAC SURGICAL PATIENT

Octogenarians (and even nonagenarians) are commonly being treated for advanced cardiac disease. Surgical intervention may be considered in this high-risk group of patients to relieve symptoms or improve quality of life. As few as 3% of octogenarians who ulti-mately require treatment for coronary artery disease may present with typical angina. [101] The elderly patients may present with low energy level or heart failure, and cardiac workup is initiated. Ricou et al reported that of 115 octogenarians with angina who under-went coronary angiography between 1988 and 1992, 54% underwent revascularization by angioplasty or CABG. [102]

The benefits of myocardial revascularization in this specific group of patients have been demonstrated by several studies. Kaul et al noted that among octogenarians, a significantly greater actuarial survival at 5 years was achieved after CABG than after angioplasty (66% versus 55%). [103] Craver et al compared 601 octogenarians undergoing cardiac surgery with two younger cohorts of patients who received similar operative intervention. [104] The octogenarians in this study, however, did demonstrate a higher incidence of NYHA class IV angina and congestive heart failure. In-hospital death rates and stroke rates were sig-nificantly higher for these elderly patients than for the younger groups (9.1% versus 3.4% and 5.7% versus 2.6%, respectively).

In one of the largest studies of octogenarians undergoing cardiac surgery, Alexander et al analyzed results from 22 centers in the National Cardiovascular Network. [105] They found that preoperative predictors for mortality in the older patients are similar to factors in younger patients and that, when comorbidities are not present in the elderly patients, mortality rates are acceptable (4.2% CABG, 7% CABG with AVR, and 18.2% CABG with mitral valve replacement). The mortality rates reported are varied, however, with a typical recent study showing 14.7% mortality rate among 76 octogenarians undergoing cardiac surgery. [106]

Among predictors of hospital death for patients 80 years and older undergoing cardiac operations, Akins et al identified chronic lung disease, postoperative stroke, preoperative use of intra-aortic balloon pump, and congestive heart failure. [107] Risk factors for poor outcome in octogenarians undergoing CABG include pre- or postoperative renal dysfunc-tion, postoperative pulmonary insufficiency, and sternal wound infection, [108] and still an-other research group found that the only independent predictor of operative mortality is preoperative intensive care unit stay. [109]

In a study of 140 octogenarians undergoing AVR, Bessou et al noted a 56.5% probabil-ity of surviving 5 years after operation. [110] Gehlot et al studied early and long-term results of AVR in 322 octogenarians and observed that significant risk factors for mortality in-clude female gender, renal impairment, concomitant bypass grafting, poor ventricular function, and chronic obstructive pulmonary disease. [111] The use of the internal mammary artery as a conduit in octogenarians undergoing CABG was found to have slightly benefi-cial effects on survival in comparison with the use of saphenous veins alone. [112]

In a comparison of octogenarians and a younger cohort of patients undergoing beating-heart coronary surgery, the older patients were found to have significantly higher complication rates for pneumonia (6% versus 0.8%), atrial fibrillation (47% versus 26%), and need for inotropic support (21% versus 7%). [113] However, in a study of 269 patients by Ricci et al, stroke incidence among octogenarians undergoing off-pump coronary by-pass operations was found to be significantly lower than it was among octogenarians undergoing conventional CABG with cardiopulmonary bypass. [114]

The issue of specific surgical management of the octogenarian undergoing CABG is as yet unresolved. The selection criteria for patients who would benefit from beating-heart surgery need further clarification, particularly as the newer operative techniques become more widely used by cardiac surgeons. Furthermore, randomized controlled trials comparing beating-heart and conventional CABG in octogenarians may elicit data to identify indications for specific techniques in this group of patients. The potential for reduced length of hospital stay and fewer complications may be resolved by trials that address operative strategies in this patient group.

Octogenarians undergoing CABG have been shown to perform well under rapid-recovery protocols. Ott et al noted that 71% of these patients could be discharged in under 10 days following surgery and that other factors such as obesity, vascular disease, and prior ambulatory difficulties delay patient recovery and rehabilitation. [115]

Significant improvements in quality of life were observed in octogenarians undergoing cardiac operations by Kumar et al. [116] They showed in a retrospective analysis of two cohorts (1986 and 1991) that both groups demonstrated clinical and quality-of-life improvements and that over 70% of both patient groups had no regret over the decision to undergo surgery. Tsai et al studied 528 consecutive patients aged 80 and over who underwent cardiac operations; at a mean follow-up of 2 years, 70% of the patients reported improvement in their health status. [117]

Cardiac treatment protocols for angina, acute myocardial infarction, and congestive heart failure must be developed to encompass patients greater than 80 years of age. Trials need to begin at the earliest stages of evaluation. For coronary disease, this would involve randomized clinical trials comparing medical and surgical treatment among patients aged 80 and over. The purpose of the trials would be to negate selection criteria, which may have excluded patients for CABG on the basis of age alone. Similarly, randomized trials of conventional versus beating-heart surgery need to be performed in this patient group. Currently, beating-heart surgery is selected on the basis of the surgeon's familiarity with techniques and patients' cardiac anatomy. The outcomes may, therefore, be related to learning curve in this rapidly evolving method. Does selection for beating-heart surgery indicate the surgeon's perception of increased risk for morbidity or simply a preference for the technique? Multicenter trials should be clear in their selection criteria as well as relative uniformity of operative methods.

The long-term outcomes of patients aged 80 years and over who undergo cardiac surgery should also be investigated. Studies to identify rates and reasons for hospital readmission, deterioration in neurologic status, and objective functional recovery of patients after heart surgery should be performed. Age-matched cohort studies to compare neurologic and functional studies between patients who undergo heart surgery and those who are treated medically may be useful in determining the utility of operation for elderly patients. Future investigations should include the following:

> *CardiacSurg 36 (Level A)*: **Randomized clinical trials comparing percutaneous coronary intervention techniques (angioplasty plus stenting) and coronary artery bypass grafting in patients aged 80 and over are needed, with emphasis on the presentation of acute myocardial infarction or congestive heart failure, or both, to clarify selection criteria for this patient group.**

> *CardiacSurg 37 (Level A)*: **Randomized clinical trials are needed that compare outcomes with conventional and beating-heart coronary artery bypass grafting in patients aged 80 and over.**

CardiacSurg 38 (Level B): **Longitudinal outcome studies are needed of octogenarians who are treated by surgery, percutaneous interventions, or medically only to suggest the functional and neurologic long-term results and the need for reintervention.**

CardiacSurg 39 (Level B): **Follow-up studies should be performed to determine the need for readmission, repeat intervention, and functional outcomes in patients aged 80 and over who have undergone cardiac surgery.**

CardiacSurg 40 (Level B): **The development of cardiac treatment protocols specifically aimed at patients aged 80 and over is a critical need. This might include prospective trials to allow earlier surgical intervention when risk profile is favorable for good outcomes, particularly for coronary artery bypass grafting.**

QUALITY OF LIFE AFTER CARDIAC SURGERY

An important goal of any surgical intervention in the elderly person is to improve the quality of life. Cardiac surgical procedures are commonly performed under acute circumstances, with immediate survival as the near-term goal of therapy. With increased risk of morbidity and mortality for major operations in the elderly population, the decision to undergo a cardiac operation may be predicated on the perception of long-term issues of quality, and not just duration of life. Chocron et al used the Nottingham Health profile questionnaire to study patients aged 70 and over before and after open-heart operations. [118] The scores showed improvement in health perception by the elderly patients after heart surgery. In the area of physical mobility, diabetes mellitus was the only predictor for worsening scores after surgery. These researchers noted that elderly patients undergoing aortic valve operations showed greater improvement in health perception than patients undergoing CABG.

Melo et al also used the Nottingham Health Profile, as well as the Medical Outcomes Study 36-item Short Form (SF-36) health survey, to study quality of life after coronary artery bypass in 150 patients, 81% of whom were older than 50 years. [119] Surgery proved to be beneficial in improving quality of life, according to patient surveys given before and 6 months following coronary revascularization. Hunt et al in a similar analysis of 123 CABG patients (mean age = 64) used the SF-36 questionnaire at 12 months postoperatively and found improvement in perception of quality of life. [120] They noted an association between poor quality of life and patients who reported severe pain or poor quality sleep.

The Sickness Impact Profile and the Psychological Well-Being Schedule were used to study a small number of elderly patients undergoing CABG. [121] The patients were noted to have improvements in physical, social, and psychological functioning following CABG. In a study by MacDonald et al, [122] which used the SF-36 health survey and the Seattle Angina Questionnaire, quality of life at 3 months following CABG in elderly patients was shown to be improved.

In an analysis of patients aged 80 and older who underwent AVR, Sundt et al found that quality of life, as measured by a postoperative SF-36 survey, was comparable to that predicted for the elderly general population, thereby emphasizing that operative therapy should not be withheld from older patients on the basis of age alone. [123] Although the study did not include matched preoperative data, the surgically treated patients demonstrated higher scores in five of eight health concepts than did the general population.

In addition to physiologic variables that may contribute to mortality, Oxman et al found by multivariate regression analysis in a study of elderly patients following elective cardiac operations that lack of participation in social groups and absence of comfort from religion were significant predictors of mortality. [124] Using the Duke Activity Status Index, Jaeger et al studied functional capacity in cardiac surgery patients aged 70 and over and noted that smoking, female gender, older age, and prior cardiac operation are among the predictors for less improvement at 1 year after operation. [125] Yun et al prospectively studied 604 patients aged 65 and over following nonemergent cardiac operations with 100% follow-up at 2 years. [126] They observed that perception of physical health peaked at 12 months; however, measurements for mental attributes (limitations attributed to emotional problems) continued to improve with time.

For patients who develop complications following cardiac surgical procedures, Wahl et al noted that 67% of patients who required prolonged intensive care unit stay ultimately survived and that approximately 50% of these survivors progressed to functional independence. [127] The study noted that patients who develop severe cardiac or neurologic dysfunction, however, have worse outcomes, with little chance for independent recovery.

Older patients who undergo mitral valve surgery typically present with clinical deterioration as a consequence of advanced heart failure; however, despite higher morbidity and mortality in this group, survivors show significant improvement in symptoms and quality of life following surgery. [128]

Further efforts to improve quality of life after heart surgery may be aided by continued refinement of postoperative survey tools for elderly patients. Comparisons with cohorts treated medically should be performed. Quality-of-life assessment should include measures of older patients' perception of health and objective measurement of their physical and mental capabilities. These data are often lacking in retrospective analyses. The older patients who require cardiac surgery may be divided into urgent and elective groups. An older patient with stable angina who ultimately requires CABG may represent a group with the greatest potential for improvement in quality of life. Urgent operation or operations performed for advanced heart failure may predict lesser degree of functional recovery. To study these issues, surveys should compare outcomes of elective with outcomes of urgent operations. Follow-up is crucial in assessing elderly patient groups, as rehospitalization rates, requirement for nursing-home admissions, and repeat cardiac intervention may determine the need to reassess earlier decision making.

Also needed are improved means of preoperative assessment of elderly patients, to accurately describe their physical and mental capabilities. Ultimately, the surgical refinements may decrease postoperative debilities, but this can be confirmed only if more detailed information about preclinical condition is available. Future investigations should include the following:

CardiacSurg 41 (Level B): **Survey tools to assess quality of life after cardiac surgery in elderly patients need to be refined, to determine the contribution of surgical intervention to long-term disability. This should include cohort studies to clarify the impact of surgical treatment on caregivers.**

CardiacSurg 42 (Level B): **Long-term study of elderly cardiac surgical patients who had prolonged perioperative course is needed to determine the degree to which functional and symptomatic improvement occurs when operative therapy is complicated by stroke, infection, or other medical condition commonly associated with surgery in elderly patients.**

CardiacSurg 43 (Level B): **Comparison studies of outcomes of acute and elective cardiac surgery in elderly patients are needed to identify high-risk groups of elderly patients and to develop potential exclusion criteria for operative therapy.**

SUMMARY

The current trends in cardiac surgery show that more operations are being performed on elderly patients. This has coincided with advances in the medical management of CAD and heart failure. Operative interventions are nevertheless an integral part of advanced cardiac therapy with our aging population. Technical improvements in the operations continue to be investigated. Coronary artery bypass and valvular operations are performed routinely on older patients with excellent results.

Accurate data are needed to determine the population at risk for heart disease and those who benefit from surgical intervention. At the primary care level, surveys to identify age bias or aberration from cardiac protocols must be performed to determine that cardiac surgical candidates are appropriately referred. At the next level, the cardiologist and cardiac surgeon must collaborate on the management of advanced heart disease. Medical versus surgical intervention trials are warranted across multiple disease entities. For CAD, further randomized prospective trials specific to the elderly population are indicated. Trials in the area of angioplasty or stent versus CABG, medical versus laser therapy or gene therapy for inoperable CAD, or angioplasty versus beating-heart surgery for single or double vessel CAD are examples of other needed trials. In the surgically treated elderly patients, further trials to define long-term results of beating-heart and minimal access valve surgery are recommended. Randomized trials are especially important for CAD in the area of beating-heart surgery to identify the potential advantages of performing CABG without the use of cardiopulmonary bypass. The degree to which these techniques may decrease stroke rate, reduce hospital stay, and improve functional recovery is still undetermined.

Older patients undergoing operations require more advanced techniques to reduce morbidity. Safer anesthetic techniques, better myocardial protection methods, and perhaps greater use of minimally invasive operations may yield better outcomes. The postoperative phase, which includes intensive care, in-hospital stay, and rehabilitation periods, require refinement in protocols and procedures to afford the best results. Cardiac surgeons require the latest data and educational support to be able to treat their older patients optimally.

KEY RESEARCH QUESTIONS IN GERIATRIC CARDIAC SURGERY

The three most important research areas identified in the specialty of geriatric cardiac surgery are the analysis and investigation of functional outcomes among geriatric cardiac surgical patients, the impact of stroke and neurocognitive deterioration among elderly surgically treated patients, and the design and assessment of geriatric clinical management programs to accommodate the increasingly older and sicker patients who may require cardiac operations. Studies to address these needs include clinical trials, observational studies, subgroup analyses, and expansion of databases to address key questions about the care of elderly cardiac surgical patients.

CardiacSurg KQ1: **To what extent do cardiac surgical operations improve functional outcomes in an elderly patient population?**

Hypothesis-generating research should include the expansion of current clinical databases to include long-term and functional outcomes of elderly cardiac surgical patients. The ability to satisfactorily gauge the success of cardiac operations in improving quality of life for elderly patients depends heavily on the accurate measure of preoperative and perioperative functional capabilities. Observational studies and database analysis should focus on refinement of risk factors for poor outcome in elderly surgically treated patients.

Hypothesis-testing research studies to address this question would be aimed at defining the benefits of surgical over medical therapy for coronary and valvular disease in older patients. Randomized trials of elderly patients treated for specific disease entities (eg, advanced CAD, mitral insufficiency with significant heart failure) are needed to clarify the role of operative therapy in improving survival and quality of life.

CardiacSurg KQ2: **How can stroke and neurocognitive deterioration following cardiac surgical procedures be reduced among elderly patients?**

Hypothesis-generating research studies should focus on the technical aspects of specific cardiac operations. Database analyses and observational studies of specific technical maneuvers currently used in operations on elderly patients should elucidate risk factors and technical contributions to cognitive impairment. Further hypothesis-generating research should focus on the development of widely acceptable neurobehavioral assessment tools (eg, cognitive tests) to be used as benchmarks in the evaluation of elderly patients before and after cardiac surgery. The newer methods of assessment may ultimately shape management decisions in cardiac surgery for the elderly patient, as they may alter technical practices of heart surgeons, revise risk stratification, and further clarify the expectations of postoperative recovery from heart surgery in the geriatric patient.

Hypothesis-testing research may include randomized trials of CABG performed with or without the use of cardiopulmonary bypass in elderly patients. Cohort studies to describe neurocognitive deterioration among nonsurgically treated elderly patients with cardiac disease are needed. Multivariate analyses for such studies may clarify the role of operative characteristics versus the presence of specific diseases in predicting cognitive decline in older patients.

CardiacSurg KQ3: **What changes in perioperative care are needed to improve outcomes in the elderly cardiac surgical patient?**

Hypothesis-generating research should include methodologic studies to identify high-risk elderly patients and devise clinical pathways for their care. Database analyses of the pre-hospital, in-hospital, and rehabilitative periods of elderly surgically treated patients should be performed to identify clinical management strategies that result in decreased morbidity and improved functional recovery.

Hypothesis-testing research studies include randomized trials of CABG with and without the use of cardiopulmonary bypass, with emphasis on reduction in morbidity. Prospective cohort studies of surgically and nonsurgically treated cardiac patients aged 75 and over are needed to clarify the potential beneficial effects of nonoperative therapy. Case-control or randomized studies of elder-specific pathways to elucidate the benefit of pathways in obtaining better functional outcomes and reducing in-hospital adverse events are needed. The aim of these studies would also be to identify treatment strategies that reduce the incidence of perioperative pulmonary complications, wound-related problems, and arrhythmias, which have been shown to be especially prevalent in elderly cardiac patients.

REFERENCES

1. American Heart Association. 2001 Heart and Stroke Statistical Update. Dallas, TX. 2000.
2. Warner CD, Weintraub WS, Craver JM, et al. Effect of cardiac surgery patient characteristics on patient outcomes from 1981 through 1995. Circulation 1997;96:1575-1579.
3. Rao V, Christakis GT, Weisel RD, et al. Changing pattern of valve surgery. Circulation 1996;94:II113-120.
4. Abramov D, Tamariz MG, Fremes SE, et al. Trends in coronary artery bypass surgery results: a recent, 9-year study. Ann Thorac Surg 2000;70:84-90.
5. Fernandez J, Chen C, Anolik G, et al. Perioperative risk factors affecting hospital stay and hospital costs in open heart surgery for patients > or = 65 years old. Eur J Cardiothorac Surg 1997;11:1133-1140.
6. Maharajh GS, Masters RG, Keon WJ. Cardiac operations in the elderly: who is at risk? Ann Thorac Surg 1998;66:1670-1673.
7. Culler SD, Weintraub WS, Shaw LJ, Becker ER. Hospital resource consumption in patients with diabetes and multivessel coronary disease undergoing revascularization. Am J Manag Care 2000;6:217-229.
8. Bearden D, Allman R, McDonald R, et al. Age, race, and gender variation in the utilization of coronary artery bypass surgery and angioplasty in SHEP. SHEP Cooperative Research Group. Systolic Hypertension in the Elderly Program. J Am Geriatr Soc 1994;42:1143-1149.
9. Paul SD, O'Gara PT, Mahjoub ZA, et al. Geriatric patients with acute myocardial infarction: Cardiac risk factor profiles, presentation, thrombolysis, coronary interventions, and prognosis. Am Heart J 1996;131:710-715.
10. Choudhary SK, Bhan A, Sharma R, et al. Aortic atherosclerosis and perioperative stroke in patients undergoing coronary artery bypass: role of intra-operative transesophageal echocardiography. Int J Cardiol 1997;61:31-38.

11. Trehan N, Mishra M, Kasliwal RR, Mishra A. Surgical strategies in patients at high risk for stroke undergoing coronary artery bypass grafting. Ann Thorac Surg 2000;70:1037-1045.

12. Pennington DG, Oaks TE, Lohmann DP. Permanent ventricular assist device support versus cardiac transplantation. Ann Thorac Surg 1999;68:729-733.

13. Vigorito C, Giordano A, Ferraro P, et al. Reduced left ventricular mechanical efficiency in elderly patients with coronary artery disease. Aging (Milano) 1995;7:205-209.

14. Uren NG, Camici PG, Melin JA, et al. Effect of aging on myocardial perfusion reserve. J Nucl Med 1995;36:2032-2036.

15. Abete P, Ferrara N, Cacciatore F, et al. Angina-induced protection against myocardial infarction in adult and elderly patients: a loss of preconditioning mechanism in the aging heart? J Am Coll Cardiol 1997;30:947-954.

16. Caldarone CA, Krukenkamp IB, Burns PG, et al. Blood cardioplegia in the senescent heart. J Thorac Cardiovasc Surg 1995;109:269-274.

17. Gottlieb S, Goldbourt U, Boyko V, et al. Improved outcome of elderly patients ($>$ or $=$ 75 years of age) with acute myocardial infarction from 1981-1983 to 1992-1994 in Israel. The SPRINT and Thrombolytic Survey Groups. Secondary Prevention Reinfarction Israel Nifedipine Trial. Circulation 1997;95:342-350.

18. Stouffer GA, Mott L, Brizolara A, Subbarao V. Left main coronary artery disease in adults younger than 50 years: a comparison with older patients. Catheter Cardiovasc Interv 2000;51:11-17.

19. Nguyen TD, de Virgilio C, Kakuda J, et al. Characteristics of patients less than 45 years of age compared with older patients undergoing coronary artery bypass grafting. Clin Cardiol 1998;21:913-916.

20. Aldea GS, Gaudiani JA, Shapira OM, et al. Comparison of risk profile and outcomes in patients undergoing surgical and catheter-based revascularization. J Card Surg 1998;13:81-89; discussion 90-82.

21. Harris WO, Mock MB, Orszulak TA, et al. Use of coronary artery bypass surgical procedure and coronary angioplasty in treatment of coronary artery disease: changes during a 10-year period at Mayo Clinic Rochester. Mayo Clin Proc 1996;71:927-935.

22. O'Keefe JH, Sutton MB, McCallister BD, et al. Coronary angioplasty versus bypass surgery in patients $>$ 70 years old matched for ventricular function. J Am Coll Cardiol 1994;24:425-430.

23. Vassilikos VP, Lim R, Kreidieh I, et al. Myocardial revascularisation in elderly patients with refractory or unstable angina and advanced coronary disease. Coron Artery Dis 1997;8:705-709.

24. Mullany CJ, Mock MB, Brooks MM, et al. Effect of age in the Bypass Angioplasty Revascularization Investigation (BARI) randomized trial. Ann Thorac Surg 1999;67:396-403.

25. Serruys PW, Unger F, Sousa JE, et al. Comparison of coronary-artery bypass surgery and stenting for the treatment of multivessel disease. N Engl J Med 2001;344:1117-1124.

26. Kim SW, Hong MK, Lee CW, et al. Multivessel coronary stenting versus bypass surgery in patients with multivessel coronary artery disease and normal left ventricular function: immediate and 2-year long-term follow-up. Am Heart J 2000;139:638-642.

27. Ritchie JL, Maynard C, Every NR, Chapko MK. Coronary artery stent outcomes in a Medicare population: less emergency bypass surgery and lower mortality rates in patients with stents. Am Heart J 1999;138:437-440.

28. Munoz JC, Alonso JJ, Duran JM, et al. Coronary stent implantation in patients older than 75 years of age: clinical profile and initial and long-term (3 years) outcome. Am Heart J 2002;143:620-626.

29. Haraphongse M, Na-Ayudhya RK, Teo KK, et al. The changing clinical profile of coronary artery bypass graft patients, 1970-89. Can J Cardiol 1994;10:71-76.

30. Christenson JT, Simonet F, Schmuziger M. The influence of age on the outcome of primary coronary artery bypass grafting. J Cardiovasc Surg (Torino) 1999;40:333-338.

31. Ivanov J, Weisel RD, David TE, Naylor CD. Fifteen-year trends in risk severity and operative mortality in elderly patients undergoing coronary artery bypass graft surgery. Circulation 1998;97:673-680.

32. Hannan EL, Burke J. Effect of age on mortality in coronary artery bypass surgery in New York, 1991-1992. Am Heart J 1994;128:1184-1191.

33. Peigh PS, Swartz MT, Vaca KJ, et al. Effect of advancing age on cost and outcome of coronary artery bypass grafting. Ann Thorac Surg 1994;58:1362-1366; discussion 1366-1367.

34. Ott RA, Gutfinger DE, Miller MP, et al. Rapid recovery after coronary artery bypass grafting: is the elderly patient eligible? Ann Thorac Surg 1997;63:634-639.

35. Yau TM, Fedak PW, Weisel RD, et al. Predictors of operative risk for coronary bypass operations in patients with left ventricular dysfunction. J Thorac Cardiovasc Surg 1999;118:1006-1013.

36. Kaul TK, Fields BL, Riggins SL, et al. Coronary artery bypass grafting within 30 days of an acute myocardial infarction. Ann Thorac Surg 1995;59:1169-1176.

37. Rao V, Ivanov J, Weisel RD, et al. Predictors of low cardiac output syndrome after coronary artery bypass. J Thorac Cardiovasc Surg 1996;112:38-51.

38. Del Rizzo DF, Fremes SE, Christakis GT, et al. The current status of myocardial revascularization: changing trends and risk factor analysis. J Card Surg 1996;11:18-29.

39. Busch T, Friedrich M, Sirbu H, et al. Coronary artery bypass procedures in septuagenarians are justified. Short and long-term results. J Cardiovasc Surg (Torino) 1999;40:83-91.

40. Kramer A, Mastsa M, Paz Y, et al. Bilateral skeletonized internal thoracic artery grafting in 303 patients seventy years and older. J Thorac Cardiovasc Surg 2000;120:290-297.

41. He GW, Acuff TE, Ryan WH, et al. Determinants of operative mortality in elderly patients undergoing coronary artery bypass grafting. Emphasis on the influence of internal mammary artery grafting on mortality and morbidity. J Thorac Cardiovasc Surg 1994;108:73-81.

42. He GW, Acuff TE, Ryan WH, Mack MJ. Risk factors for operative mortality in elderly patients undergoing internal mammary artery grafting. Ann Thorac Surg 1994;57:1453-1460; discussion 1460-1451.

43. Gutfinger DE, Ott RA, Miller M, et al. Aggressive preoperative use of intraaortic balloon pump in elderly patients undergoing coronary artery bypass grafting. Ann Thorac Surg 1999;67:610-613.

44. Paone G, Higgins RS, Havstad SL, Silverman NA. Does age limit the effectiveness of clinical pathways after coronary artery bypass graft surgery? Circulation 1998;98:II41-45.

45. Stewart RD, Campos CT, Jennings B, et al. Predictors of 30-day hospital readmission after coronary artery bypass. Ann Thorac Surg 2000;70:169-174.

46. Samuels LE, Kaufman MS, Morris RJ, et al. Coronary artery bypass grafting in patients with COPD. Chest 1998;113:878-882.

47. Boyd WD, Desai ND, Del Rizzo DF, et al. Off-pump surgery decreases postoperative complications and resource utilization in the elderly. Ann Thorac Surg 1999;68:1490-1493.

48. Koutlas TC, Elbeery JR, Williams JM, et al. Myocardial revascularization in the elderly using beating heart coronary artery bypass surgery. Ann Thorac Surg 2000;69:1042-1047.

49. Yokoyama T, Baumgartner FJ, Gheissari A, et al. Off-pump versus on-pump coronary bypass in high-risk subgroups. Ann Thorac Surg 2000;70:1546-1550.

50. Stahle E, Kvidal P, Nystrom SO, Bergstrom R. Long-term relative survival after primary heart valve replacement. Eur J Cardiothorac Surg 1997;11:81-91.

51. Hannan EL, Racz MJ, Jones RH, et al. Predictors of mortality for patients undergoing cardiac valve replacements in New York State. Ann Thorac Surg 2000;70:1212-1218.

52. Lee EM, Porter JN, Shapiro LM, Wells FC. Mitral valve surgery in the elderly. J Heart Valve Dis 1997;6:22-31.

53. Kvidal P, Bergstrom R, Horte LG, Stahle E. Observed and relative survival after aortic valve replacement. J Am Coll Cardiol 2000;35:747-756.

54. Logeais Y, Langanay T, Roussin R, et al. Surgery for aortic stenosis in elderly patients. A study of surgical risk and predictive factors. Circulation 1994;90:2891-2898.

55. Morell VO, Daggett WM, Pezzella AT, et al. Aortic stenosis in the elderly: result of aortic valve replacement. J Cardiovasc Surg (Torino) 1996;37:33-35.

56. Grossi EA, Zakow PK, Sussman M, et al. Late results of mitral valve reconstruction in the elderly. Ann Thorac Surg 2000;70:1224-1226.

57. Vincens JJ, Temizer D, Post JR, et al. Long-term outcome of cardiac surgery in patients with mitral stenosis and severe pulmonary hypertension. Circulation 1995;92:II137-142.

58. Hammermeister K, Sethi GK, Henderson WG, et al. Outcomes 15 years after valve replacement with a mechanical versus a bioprosthetic valve: final report of the Veterans Affairs randomized trial. J Am Coll Cardiol 2000;36:1152-1158.

59. Helft G, Tabone X, Georges JL, et al. Late results with bioprosthetic valves in the elderly. J Card Surg 1999;14:252-258.

60. Kobayashi Y, Eishi K, Nagata S, et al. Choice of replacement valve in the elderly. J Heart Valve Dis 1997;6:404-409.

61. Banbury MK, Cosgrove DM, Lytle BW, et al. Long-term results of the Carpentier-Edwards pericardial aortic valve: a 12-year follow-up. Ann Thorac Surg 1998;66:S73-76.

62. Santini F, Bertolini P, Montalbano G, et al. Hancock versus stentless bioprosthesis for aortic valve replacement in patients older than 75 years. Ann Thorac Surg 1998;66:S99-S103.

63. Larsen SS, Lund O, Hemmert-Lund H, et al. Short-term results after aortic valve replacement with stentless xenografts in elderly patients. Scand Cardiovasc J 2000;34:511-515.

64. Schmidtke C, Bechtel JF, Noetzold A, Sievers HH. Up to seven years of experience with the Ross procedure in patients >60 years of age. J Am Coll Cardiol 2000;36:1173-1177.

65. Milano A, Guglielmi C, De Carlo M, et al. Valve-related complications in elderly patients with biological and mechanical aortic valves. Ann Thorac Surg 1998;66:S82-S87.

66. Jamieson WR, Miyagishima RT, Grunkemeier GL, et al. Bileaflet mechanical prostheses for aortic valve replacement in patients younger than 65 years and 65 years of age or older: major thromboembolic and hemorrhagic complications. Can J Surg 1999;42:27-36.

67. Masters RG, Semelhago LC, Pipe AL, Keon WJ. Are older patients with mechanical heart valves at increased risk? Ann Thorac Surg 1999;68:2169-2172.

68. Jones EL, Weintraub WS, Craver JM, et al. Interaction of age and coronary disease after valve replacement: implications for valve selection. Ann Thorac Surg 1994;58:378-384; discussion 384-375.

69. Shapira OM, Kelleher RM, Zelingher J, et al. Prognosis and quality of life after valve surgery in patients older than 75 years. Chest 1997;112:885-894.

70. Christenson JT, Simonet F, Schmuziger M. The influence of age on the results of reoperative coronary artery bypass grafting. Coron Artery Dis 1997;8:91-96.

71. Christenson JT, Schmuziger M, Simonet F. Reoperative coronary artery bypass procedures: risk factors for early mortality and late survival. Eur J Cardiothorac Surg 1997;11:129-133.

72. Weintraub WS, Jones EL, Craver JM, et al. In-hospital and long-term outcome after reoperative coronary artery bypass graft surgery. Circulation 1995;92:II50-57.

73. Pellegrini RV, Di Marco RF, Werner AM, Marrangoni AG. Recurrent ischemic heart disease: the effect of advancing age. J Cardiovasc Surg (Torino) 1994;35:371-376.

74. Ehrlich MP, Ergin MA, McCullough JN, et al. Results of immediate surgical treatment of all acute type A dissections. Circulation 2000;102:III248-252.

75. Ehrlich M, Fang WC, Grabenwoger M, et al. Perioperative risk factors for mortality in patients with acute type A aortic dissection. Circulation 1998;98:II294-298.

76. Bachet J, Goudot B, Dreyfus G, et al. Surgery of acute type A dissection: what have we learned during the past 25 years? Z Kardiol 2000;89 Suppl 7:47-54.

77. Aranki SF, Shaw DP, Adams DH, et al. Predictors of atrial fibrillation after coronary artery surgery. Current trends and impact on hospital resources. Circulation 1996;94:390-397.

78. Dacey LJ, Munoz JJ, Baribeau YR, et al. Reexploration for hemorrhage following coronary artery bypass grafting: incidence and risk factors. Northern New England Cardiovascular Disease Study Group. Arch Surg 1998;133:442-447.

79. Christenson JT, Schmuziger M, Maurice J, et al. Gastrointestinal complications after coronary artery bypass grafting. J Thorac Cardiovasc Surg 1994;108:899-906.

80. Lazar HL, Hudson H, McCann J, et al. Gastrointestinal complications following cardiac surgery. Cardiovasc Surg 1995;3:341-344.

81. Perugini RA, Orr RK, Porter D, et al. Gastrointestinal complications following cardiac surgery. An analysis of 1477 cardiac surgery patients. Arch Surg 1997;132:352-357.

82. Visser T, Bove P, Barkel D, et al. Colorectal complications following cardiac surgery. Six-year experience. Dis Colon Rectum 1995;38:1210-1213.

83. Ostermann ME, Taube D, Morgan CJ, Evans TW. Acute renal failure following cardiopulmonary bypass: a changing picture. Intensive Care Med 2000;26:565-571.

84. Borger MA, Rao V, Weisel RD, et al. Deep sternal wound infection: risk factors and outcomes. Ann Thorac Surg 1998;65:1050-1056.

85. Munoz P, Menasalvas A, Bernaldo de Quiros JC, et al. Postsurgical mediastinitis: a case-control study. Clin Infect Dis 1997;25:1060-1064.

86. Michalopoulos A, Stavridis G, Geroulanos S. Severe sepsis in cardiac surgical patients. Eur J Surg 1998;164:217-222.

87. Harrington OB, Duckworth JK, Starnes CL, et al. Silent aspiration after coronary artery bypass grafting. Ann Thorac Surg 1998;65:1599-1603.

88. Rolfson DB, McElhaney JE, Jhangri GS, Rockwood K. Validity of the confusion assessment method in detecting postoperative delirium in the elderly. Int Psychogeriatr 1999;11:431-438.

89. Hogue CW, Murphy SF, Schechtman KB, D?avila-Rom?an VG. Risk factors for early or delayed stroke after cardiac surgery. Circulation 1999;100:642-647.

90. Roach GW, Kanchuger M, Mangano CM, et al. Adverse cerebral outcomes after coronary bypass surgery. Multicenter Study of Perioperative Ischemia Research Group and the Ischemia Research and Education Foundation Investigators. N Engl J Med 1996;335:1857-1863.

91. Janssen DP, Noyez L, van Druten JA, et al. Predictors of neurological morbidity after coronary artery bypass surgery. Eur J Cardiothorac Surg 1999;15:166-172.

92. D'Agostino RS, Svensson LG, Neumann DJ, et al. Screening carotid ultrasonography and risk factors for stroke in coronary artery surgery patients. Ann Thorac Surg 1996;62:1714-1723.

93. Morino Y, Hara K, Tanabe K, et al. Retrospective analysis of cerebral complications after coronary artery bypass grafting in elderly patients. Jpn Circ J 2000;64:46-50.

94. McKhann GM, Goldsborough MA, Borowicz LM, et al. Cognitive outcome after coronary artery bypass: a one-year prospective study. Ann Thorac Surg 1997;63:510-515.

95. Mickleborough LL, Walker PM, Takagi Y, et al. Risk factors for stroke in patients undergoing coronary artery bypass grafting. J Thorac Cardiovasc Surg 1996;112:1250-1258; discussion 1258-1259.

96. Rao V, Christakis GT, Weisel RD, et al. Risk factors for stroke following coronary bypass surgery. J Card Surg 1995;10:468-474.

97. Almassi GH, Sommers T, Moritz TE, et al. Stroke in cardiac surgical patients: determinants and outcome. Ann Thorac Surg 1999;68:391-397; discussion 397-398.

98. John R, Choudhri AF, Weinberg AD, et al. Multicenter review of preoperative risk factors for stroke after coronary artery bypass grafting. Ann Thorac Surg 2000;69:30-35; discussion 35-36.

99. Hammon JW, Stump DA, Kon ND, et al. Risk factors and solutions for the development of neurobehavioral changes after coronary artery bypass grafting. Ann Thorac Surg 1997;63:1613-1618.

100. Ahlgren E, Aren C. Cerebral complications after coronary artery bypass and heart valve surgery: risk factors and onset of symptoms. J Cardiothorac Vasc Anesth 1998;12:270-273.

101. Talwalkar NG, Damus PS, Durban LH, et al. Outcome of isolated coronary artery bypass surgery in octogenarians. J Card Surg 1996;11:172-179.

102. Ricou FJ, Suilen C, Rothmeier C, et al. Coronary angiography in octogenarians: results and implications for revascularization. Am J Med 1995;99:16-21.

103. Kaul TK, Fields BL, Wyatt DA, et al. Angioplasty versus coronary artery bypass in octogenarians. Ann Thorac Surg 1994;58:1419-1426.

104. Craver JM, Puskas JD, Weintraub WW, et al. 601 octogenarians undergoing cardiac surgery: outcome and comparison with younger age groups. Ann Thorac Surg 1999;67:1104-1110.

105. Alexander KP, Anstrom KJ, Muhlbaier LH, et al. Outcomes of cardiac surgery in patients > or = 80 years: results from the National Cardiovascular Network. J Am Coll Cardiol 2000;35:731-738.

106. Colon G, Perez CM, Guzman M. Perioperative outcomes in octogenarians undergoing cardiac surgery in Puerto Rico. P R Health Sci J 2000;19:115-122.

107. Akins CW, Daggett WM, Vlahakes GJ, et al. Cardiac operations in patients 80 years old and older. Ann Thorac Surg 1997;64:606-614; discussion 614-605.

108. Williams DB, Carrillo RG, Traad EA, et al. Determinants of operative mortality in octogenarians undergoing coronary bypass. Ann Thorac Surg 1995;60:1038-1043.

109. Deiwick M, Tandler R, Mollhoff T, et al. Heart surgery in patients aged eighty years and above: determinants of morbidity and mortality. Thorac Cardiovasc Surg 1997;45:119-126.

110. Bessou JP, Bouchart F, Angha S, et al. Aortic valvular replacement in octogenarians. Short-term and mid-term results in 140 patients. Cardiovasc Surg 1999;7:355-362.

111. Gehlot A, Mullany CJ, Ilstrup D, et al. Aortic valve replacement in patients aged eighty years and older: early and long-term results. J Thorac Cardiovasc Surg 1996;111:1026-1036.

112. Morris RJ, Strong MD, Grunewald KE, et al. Internal thoracic artery for coronary artery grafting in octogenarians. Ann Thorac Surg 1996;62:16-22.

113. Stamou SC, Dangas G, Dullum MK, et al. Beating heart surgery in octogenarians: perioperative outcome and comparison with younger age groups. Ann Thorac Surg 2000;69:1140-1145.

114. Ricci M, Karamanoukian HL, Abraham R, et al. Stroke in octogenarians undergoing coronary artery surgery with and without cardiopulmonary bypass. Ann Thorac Surg 2000;69: 1471-1475.

115. Ott RA, Gutfinger DE, Miller M, et al. Rapid recovery of octogenarians following coronary artery bypass grafting. J Card Surg 1997;12:309-313.

116. Kumar P, Zehr KJ, Chang A, et al. Quality of life in octogenarians after open heart surgery. Chest 1995;108:919-926.

117. Tsai TP, Chaux A, Matloff JM, et al. Ten-year experience of cardiac surgery in patients aged 80 years and over. Ann Thorac Surg 1994;58:445-450; discussion 450-441.

118. Chocron S, Tatou E, Schjoth B, et al. Perceived health status in patients over 70 before and after open-heart operations. Age Ageing 2000;29:329-334.

119. Melo E, Antunes M, Ferreira PL. Quality of life in patients undergoing coronary revascularization. Rev Port Cardiol 2000;19:889-906.

120. Hunt JO, Hendrata MV, Myles PS. Quality of life 12 months after coronary artery bypass graft surgery. Heart Lung 2000;29:401-411.

176   CHAPTER 6

121. Page SA, Verhoef MJ, Emes CG. Quality of life, bypass surgery and the elderly. Can J Cardiol 1995;11:777-782.
122. MacDonald P, Stadnyk K, Cossett J, et al. Outcomes of coronary artery bypass surgery in elderly people. Can J Cardiol 1998;14:1215-1222.
123. Sundt TM, Bailey MS, Moon MR, et al. Quality of life after aortic valve replacement at the age of >80 years. Circulation 2000;102:III70-74.
124. Oxman TE, Freeman DH, Manheimer ED. Lack of social participation or religious strength and comfort as risk factors for death after cardiac surgery in the elderly. Psychosom Med 1995;57:5-15.
125. Jaeger AA, Hlatky MA, Paul SM, Gortner SR. Functional capacity after cardiac surgery in elderly patients. J Am Coll Cardiol 1994;24:104-108.
126. Yun KL, Sintek CF, Fletcher AD, et al. Time related quality of life after elective cardiac operation. Ann Thorac Surg 1999;68:1314-1320.
127. Wahl GW, Swinburne AJ, Fedullo AJ, et al. Long-term outcome when major complications follow coronary artery bypass graft surgery. Recovery after complicated coronary artery bypass graft surgery. Chest 1996;110:1394-1398.
128. Goldsmith I, Lip GY, Kaukuntla H, Patel RL. Hospital morbidity and mortality and changes in quality of life following mitral valve surgery in the elderly. J Heart Valve Dis 1999;8:702-707.

7

GERIATRIC OPHTHALMOLOGY

Andrew G. Lee, MD; Anne Louise Coleman, MD, PhD*

The aging of the baby boomers has created a dramatic demographic shift toward an older population in the United States. The health care needs of this aging population will impact ophthalmology disproportionately. [1] Although ophthalmologists are accustomed to caring for elderly patients, they may not be familiar with some of the issues associated with visual loss in the geriatric population. Traditional clinical measures of visual function (eg, Snellen acuity, perimetry) are not adequate to determine the functional impact of visual impairment or the satisfaction or dissatisfaction with therapy of older patients. [1–33] Most ophthalmologists recognize that with age, visual impairment and blinding disorders occur with increasing frequency. [34–56] However, they should also recognize that poor visual function affects other quality-of-life parameters, including disability, [11,32,57] falls and fractures, [58–75] activities of daily living (ADLs) and independence, [76–84] use of community support services, sense of well-being, [85–87] and mortality. [88]

This chapter reviews the available pertinent literature in geriatric ophthalmology, identifies gaps in the current knowledge base, and provides a needs assessment that is the basis for the recommended research agenda.

METHODS

Two searches were conducted on this topic, both on the National Library of Medicine's PubMed database. The time period covered was from 1980 through March 2, 2001. The first search strategy combined terms for ophthalmologic surgical procedures or low vision with terms for risk factors, age factors, postoperative complications, or outcomes. This search generated 2235 references, but only a sampling of the most current 300 were sent to the authors. The second search combined terms for vision disorders or eye diseases with terms for functional status or ADLs. This search resulted in 779 references, all of which were sent to the authors. The titles were reviewed for topicality, currency, and appropriateness. Relevant full articles were retrieved from the refined list. Papers that addressed the following issues were identified:

- age as a risk factor for ophthalmic diseases;

- age as a prognostic indicator for treatment outcome;

- age-related risk factors for poor outcomes, including comorbidity, functional status, cognitive impairment, emotional status, self-assessed heath, socioeconomic level, and social support;

* Lee: Associate Professor of Ophthalmology, Neurology, and Neurosurgery, University of Iowa Hospitals and Clinics, Iowa City, IA; Coleman: Professor of Ophthalmology, Jules Stein Eye Institute, University of California, Los Angeles, CA.

Acknowledgment: This work was reviewed by the American Academy of Ophthalmology, Committee on Aging and the Inter-specialty Education Committee.

- the impact of vision on positive and negative outcomes, eg, hospitalization, length of stay, delirium, falls, and depression;

- specific diseases or surgical procedures or risks in elderly adults.

Case reports and letters were excluded unless they added significant information. Pre-1990 articles were included only if they added significant historical or other information.

In the discussion that follows, we give particular emphasis to randomized clinical trials, when available, and to meta-analyses of such trials. We also highlight the four ocular pathologies that have the highest impact and highest incidence among elderly people: cataract, glaucoma, age-related macular degeneration or ARMD, and diabetic retinopathy. The focus is on the research regarding geriatric issues specific to these disorders.

ASSESSING VISUAL LOSS IN AGE

SCOPE OF THE PROBLEM

Ophthalmologists are aware that visual loss is common in the elderly population and that the incidence rates of blinding disorders (eg, cataract, ARMD, glaucoma, and diabetic retinopathy) increase with increasing age. [34–56] Visual impairment defined by Snellen acuity worse than 20/40 occurs in as many as 21% of persons aged 75 years or older. The Salisbury Eye Evaluation (SEE) project, which studied 2520 individuals aged 65 to 84, found the prevalence of visual acuity worse than 20/40 but better than 20/200 to be 11.4% in the white Americans and 16.4% in the black Americans studied. [33] The Beaver Dam Eye Study, which examined 4926 persons aged 43 to 86 years, found that a best-corrected visual acuity worse than 20/40 occurred in 21.1% of those aged 75 years and older, in 5.0% of those between 64 and 74, in 0.9% of those between 55 and 64, and in 0.8% of those between 43 and 54. [7,49–51] Female gender was found to be an independent predictor of poor visual acuity. The Melbourne (Australia) Visual Impairment Project reported visual acuity less than 20/60 in 1.34% of 3271 persons. Of those with visual impairment, 89% were 60 years or older, and in the multiple regression analysis, age was found to be the only significant predictor of visual impairment. [89]

MEASURES AND LEVELS OF VISUAL LOSS

Although Snellen testing is the standard measure of visual acuity in most ophthalmology clinics, there are other quantitative measures of visual acuity. In the Snellen system, letter size is defined as the distance at which the overall letter height subtends 5 minutes of arc. Snellen acuity can be converted to decimal acuity. Visual acuity can be specified in terms of minimum angle of resolution (MAR), calculated by dividing the letter size by the test distance. A derivative of MAR is the logarithm of MAR (logMAR). Other non-Snellen measures include the Bailey-Lovie logMAR chart and the early treatment diabetic retinopathy study (ETDRS) chart. [2] Many ophthalmologic clinical trials have adopted these non-Snellen measures of acuity because they can provide more quantitative and comparative data in studies of visual function.

The Snellen measure of visual acuity has also been used to define levels of visual impairment, blindness, and low vision. *Visual impairment* is usually defined as best-corrected Snellen visual acuity worse than 20/40 but better than 20/200. *Legal blindness* is defined as best-corrected visual acuity of 20/200 or worse or a visual field diameter less than 10 degrees. *Low vision* is defined as visual acuity less than 20/60 in the better eye. [3–5]

MEASURING IMPACT OF LOSS ON VISUAL FUNCTION

The most common causes of visual impairment in elderly persons are age-related cataract, ARMD, glaucoma, and diabetic retinopathy. Of all persons aged 75 years and over, 52% have advanced cataracts, [6,7] 25% have nonexudative ARMD, 5% have exudative ARMD, and 2% to 10% have glaucoma. [6–8] Many studies have devised measures of functional outcome following cataract extraction. [9–30] Although the standard measure of visual function in eye research has been Snellen visual acuity, other non-Snellen measures of visual function may be more important in determining the functional impact of visual loss in elderly persons.

Rumsey correlated visual complaints with objective visual tests in 50 older adults and in 20 middle-aged adults and found that decrements in visual acuity, decreased contrast sensitivity, increased glare sensitivity, diminished color vision, and loss of stereopsis were all more apparent in the older group. [31] These results indicate that answers to task-specific questions may provide greater insight into older adults' visual performance in their normal environment than simple measurement of Snellen visual acuity alone can provide.

Using a visual-functioning index (VF-7), Uusitalo et al measured functional impairment in 168 patients with cataracts. [30] The functional items were nighttime driving; reading small print; watching television; seeing steps, stairs, or curbs; reading traffic, street, or store signs; cooking; and doing fine handwork. The correlation among changes in the VF-7 score and visual acuity in the operated eye was 0.17. The correlation between changes in the VF-7 and patient satisfaction after cataract surgery was high ($r = 0.56$), and the VF-7 was a strong predictor of patient satisfaction after cataract surgery. Improved Snellen acuity has been the traditional outcome measure for successful cataract surgery, but these researchers' findings support the use of measures of postoperative functional outcomes and of patient satisfaction.

Rubin et al described the correlation between psychophysical measures of visual impairment and self-reported difficulty with everyday visual tasks in a population-based sample of persons aged 65 years and older. [32,33] Visual acuity, contrast and glare sensitivity, stereoacuity, and visual fields were found to be significant independent risk factors for self-reported visual disability. Visual impairment defined by Snellen acuity alone was not the only association with subjective disability, and additional vision measures were recommended to better understand the functional impact of vision loss.

MEASURING IMPACT OF LOSS ON FUNCTIONAL ABILITY

In a study of 1210 community-dwelling women aged 75 years and older that compared women with low visual acuity or low contrast sensitivity and women with good vision, the women with poor vision were found to be significantly more likely to be physically dependent. [90] The researchers concluded that testing contrast sensitivity in addition to Snellen acuity would allow better prediction of impairment in ADLs. McClure et al demonstrated that specific levels of objective vision loss measured by acuity, reading index, and contrast sensitivity corresponds with subjective functional difficulty in the performance of daily living tasks. [91]

Assessment instruments that provide more information about visual function than the standard Snellen acuity testing can provide have been developed. For example, a health-related quality-of-life (HRQOL) instrument measures the ability to engage in ADLs (eg, self-care, driving, working) and the self-perception of well-being (eg, pain, energy, and self-image). The Medical Outcomes Study Short Form 36-item health survey (SF-36) is the most widely used HRQOL instrument. The SF-36 measures eight aspects of HRQOL, including general health perceptions, physical functioning, role limitations, bodily pain, mental functioning (eg, mental health, energy or fatigue), and emotional function (eg, role limitations, social functioning). [92] Targeted HRQOL measures specific for ocular diseases have been developed. These include the Visual Functioning Scale (VF-14), which measures the person's ability to perform 14 vision-dependent activities. The Activities of Daily Vision Scale (ADVS), developed for evaluating cataracts, rates difficulty with 20 common visual activities (eg driving at night, reading newsprint, reading labels). The National Eye Institute Visual Functioning Questionnaire (NEI-VFQ) was developed to assess functional impairment in eye disorders and is similar to the ADVS in content. This instrument is a 25-item questionnaire that includes items for distance and near vision, eye pain, driving, emotional well-being, social and role functioning, and dependency. These instruments define overall functioning in patients with ocular disease, and assessments of treatment outcome should include at least one of them. [17,18,93,94]

Some researchers have used these instruments to measure the impact of vision loss on function. Mangione et al reported that NEI-VFQ scores were the lowest for 90 persons with low vision and 108 with ARMD. [93] The median Snellen binocular visual acuity in those with low vision was 20/252 and in those with ARMD was 20/63. The scores for vision-specific difficulties, dependency, social function, and mental health were lowest in the low-vision group. Visual impairment was found to be associated with decreased overall function. Scott et al studied 156 low-vision patients using the NEI-VFQ, VF-14, and the SF-36. [95] These researchers found that patients' scores on four subscales of the NEI-VFQ improved after low-vision aids were prescribed and refractive error was corrected. Although the SF-36 was unchanged, the VF-14 score improved after treatment. Many researchers have suggested that at least one of the functional outcome tools (eg, NEI-VFQ, SF-36, VF-14) should be included in studies of visual intervention or treatment. [93,94,96–102]

> ***Ophth 1 (Level B)***: **Future research in the treatment of ocular disease in the older person or rehabilitation for older persons with low vision should, wherever possible, make use of tools for assessing functional outcomes.**

VISUAL LOSS AND SPECIFIC GERIATRIC CONDITIONS

VISUAL LOSS AND FALLS

Falls are a common cause of morbidity and mortality in the elderly population. Each year approximately 25% to 35% of older persons fall, [64,73,74] and each year up to 7% of patients aged 75 and older require an emergency room visit after a fall. [58–75] Falls by elderly persons can be devastating, and more than 40% result in hospitalization. [67,68]

Studies have established that poor vision is a risk factor for falls. [6,58–74] Nevitt et al reported a threefold risk for multiple falls with poor vision. [64] Decreased contrast sensitivity and poor depth perception are associated with an increased risk of falls and hip fractures, [58] and impaired visual acuity is associated with an increased risk of wrist and humerus fractures. [60] The Beaver Dam Eye Study found that 11% (943) of 2365 persons aged 60 years or older with acuity less than 20/25 but only 4.4% of those with normal visual acuity had experienced a fall in the prior year. [6]

> *Ophth 2 (Level A)*: **Elderly patients with visual impairment treated with low-vision rehabilitation or whose vision has improved following a specific intervention (eg, cataract surgery, refraction) should be compared with an untreated group or a treated group without visual improvement. The change in incidence of falls over time in the two groups should be prospectively studied.**

> *Ophth 3 (Level B)*: **Cross-sectional or prospective cohort studies should be performed to determine if certain ocular disorders are more or less likely to be associated with falls by elderly persons and whether multiple ocular disorders are synergistic or additive risk factors.**

> *Ophth 4 (Level B)*: **Time-series studies of correlations between level of visual function and likelihood of falls should be carried out in cohort studies.**

Since visual impairment increases the risk of falls, elderly patients with known visual impairment should have access to services to make their home environment safer. Ophthalmologists should be aware of these measures, including:

- increasing lighting and decreasing glare;

- increasing contrast at danger areas such as corners and on stair steps;

- removing floor obstacles, minimizing clutter, and reducing floor hazards (eg, anchoring loose rugs and eliminating uneven surfaces);

- utilizing well-designed hand rails and assistive furnishings (eg, use of non-skid flooring);

- using appropriate walking devices (stable walker and cane types);

- avoiding improper footwear (eg, high-heeled shoes). [16]

> *Ophth 5 (Levels B, A)*: **Prospective interventional studies are needed to establish whether interventions to reduce environmental hazards are cost-effective and practical. Prospective interventional randomized or nonrandomized studies should be performed to determine if the incidence of falls in older patients with visual impairment decreases among those for whom home safety improvements are performed.**

VISUAL LOSS AND HEARING LOSS

In elderly persons, visual impairment commonly occurs with other impairments. For example, visual and hearing loss may both occur in the same patient, and the presence of both sensory impairments increases their functional impact. Appollonio et al demonstrated the predictive value of hearing and visual impairments for mortality in 1140 noninstitutionalized elderly persons. [38] Keller et al in a prospective study of 576 older persons demonstrated that visual and auditory impairment impacts functional status, and that combined vision and hearing impairments have a greater effect on function than do single sensory impairments. Moreover, they found that these two sensory impairments, hearing and visual loss, influence functional status independently of mental status and comorbid illness. [83] Klein et al in the Beaver Dam Study documented the common coexistence of ARMD and hearing loss. [103] Multiple studies have demonstrated that hearing loss and visual loss are interrelated deficits that may increase the functional impact of either sensory deficit alone. [103–107] Overall, these results suggest that interventions to improve sensory function may improve functional independence as well.

> **Ophth 6 (Level B)**: **Research is needed to quantify the effect of multisensory loss in elderly patients (eg, hearing and vision) on functional outcomes. Observational cohort studies should be performed to determine which ocular disorders (eg, age-related macular degeneration, cataract glaucoma) are more likely to be associated with hearing loss and whether or not these ocular disorders have an additive or synergistic effect on functional outcome.**

> **Ophth 7 (Level A)**: **Prospective, focused cohort studies with appropriate comparison groups or nonrandomizd controlled trials of interventions for multisensory loss, including visual or hearing rehabilitation, should be performed to test for improved functional outcomes.**

VISUAL LOSS AND DEPRESSION

Visual disability can cause secondary grief, anxiety, and depressed mood. These nonvisual consequences of visual impairment can worsen or precipitate clinical depression in the elderly person. Appollonio et al showed that an uncorrected sensory deprivation is associated with a significant and independent impairment of mood, decreased self-sufficiency in instrumental ADLs, and impaired social relationships. [108] In men with uncorrected sensory impairment, the unadjusted 6-year mortality rate was found to be almost twice that of the other two study groups. Rovner et al reported a correlation between disability, depression, and impaired vision in a small sample of community-dwelling older persons. [109] Rovner and Ganguli further assessed the relationship of depression, impaired vision, and disability in a later study of 872 noninstitutionalized older patients. [110] They found impaired vision and depression both to be associated strongly with functional impairment and concluded that treating depression might reduce excess disability associated with impaired vision. Carabellese studied vision and depression in 1191 noninstitutionalized persons aged 70 to 75 years and found that visual impairment is significantly and independently associated with an increased risk for depression, decreased self-sufficiency in ADLs, and impaired social relationships. [80]

Ophth 8 (Level B): **Research is needed to establish what types and what level of visual impairment might be associated with clinical depression in elderly patients. Observational cohort studies should be performed to determine the interaction of visual impairment and depression on the health-related quality of life or other studies of function in older persons.**

Ophth 9 (Level B): **Interventional studies of the evaluation and treatment of depression in older patients with visual impairment should be performed to determine the best timing for intervention.**

Ophth 10 (Level A): **Interventional studies of the effect in elderly patients of specific treatments of visual loss on depression should be performed to determine if improvement in the vision-related depression might lead to improved health-related quality of life and overall functioning.**

VISUAL LOSS AND DEMENTIA

Visual loss is associated with and may worsen dementia or delirium. [111–113] Uhlman et al studied 87 older patients with mild-to-moderate Alzheimer's disease and 87 nondemented age- and sex-matched control patients. [111] The researchers found the prevalence of visual impairment to be higher in cases than in controls and visual impairment to be associated with both an increased risk for and an increased clinical severity of Alzheimer's disease. The increased risk of dementia in the existing cohort studies for Alzheimer's disease did not demonstrate a progressive dose-response relationship, and a cohort study alone does not establish a cause-and-effect relation.

Ophth 11 (Level B): **Observational cohort studies should be performed to determine if there is any association between type or severity of visual loss and the major causes of dementia (eg, Alzheimer's disease, multi-infarct dementia).**

Ophth 12 (Level B): **Large population studies should be performed to determine if dementia and visual loss are associated in elderly persons and if the association is independent of other important variables (eg, age could explain the entire association).**

Ophth 13 (Level A): **If an association between dementia and visual loss is found (Ophth 12), especially a severity-related one, then interventional studies should be performed to determine if improvement or stabilization of vision might reduce the incidence or severity of dementia in older persons.**

Ophth 14 (Level A): **In elderly patients with visual loss and dementia, the type and timing of specific interventions should be compared to determine the most effective for improving visual function that leads to improved health-related quality of life or overall functioning.**

VISUAL LOSS AND OVERALL FUNCTION

Several population-based studies have shown an association between visual impairment and overall function. In Established Populations for the Epidemiologic Studies of the Elderly, a population-based study of 5143 elderly persons, 26% of 577 individuals with limitation in ADLs were found to be visually impaired. [114] The Massachusetts Health Care Panel Study of noninstitutionalized elderly persons reported 289 with good vision and 207 with self-perceived visual impairment. [79] The poor-vision group was 2.3 times more likely than the group with good vision to need help grocery shopping and 1.68 times more likely to need help paying bills. In the Salisbury Eye Evaluation project, researchers found visual impairment to be an important predictor of lack of social or religious activities. [115] They also found visual loss to be associated with 1.82 times greater odds of significant difficulty on any ADL and to be associated with 2.45 greater odds of significant difficulty on any instrumental ADL. The Blue Mountains Eye Study found that visual impairment affects the independence of elderly persons, especially women. [77,78] Visually impaired individuals were found to be more likely to rely on community support services, more likely to rely on regular help for cleaning or shopping, and five times more likely to be unable to go out alone.

Marx et al surveyed 103 nursing-home residents for ADL function and found a strong link between low vision and ADL disability; they also found that residents' ADL dependency was significantly related to the presence of eye disorders. [116] Pillar et al evaluated hospitalized elderly blind patients with motor impairments admitted for physical rehabilitation and found functional independence to be less common in these patients than in those who were visually intact. [117] Maino reported that visually impaired elders are much more likely than their normal-sighted peers to have mobility restrictions. [118] Older persons with visual impairment were found to be three to four times more likely to have difficulty walking, going outside, and getting in and out of bed. These and other studies have shown that there is a relationship between visual impairment and loss of independence. [117-130] Research is now needed to determine if there is a relationship between the type and severity of visual loss and loss of overall function.

> *Ophth 15 (Level B)*: **Single-time observational or time-series observational studies should be performed in elderly patients to determine the relationship between loss of independence or decreases in measures of overall function and the type (eg, cataract, glaucoma), timing of onset (eg, early or late), and severity of loss of vision.**

> *Ophth 16 (Level A)*: **Interventional studies should be performed to determine whether stabilization or improvement in vision or visual function (eg, with low-vision rehabilitation) in elderly patients leads to increased independence and improved overall functioning.**

VISUAL LOSS AND DRIVING IMPAIRMENT

Visual loss impairs the older person's ability to drive. [7,20,131-136] As people age, visual functions such as acuity, visual field, and night vision deteriorate. This decline in vision is associated in part with the elderly age group's increase in vehicular accidents per mile driven. Kosnik et al showed that older persons who have recently given up driving report more visual problems than do their driving counterparts. [131] These researchers found driving problems to be related not only to decreased Snellen acuity but also to difficulties in dynamic vision, visual processing speed, visual search, light sensitivity, and near vision. Ball et al examined the association between visual impairment in 257 older drivers and the avoidance of challenging driving situations; they found that drivers with visual impairment report more avoidance behavior than do visually normal drivers. [133]

There is a need for evidence of a significant predictive relationship between changes in vision function and automobile crashes. [136] Although most states require vision screening for driver's license renewal, some do not. Among those states requiring vision screening, there is considerable variation in the frequency and level of testing. Efforts to determine the role of vision in driving, though suggestive, have not been useful in identifying at-risk older drivers. Researchers have observed that older drivers are often aware of their decreased functional capacity and voluntarily adjust their driving patterns by driving less frequently, for shorter distances, during daylight hours, more slowly, and during non-rush hours. Although not statistically significant, the decline in annual traffic fatality rates with increased state vision screening requirements suggests a possible beneficial effect of vision screening.

> *Ophth 17 (Level B)*: **Single-time or time-series observational studies are needed to determine if mandatory vision screening of elderly drivers appears beneficial in decreasing or preventing traffic accidents.**

> *Ophth 18 (Level A)*: **Interventional cohort studies should be performed to determine whether improvement in vision decreases the frequency and severity of traffic accidents by elderly drivers.**

Traditional measures of visual screening for driving ability (eg, Snellen acuity and perimetry) may not be sufficient to assess the elderly driver's predilection for traffic accidents. The useful field of view is one functional measure of visual field that correlates with driving ability and may be predictive of future vehicular accidents. Owsley et al in a comparison of 279 older adults with cataract and 105 patients without cataract showed that cataract adversely affects driving ability. [20] As with previous studies of elderly drivers with visual impairment, these patients were found to be avoiding potentially dangerous or challenging driving situations. The drivers with cataract were twice as likely to report reductions in days driven and number of destinations per week, driving slower than the general traffic flow, and preferring someone else to drive. They were five times more likely to have received advice about limiting their driving, four times more likely to report difficulty with challenging driving situations, and two times more likely to reduce their driving exposure. Cataract patients were also found to be 2.5 times more likely to have had an at-fault crash in the prior 5 years. McGwin et al found that impairment of useful field of view is associated with both self-reported and state-recorded car accidents; glaucoma was identified as a significant risk factor for state-recorded crashes. [134] Kline et al reported age-related visual problems that are related to types of automobile accidents more common among older drivers. [132] Although central visual loss and impaired driving have been well studied, peripheral vision loss also appears to be associated with impaired driving. There is a need to define the types and extent of peripheral vision loss that might impair driving.

> *Ophth 19 (Level B)*: **Single-time or cross-sectional observational studies of a suitable cohort are needed to determine whether there is a**

relationship between the older person's driving performance and the type, severity, and onset of loss of vision.

Ophth 20 (Level B): Observational cohort studies should be performed to determine the interaction between visual loss and other comorbidities or risk factors for unsafe driving such as physical impairments, decreased hearing, and decreased cognition.

Ophth 21 (Level A): Interventional studies of treatments to improve vision or stabilize vision loss in older patients with visual impairment should be performed to determine whether improvement in vision decreases the frequency and severity of traffic accidents among elderly drivers.

VISUAL LOSS AND HOSPITALIZATION

It has been determined that impaired vision contributes to an increase in the average length of hospital stay of elderly patients. One study found that the average length of stay for visually impaired patients was 11.9 days but only 8.2 days for those without visual impairment. [137] Visually impaired patients also experience more problems after discharge. [119] In hospitalized patients, vision impairment was found to be significantly more common among patients with delirium, and those with delirium were found to have increased mortality, institutionalization, and readmission rates after 1 year. [112] See also the discussion of delirium in the chapter on cross-cutting issues (Chapter 13).

Ophth 22 (Level B): Single-time or time-series observational studies are needed to establish the relationship in elderly patients of the type and severity of visual loss to the length of hospital stay and to the incidence and severity of in-hospital comorbidities (eg, delirium and depression).

Ophth 23 (Level A): Interventional studies of treatments to improve or stabilize vision prior to or during hospitalization should be performed to determine if such treatments decrease the length of hospital stay or reduce the incidence or severity of delirium in hospitalized elderly patients.

COMPREHENSIVE EYE EVALUATION AND SCREENING

Up to 40% of blindness among elderly persons is either preventable or treatable. [138] However, no randomized controlled trials or cohort studies have addressed the timing of evaluations for visual impairment or the efficacy of interventions following screening. A meta-analysis of the literature on visual screening of elderly persons revealed no benefit to screening persons aged 65 years and older. [139] The American Academy of Ophthalmology (AAO) Preferred Practice Pattern (PPP) for Comprehensive Adult Eye Evaluation nevertheless recommends an eye examination every 1 to 2 years for patients aged 65 years and older. [140] The U.S. Preventive Services Task Force also recommends screening elderly persons for visual impairment with Snellen visual acuity. [141] These recommendations are based upon the well-documented high prevalence rate of common and often asymptomatic eye pathology in the elderly age group, including cataract, ARMD, glaucoma, and diabetic retinopathy. [142]

Ariyasu et al studied vision screening in 317 patients and found that near visual acuity of 20/40 or worse and distance visual acuity worse than 20/30 is significantly associated with eye pathology. [143] These two vision tests were found to have a sensitivity and specificity of 0.73 to 0.75. The likelihood ratios for pathology were 2.8 for the near vision test and 2.7 for the distance vision test.

> **Ophth 24 (Level B)**: Prospective observational studies are needed to validate the current recommendations for visual screening and to establish the most cost-effective and reliable means for detecting treatable pathology in elderly persons. Prospective cost-effectiveness studies of vision screening of elderly populations at risk are needed to establish the efficacy of such programs. Prospective observational studies should define the leading approaches to screening (eg, Snellen testing, J-scale, visual function scales, comprehensive examinations), and comparative studies should be performed to determine cost-effectiveness, validity, reliability, and feasibility.

> **Ophth 25 (Level A)**: Interventional studies should be performed in elderly persons to compare no screening with different screening methods, measuring efficacy on the basis of visual and functional outcome.

IMPORTANT EYE DISORDERS IN GERIATRIC POPULATIONS

CATARACT

Definition and Treatment

Cataract, defined as opacity in the lens, is the leading cause of blindness worldwide. Cataract is present in 14.3% of men and 23.5% of women between the ages of 65 and 74 years. [49]

No effective medical therapy of cataract exists, but ongoing research studies are addressing the question. Current studies have focused on the indications, techniques, and timing for surgical treatment. Surgical removal of a cataract, however, is not mandated by the mere presence of a lens opacity. The AAO PPP for cataract summarizes the indications for surgery. [10] Cataract surgery is generally indicated if vision is impaired by cataract, if that vision no longer meets the patient's needs, and if surgery provides a reasonable likelihood of improved visual function. Thus, the need for cataract surgery should be determined primarily by the functional status of the patient, and preoperative assessment should include the needs and preferences of the patient. Other specific indications for surgery are lens-induced disease such as phacomorphic or phacolytic glaucoma and cases when visualization of the fundus is necessary (eg, diabetic retinopathy) for adequate treatment of intraocular pathology.

Cataract Surgery and Functional Decline

There is a demonstrated association between decreased visual acuity from cataract and decreased overall well-being. [85,87] Bernth-Petersen interviewed patients with the Visual Function Index before and after cataract extraction and noted that at 1 year after surgery their reading capacity, distance vision, television watching, and other activities had significantly improved. [144] This was the first study to assess the effect of other eye diseases on the functional outcome after cataract surgery. Applegate et al measured outcome after cataract surgery with multiple vision-specific and generic instruments. In this study, patients' ADLs were not found to have improved. [11]

The inability of these early studies to demonstrate improvement in functional status after cataract surgery may have been due to the insensitivity of generic health status instruments to change in vision-specific areas of functional improvement. The subsequent development of the ADVS, which asks persons to rate their difficulty with 20 common visual activities, addresses this problem for researchers interested in measuring visual function. Examples of visual activities included in the ADVS are ability to drive at night and ability to read ordinary newsprint and labels on medications. Open-ended interviews using the ADVS were performed with elderly persons with bilateral cataracts. [94] Improvements in ADVS scores after cataract extraction have been reported. [17,18]

Two observational studies of outcome after cataract extraction used standardized questionnaires and reported improvements in vision-targeted functioning and generic health-related quality of life. [26,39] Javitt et al reported that 75% to 92% of patients with cataract improved in self-reported visual function after cataract surgery; the percentage who improved depended on whether patients had cataract extraction in their first, second, or both eyes during the period of study. [122] A second multicenter study found that 89% of patients reported improvement on the VF-14 after cataract extraction. [25] Even though the ADVS and VF-14 cover similar content, only 77% of the patients in a study by Mangione et al had a positive change on the ADVS. [18] The proportion of patients who improved in the latter study may have been lower because of greater ocular and medical comorbidity and older age of the patients.

Brenner et al reported a positive correlation between visual function and improvements in mental health, current life satisfaction, and social functioning. [39] Steinberg et al administered the Sickness Impact Profile (SIP), a multidimensional survey designed to measure the behavioral impact of illness, [125] to cataract patients. [26] Although 89% had improved vision-targeted VF-14 scores, only 67% had improved SIP scores. Monestam and Wachtmeister found that visual problems while driving declined from 82% preoperatively to 5% after surgery and that problems estimating distance decreased from 37% to 6%. [19] These researchers assessed the impact of cataract surgery on low-vision patients; 81% reported an improved ability to perform visually demanding tasks after cataract surgery. The number of patients who were unable to read newspaper-size print decreased from 44% to 21% after surgery. Patients with loss of peripheral visual fields also gained orientation ability.

Keeffe et al developed an instrument to describe and quantify handicap caused by vision impairment. [82] They used an item pool derived from focus groups and from a review of vision-related quality-of-life questionnaires. They administered the 76-item Impact of Vision Impairment to 95 people and found an association between visual acuity and the type and degree of handicap on subscales. The findings from numerous studies suggest that there is a functional benefit from cataract extraction: Those with the greatest improvement in visual functional status have less decline in generic health-related quality of life.

> ***Ophth 26 (Level A)***: **Interventional studies with elderly patients are needed to determine if there are differences in the amount of functional improvement that are based on the timing of cataract surgery, the initial and final visual outcome, whether one or both eyes are operated on, and the age of the patient at the time of the surgery.**

> ***Ophth 27 (Level B)***: **Meta-analyses of existing data from previously performed interventional studies and clinical trials of cataract extraction should be performed to provide age-specific and age-stratified data for the elderly age group and to identify any age-specific differences in functional outcome.**

AGE-RELATED MACULAR DEGENERATION

Definition and Treatment

ARMD is defined by the AAO PPP as a disorder of the macular that most often occurs in patients older than 50 years. Of persons aged 75 years and older, 25% have nonexudative ARMD and 5% have exudative. [6-8] ARMD is characterized by the following:

- the presence of drusen;

- retinal pigment epithelial (RPE) hypopigmentation or hyperpigmentation;

- geographic atrophy of the RPE and choriocapillaris;

- exudative neovascular maculopathy with choroidal neovascularization, serous or hemorrhagic detachments of the sensory retina or RPE, hard exudates, and subretinal or sub-RPE fibrovascular proliferation and disciform scar;

- the presence of no other cause for these findings. [34]

There is no known effective medical or surgical treatment for the nonexudative form of ARMD. [91,145-153] Current research is focusing on the pathogenesis, prevention, and treatment of ARMD. The exudative form of ARMD may benefit from laser therapy to treat the underlying subretinal neovascularization. [150-153]

Functional Impairment

Williams et al studied 86 elderly patients with ARMD and legal blindness in at least one eye. [154] Participants completed the Quality of Well-being Scale, the Instrumental Activities of Daily Living index, self-rated general health status questionnaire, and the Profile of Mood States. Persons with ARMD were found to suffer significant emotional distress and profoundly reduced quality of life, and they required assistance with key ADLs.

The effects of ARMD in one eye may affect binocular function. Faubert and Overbury studied 59 older adults with ARMD and found that in almost half the cases spatial contrast sensitivity is worse when both eyes are used together. [155] "Binocular inhibition" was not found to be related to the contrast sensitivity of the better eye or to visual acuity.

Mangione et al studied 201 RMD patients and found that severity of ARMD is associated with poorer scores on the ADVS and is most significant for near vision and driving. [53]

Although there are good data on the potential for treating ARMD with laser photocoagulation, data on the visual outcomes from therapy, particularly for subfoveal neovascularization, have been limited. Research on the cause, prevention, and treatment of ARMD is ongoing. Although visual improvement may be limited currently for the treatments for ARMD, visual preservation or stabilization may be helpful.

> *Ophth 28 (Level A)*: **Interventional studies are needed to define the efficacy, cost-effectiveness, and functional outcomes of specific treatments for age-related macular degeneration.**

> *Ophth 29 (Level A)*: **Interventional studies are needed to determine the differences made, if any, by the timing of the treatment of age-related macular degeneration, with results stratified by age of the patient or timing of onset.**

> *Ophth 30 (Level B)*: **Meta-analyses of existing data from interventional and clinical studies on age-related macular degeneration should be performed to provide age-specific and age-stratified data regarding type, timing of therapy, and visual and functional outcome.**

> *Ophth 31 (Level B)*: **All interventional studies of age-related macular degeneration should include demonstration of improvement in function as well as in visual acuity.**

GLAUCOMA

Definition and Treatment

Glaucoma is a term used to describe a number of disorders that result in optic nerve damage due in part to elevated intra-ocular pressure. [35,156] This damage produces gradual and progressive visual field loss. Glaucoma is the third most common cause of visual loss and affects 2.5% of the population aged 40 years or over. The incidence of glaucoma increases with age and disproportionately affects elderly black Americans; 10% of black Americans but only 2% of white Americans have glaucoma. The most common type of glaucoma is primary open-angle glaucoma (POAG).

The AAO PPP defines POAG as a multifactorial optic neuropathy in which there is characteristic acquired loss of retinal ganglion cells and atrophy of the optic nerve. The disease is generally adult onset, chronic, and bilateral but often asymmetric. The angle is open and normal appearing, and there is no secondary cause for glaucoma. There is evidence of progressive optic nerve damage from changes in the optic disc and retinal nerve fiber layer, and visual field defects are characteristic.

There is no cure for POAG. Medical treatment with topical or systemic agents to lower intra-ocular pressure in POAG is the first line of therapy. The AAO PPP for POAG, derived from an expert consensus panel review of the available literature, recommends a 20% reduction in intra-ocular pressure for POAG patients with progressive visual field loss or optic nerve damage. [35] The recommended follow-up schedule should be based upon stabilization of intra-ocular pressure within a 3-month maximum, with adjustment of therapy until the target intra-ocular pressure is reached. The goals of medical treatment are to slow or halt progression of visual loss, to prevent further damage to the optic nerve, and to lower intraocular pressure. Although most patients with POAG have elevated intra-ocular pressure, some do not but still sustain visual loss and optic nerve cupping. This condition is known as *normal* or *low-tension* glaucoma. The Collaborative Normal-Tension Glaucoma Study Group demonstrated in a multicenter randomized controlled trial that treatment of intra-ocular pressure is helpful. This study found a 20% reduction in rate of visual field loss at 3 years and a 40% reduction at 5 years if intra-ocular pressure was reduced by 30% in comparison with untreated eyes. [42,43] The AAO PPP recommends that the choice of treatment take into consideration quality of life, patient's physical, visual, medical, psychologic, and social circumstances. [35]

POAG patients who fail, are intolerant to, or are nonadherent with medical therapy may require surgical treatment. The goal of surgical therapy in glaucoma is to lower the intra-ocular pressure of an eye. Although surgery may result in lower eye pressures, eyes may continue to have progressive glaucomatous damage after surgery.

Functional Impact

The older person's HRQOL is affected by glaucoma. Sherwood et al reported the negative impact of glaucoma on quality of life. [128] Wilson et al measured functional status and well-being of glaucoma patients with the SF-36 questionnaire. [76] Both studies reported lower scores on general health instruments and quality of life in glaucoma patients than in control patients. Parrish et al and Guttierrez et al described decreased scores on the NEI-VFQ, the VF-14, and the ADVS. [99,121] Scores on the VF-14 and the NEI-VFQ were associated with visual field impairment. ADVS scores were worse in glaucoma patients. All these studies indicate loss of function in multiple domains.

> *Ophth 32 (Level A)*: **Interventional studies are needed to determine if the type and timing of treatments of glaucoma alters efficacy and if efficacy in elderly patients improves functional outcome.**

> *Ophth 33 (Level A)*: **Interventional studies are needed to determine the cost-effectiveness and durability of stabilization or improvement of vision in elderly glaucoma patents.**

> *Ophth 34 (Level A)*: **Interventional studies should be performed to determine if preventive measures or screening for glaucoma in older persons is effective and improves functional outcome.**

> *Ophth 35 (Level B)*: **Observational studies are needed to determine if treatment efficacy and functional outcome for glaucoma therapy differ by age.**

> *Ophth 36 (Level B)*: **Meta-analyses of existing data from interventional and clinical studies on surgical and medical treatment for glaucoma should be performed to provide age-specific and age-stratified data on functional outcome.**

DIABETIC RETINOPATHY

Diabetic retinopathy is defined as the retinal changes caused by diabetes mellitus. Diabetes type 1 or 2 may produce diabetic retinopathy, and the incidence of diabetic retinopathy increases with the duration of systemic disease. There are two types of diabetic retinopathy, nonproliferative and proliferative. The nonproliferative form causes retinal hemorrhages and exudates. Leakage of fluid from microaneurysms may produce visual loss as a consequence of diabetic macular edema. Type 2 diabetes is more likely to have macular edema. The proliferative form occurs as a result of new blood vessel formation (neovascularization) in response to retinal ischemia. These new blood vessels are friable and may bleed, leading to vitreous hemorrhage and secondary visual loss. Traction may develop on the underlying retina and result in a tractional retinal detachment. Neovascularization may develop on the iris or the angle and lead to neovascular glaucoma.

Diabetic retinopathy is the fourth most common cause of visual loss in the elderly age group. [44–48,157–159] Good control of blood glucose is important in the treatment and prevention of diabetic retinopathy. In the Diabetes Control and Complications Trial, patients with type 1 diabetes mellitus were randomized to conventional therapy or to intensive therapy with the aim of achieving near-normal blood glucose and glycosylated hemoglobin concentrations. [44] An average of 4 years after randomization, the proportion of patients who had worsening retinopathy, including proliferative retinopathy, macular edema, and the need for laser therapy, was lower in the intensive-therapy group than in the conventional-therapy group. Comorbid conditions such as hypertension and hyperlipidemia can worsen diabetic retinopathy and should also be treated. [159]

Multiple studies have demonstrated that laser treatment significantly reduces the incidence and severity of visual loss and blindness due to proliferative diabetic retinopathy and macular edema. [44–48] The Diabetic Retinopathy Study showed that laser treatment with panretinal photocoagulation for proliferative diabetic retinopathy reduces blindness by up to 60%. [45] Miller et al studied the impact of diabetes on disability and physical functioning in 116 diabetic inner-city black Americans aged 70 years and older and found that impairments in visual function explains part of the association between diabetic status and poor general health, disability, and falls. [160]

> *Ophth 37 (Level B)*: **Observational studies should be performed to determine the functional impact of diabetic retinopathy on the health-related quality of life of older diabetic patients.**

> *Ophth 38 (Level A)*: **Interventional studies are needed to determine whether specific preventive strategies (eg, tight diabetic control measures or diabetic retinopathy screening programs) and treatment measures improve functional outcomes in older diabetic patients.**

> *Ophth 39 (Level B)*: **Observational studies are needed to determine if the age of the patient, age at onset of diagnosis, and age at initiation of treatment are important factors in functional outcome in diabetic retinopathy.**

> *Ophth 40 (Level B)*: **Meta-analyses of data from existing and future interventional studies on the treatment of diabetes, including diabetic control, laser treatment for proliferative diabetic retinopathy**

and diabetic macular edema, and surgical treatment, should be performed to provide age-specific and age-stratified data on functional
outcome.

LOW VISION

The AAO PPP on low vision defines moderate visual impairment as best corrected vision
of less than 20/60 and profound visual loss as less than 20/400 or visual field diameter less
than 10 degrees. [36] Low vision is defined as profound visual impairment in one eye or at
least moderate visual impairment in both eyes. Studies have shown that profound visual
loss is a significant psychologic loss for patients. Low vision ranks only behind arthritis
and heart disease for impact on function in the elderly age group. Visual loss is often rated
as the elderly patient's worst problem, even in the context of other chronic disabling
conditions such as cardiac disease. Fletcher et al have emphasized that comprehensive
low-vision rehabilitation programs can have dramatic results in increasing the independence and productivity of affected persons; numerous studies document that low-vision
rehabilitation improves patient independence, performance of ADLs, and quality of
life. [3-5,161,162] The ACOVE (Assessing Care of Vulnerable Elders) report documented that
74% of patients undergoing low-vision services improve their overall functioning, including their ability to cook, read, drive, decrease their dependence on others, and improve
productivity at work. [138] Scott et al investigated the functional status and quality of life of
patients at a low-vision clinic and evaluated the impact of low-vision services. [95] Using
the SF-36, VF-14, and NEI-VFQ, these researchers demonstrated that low-vision clinic
patients perceive marked impairment of functional status and quality of life. Elliott et al
studied the demographic characteristics of 4744 low-vision patients, of whom 71% were
aged 65 or over and 55% were aged 75 or over; ARMD was the primary diagnosis in 75%,
and 46% had cataract. [163]

> *Ophth 41 (Level A)*: **Interventional studies should be performed in eld-
> erly persons to determine if the types and visual outcome effective-
> ness of low-vision therapies are important factors in functional
> outcomes.**

RECOMMENDED RESEARCH STRATEGIES

This review of recent literature on geriatric ophthalmology emphasizes functional outcomes, especially with regard to the four major causes of visual impairment in elderly
persons. In setting their own research agendas, researchers in ophthalmology are invited to
use this needs assessment to identify the types and scope of studies needed to improve the
ophthalmic care of elderly patients. The following recommendations are based upon this
review of the literature:

■ Existing data from interventional studies and clinical trials in ophthalmology should
  be systematically "mined" for age-specific and age-stratified information in outcomes
  among elderly patients. The timing or efficacy for specific interventions may be partly
  dependent on age.

■ All new research should be aimed at producing age-specific and age-stratified data. In addition, editors and editorial boards of the major ophthalmology journals should consider requiring such data in reports of ongoing publications and research.

■ Studies should be directed at age-specific and age-stratified outcomes. Interventional studies should include functional assessment and functional outcomes in addition to visual assessment and visual outcomes.

KEY RESEARCH QUESTIONS IN GERIATRIC OPHTHALMOLOGY

Ophth KQ1: **Does visual improvement or stabilization, including low-vision rehabilitation, reduce the severity, incidence, and prevalence of depression, dementia, delirium, falls, driving accidents, loss of function or quality of life, and hospital complications in the elderly population?**

Hypothesis-generating: Observational cohort studies would document whether visual loss impacts these conditions and disorders of elderly persons. This could be achieved through surveys of existing patients with visual loss prospectively.

Hypothesis-testing: We recommend that interventional studies be performed to determine if visual improvement or low-vision rehabilitation reduces the severity of, the incidence of, and the prevalence of the listed disorders in the elderly population. These studies could be nonrandomized controlled trials using nonresponders as a comparison group. Ethical issues regarding the withholding of treatments to improve visual function might exclude the feasibility of a randomized trial. In the case of low-vision rehabilitation, because these services are currently not universally available or accepted, comparison groups of treated and untreated patients would be readily available.

Ophth KQ2: **What is the best timing for and what are the best methods for intervention in visual loss in the elderly person, and what are the best outcome measures for documenting success?**

Hypothesis-generating: We recommend that existing data from clinical trials and interventional studies be re-examined by meta-analysis to determine if age-specific and age-stratified recommendations from these trials are valid for elderly persons.

Hypothesis-testing: We recommend interventional studies to determine the best timing for and the specific methods for intervention in visual loss, and we recommend the use of outcome measures that include the functional impact of visual loss or visual improvement in elderly persons. Interventional studies on the efficacy of preoperative and prehospitalization visual screening and subsequent vision treatments should be performed. Functional measures should be included as primary or secondary outcome measures for these studies.

Ophth KQ3: **What are the risk factors for functional vision impairment in the elderly person and what screening intervals and methods and what instruments for measuring visual function would be best for identifying an older person's risks for such impairment?**

Hypothesis-generating: We recommend observational cohort studies to determine the risk factors for functional visual impairment in the elderly person.

Hypothesis-testing: We recommend interventional studies in elderly persons to determine the best intervals for visual screening, the best methods for visual screening, the best measures of visual function, and the most valid and reliable instruments for measuring function.

REFERENCES

1. Bierman A, Spector W, Atkins D, et al. Improving the Health Care of Older Americans. A Report of the AHRQ Task Force on Aging. Rockville, MD: Agency for Healthcare Research and Quality, 2001. AHRQ Publication No. 01-0030.

2. Bailey IL. New procedures for detecting early vision losses in the elderly. Optom Vis Sci 1993;70:299-305.

3. Castor TD, Carter TL. Low vision: physician screening helps to improve patient function. Geriatrics 1995;50:51-52, 55-57; quiz 58-59.

4. Fletcher DC, Shindell S, Hindman T, Schaffrath M. Low vision rehabilitation. Finding capable people behind damaged eyeballs. West J Med 1991;154:554-556.

5. Fletcher DC. Low vision: the physician's role in rehabilitation and referral. Geriatrics 1994;49:50-53.

6. Klein BE, Klein R, Lee KE, Cruickshanks KJ. Performance-based and self-assessed measures of visual function as related to history of falls, hip fractures, and measured gait time. The Beaver Dam Eye Study. Ophthalmology 1998;105:160-164.

7. Klein R, Klein BE, Linton KL, De Mets DL. The Beaver Dam Eye Study: visual acuity. Ophthalmology 1991;98:1310-1315.

8. Tielsch JM, Javitt JC, Coleman A, et al. The prevalence of blindness and visual impairment among nursing home residents in Baltimore. N Engl J Med 1995;332:1205-1209.

9. Tielsch JM, Steinberg EP, Cassard SD, et al. Preoperative functional expectations and postoperative outcomes among patients undergoing first eye cataract surgery. Arch Ophthalmol 1995;113:1312-1318.

10. American Academy of Ophthalmology. Preferred Practice Patterns. Cataract in the Adult Eye. 1996.

11. Applegate WB, Miller ST, Elam JT, et al. Impact of cataract surgery with lens implantation on vision and physical function in elderly patients. JAMA 1987;257:1064-1066.

12. Bruce DW, Gray CS. Beyond the cataract: visual and functional disability in elderly people. Age Ageing 1991;20:389-391.

13. Cataract Management Guideline Panel. Clinical Practice Guideline Number 4. Cataract in adults: management of functional impairment. Rockville MD: Department of Health and Human Services, Public Health Service, 1993. AHCPR Pub 93-0542.

14. Crabtree HL, Hildreth AJ, O'Connell JE, et al. Measuring visual symptoms in British cataract patients: the cataract symptom scale. Br J Ophthalmol 1999;83:519-523.

15. Javitt JC, Steinberg EP, Sharkey P, et al. Cataract surgery in one eye or both. A billion dollar per year issue. Ophthalmology 1995;102:1583-1592; discussion 1592-1583.

16. Lee AG, Beaver HA, Teasdale T. The Aging Eye (CD-ROM). Houston, TX: Baylor College of Medicine, 2001.

17. Mangione CM, Orav EJ, Lawrence MG, et al. Prediction of visual function after cataract surgery. A prospectively validated model. Arch Ophthalmol 1995;113:1305-1311.

18. Mangione CM, Phillips RS, Lawrence MG, et al. Improved visual function and attenuation of declines in health-related quality of life after cataract extraction. Arch Ophthalmol 1994;112:1419-1425.

19. Monestam E, Wachtmeister L. Impact of cataract surgery on car driving: a population based study in Sweden. Br J Ophthalmol 1997;81:16-22.

20. Owsley C, Stalvey B, Wells J, Sloane ME. Older drivers and cataract: driving habits and crash risk. J Gerontol A Biol Sci Med Sci 1999;54:M203-M211.

21. Powe NR, Schein OD, Gieser SC, et al. Synthesis of the literature on visual acuity and complications following cataract extraction with intraocular lens implantation. Cataract Patient Outcome Research Team. Arch Ophthalmol 1994;112:239-252.

22. Powe NR, Tielsch JM, Schein OD, et al. Rigor of research methods in studies of the effectiveness and safety of cataract extraction with intraocular lens implantation. Cataract Patient Outcome Research Team. Arch Ophthalmol 1994;112:228-238.

23. Schein OD, Steinberg EP, Cassard SD, et al. Predictors of outcome in patients who underwent cataract surgery. Ophthalmology 1995;102:817-823.

24. Schein OD, Bass EB, Sharkey P, et al. Cataract surgical techniques. Preferences and underlying beliefs. Arch Ophthalmol 1995;113:1108-1112.

25. Steinberg EP, Tielsch JM, Schein OD, et al. National study of cataract surgery outcomes. Variation in 4-month postoperative outcomes as reflected in multiple outcome measures. Ophthalmology 1994;101:1131-1140; discussion 1140-1131.

26. Steinberg EP, Tielsch JM, Schein OD, et al. The VF-14. An index of functional impairment in patients with cataract. Arch Ophthalmol 1994;112:630-638.

27. Bass EB, Steinberg EP, Luthra R, et al. Do ophthalmologists, anesthesiologists, and internists agree about preoperative testing in healthy patients undergoing cataract surgery? Arch Ophthalmol 1995;113:1248-1256.

28. Superstein R, Boyaner D, Overbury O. Functional complaints, visual acuity, spatial contrast sensitivity, and glare disability in preoperative and postoperative cataract patients. J Cataract Refract Surg 1999;25:575-581.

29. Tobacman JK, Zimmerman B, Lee P, et al. Visual function impairments in relation to gender, age, and visual acuity in patients who undergo cataract surgery. Ophthalmology 1998;105:1745-1750.

30. Uusitalo RJ, Brans T, Pessi T, Tarkkanen A. Evaluating cataract surgery gains by assessing patients' quality of life using the VF-7. J Cataract Refract Surg 1999;25:989-994.

31. Rumsey KE. Redefining the optometric examination: addressing the vision needs of older adults. Optom Vis Sci 1993;70:587-591.

32. Rubin GS, Roche KB, Prasada-Rao P, Fried LP. Visual impairment and disability in older adults. Optom Vis Sci 1994;71:750-760.

33. Rubin GS, West SK, Munoz B, et al. A comprehensive assessment of visual impairment in a population of older Americans. The SEE Study. Salisbury Eye Evaluation Project. Invest Ophthalmol Vis Sci 1997;38:557-568.

34. American Academy of Ophthalmology. Preferred Practice Patterns. Age-related Macular Degeneration. Limited Revision. 2001.

35. American Academy of Ophthalmology. Preferred Practice Patterns. Primary Open Angle Glaucoma. 2000.

36. American Academy of Ophthalmology. Preferred Practice Patterns. Vision Rehabilitation for Adults. 2001.

37. Albrecht KG, Lee PP. Conformance with preferred practice patterns in caring for patients with glaucoma. Ophthalmology 1994;101:1668-1671.

38. Appollonio I, Carabellese C, Magni E, et al. Sensory impairments and mortality in an elderly community population: a six-year follow-up study. Age Ageing 1995;24:30-36.

39. Brenner MH, Curbow B, Javitt JC, et al. Vision change and quality of life in the elderly. Response to cataract surgery and treatment of other chronic ocular conditions. Arch Ophthalmol 1993;111:680-685.

40. Campbell VA, Crews JE, Moriarty DG, et al. Surveillance for sensory impairment, activity limitation, and health-related quality of life among older adults—United States, 1993-1997. Mor Mortal Wkly Rep CDC Surveill Summ 1999;48:131-156.

41. Carter TL. Age-related vision changes: a primary care guide. Geriatrics 1994;49:37-42, 45; quiz 46-37.

42. Collaborative Normal-Tension Glaucoma Study Group. Comparison of glaucomatous progression between untreated patients with normal-tension glaucoma and patients with therapeutically reduced intraocular pressures. Am J Ophthalmol 1998;126:487-497.

43. Collaborative Normal-Tension Glaucoma Study Group. The effectiveness of intraocular pressure reduction in the treatment of normal-tension glaucoma. Am J Ophthalmol 1998;126:498-505.

44. The Diabetes Control and Complications Trial/Epidemiology of Diabetes Interventions and Complications Research Group. Retinopathy and nephropathy in patients with type 1 diabetes four years after a trial of intensive therapy. N Engl J Med 2000;342:381-389.

45. The Diabetic Retinopathy Study Research Group. Indications for photocoagulation treatment of diabetic retinopathy: Diabetic Retinopathy Study Report No. 14. Int Ophthalmol Clin 1987;27:239-253.

46. The Diabetic Retinopathy Study Research Group. Photocoagulation treatment of proliferative diabetic retinopathy. Clinical application of Diabetic Retinopathy Study (DRS) findings, DRS Report No. 8. Ophthalmology 1981;88:583-600.

47. The Early Treatment Diabetic Retinopathy Study Research Group. Photocoagulation for diabetic macular edema: Early Treatment Diabetic Retinopathy Study Report No. 4. Int Ophthalmol Clin 1987;27:265-272.

48. The Early Treatment Diabetic Retinopathy Study Research Group. Early photocoagulation for diabetic retinopathy. ETDRS Report No. 9. Ophthalmology 1991;98:766-785.

49. Klein BE, Klein R, Linton KL. Prevalence of age-related lens opacities in a population. The Beaver Dam Eye Study. Ophthalmology 1992;99:546-552.

50. Klein R, Klein BE, Linton KL. Prevalence of age-related maculopathy. The Beaver Dam Eye Study. Ophthalmology 1992;99:933-943.

51. Klein R. Age-related eye disease, visual impairment, and driving in the elderly. Hum Factors 1991;33:521-525.

52. Tielsch JM, Sommer A, Katz J, et al. Socioeconomic status and visual impairment among urban Americans. Baltimore Eye Survey Research Group. Arch Ophthalmol 1991;109:637-641.

53. Mangione CM, Gutierrez PR, Lowe G, et al. Influence of age-related maculopathy on visual functioning and health-related quality of life. Am J Ophthalmol 1999;128:45-53.

54. Olsen CL, Kassoff A, Gerber T. The care of diabetic patients by ophthalmologists in New York State. Ophthalmology 1989;96:739-745.

55. Perry DP. ARMD is robbing older people blind–and stealing their independence, too. J Am Optom Assoc 1999;70:7-9.

56. Salive ME, Guralnik J, Christen W, et al. Functional blindness and visual impairment in older adults from three communities. Ophthalmology 1992;99:1840-1847.

57. Jette AM, Branch LG. Impairment and disability in the aged. J Chronic Dis 1985;38:59-65.

58. Cummings SR, Nevitt MC, Browner WS, et al. Risk factors for hip fracture in white women. Study of Osteoporotic Fractures Research Group. N Engl J Med 1995;332:767-773.

59. Cwikel J. Falls among elderly people living at home: medical and social factors in a national sample. Isr J Med Sci 1992;28:446-453.

60. Kelsey JL, Browner WS, Seeley DG, et al. Risk factors for fractures of the distal forearm and proximal humerus. The Study of Osteoporotic Fractures Research Group (published erratum appears in Am J Epidemiol 1992 135:1183). Am J Epidemiol 1992;135:477-489.

61. Lord SR, McLean D, Stathers G. Physiological factors associated with injurious falls in older people living in the community. Gerontology 1992;38:338-346.

62. Melton LJ, 3rd, Riggs BL. Risk factors for injury after a fall. Clin Geriatr Med 1985;1: 525-539.

63. Myers AH, Robinson EG, Van Natta ML, et al. Hip fractures among the elderly: factors associated with in-hospital mortality. Am J Epidemiol 1991;134:1128-1137.

64. Nevitt MC, Cummings SR, Kidd S, Black D. Risk factors for recurrent nonsyncopal falls. A prospective study. JAMA 1989;261:2663-2668.

65. Nevitt MC, Cummings SR, Hudes ES. Risk factors for injurious falls: a prospective study. J Gerontol 1991;46:M164-M170.

66. O'Loughlin JL, Robitaille Y, Boivin JF, Suissa S. Incidence of and risk factors for falls and injurious falls among the community-dwelling elderly. Am J Epidemiol 1993;137:342-354.

67. Sattin RW, Lambert Huber DA, DeVito CA, et al. The incidence of fall injury events among the elderly in a defined population. Am J Epidemiol 1990;131:1028-1037.

68. Sattin RW. Falls among older persons: a public health perspective. Annu Rev Public Health 1992;13:489-508.

69. Sorock GS. Falls among the elderly: epidemiology and prevention. Am J Prev Med 1988;4: 282-288.

70. Speechley M, Tinetti M. Falls and injuries in frail and vigorous community elderly persons. J Am Geriatr Soc 1991;39:46-52.

71. Tinetti ME. Instability and falling in elderly patients. Semin Neurol 1989;9:39-45.

72. Tinetti ME, Powell L. Fear of falling and low self-efficacy: a case of dependence in elderly persons. J Gerontol 1993;48 Spec No:35-38.

73. Tinetti ME, Doucette J, Claus E, Marottoli R. Risk factors for serious injury during falls by older persons in the community. J Am Geriatr Soc 1995;43:1214-1221.

74. Tinetti ME, McAvay G, Claus E. Does multiple risk factor reduction explain the reduction in fall rate in the Yale FICSIT Trial? Frailty and Injuries Cooperative Studies of Intervention Techniques. Am J Epidemiol 1996;144:389-399.

75. Tobis JS, Block M, Steinhaus-Donham C, et al. Falling among the sensorially impaired elderly. Arch Phys Med Rehabil 1990;71:144-147.

76. Wilson MR, Coleman AL, Yu F, et al. Functional status and well-being in patients with glaucoma as measured by the Medical Outcomes Study Short Form-36 questionnaire. Ophthalmology 1998;105:2112-2116.

77. Wang JJ, Mitchell P, Smith W, et al. Impact of visual impairment on use of community support services by elderly persons: the Blue Mountains Eye Study. Invest Ophthalmol Vis Sci 1999;40:12-19.

78. Wang JJ, Mitchell P, Smith W. Vision and low self-rated health: the Blue Mountains Eye Study. Invest Ophthalmol Vis Sci 2000;41:49-54.

79. Branch LG, Horowitz A, Carr C. The implications for everyday life of incident self-reported visual decline among people over age 65 living in the community. Gerontologist 1989;29: 359-365.

80. Carabellese C, Appollonio I, Rozzini R, et al. Sensory impairment and quality of life in a community elderly population. J Am Geriatr Soc 1993;41:401-407.

81. Keeffe JE, Lam D, Cheung A, et al. Impact of vision impairment on functioning. Aust N Z J Ophthalmol 1998;26 Suppl 1:S16-S18.

82. Keeffe JE, McCarty CA, Hassell JB, Gilbert AG. Description and measurement of handicap caused by vision impairment. Aust N Z J Ophthalmol 1999;27:184-186.

83. Keller BK, Morton JL, Thomas VS, Potter JF. The effect of visual and hearing impairments on functional status. J Am Geriatr Soc 1999;47:1319-1325.

84. Kelly M. Consequences of visual impairment on leisure activities of the elderly. Geriatr Nurs 1995;16:273-275.

85. Lee PP, Smith JP, Kington R. The relationship of self-rated vision and hearing to functional status and well-being among seniors 70 years and older. Am J Ophthalmol 1999;127:447-452.

86. Lee PP, Spritzer K, Hays RD. The impact of blurred vision on functioning and well-being. Ophthalmology 1997;104:390-396.

87. Lee PP, Whitcup SM, Hays RD, et al. The relationship between visual acuity and functioning and well-being among diabetics. Qual Life Res 1995;4:319-323.

88. Thompson JR, Gibson JM, Jagger C. The association between visual impairment and mortality in elderly people. Age Ageing 1989;18:83-88.

89. Livingston PM, Lee SE, McCarty CA, Taylor HR. A comparison of participants with non-participants in a population-based epidemiologic study: the Melbourne Visual Impairment Project. Ophthalmic Epidemiol 1997;4:73-81.

90. Dargent-Molina P, Hays M, Breart G. Sensory impairments and physical disability in aged women living at home. Int J Epidemiol 1996;25:621-629.

91. McClure ME, Hart PM, Jackson AJ, et al. Macular degeneration: do conventional measurements of impaired visual function equate with visual disability? Br J Ophthalmol 2000;84:244-250.

92. Ware JE, Jr., Sherbourne CD. The MOS 36-item short-form health survey (SF-36). I. Conceptual framework and item selection. Med Care 1992;30:473-483.

93. Mangione CM, Berry S, Spritzer K, et al. Identifying the content area for the 51-item National Eye Institute Visual Function Questionnaire: results from focus groups with visually impaired persons. Arch Ophthalmol 1998;116:227-233.

94. Mangione CM, Phillips RS, Seddon JM, et al. Development of the 'Activities of Daily Vision Scale'. A measure of visual functional status. Med Care 1992;30:1111-1126.

95. Scott IU, Smiddy WE, Schiffman J, et al. Quality of life of low-vision patients and the impact of low-vision services. Am J Ophthalmol 1999;128:54-62.

96. Cassard SD, Patrick DL, Damiano AM, et al. Reproducibility and responsiveness of the VF-14. An index of functional impairment in patients with cataracts. Arch Ophthalmol 1995;113:1508-1513.

97. Hart PM, Chakravarthy U, Stevenson MR, Jamison JQ. A vision specific functional index for use in patients with age related macular degeneration. Br J Ophthalmol 1999;83:1115-1120.

98. Horowitz A. Vision impairment and functional disability among nursing home residents. Gerontologist 1994;34:316-323.

99. Parrish RK, Gedde SJ, Scott IU, et al. Visual function and quality of life among patients with glaucoma. Arch Ophthalmol 1997;115:1447-1455.

100. Ross CK, Stelmack JA, Stelmack TR, et al. Development and sensitivity to visual impairment of the Low Vision Functional Status Evaluation (LVFSE). Optom Vis Sci 1999;76:212-220.

101. Turco PD, Connolly J, McCabe P, Glynn RJ. Assessment of functional vision performance: a new test for low vision patients. Ophthalmic Epidemiol 1994;1:15-25.

102. Lawton MP, Brody EM. Assessment of older people: self-maintaining and instrumental activities of daily living. Gerontologist 1969;9:179-186.

103. Klein R, Cruickshanks KJ, Klein BE, et al. Is age-related maculopathy related to hearing loss? Arch Ophthalmol 1998;116:360-365.

104. Bagley M. Helping older adults to live better with hearing and vision losses. J Case Manag 1998;7:147-152.
105. Guralnik JM. The impact of vision and hearing impairments on health in old age. J Am Geriatr Soc 1999;47:1029-1031.
106. Rudberg MA, Furner SE, Dunn JE, Cassel CK. The relationship of visual and hearing impairments to disability: an analysis using the longitudinal study of aging. J Gerontol 1993;48:M261-M265.
107. Rubin GS, Bandeen-Roche K, Huang GH, et al. The association of multiple visual impairments with self-reported visual disability: SEE project. Invest Ophthalmol Vis Sci 2001;42: 64-72.
108. Appollonio I, Carabellese C, Frattola L, Trabucchi M. Effects of sensory aids on the quality of life and mortality of elderly people: a multivariate analysis. Age Ageing 1996;25:89-96.
109. Rovner BW, Zisselman PM, Shmuely-Dulitzki Y. Depression and disability in older people with impaired vision: a follow-up study. J Am Geriatr Soc 1996;44:181-184.
110. Rovner BW, Ganguli M. Depression and disability associated with impaired vision: the MoVies Project. J Am Geriatr Soc 1998;46:617-619.
111. Uhlmann RF, Larson EB, Koepsell TD, et al. Visual impairment and cognitive dysfunction in Alzheimer's disease. J Gen Intern Med 1991;6:126-132.
112. George J, Bleasdale S, Singleton SJ. Causes and prognosis of delirium in elderly patients admitted to a district general hospital. Age Ageing 1997;26:423-427.
113. Steinman SB, Steinman BA, Trick GL, Lehmkuhle S. A sensory explanation for visual attention deficits in the elderly. Optom Vis Sci 1994;71:743-749.
114. Salive ME, Guralnik J, Glynn RJ, et al. Association of visual impairment with mobility and physical function. J Am Geriatr Soc 1994;42:287-292.
115. West SK, Munoz B, Rubin GS, et al. Function and visual impairment in a population-based study of older adults. The SEE project. Salisbury Eye Evaluation. Invest Ophthalmol Vis Sci 1997;38:72-82.
116. Marx MS, Werner P, Cohen-Mansfield J, Feldman R. The relationship between low vision and performance of activities of daily living in nursing home residents. J Am Geriatr Soc 1992;40:1018-1020.
117. Pillar T, Gaspar E, Dickstein R. Physical rehabilitation of the elderly blind patient. Int Disabil Stud 1990;12:75-77.
118. Maino JH. Visual deficits and mobility. Evaluation and management. Clin Geriatr Med 1996;12:803-823.
119. Boter H, Mistiaen P, Duijnhouwer E, Groenewegen I. The problems of elderly patients at home after ophthalmic treatment. J Ophthalmic Nurs Technol 1998;17:59-65.
120. Cate Y, Baker SS, Gilbert MP. Occupational therapy and the person with diabetes and vision impairment. Am J Occup Ther 1995;49:905-911.
121. Gutierrez P, Wilson MR, Johnson C, et al. Influence of glaucomatous visual field loss on health-related quality of life. Arch Ophthalmol 1997;115:777-784.
122. Javitt JC, Brenner MH, Curbow B, et al. Outcomes of cataract surgery. Improvement in visual acuity and subjective visual function after surgery in the first, second, and both eyes. Arch Ophthalmol 1993;111:686-691.
123. Jayamanne DG, Allen ED, Wood CM, Currie S. Correlation between early, measurable improvement in quality of life and speed of visual rehabilitation after phacoemulsification. J Cataract Refract Surg 1999;25:1135-1139.
124. Lundstrom M, Fregell G, Sjoblom A. Vision related daily life problems in patients waiting for a cataract extraction. Br J Ophthalmol 1994;78:608-611.
125. Bergner M, Bobbitt RA, Carter WB, Gilson BS. The Sickness Impact Profile: development and final revision of a health status measure. Med Care 1981;19:787-805.

126. Nelson P, Aspinall P, O'Brien C. Patients' perception of visual impairment in glaucoma: a pilot study. Br J Ophthalmol 1999;83:546-552.

127. Phillips KE, Russello SM, Bonesi J, Garcon R. Functional visual problems: training home care aides to identify early signs. Caring 1997;16:54, 56-60, 62-54.

128. Sherwood MB, Garcia-Siekavizza A, Meltzer MI, et al. Glaucoma's impact on quality of life and its relation to clinical indicators. A pilot study. Ophthalmology 1998;105:561-566.

129. Swagerty DL. The impact of age-related visual impairment on functional independence in the elderly. Kans Med 1995;96:24-26.

130. Wahl HW, Schilling O, Oswald F, Heyl V. Psychosocial consequences of age-related visual impairment: comparison with mobility-impaired older adults and long-term outcome. J Gerontol B Psychol Sci Soc Sci 1999;54:P304-P316.

131. Kosnik WD, Sekuler R, Kline DW. Self-reported visual problems of older drivers. Hum Factors 1990;32:597-608.

132. Kline DW, Kline TJ, Fozard JL, et al. Vision, aging, and driving: the problems of older drivers. J Gerontol 1992;47:P27-P34.

133. Ball K, Owsley C, Stalvey B, et al. Driving avoidance and functional impairment in older drivers. Accid Anal Prev 1998;30:313-322.

134. McGwin G, Owsley C, Ball K. Identifying crash involvement among older drivers: agreement between self-report and state records. Accid Anal Prev 1998;30:781-791.

135. Owsley C, Ball K, McGwin G, Jr., et al. Visual processing impairment and risk of motor vehicle crash among older adults. JAMA 1998;279:1083-1088.

136. Shipp MD, Penchansky R. Vision testing and the elderly driver: is there a problem meriting policy change? J Am Optom Assoc 1995;66:343-351.

137. Morse AR, Yatzkan E, Berberich B, Arons RR. Acute care hospital utilization by patients with visual impairment. Arch Ophthalmol 1999;117:943-949.

138. Wenger NS, Shekelle PG. Assessing care of vulnerable elders: ACOVE project overview. Ann Intern Med 2001;135:642-646.

139. Smeeth L, Iliffe S. Community screening for visual impairment in the elderly. Cochrane Database Syst Rev 2000:CD001054.

140. American Academy of Ophthalmology. Preferred Practice Patterns. Comprehensive Adult Medical Eye Evaluation. 2000.

141. U.S. Preventive Services Task Force. Recommendations for screening for visual impairment. In Guide to Clinical Preventive Services, 2nd ed. Baltimore MD: Williams & Wilkins, 1996, pp 373-382.

142. Rahmani B, Tielsch JM, Katz J, et al. The cause-specific prevalence of visual impairment in an urban population. The Baltimore Eye Survey. Ophthalmology 1996;103:1721-1726.

143. Ariyasu RG, Lee PP, Linton KP, et al. Sensitivity, specificity, and predictive values of screening tests for eye conditions in a clinic-based population. Ophthalmology 1996;103:1751-1760.

144. Bernth-Petersen P. Visual functioning in cataract patients. Methods of measuring and results. Acta Ophthalmol (Copenh) 1981;59:198-205.

145. Verteporfin Study Group. Verteporfin therapy of subfoveal choroidal neovascularization in age-related macular degeneration: two-year results of a randomized clinical trial including lesions with occult with no classic choroidal neovascularization–verteporfin in photodynamic therapy report 2. Am J Ophthalmol 2001;131:541-560.

146. Verteporfin Study Group. Photodynamic therapy with verteporfin for age-related macular degeneration. American Academy of Ophthalmology. Ophthalmology 2000;107:2314-2317.

147. Dahlin-Ivanoff S, Klepp KI, Sjostrand J. Development of a health education programme for elderly with age-related macular degeneration: a focus group study. Patient Educ Couns 1998;34:63-73.

148. Fine AM, Elman MJ, Ebert JE, et al. Earliest symptoms caused by neovascular membranes in the macula. Arch Ophthalmol 1986;104:513-514.

149. Fine SL. Early detection of extrafoveal neovascular membranes by daily central field evaluation. Ophthalmology 1985;92:603-609.

150. Gelfand YA, Linn S, Miller B. The application of the macular photocoagulation study eligibility criteria for laser treatment in age-related macular degeneration. Ophthalmic Surg Lasers 1997;28:823-827.

151. Klein ML, Jorizzo PA, Watzke RC. Growth features of choroidal neovascular membranes in age-related macular degeneration. Ophthalmology 1989;96:1416-1419; discussion 1420-1411.

152. Macular Photocoagulation Study Group. Visual outcome after laser photocoagulation for subfoveal choroidal neovascularization secondary to age-related macular degeneration. The influence of initial lesion size and initial visual acuity. Arch Ophthalmol 1994;112:480-488.

153. Vander JF, Morgan CM, Schatz H. Growth rate of subretinal neovascularization in age-related macular degeneration. Ophthalmology 1989;96:1422-1426; discussion 1426-1429.

154. Williams RA, Brody BL, Thomas RG, et al. The psychosocial impact of macular degeneration. Arch Ophthalmol 1998;116:514-520.

155. Faubert J, Overbury O. Binocular vision in older people with adventitious visual impairment: sometimes one eye is better than two. J Am Geriatr Soc 2000;48:375-380.

156. Hertzog LH, Albrecht KG, LaBree L, Lee PP. Glaucoma care and conformance with preferred practice patterns. Examination of the private, community-based ophthalmologist. Ophthalmology 1996;103:1009-1013.

157. Ferris F. Early photocoagulation in patients with either type I or type II diabetes. Trans Am Ophthalmol Soc 1996;94:505-537.

158. Ferris FL, 3rd. How effective are treatments for diabetic retinopathy? JAMA 1993;269:1290-1291.

159. Lee ET, Keen H, Bennett PH, et al. Follow-up of the WHO Multinational Study of Vascular Disease in Diabetes: general description and morbidity. Diabetologia 2001;44 Suppl 2:S3-S13.

160. Miller DK, Lui LY, Perry HM, et al. Reported and measured physical functioning in older inner-city diabetic African Americans. J Gerontol A Biol Sci Med Sci 1999;54:M230-M236.

161. D'Ilura T, McInerney R, Horowitz A. An evaluation of low vision services. J Vis Impair Blindness 1995;Nov-Dec:487-493.

162. Monestam E, Wachtmeister L. The impact of cataract surgery on low vision patients. A population based study. Acta Ophthalmol Scand 1997b;75:569-576.

163. Elliott DB, Trukolo-Ilic M, Strong JG, et al. Demographic characteristics of the vision-disabled elderly. Invest Ophthalmol Vis Sci 1997;38:2566-2575.

8

GERIATRIC OTOLARYNGOLOGY

Hinrich Staecker, MD, PhD*

Otolaryngology deals with a wide variety of disorders, from communication disorders, allergies, and sinusitis to complex head and neck malignancies. Up to one third of patients seen by the average otolaryngologist are aged 65 or over. With an aging population, health care of the elderly population is becoming increasingly important, but the importance of the older patient has been only partially recognized. Otolaryngology textbooks typically feature a section devoted to the care of the elderly patient; however, the principles of geriatric medicine and issues of concern specific to geriatric otolaryngologic patients have not been widely applied. Furthermore, a significant portion of the literature dealing with geriatric issues in otolaryngology consists of case reports and uncontrolled case series. The purpose of this review is to assess the current knowledge in geriatric otolaryngology and to define important areas for future development.

METHODS

The search was conducted on the National Library of Medicine's PubMed database. The time period covered was from 1980 to April 2001. The search strategy combined various terms for otolaryngology, hearing, balance, head and neck cancer, swallowing, allergy, sinusitis, voice, larynx, smell, and olfaction. Individual hits were refined by using the "related articles" button. Otolaryngology textbooks with chapters on geriatrics were reviewed, and their bibliographies were added to the database. Additional requirements were either that the publication be a review, clinical trial, randomized controlled trial, or meta-analysis, or that terms for risk or age factors be present as title words or MeSH headings. Terms denoting age were *age factors, age, aging, elderly, geriatric, gerontologic, older,* or *octogenarian, nonagenarian,* or *centenarian.*

THE AUDITORY SYSTEM

EPIDEMIOLOGY

Hearing loss is the most common otolaryngologic disability affecting elderly persons. Our understanding of age-related hearing degeneration has increased significantly through several large population-based studies. A wide variety of age-specific changes as well as common otologic diseases occur in elderly persons. Among the best-characterized longitudinally studied populations is the Framingham cohort. A study of 1662 patients from the cohort aged 60 to 90 showed an age-related increase in pure-tone thresholds and a concurrent decrease in speech discrimination. The rate of hearing decline was found to be equal in men and women, but on average, men started with worse hearing. Interestingly, there was also a slight change in contralateral acoustic reflex thresholds in both the men and the women. A further observation of the study was that only 10% of patients who were

---

* Associate Professor of Otolaryngology, Head and Neck Surgery, Division of Otolaryngology, University of Maryland School of Medicine, Baltimore, MD.

candidates for hearing aids used them. [1] The rate of hearing decline has also been estimated by following a clinic population over a 6-year period. Having the measurements taken by the same audiologist reduced variability in results. In a study of 1475 patients over 6 years, an average decline in hearing of 1 to 8 dB was seen at 250 Hz, and a 10- to 15-dB decline in hearing was noted at 8 kHz. There appeared to be two main patterns of hearing degeneration. The low-frequency pattern of hearing loss appeared to be age dependent, and women had worse thresholds than men. The high-frequency pattern of hearing loss had a different pattern of progression; the rate of threshold change decreased with age. This difference in pattern is interpreted as possibly representing a disorder of the stria vascularis (the organ that generates the endocochlear potential) for the low-frequency loss and a hair cell disorder for the high-frequency loss. [2]

The Baltimore Longitudinal Study of Aging examined 681 men and 416 women from 1965 to 1995 using standard pure-tone audiometry. The individuals were screened for prior otologic disease and noise exposure. This study demonstrated that the rate of loss in hearing sensitivity is greater in women than in men. In men, a decrease in hearing sensitivity is detectable from age 30 on. Women tend to have better high-frequency hearing than men do, and men have better low-frequency hearing. Overall, there was significant variation within the study group. A conclusion of this study was that age-related declines in hearing (with the aforementioned gender factors) occur in persons with no history of noise exposure or evidence of noise exposure on their audiograms. [3] This differs somewhat from the interpretation of the Framingham data, which suggested that the preponderance of male high-frequency hearing loss is related to occupational noise exposure. Epidemiologic studies have consistently shown a 30% to 70% incidence of age-related hearing loss but widely variable assessment of the degree of impairment induced by the hearing loss. Overall, the degree of hearing loss increases with increasing age and is more prevalent in geriatric patients who are institutionalized. [4,5]

DISEASES OF THE PINNA AND EXTERNAL AUDITORY CANAL

Cerumen impaction can have a significant effect on the hearing of elderly patients. In a random sampling of hospitalized elderly patients over a 1-year period, 30% were found to have cerumen impaction. Improved hearing was obtained in 75% of ears that underwent removal of cerumen. [6]

DISEASES OF THE TYMPANIC MEMBRANE AND MIDDLE EAR

Numerous studies have examined the age-related risk of otologic surgery for tympanic membrane perforations, both in terms of complications and surgical outcome. Age over 65 has no impact on graft success rate in tympanoplasty. [7] In a study comparing 42 elderly otosclerosis patients (age > 65) with 275 younger adult patients with otosclerosis, Vartiainen [8] determined that there was no significant increase in surgical complications in the older patients and that recovery of hearing was similar in the two groups. The conclusion was that age is not a contraindication to middle ear surgery. There have been no controlled intervention trials comparing quality of life after surgery with hearing aid placement in older patients with otosclerosis.

Eustachian tube dysfunction has been described in the elderly population, but few studies have attempted to establish a clear etiology. When 36 temporal bones of younger adult and elderly patients were examined, calcifications of the eustachian tube cartilage and atrophy of the tensor veli palatini were found to increase in prevalence and severity with age. [9] Another study also found functional compliance to change with aging, which affects the overall function of the eustachian tube. [10] No studies have examined the prevalence of serous otitis media in elderly persons, and the contribution of eustachian tube dysfunction to hearing loss in older people has not been defined.

Otolaryn 1 (Levels B, A): **Randomized controlled trials or prospective cohort studies of otosclerosis patients are needed to compare the effects of surgery or amplification on function and quality of life.**

Otolaryn 2 (Level B): **Patients with unilateral hearing loss of any cause should be compared with those who have bilateral hearing loss in an observational study, either at a single time or longitudinally to assess functional and quality-of-life outcomes.**

Otolaryn 3 (Level A): **The effects of bilateral surgery should be compared with those of unilateral surgery in randomized controlled trials or prospective cohort studies of elderly patients with otosclerosis.**

Otolaryn 4 (Level B): **In order to better define the contribution in older people of eustachian tube dysfunction to hearing loss, an observational study, at a single time or longitudinally, should be carried out in which audiogram and tympanogram findings are correlated with symptoms and signs of eustachian tube dysfunction.**

Otolaryn 5 (Levels, B, A): **If a strong correlation between eustachian tube dysfunction and hearing loss is found (see Otolaryn 4), interventions to improve eustachian tube dysfunction should be tested in preliminary studies and ultimately in a randomized controlled trial to determine if improving eustachian tube function improves hearing in older people with and without presbycusis.**

PRESBYCUSIS OR SENSORINEURAL HEARING LOSS

The incidence and impact of age-related sensorineural hearing loss is well established. Recent studies are beginning to define deficits in addition to the previously described degeneration of the auditory hair cells, auditory neurons, and stria vascularis. Schuknecht and Gacek [11] classified presbycusis on the basis of histologic criteria. In this review of the subject, they reported that the four diagnostic criteria of age-related hearing loss (sensory cell degeneration, neural degeneration, strial atrophy, and cochlear conductive loss) held up in a review of 21 cases that met the clinical diagnosis of presbycusis. Of note was the observation that most cases seemed to have a mixed pathologic pattern. More recent analysis of temporal bone specimens has shown a high incidence of mutations of mitochondrial DNA within the peripheral auditory system. [12]

Age-related changes in the central nervous system (central presbycusis) also play an important role in hearing deficits in older patients. Clearly documented auditory brain-stem response (ABR) changes occur with aging. Standard testing of ABR examines the auditory pathway from the cochlea to the inferior colliculus. In a study of 92 persons aged 50 to 90 and 30 control persons aged 20 to 29, a progressive delay in wave l, wave III, and wave V of the ABR was found. Interestingly, there was a lengthening in I–V and II–V interpeak intervals observed in the cohort aged 70 to 79 years old that was not present in the oldest subjects. [13] This suggests that there is a cohort of the very aged that has better than average central (brain-stem level) auditory processing. ABR and a central auditory test battery were used to study patients matched for peripheral hearing loss. Patients classified as having a retrocochlear loss (by ABR criteria) overall were found to be poorer performers on the central auditory test battery. [14]

A number of significant changes occur in central processing of auditory information in elderly patients. In a study that compared a cohort of young (average age of 26) with a group of older (average age of 70) men, monaural and binaural temporal thresholds were measured. The elderly group showed poorer performance on both monaural and binaural processing tasks. These measurements were independent of peripheral system disease. [15]

Stach et al [16] investigated the prevalence of central presbycusis in a study of 700 patients aged 50 and older. From each 5-year cohort, 100 consecutive patients with a complaint of hearing loss were enrolled and studied for the effects of central auditory processing on hearing. An age-related increase in central presbycusis that reached an incidence of 95% by the 70s was found. The results were controlled for absolute hearing threshold. This study also examined an age-matched group of persons without complaints of hearing loss. This population also demonstrated the presence of central auditory processing disorders, but at a lower rate. A study of 25 cognitively intact adults with normal hearing revealed central auditory processing declines despite normal cognition, peripheral hearing sensitivity, and linguistic capability. The synthetic sentence identification–ipsilateral competing message test appeared to be the most sensitive measure of central auditory dysfunction. [17] There are no clear data on the significance or the functional impact of these findings.

Impact of Presbycusis on Quality of Life

A number of studies have examined the impact of hearing loss on elderly persons. [5,18–26] A patient-based outcomes study was carried out on 2466 patients between the ages of 17 and 80. Patients were tested with standard audiologic measures as well as with sentences in noise. The researchers found an age-related decrease in performance of auditory tasks such as sentence identification that correlated with increasing hearing thresholds. They also found a matched increase in disability outcomes as measured by validated subjective outcomes tools that identified features of communication disability that led to feelings of isolation and depression. [18] In a study of more than 18,000 nursing-home residents, sensory deprivation due to hearing loss was found to have a significant impact on social interaction. This was compounded when there was associated visual loss. [19] Studies carried out on a cohort of 472 patients with mild to moderate hearing loss with disease-specific outcome measures revealed that even mild hearing losses have a significant impact on perceived emotional, social, and communication function. Sixty-six percent of individuals tested found that this represented a severe handicap for them despite hearing losses starting from only 27 to 55 dB. [20] In a follow-up study, 194 elderly patients were randomized into two groups, one receiving hearing aids immediately and one being placed on a waiting list. The effect of hearing aid use on quality of life was documented by a variety of outcome tools. A statistically significant effect on quality of life and cognitive function was demonstrated in the patients who received treatment immediately. [21]

Several studies have explored the association of hearing loss and depression or cognitive impairment. [22–26] A study on a population of more than 1100 elderly persons found that hearing loss is correlated with depression and decreased independence. [22] A small (N = 100) case-control study of normal persons and patients with Alzheimer's disease did show an increase in the odds of having dementia with increasing hearing loss. Increasing degree of hearing loss correlated with increased cognitive impairment in this population. [24] There is some evidence to suggest that more accurate assessments of impairment can be derived from the patient's spouse and that discrepancies between hearing level and perceived deficit may be explained by the presence of central auditory processing deficits. [25] Another interesting observation is that hearing loss in the elderly person may be associated with depression. In a study of 43 geriatric patients with major depression, the age of onset of depression correlated with decreased acuity of hearing. It was unclear from this study if the associated hearing loss could be purely related to greater age of the patient, but it does suggest that the association between hearing loss and depression in the elderly population should be investigated. [26]

Inheritance of Presbycusis

The inheritance patterns of presbycusis were studied in the Framingham cohort. Hearing levels in unrelated spouse pairs were compared with those of sibling pairs and parent-child pairs. Pure-tone averages for low-, middle-, and high-frequency hearing were calculated to generate an audiometric pattern that was graded as normal, flat loss (consistent with strial atrophy), or high-frequency loss (consistent with sensory pathology). Hearing levels were correlated between the aforementioned groups. A grouping of hearing threshold changes within parent-child groups and within sibling groups was found. Sisters and mother-daughter and mother-son pairs showed an association of hearing threshold changes at all three frequency sets. The strial pattern of loss showed stronger aggregation and association among female relatives. The sensory pattern of hearing loss was found to aggregate in all related pairs except father-child pairs. This was interpreted as showing that there is a stronger heritable component to the strial pattern of sensory loss and that the inheritance of presbycusis has a genetic component in women and mixed causes in men. [27] The Framingham study also suggested that patients with a history of noise exposure continue to be at greater risk of progressive hearing loss. This may offer an opportunity for intervention. [28]

The Impact of Hearing Loss on Dementia

A number of studies have suggested that there is link or at least an association between hearing loss and dementia. [29] In a study of 30 patients with Alzheimer's disease and 22 patients with generalized cognitive impairment who presented to a memory disorders clinic, 98% of patients failed a pure-tone hearing test. [30] This indicates that certain populations may have extremely high rates of hearing loss. Gates et al [31] examined hearing in a cohort of 82 elderly patients enrolled in a prospective Alzheimer's disease research program. Forty patients were judged to be nondemented (on the basis of the clinical dementia rating scale scores), and 42 were judged to have probable Alzheimer's disease, also on the basis of dementia rating scores. Pure-tone testing showed no difference in the incidence of hearing loss in the two groups, but the probable Alzheimer's disease group had a much higher incidence of central auditory processing abnormalities. In a follow-up study Gates et al [32] examined patients from the Framingham study and found that hearing loss significantly lowers performance on the verbal portions of the Mini–Mental State Examination. Patients were also tested with synthetic sentence identification with ipsilateral competing message (a test for central auditory dysfunction). A poor score in both ears was associated with a high relative risk of subsequent clinical dementia. This finding suggests that central auditory processing dysfunction may precede or be an early sign of some dementia.

Treatment of Presbycusis

It is well accepted that hearing aids are the treatment of choice for those with moderate hearing impairment. The choice of hearing aids for the elderly patient needs careful consideration. A study of in-the-canal (ITC) hearing aid use in 220 patients with an average age of 69 found significant benefit from amplification. Yet elderly patients found ITC aids difficult to manipulate. [33] It is important to take into account central processing as well as cognitive impairment in assessing the impact of these devices on the aging listener. Currently, no hearing aids provide clear transmission of sound in a noisy background, and furthermore, they do little to improve the function of persons with poor speech discrimination.

Despite the demonstrated impact of hearing loss on quality of life, only 14 % of older persons with hearing loss are fitted with and use hearing aids. No clearly identifiable variables (eg, age, degree of hearing loss, educational status, financial status) have been found to consistently correlate with hearing aid use. [20,21] The newer implantable hearing aids may help with problems of high-frequency gain and feedback, and cochlear implantation is beneficial for patients with very poor speech discrimination. Additional ways of improving the function of those with hearing impairment is the use of assistive listening devices. Amplified doorbells and phones and headphones for television viewing can improve the function of both the independent and dependent older person. For patients with profound hearing loss, cochlear implantation has become the treatment of choice. Shin et al [34] compared the complication rates and outcomes of 27 patients older than 60 with those of a group of younger adult patients. This retrospective study showed no increased incidence of complications in the older group and no significantly different outcome in auditory function between the two groups. Recent studies have begun to examine the cost-effectiveness of cochlear implantation in elderly patients. Francis et al examined the improvement in quality of life in a cohort of adults aged 50 to 80. Using the Ontario Health Utilities Index, this study determined that cochlear implantation improves quality of life and is cost-effective. [35]

Neurotology

A limited number of papers are devoted to neurotologic surgery for the elderly patient. Age was not found to be predictive of return to premorbid function in a series of Ménière's patients treated with labyrinthectomy. [36] There are no large studies of elderly patients treated with gentamicin for Ménière's disease. Treatment of acoustic neuroma has been rapidly evolving over the past 10 years. Currently, age is not considered a contraindication for surgical management of the tumor. Some studies do, however, suggest that patient age may affect postoperative complications to some degree. Age over 55 was found to be a statistically significant risk factor for the development of postoperative disequilibrium. [37] One series of papers has examined the growth rate of acoustic neuroma and has concluded that a selected group of patients may be candidates for observation rather than surgical excision or radiation. Studies suggest that in growing tumors (30% to 40%), the average growth rate is 1 mm per year, making no treatment other than observation with serial magnetic resonance imaging possible in a selected patient population. [38,39] da Cruz et al [40] examined the quality of life in postoperative acoustic neuroma patients and found no statistically significant effect of age on patient-based outcome data.

Summary

Hearing loss, especially age-related hearing loss, is probably the most common otolaryngologic disorder afflicting the elderly age group. Treatment of presbycusis is currently limited to amplification. The overall low level of use and dissatisfaction with hearing aids is not thoroughly addressed in the literature.

Review of the literature reveals that there are no age-related contraindications to middle-ear surgery. No significant data are available for neurotologic surgery. Recent developments in treating acoustic neuroma have shown that observation may be a reasonable treatment choice for nongrowing or slow-growing tumors in elderly patients.

The past 10 years have shown that central auditory processing disorder, as distinguished from peripheral auditory degeneration, affects the hearing of elderly persons. It is unclear what the impact of this disorder is on communication by older persons. Advances are being made in the understanding of peripheral age-related auditory dysfunction, with large cohort studies identifying both genetic and environmental factors. Thus far, even though there have been tremendous advances in molecular biology of presbycusis in animal models, no human "presbycusis" genes have been identified.

> *Otolaryn 6 (Level B)*: **An instrument that would test hearing in small groups set in a noisy environment needs to be developed and validated. Such an instrument would be helpful in all the following recommended studies.**

> *Otolaryn 7 (Levels B, A)*: **There is a need for a definitive test of the widely accepted belief that bilateral hearing aids are better than unilateral aids. This could be done by prospective cohort study or by randomized controlled trial. Such studies are needed both for implantable and external-ear hearing aids. Outcome measures should include hearing, speech discrimination, quality of life, and cost-benefit analysis. In the case of unilateral implantation, the unoperated ear can serve as an additional control regarding hearing.**

> *Otolaryn 8 (Level B)*: **The value of unilateral and bilateral implantable hearing aids needs to be assessed. A preliminary evaluation would require only measures of hearing and quality of life in the preoperative period with removable hearing aids in use, comparing these with similar measures taken after unilateral or bilateral implantation.**

Otolaryn 9 (Level B): Studies of elderly patients with profound sensorineural hearing loss are needed that resemble trials for moderate to severe hearing loss in the same age group. The economic benefits of cochlear implantation in the geriatric population is beginning to be defined. Prospective observational studies are now needed that will take into account issues such as loss of independence and cost-benefit ratios.

Otolaryn 10 (Level B): An observational study comparing temporal bone pathology, pertinent molecular markers, and audiometric data would significantly aid our understanding of age-related hearing loss.

Otolaryn 11 (Level B): Research has linked hearing loss with reduced quality of life, loss of independence, and depression. Observational studies are needed that would correlate patient-based outcome measures and degree of hearing loss. These data should be used to develop guidelines for otolaryngologists to consider in obtaining geriatric consultation for at-risk patients.

Otolaryn 12 (Level B): Studies have defined impaired central auditory processing and identified its importance in aging. Central auditory testing is currently performed only in tertiary care centers and takes up to half a day for a single patient. Briefer test panels need to be developed and validated to aid the screening of older patients. This can be carried out as an observational trial for hypothesis generation.

VESTIBULAR SYSTEM

Balance disorders, though probably as common as auditory problems in elderly persons, are complex and have not been as fully studied. A large percentage of balance disorders can be attributed to cardiovascular disease, neurologic disease, or medication effects, but a significant number can nonetheless be ascribed to disorders of the peripheral vestibular system.

HISTOLOGIC STUDIES

Recent temporal bone studies have shown that there is an age-related decline in both vestibular sensory and ganglion cells. Type I hair cells show a significant decline in the cristae, whereas type II hair cells are lost in both the cristae and the macular organs. [41] There is also a decline of vestibular ganglion cells with age. [42] In a histologic study of human brain stems, Alvarez et al [43] demonstrated that there is an age-related loss of neurons in the descending medial and lateral vestibular nuclei but that the neurons of the superior vestibular nucleus are preserved.

ETIOLOGY OF DIZZINESS

A study by Davis [44] determined the cause of dizziness in 117 consecutive older men aged 50 and over. The average duration of the complaint was 45 weeks. Seventy-one percent of patients had peripheral vestibular system dysfunction, and benign paroxysmal positional vertigo (BPPV) was the cause of vertigo in one third of these patients. Visual system disturbances were the primary diagnosis in 1%, and proprioceptive disorders the primary diagnosis in 7%. Metabolic or structural lesions of the brain stem were found in 22% of the patients. Psychiatric causes of dizziness were rare. [44]

A study of 50 consecutive patients aged 60 and over found symptoms of lightheadedness and syncope to be associated with cardiovascular causes of dizziness but the symptom of vertigo to be associated with peripheral vestibular disorders. [45] Most patients in this study complained of their presenting symptoms for more than 1 year, suggesting that diagnosis and treatment of many of these complaints is ineffective.

Among the most common peripheral vestibular system pathologies is BPPV. In a cross-sectional study of patients complaining either of dizziness or balance disorders, unrecognized BPPV was found in 9% of patients. This diagnosis was associated with a history of prior falls, depression, and low activities of daily living scores. [46] In a retrospective study from a balance disorder clinic of 1194 patients aged 70 years or older, 39% of patients were found to have BPPV. [47] This combination of findings suggests that all elderly patients complaining of dizziness, even when not complaining of the classic signs of BPPV, should be examined with a Dix-Hallpike maneuver. BPPV is easily treatable with either an Epley maneuver or a variety of home exercises. Comparisons of outcomes of the use of the Epley maneuver versus more conservative treatment for elderly patients have not been conducted.

DEVELOPMENTS IN VESTIBULAR TESTING

Changes in vestibular test results with age are well documented. This would be expected, given the histologic data cited above. Posturography has recently been used to investigate functional balance in elderly persons. Wolfson et al [48] examined 234 elderly persons (average age 76) and compared them with 34 young control persons. The response to conflicting balance information of the two groups was found to differ significantly. Cohen et al [49] evaluated four age cohorts (< 44, 45 to 69, 70 to 79, and 80 to 89); these researchers found a continual age-related decline in sensory organization test scores that persisted into the 80s. These changes were not, however, directly associated with decrease in independence. Baloh et al [50] prospectively examined 72 subjects (aged 79 to 91) with normal neurologic examinations and followed repeated posturography examinations yearly; these researchers found that over time there is a significant increase in sway velocity and degree of sway with dynamic stimulation of balance. Borger et al [51] found that a standardized movement in the visual surround appears to increase sway and perturb balance to a greater degree in elderly subjects. Specific testing needs to be developed to diagnose neurovestibular causes of dizziness and to determine fall risk.

TREATMENT OF AGE-RELATED BALANCE PROBLEMS

Few studies have rigorously looked at methods to improve balance in elderly persons. Generally, balance disorders have been treated with physical therapy. The effect of Tai Chi was recently evaluated by the use of posturography. Twenty-five test persons who practiced Tai Chi were compared with 14 control persons and were found to have statistically better outcomes on dynamic posturography. [52] No long-term studies have correlated diagnosed peripheral vestibular system disease with treatment modality and outcome. Also, no prospective studies have been performed to evaluate the pharmacologic treatment of vertigo.

SUMMARY

Balance disorders are common and have a complex etiology. Even though balance disorders in elderly persons can be related to many causes, histologic and epidemiologic data suggest that a significant portion of balance disorders can be ascribed to disorders of the peripheral auditory system. No long-term prospective studies have combined the improvements in diagnostic techniques seen in the past 10 years with patient-based outcome measures. Also, little to no data are available on the correlation between histologic patterns of degeneration and changes seen in vestibular testing.

> *Otolaryn 13 (Level B)*: **The available literature supports the idea that vestibular disease is commonly misdiagnosed. An observational study is needed to determine how different practitioners evaluate and treat the chief complaint of dizziness that is assumed to be of vestibular or undefined origin. This study should also determine the prevalence of the use of medications such as meclizine and the prevalence of physical therapy referral. Findings should then be used to develop best practice guidelines.**

> *Otolaryn 14 (Level A)*: **Currently, several patient-based outcomes questionnaires for vestibular disorders are available. Vestibular testing can consist of a combination of very different test modalities, including electronystagmography, rotary chair testing, testing of positional nystagmus, and posturography. A prospective randomized controlled study is needed to define which modality or combination of modalities is optimal for evaluating the elderly patient and determining level of vestibular system impairment and impact on quality of life.**

> *Otolaryn 15 (Level B)*: **Currently, no data exist correlating aging, vestibular function, and vestibular system histopathology. A collection of temporal bones of different aged patients with vestibular test results is needed to achieve a level of understanding similar to that we have for the auditory system.**

THE NOSE AND SINUSES

SMELL

There has been little recent specific study of sinonasal disease in elderly persons. Olfactory sensitivity has been found to decline with aging. [53,54] This may potentially be related to degeneration of both peripheral and central olfactory pathways. [55,56] One recent study has examined the smell sensitivity in normal elderly persons and patients with Alzheimer's disease. [57] The 80 patients with Alzheimer's disease who were examined had awareness of olfactory sensitivity that was similar to that of chronic sinusitis patients (ninefold less than that of normal elderly persons). Interestingly, 74% of the Alzheimer's disease patients and 77% of the normal elderly persons who were found to have abnormal smell sensitivity rated themselves as having normal smell sensitivity on a questionnaire.

SINUSITIS AND NASAL DISCHARGE

A common symptom among elderly patients is postnasal drip, which may be constant or induced by food (gustatory rhinitis). It is thought that this may be due to loss of autonomic control, [58] but it is more commonly the result of dehydration from poor fluid intake or a side effect of medications. Few studies have specifically examined the incidence or prevalence of sinusitis in the elderly population. Knutson et al noted that sinusitis is common in elderly persons and may have more subtle presenting signs and that when sinusitis is properly treated, the management of asthma can be improved. [59] The results of sinus surgery for chronic sinusitis has been examined. In a study of 1112 patients who underwent endoscopic sinus surgery, patients older than 65 made up 15% of the patient population. This group had a higher incidence of minor complications but final outcomes that were similar to those for the other age groups. [60]

> *Otolaryn 16 (Level B)*: **An observational study is needed to define the incidence of sinusitis in older people and to learn whether diagnostic and treatment approaches to the elderly patient are different. Most studies of sinusitis give an average age but have not assessed their data in terms of age cohorts. If age-related differences are identified, risk-factor assessment (elderly versus nonelderly) will have to be carried out by means of prospective cohort studies.**

> *Otolaryn 17 (Level B)*: **Depending on the outcome of the research recommended in Otolaryn 16, a prospective study on the risk factors for sinusitis in the elderly person is needed. This would examine the incidence of allergic and nonallergic rhinitis, as well as the environmental factors that predispose the older person to sinusitis.**

SWALLOWING

In a study of normal volunteers (N = 80) divided into four age cohorts, liquid and semisolid swallows were studied with manometry and videofluoroscopy. Total swallowing time and time to initiation of oropharyngeal swallowing was found to be prolonged in advanced age. Upper esophageal sphincter pressure, peak pressure, and rate of bolus propagation did not appear to be affected by age above 65. [61] Other studies at least partially contradict these data, showing an overall slowing of pharyngeal swallowing time but also confirming an impairment in the opening of the upper esophageal sphincter. [62] In a study of 53 asymptomatic persons with an average age of 75, the repetitive oral suction test was applied to noninvasively evaluate swallowing function. Significant abnormalities in peak suction pressure, frequency of multiple swallows after one ingestion, frequency of polyphasic laryngeal movements, frequency of inspiration after swallowing, and frequency of coughing during or after swallowing were demonstrated. [63] This suggests that a normal (nondysphagic) population of patients has an increased incidence of a variety of physiologic abnormalities in the swallowing process and that concomitant disease may be more likely to result in pathologic dysphagia in older individuals who develop additional neurologic diseases. [63-65] A series of elderly volunteers without symptoms of dysphagia were examined by endoscopy and fluoroscopy and were found to require a much larger pharyngeal bolus to initiate swallowing. [66] Other researchers have shown that with age there is an increase in pharyngeal swallow delay, a decrease in the duration of swallow, decreased cricopharyngeal swallowing, and decreased peristaltic amplitude and velocity. [67] No studies have linked these changes or targeted treatment of these changes to improved nutritional status and quality of life in elderly persons.

Despite the fact that swallowing pressure remains constant across aging, the reserve capacity of pressure generation within the oral cavity is reduced. It has been argued that concomitant illness might thus put elderly patients more at risk of dysphagia because of reduced reserves. [68] Normal aging does not appear to result in problems with the coordination of swallowing and protective deglutitive vocal cord closure. [69] However, pressure sensitivity in the supraglottis of normal aging volunteers appears to decrease with age. [70] This loss of sensory function may contribute both to dysphagia and aspiration in elderly persons. More recent studies have looked at healthy persons between the ages of 80 and 94. Again, increases in pharyngeal delay as well as a decrease in muscular reserve were demonstrated. Researchers conclude that there may be a role for exercise to improve reserve and possibly prevent later swallowing disorders. [71]

In the population aged 65 and older, 10% to 30% are estimated to have dysphagia, although this number is largely unsubstantiated. [72] Some studies are beginning to address components of the swallowing system in a prospective fashion, allowing the establishment of measurement norms. Using four age cohorts (< 50, 51 to 70, 71 to 85, and > 85) with a sample of 30 in each, Jego et al [73] studied by electromyography the activity of the mylohyoid muscle during swallowing. No significant differences among the groups were found. Rehabilitation of swallowing after head and neck cancer is vital for restoring the patient to a satisfactory functional state. A study of 32 patients with moderate to severe aspiration after resection of a head and neck malignancy showed that prognosis for restoration of function was related to initial tumor size, but age was not a statistically significant variable. [74]

Xerostomia may significantly contribute to dysphagia and is common among elderly persons. The incidence of this problem is estimated to be as high as 1 in 5 elderly noninstitutionalized adults. A study of 67 randomly selected elderly persons (institutionalized and noninstitutionalized) showed that there is a statistically significant ($P < .001$) association between xerostomia (measured by sialometry and questionnaire) and inadequacy of nutritional intake. [75] There is evidence that there is a normal degeneration in salivary gland function with age. [76] However, several studies based on actual measurements of salivary flow suggest that, despite this histologic evidence of loss of salivary acinar structure, flow rates do not decrease with age. Fischer and Ship [77] examined unstimulated and stimulated salivary flow rates in healthy persons (no xerostomia) aged 20 to 40 and 60 to 80 years old. No differences in unstimulated or stimulated parotid flow rates were seen between the two groups. The same researchers have found that dehydration and recovery from dehydration do not have an age-related differential effect on salivary flow. [78] The largest study completed examined 1493 persons between ages 5 and 88 using the whole saliva test rather than just isolating parotid salivary flows. Resting salivary flow was demonstrated to decline in an age-related fashion, thus contradicting studies based on parotid salivary flow alone. [79]

Besides functioning in lubrication during mastication, saliva also produces substances that are important for protecting the mucosal and dental surfaces of the mouth from infection. A recent study of 45 nonhospitalized dentate elderly persons (aged 79 to 89) and 22 nonelderly persons (aged 21 to 51) demonstrated that there is an age-related decline in secretory leukocyte protease inhibitor and lysozyme (antimicrobial proteins found in saliva). Overall, protein levels and electrolytes in the saliva have been shown not to change with age. [80,81] Astor et al [82] observed that medication (particularly anticholinergics and antipsychotics) and systemic illness are probably the most common causes of xerostomia. In an analysis of 100 consecutive patients aged > 60 presenting at a xerostomia clinic, 60% were found to have salivary gland hypofunction. Of these, two thirds were found to suffer from Sjögren's syndrome. [83]

There are clear age-related changes in the physiology of swallowing. Yet for the most part this does not appear to result in clinically significant dysphagia.

> *Otolaryn 18 (Level B)*: **Currently, there is no consensus on the optimal evaluation of the dysphagia patient. A comparison of functional endoscopic evaluation of swallowing with modified barium swallow is needed to evaluate swallowing function and outcome of therapy in patients with dysphagia. Specificity and sensitivity should be determined, and cost-benefit analysis should be carried out.**

LARYNX

VOICE

Many studies have looked at the effect of aging on voice quality. [84] A basic description of age-related voice changes includes any alteration in voice pitch and increased variability in pitch. With age, the fundamental frequency of the male voice increases and of the female voice decreases. Estimated subglottic pressure increases with increasing age. Overall, for unclear reasons, women have fewer age-related degeneration effects. [85] In a longitudinal study of 20 patients, voice onset time and spectral features of the voice over 30 years were compared. The men tested showed a decrease in output in the 2- to 4-kHz part of the vocal spectrum. The voice onset time also was found to become prolonged with age. [86]

The histologic changes in aging vocal cords have been studied. Fatty degeneration of the laryngeal muscles increases, and fiber density and elastin fibers in the vocal folds decrease. [87] Increasing ossification of the larynx with aging alters the elastic and biomechanical properties of the insertion points of the vocal cords. A concomitant loss of sulfated glycosaminoglycans in the vocal ligament tendon results in stiffening of the insertion zones. [88]

Several studies suggest that it is important to exclude a variety of disorders prior to making the diagnosis of presbylarynges. Woo et al [89] retrospectively reviewed 151 patients over the age of 60 presenting for evaluation at a voice clinic with a complaint of dysphonia. Only 6 patients were found to fit the diagnosis of presbylarynges, with vocal fold bowing and breathiness. The remaining patients were found to have voice changes related to central nervous system dysfunction (eg, stroke, Parkinson's disease), benign vocal cord lesions, inflammatory disorders, neoplasia, or vocal cord paralysis. In contrast, Hagen et al [90] retrospectively reviewed 47 patients over the age of 60 presenting with dysphonia. This study found that up to 30% of these patients could be diagnosed with presbylarynges. Treatment for this disorder was speech therapy; phonosurgery was reserved for failures of speech therapy.

Tucker [91] reported the results of vocal fold medialization using a modification of the Isshiki technique in 6 patients with the diagnosis of presbylarynges. The report claims that there are significant short-term benefits in terms of voice improvement; however, progressive relaxation of laryngeal tissues makes the long-term results of this procedure unsatisfactory. No studies using more current concepts of laryngeal framework surgery have focused on the elderly voice.

> ***Otolaryn 19 (Levels B, A)***: **An epidemiologic study of the true incidence and etiology of age-related voice disorders is needed. For this purpose, a normal population (ie, not referred or otherwise selected patients) needs to be identified and screened for voice disorders. New surgical methods of treatment should be explored. Prospective randomized studies comparing conservative with surgical treatment for presbylarynges would follow.**

MALIGNANCIES

In a retrospective study of 414 patients who underwent total laryngectomy, age greater than 65 or even age greater than 80 was found not to be a variable contributing to medical or surgical complications. [92] Pera et al [93] as well as other retrospective studies have confirmed these findings. In a study of 371 patients, Huygen et al [94] also showed no increase in complication with age; however, age above 70 was found to be significantly predictive of death within 3 years after treatment. Patients older than 70 have also been found to have a higher incidence of developing a second primary neoplasm after surgical or radiotherapeutic treatment of laryngeal cancer. [95] Laryngectomy, though safe for elderly patients, may have different long-term consequences. In a study of 58 patients following laryngectomy, a decrease in long-term expiratory function was found. This was more pronounced in patients over age 65, even when age-related decrease in pulmonary function was considered. Treatment with bronchodilators reversed this trend. [96]

HEAD AND NECK CANCER

The effect of aging on head and neck cancer has been assessed in a number of retrospective studies. The most common complications surveyed in these studies were mortality, myocardial infarction, pneumonia, pulmonary embolus, wound infection, postoperative urinary tract infection, and postoperative bleeding. Generally not examined were change in mental status, percentage of patients who were converted from an independence to an institutionalized status, and the incidence of decubitus ulcers.

The management of cancers of the oral cavity is challenging from both an oncologic and a rehabilitative standpoint. A retrospective study in the *British Journal of Cancer* examined prognostic factors in the treatment of squamous cell carcinoma of the tongue. In stage I and II cancers, age above 65 was found to be a significant negative prognostic factor for survival. Age was not found to influence the prognosis of stage III and IV cancers. [97] In a series of 187 poor-prognosis patients (recurrence of tongue cancer after radiotherapy), age at tumor presentation was found to be significant in determining outcome in men. Older men (age range 50 to 80) were statistically more likely to have shorter survival than age-matched women or younger persons. [98] Barzan et al [99] examined prognostic factors in 438 patients with a variety of head and neck malignancies. Patients were divided into three groups by age. Age was not found to be correlated with outcome. In a comparative study of major head and neck surgery in 115 patients older than 70, Kowalski et al [100] demonstrated that there is no age-related effect on surgical mortality. This was interpreted as an indication to treat elderly patients with standard oncologic protocols. McGuirt and Davis [101] found an increased incidence of complications in head and neck cancer patients aged over 80 but also found that this group and younger patients had a similar prognosis for survival and function. In a retrospective cohort study, age over 65 or age over 80 was not found to be a risk factor for the development of distant metastasis after resection of stage III or IV head and neck cancer. Screening for distant metastasis in geriatric patients should therefore depend on disease-based risk factors rather than age. [102] Janot et al [103] prospectively compared the predictive effects of clinical information and pathologic information in 108 patients presenting with head and neck cancer. Multivariate analysis showed that age and nodal status are prognostic for survival. Age, tumor status, and histologic differentiation are predictive of metastatic disease. In a retrospective study of 207 patients, Magnano et al [104] found no effect of age on the incidence of metastatic disease. Age also does not appear to have an effect on the radiosensitivity of tumors. [105] Recent attempts at curative radiotherapy for head and neck cancer have used an accelerated dosing schedule. Age above 70 years as an independent variable was not found to be associated with an increased incidence of radiotherapy complications such as mucositis and weight loss. [106]

Age does not appear to play a role in the defects and physical disabilities induced by aggressive resection of head and neck cancer. The development of microvascular techniques for reconstruction of defects of the oral cavity, pharynx, and hypopharynx has significantly improved the rehabilitation of these patients. Bridger et al [107] retrospectively studied 26 patients older than 70 years and 91 patients younger than 70 years and found no differences in the postoperative complication rates for these two groups. Distribution of the type of cancer resected and the size of the defect were similar in the two groups. Shestak et al [108] studied 72 patients in 10-year age cohorts ranging from 50 to 80 years old who underwent microvascular free-flap reconstruction; they found no statistically significant difference in complication rates in the patients ranging from age 70 to 79. Some older studies suggested that poor nutritional status may have more of an adverse affect on surgical outcome in older than in young patients. A retrospective study also demonstrated a significant difference in evaluation and preoperative treatment of malnutrition in elderly and younger patients. Elderly patients were found to have a higher complication rate when in poor nutritional status, but younger patients were found to be more likely to receive pre- and perioperative nutrition treatment. [109] For further discussion, see the section on preoperative nutrition in Chapter 13, Cross-Cutting Issues.

From retrospective studies there appears to be no contraindication to standard oncologic treatment for head and neck cancer in older patients. Prospective studies are needed to confirm this. There is also little information on surgical decision making with regard to age.

> *Otolaryn 20 (Level B)*: **We need to understand better the present practice regarding head and neck cancer care. For this purpose, we recommend a prospective, multi-institutional study of a cohort of older patients with head and neck cancer. Observations would include comorbidity, functional status, advance directives, and physician recommendations, followed by description of the perioperative and postoperative course, complications, recovery, and rehabilitation. The outcome would be a regression-based model of preoperative, perioperative, and postoperative risk factors predicting outcomes, as well as a description of present practice.**

> *Otolaryn 21 (Level B)*: **We need to know the outcomes to be expected in older patients with head and neck cancer who are surgical candidates. A prospective multi-institutional study is needed that measures functional status, quality of life, social functioning, and depression as outcomes. Preoperative data should be compared with follow-up data for 1 to 3 years. Observations should be stratified by the scope of the surgery performed.**

> *Otolaryn 22 (Level A)*: **Depending on the outcome of the study recommended in Otolaryn 21, a prospective, possibly randomized controlled study comparing different surgical approaches for individual cancers (eg, tongue, pharynx) should be designed and performed.**

> *Otolaryn 23 (Level B)*: **The wealth of data emerging from molecular biology studies of head and neck cancer needs to be explored in terms of age. Prospective observational studies are needed to determine if the markers and molecular genetics of head and neck cancer are different in the elderly person and if this impacts treatment decisions.**

KEY RESEARCH QUESTIONS IN GERIATRIC OTOLARYNGOLOGY

Otolaryn KQ1: **How can research be used to improve hearing-related quality of life for elderly persons?**

Hypothesis-testing: There is a need for a definitive test of the widely held belief that bilateral hearing aids are better than unilateral. This can be done by a well-designed prospective cohort study or by a randomized controlled trial. The quality-of-life impact and cost-benefit ratios of hearing rehabilitation should be studied for new hearing aids, implantable hearing aids, and cochlear implants. Outcome measures should include hearing, speech discrimination, quality of life, and cost-benefit analysis. The design could be a targeted cohort study or a randomized controlled trial.

Otolaryn KQ2: Can disorders of the peripheral vestibular system be accurately recognized and their causes determined, and does targeted treatment benefit elderly patients with balance disorders or dizziness?

Hypothesis-generating: Diagnostic techniques have improved in the past 10 years. We now need large prospective cohort studies to determine the prevalence of the various major causes of dizziness and balance disorders and the prevalence of the use of nonspecific drugs like meclizine and of physical therapy.

Hypothesis-testing: Subsequently, researchers should identify patients suffering dizziness or balance disorders due to particular causes and run randomized controlled trials on each type of patient, comparing outcomes after various treatment regimens. Quality of life would be an important outcome measure in these randomized controlled trials. Thus, a comprehensive set of guidelines could be developed for classification of patients by cause and for treatment of each class.

Otolaryn KQ3: **Does standard management of head and neck cancer compromise quality of life in the elderly patient to a greater degree than in the younger patient?**

Hypothesis-generating: From retrospective studies there appears to be no contraindication to standard oncologic treatment for head and neck cancer on the basis of incidence of complications. Prospective studies are needed to confirm this. There is also little information on surgical decision making with regard to age. A prospective multicenter study is needed to determine if young and old patients are treated differently.

There is little or no information on the impact of head and neck surgery on independence. For this purpose, we recommend a prospective, multi-institutional cohort study of patients with head and neck cancer. Observations would include age, comorbidity, functional status, advance directives, and physician recommendations, followed by description of the perioperative and postoperative course, complications, recovery, and rehabilitation. The outcome would be a regression-based model of preoperative factors predicting outcomes, as well as a description of present practice.

REFERENCES

1. Gates GA, Cooper JC, Jr., Kannel WB, Miller NJ. Hearing in the elderly: the Framingham cohort, 1983-1985. Part I. Basic audiometric test results. Ear Hear 1990;11:247-256.
2. Gates GA, Cooper JC. Incidence of hearing decline in the elderly. Acta Otolaryngol 1991;111:240-248.
3. Pearson JD, Morrell CH, Gordon-Salant S, et al. Gender differences in a longitudinal study of age-associated hearing loss. J Acoust Soc Am 1995;97:1196-1205.
4. Parving A, Biering-Sorenson M, Bech B, et al. Hearing in the elderly > or = 80 years of age: prevalence of problems and sensitivity. Scand Audiol 1997;26:99-106.
5. Stumer J, Hickson L, Worrall L. Hearing impairment, disability and handicap in elderly people living in residential care and in the community. Disabil Rehabil 1996;18:76-82.
6. Lewis-Cullinan C, Janken JK. Effect of cerumen removal on the hearing ability of geriatric patients. J Adv Nurs 1990;15:594-600.

7. Emmett JR. Age as a factor in the success of tympanoplasty: a comparison of outcomes in the young and old. Ear Nose Throat J 1999;78:480, 483.
8. Vartiainen E. Surgery in elderly patients with otosclerosis. Am J Otol 1995;16:536-538.
9. Takasaki K, Sando I, Balaban CD, et al. Histopathological changes of the eustachian tube cartilage and the tensor veli palatini muscle with aging. Laryngoscope 1999;109:1679-1683.
10. Kaneko A, Hosoda Y, Doi T, et al. Tubal compliance—changes with age and in tubal malfunction. Auris Nasus Larynx 2001;28:121-124.
11. Schuknecht HF, Gacek MR. Cochlear pathology in presbycusis. Ann Otol Rhinol Laryngol 1993;102:1-16.
12. Fischel-Ghodsian N, Bykhovskaya Y, Taylor K, et al. Temporal bone analysis of patients with presbycusis reveals high frequency of mitochondrial mutations. Hear Res 1997;110:147-154.
13. Oku T, Hasegewa M. The influence of aging on auditory brainstem response and electro-cochleography in the elderly. ORL J Otorhinolaryngol Relat Spec 1997;59:141-146.
14. Rizzo SR, Jr., Gutnick HN. Cochlear versus retrocochlear presbyacusis: clinical correlates. Ear Hear 1991;12:61-63.
15. Strouse A, Ashmead DH, Ohde RN, Grantham DW. Temporal processing in the aging auditory system. J Acoust Soc Am 1998;104:2385-2399.
16. Stach BA, Spretnjak ML, Jerger J. The prevalence of central presbyacusis in a clinical population. J Am Acad Audiol 1990;1:109-115.
17. Rodriguez GP, DiSarno NJ, Hardiman CJ. Central auditory processing in normal-hearing elderly adults. Audiology 1990;29:85-92.
18. Lutman ME. Hearing disability in the elderly. Acta Otolaryngol Suppl 1990;476:239-248.
19. Resnick HE, Fries BE, Verbrugge LM. Windows to their world: the effect of sensory impairments on social engagement and activity time in nursing home residents. J Gerontol B Psychol Sci Soc Sci 1997;52:S135-S144.
20. Mulrow CD, Aguilar C, Endicott JE, et al. Association between hearing impairment and the quality of life of elderly individuals. J Am Geriatr Soc 1990;38:45-50.
21. Mulrow CD, Aguilar C, Endicott JE, et al. Quality-of-life changes and hearing impairment: a randomized trial. Ann Intern Med 1990;113:188-194.
22. Carabellese C, Appollonio I, Rozzini R, et al. Sensory impairment and quality of life in a community elderly population. J Am Geriatr Soc 1993;41:401-407.
23. Ciurlia-Guy E, Cashman M, Lewsen B. Identifying hearing loss and hearing handicap among chronic care elderly people. Gerontologist 1993;33:644-649.
24. Uhlmann RF, Larson EB, Rees TS, et al. Relationship of hearing impairment to dementia and cognitive dysfunction in older adults. JAMA 1989;261:1916-1919.
25. Chmiel R, Jerger J. Some factors affecting assessment of hearing handicap in the elderly. J Am Acad Audiol 1993;4:249-257.
26. Kalayam B, Meyers BS, Kakuma T, et al. Age at onset of geriatric depression and sensori-neural hearing deficits. Biol Psychiatry 1995;38:649-658.
27. Gates GA, Couropmitree NN, Myers RH. Genetic associations in age-related hearing thresholds. Arch Otolaryngol Head Neck Surg 1999;125:654-659.
28. Gates GA, Schmid P, Kujawa SG, et al. Longitudinal threshold changes in older men with audiometric notches. Hear Res 2000;141:220-228.
29. Strouse AL, Hall JW, 3rd, Burger MC. Central auditory processing in Alzheimer's disease. Ear Hear 1995;16:230-238.
30. Gold M, Lightfoot LA, Hnath-Chisolm T. Hearing loss in a memory disorders clinic: a specially vulnerable population. Arch Neurol 1996;53:922-928.
31. Gates GA, Karzon RK, Garcia P, et al. Auditory dysfunction in aging and senile dementia of the Alzheimer's type. Arch Neurol 1995;52:626-634.

32. Gates GA, Cobb JL, Linn RT, et al. Central auditory dysfunction, cognitive dysfunction, and dementia in older people. Arch Otolaryngol Head Neck Surg 1996;122:161-167.

33. Parving A, Boisen G. In-the-canal hearing aids. Their use by and benefit for the younger and elderly hearing-impaired. Scand Audiol 1990;19:25-30.

34. Shin YJ, Fraysse B, Deguine O, et al. Benefits of cochlear implantation in elderly patients. Otolaryngol Head Neck Surg 2000;122:602-606.

35. Francis HW, Chee N, Yeagle J, et al. Impact of cochlear implants on the functional health status of older adults. Laryngoscope 2002;112:1482-1488.

36. Pereira KD, Kerr AG. Disability after labyrinthectomy. J Laryngol Otol 1996;110:216-218.

37. Driscoll CL, Lynn SG, Harner SG, et al. Preoperative identification of patients at risk of developing persistent dysequilibrium after acoustic neuroma removal. Am J Otol 1998;19: 491-495.

38. Rosenberg SI. Natural history of acoustic neuromas. Laryngoscope 2000;110:497-508.

39. Walsh RM, Bath AP, Bance ML, et al. The natural history of untreated vestibular schwannomas: is there a role for conservative management? Rev Laryngol Otol Rhinol (Bord) 2000;121:21-26.

40. da Cruz MJ, Moffat DA, Hardy DG. Postoperative quality of life in vestibular schwannoma patients measured by the SF36 Health Questionnaire. Laryngoscope 2000;110:151-155.

41. Merchant SN, Velazquez-Villasenor L, Tsuji K, et al. Temporal bone studies of the human peripheral vestibular system: normative vestibular hair cell data. Ann Otol Rhinol Laryngol Suppl 2000;181:3-13.

42. Velazquez-Villasenor L, Merchant SN, Tsuji K, et al. Temporal bone studies of hte human peripheral vestibular system: normative Scarpa's ganglion cell data. Ann Otol Rhinol Laryngol Suppl 2000;181:14-19.

43. Alvarez JC, Diaz C, Suarez C, et al. Aging and the human vestibular nuclei: morphometric analysis. Mech Ageing Dev 2000;114:149-172.

44. Davis LE. Dizziness in elderly men. J Am Geriatr Soc 1994;42:1184-1188.

45. Lawson J, Fitzgerald J, Birchall J, et al. Diagnosis of geriatric patients with severe dizziness. J Am Geriatr Soc 1999;47:12-17.

46. Oghalai JS, Manolidis S, Barth JL, et al. Unrecognized benign paroxysmal positional vertigo in elderly patients. Otolaryngol Head Neck Surg 2000;122:630-634.

47. Katsarkas A. Dizziness in aging: a retrospective study of 1194 cases. Otolaryngol Head Neck Surg 1994;110:296-301.

48. Wolfson L, Whipple R, Derby CA, et al. A dynamic posturography study of balance in healthy elderly. Neurology 1992;42:2069-2075.

49. Cohen H, Heaton LG, Congdon SL, Jenkins HA. Changes in sensory organization test scores with age. Age Ageing 1996;25:39-44.

50. Baloh RW, Corona S, Jacobson KM, et al. A prospective study of posturography in normal older people. J Am Geriatr Soc 1998;46:438-443.

51. Borger LL, Whitney SL, Redfern MS, Furman JM. The influence of dynamic visual environments on postural sway in the elderly. J Vestib Res 1999;9:197-205.

52. Wong AM, Lin YC, Chou SW, et al. Coordination exercise and postural stability in elderly people: effect of Tai Chi Chuan. Arch Phys Med Rehabil 2001;82:608-612.

53. Deems DA, Doty RL. Age-related changes in the phenyl ethyl alcohol odor detection threshold. Trans Pa Acad Ophthalmol Otolaryngol 1987;39:646-650.

54. Doty RL, Shaman P, Applebaum SL, et al. Smell identification ability: changes with age. Science 1984;226:1441-1443.

55. Deems DA, Doty RL, Settle RG, et al. Smell and taste disorders, a study of 750 patients from the University of Pennsylvania Smell and Taste Center. Arch Otolaryngol Head Neck Surg 1991;117:519-528.

56. Schiffman SS. Taste and smell in disease (second of two parts). N Engl J Med 1983;308: 1337-1343.

57. Nordin S, Monsch AU, Murphy C. Unawareness of smell loss in normal aging and Alzheimer's disease: discrepancy between self-reported and diagnosed smell sensitivity. J Gerontol B Psychol Sci Soc Sci 1995;50:P187-P192.

58. Edelstein DR. Aging of the normal nose in adults. Laryngoscope 1996;106:1-25.

59. Knutson JW, Slavin RG. Sinusitis in the aged: optimal management strategies. Drugs Aging 1995;7:310-316.

60. Jiang RS, Hsu CY. Endoscopic sinus surgery for the treatment of chronic sinusitis in geriatric patients. Ear Nose Throat J 2001;80:230-232.

61. Robbins J, Hamilton JW, Lof GL, Kempster GB. Oropharyngeal swallowing in normal adults of different ages. Gastroenterology 1992;103:823-829.

62. McKee GJ, Johnston BT, McBride GB, Primrose WJ. Does age or sex affect pharyngeal swallowing? Clin Otolaryngol 1998;23:100-106.

63. Nilsson H, Ekberg O, Olsson R, Hindfelt B. Quantitative aspects of swallowing in an elderly nondysphagic population. Dysphagia 1996;11:180-184.

64. Nicosia MA, Hind JA, Roecker EB, et al. Age effects on the temporal evolution of isometric and swallowing pressure. J Gerontol A Biol Sci Med Sci 2000;55:M634-M640.

65. Nilsson H, Ekberg O, Olsson R, Hindfelt B. Quantitative assessment of oral and pharyngeal function in Parkinson's disease. Dysphagia 1996;11:144-150.

66. Shaker R, Ren J, Zamir Z, et al. Effect of aging, position, and temperature on the threshold volume triggering pharyngeal swallows. Gastroenterology 1994;107:396-402.

67. Tracy JF, Logemann JA, Kahrilas PJ, et al. Preliminary observations on the effects of age on oropharyngeal deglutition. Dysphagia 1989;4:90-94.

68. Robbins J, Levine R, Wood J, et al. Age effects on lingual pressure generation as a risk factor for dysphagia. J Gerontol A Biol Sci Med Sci 1995;50:M257-M262.

69. Zamir Z, Ren J, Hogan WJ, Shaker R. Coordination of deglutitive vocal cord closure and oral-pharyngeal swallowing events in the elderly. Eur J Gastroenterol Hepatol 1996;8:425-429.

70. Aviv JE. Effects of aging on sensitivity of the pharyngeal and supraglottic areas. Am J Med 1997;103:74S-76S.

71. Logemann JA, Pauloski BR, Rademaker AW, et al. Temporal and biomechanical characteristics of oropharyngeal swallow in younger and older men. J Speech Lang Hear Res 2000;43:1264-1274.

72. Barczi SR, Sullivan PA, Robbins J. How should dysphagia care of older adults differ? establishing optimal practice patterns. Semin Speech Lang 2000;21:347-361.

73. Jego A, Chassagne P, Landrin-Dutot I, et al. Does age play a role in mylohyoideus muscle function? Neurogastroenterol Motil 2001;13:81-87.

74. Denk DM, Swoboda H, Schima W, Eibenberger K. Prognostic factors for swallowing rehabilitation following head and neck cancer surgery. Acta Otolaryngol 1997;117:769-774.

75. Rhodus NL, Brown J. The association of xerostomia and inadequate intake in older adults. J Am Diet Assoc 1990;90:1688-1692.

76. Scott J. A morphometric study of age changes in the histology of the ducts of human submandibular salivary glands. Arch Oral Biol 1977;22:243-249.

77. Fischer D, Ship JA. Effect of age on variability of parotid salivary gland flow rates over time. Age Ageing 1999;28:557-561.

78. Ship JA, Fischer DJ. The relationship between dehydration and parotid salivary gland function in young and older healthy adults. J Gerontol A Biol Sci Med Sci 1997;52:M310-M319.

79. Lopez-Jornet MP, Bermejo-Fenoll A. Is there an age-dependent decrease in resting secretion of saliva of healthy persons? a study of 1493 subjects. Braz Dent J 1994;5:93-98.

80. Shugars DC, Watkins CA, Cowen HJ. Salivary concentration of secretory leukocyte protease inhibitor, an antimicrobial protein, is decreased with advanced age. Gerontology 2001;47:246-253.

81. Wu AJ, Atkinson JC, Fox PC, et al. Cross-sectional and longitudinal analyses of stimulated parotid salivary constituents in healthy, different-aged subjects. J Gerontol 1993;48: M219-M224.

82. Astor FC, Hanft KL, Ciocon JO. Xerostomia: a prevalent condition in the elderly. Ear Nose Throat J 1999;78:476-479.

83. Longman LP, Higham SM, Rai K, et al. Salivary gland hypofunction in elderly patients attending a xerostomia clinic. Gerodontology 1995;12:67-72.

84. Slavit DH. Phonosurgery in the elderly: a review. Ear Nose Throat J 1999;78:505-509, 512.

85. Higgins MB, Saxman JH. A comparison of selected phonatory behaviors of healthy aged and young adults. J Speech Hear Res 1991;34:1000-1010.

86. Decoster W, Debruyne F. Changes in spectral measures and voice-onset time with age: a cross-sectional and a longitudinal study. Folia Phoniatr Logop 1997;49:269-280.

87. Kahane JC. Histologic structure and properties of the human vocal folds. Ear Nose Throat J 1988;67:322, 324-325, 329-330.

88. Paulsen F, Kimpel M, Lockemann U, Tillmann B. Effects of ageing on the insertion zones of the human vocal fold. J Anat 2000;196 (Pt 1):41-54.

89. Woo P, Casper J, Colton R, Brewer D. Dysphonia in the aging: physiology versus disease. Laryngoscope 1992;102:139-144.

90. Hagen P, Lyons GD, Nuss DW. Dysphonia in the elderly: diagnosis and management of age-related voice changes. South Med J 1996;89:204-207.

91. Tucker HM. Laryngeal framework surgery in the management of the aged larynx. Ann Otol Rhinol Laryngol 1988;97:534-536.

92. Arriaga MA, Kanel KT, Johnson JT, Myers EN. Medical complications in total laryngectomy: incidence and risk factors. Ann Otol Rhinol Laryngol 1990;99:611-615.

93. Pera E, Moreno A, Galindo L. Prognostic factors in laryngeal carcinoma: a multifactorial study of 416 cases. Cancer 1986;58:928-934.

94. Huygen PL, van den Broek P, Kazem I. Age and mortality in laryngeal cancer. Clin Otolaryngol 1980;5:129-137.

95. Nikolaou AC, Markou CD, Petridis DG, Daniilidis IC. Second primary neoplasms in patients with laryngeal carcinoma. Laryngoscope 2000;110:58-64.

96. Ackerstaff AH, Hilgers FJ, Balm AJ, Van Zandwijk N. Long-term pulmonary function after total laryngectomy. Clin Otolaryngol 1995;20:547-551.

97. Kantola S, Parikka M, Jokinen K, et al. Prognostic factors in tongue cancer–relative importance of demographic, clinical and histopathological factors. Br J Cancer 2000;83:614-619.

98. Llewelyn J, Mitchell R. Survival of patients who needed salvage surgery for recurrence after radiotherapy for oral carcinoma. Br J Oral Maxillofac Surg 1997;35:424-428.

99. Barzan L, Veronesi A, Caruso G, et al. Head and neck cancer and ageing: a retrospective study in 438 patients. J Laryngol Otol 1990;104:634-640.

100. Kowalski LP, Alcantara PS, Magrin J, Parise Junior O. A case-control study on complications and survival in elderly patients undergoing major head and neck surgery. Am J Surg 1994;168:485-490.

101. McGuirt WF, Davis SP, 3rd. Demographic portrayal and outcome analysis of head and neck cancer surgery in the elderly. Arch Otolaryngol Head Neck Surg 1995;121:150-154.

102. Alvi A, Johnson JT. Development of distant metastasis after treatment of advanced-stage head and neck cancer. Head Neck 1997;19:500-505.

103. Janot F, Klijanienko J, Russo A, et al. Prognostic value of clinicopathological parameters in head and neck squamous cell carcinoma: a prospective analysis. Br J Cancer 1996;73:531-538.

104. Magnano M, Bongioannini G, Lerda W, et al. Lymphnode metastasis in head and neck squamous cells carcinoma: multivariate analysis of prognostic variables. J Exp Clin Cancer Res 1999;18:79-83.
105. Stausbol-Gron B, Overgaard J. Relationship between tumour cell in vitro radiosensitivity and clinical outcome after curative radiotherapy for squamous cell carcinoma of the head and neck. Radiother Oncol 1999;50:47-55.
106. Allal AS, Maire D, Becker M, Dulguerov P. Feasibility and early results of accelerated radiotherapy for head and neck carcinoma in the elderly. Cancer 2000;88:648-652.
107. Bridger AG, O'Brien CJ, Lee KK. Advanced patient age should not preclude the use of free-flap reconstruction for head and neck cancer. Am J Surg 1994;168:425-428.
108. Shestak KC, Jones NF, Wu W, et al. Effect of advanced age and medical disease on the outcome of microvascular reconstruction for head and neck defects. Head Neck 1992;14:14-18.
109. Linn BS, Robinson DS, Klimas NG. Effects of age and nutritional status on surgical outcomes in head and neck cancer. Ann Surg 1988;207:267-273.

9

GERIATRIC GYNECOLOGY

Karen L. Miller, MD; Morton A. Stenchever, MD;
Holly E. Richter, PhD, MD; Evelyn C. Granieri, MD, MPH, MSEd;
William C. Andrews, MD, FACOG, FRCOG*

Gynecologists play three roles in the health care of women aged 65 and over: surgeon, consultant and therapist for gynecologic disorders, and provider of primary and preventive health care. The research reviewed here addresses topics related to one or more of these roles. Our review indicates that, as the population ages, our astounding lack of knowledge about caring for elderly women in these three contexts must be addressed.

METHODS

The MEDLINE database was searched via PubMed. The period covered was from 1990 to March 21, 2001. The search was limited to English language and human subjects. The search strategy combined the MeSH terms for gynecologic surgical procedures, hormone replacement therapy, cervical cancer and cervical cancer screening, breast cancer and breast cancer screening, ovarian cancers and ovarian cancer screening, pelvic organ prolapse, and postmenopausal osteoporosis with terms for age factors, risk factors, perioperative care, perioperative complications (including the specific terms *delirium, decubitus ulcer, pneumonia,* and *cerebrovascular accident*), comorbidity, outcome, quality of life, prognosis, recovery, length of stay, functional status, resuscitation status, and discharge planning. In all, 9522 items were retrieved.

The search was then narrowed to 1638 by requiring that the term *age factors* or variants of the word *age* be included in the title. During the time from March 2001 until this monograph was completed, striking studies from the Women's Health Initiative with unexpected results were published about hormone replacement therapy. Therefore, sections about hormone replacement were updated to include the more recent information.

PERIOPERATIVE MANAGEMENT FOR GYNECOLOGIC SURGERY

Topics and research questions regarding general perioperative management of elderly patients are addressed in the chapter on cross-cutting issues (see Chapter 13). For this chapter, studies focused on gynecologic surgery were sought to determine the current state of knowledge and to identify gaps that suggest the best direction of future research.

* Miller: Assistant Professor, Department of Obstetrics and Gynecology, University of Utah Health Sciences Center, Salt Lake City, UT; Stenchever: Professor and Chairman Emeritus, Department of Obstetrics and Gynecology, University of Washington School of Medicine, Seattle, WA; Richter: Associate Professor, Medical Surgical Gynecology, University of Alabama at Birmingham, Birmingham, AL; Granieri: Associate Professor of Geriatric Medicine, Mount Sinai School of Medicine, Chief of Geriatrics Services, Bronx VA Medical Center, Bronx, NY; Andrews: Professor Emeritus of Obstetrics and Gynecology, Eastern Virginia Medical School, Norfolk, VA.

QUALITY OF DATA

Few studies have been published about gynecologic surgery in elderly women. In the published studies, many common geriatric complications were not recognized or sought by the investigators. For instance, none of the case series, retrospective reviews, or case-control studies noted delirium, falls, or electrolyte imbalance. These occur commonly in hospitalized elderly patients, and it is unlikely that they were completely absent in the populations described. Furthermore, all studies on the topic of gynecologic surgery generally were retrospective chart reviews, and undoubtedly geriatric complications were not well documented and therefore were not obtainable. Finally, no studies that evaluated functional or quality-of-life outcomes in older women were found.

Studies were found regarding the incidence and prevalence in older populations of hysterectomy, [1-3] the prevalence in older women of surgery for pelvic organ prolapse (POP), [4] complications in elderly women of gynecologic surgery (including benign and malignant diseases), [5-11] and preoperative evaluation of risk factors for cardiac complications in older women. [12] No studies involved institutionalized elderly persons.

RESULTS

Epidemiology

Annually from 1988 to 1990, 4 per 1000 women aged 65 to 74 and 2 per 1000 aged 75 and over underwent hysterectomy in the United States; [2] similar rates were reported in Finland. [9] In one state, the cumulative probability of a woman's having undergone a hysterectomy was 33% by age 55 and 43% by age 85. [1] Most hysterectomies in older women were found to have been done for POP, followed by malignant disease; roughly one third of all hysterectomies fell in each category. [1,2] Bilateral salpingo-oophorectomy was performed in 87% of abdominal and 7% of vaginal hysterectomies. [2] A woman has a 10% to 11% cumulative risk to age 80 of undergoing surgery for urinary incontinence or POP. [4,13]

Morbidity and Mortality

In Finland, age was associated with mortality in 300,000 hysterectomies, not controlling for comorbidities. [9] Six-week mortality ranged from 3 per 10,000 in the age group 40 to 50 years to 209 per 10,000 in those aged 80 and over. Sixty-three percent of deaths were due primarily to cancer, and 27% to cardiovascular events. In 66,478 Medicare patients undergoing continence procedures, the 30-day mortality was 0.33%. [5] Mortality increased linearly with age, from 0.2% at age 65 to 74 to 1.6% in those aged 85 and over. Age-specific mortality rates were not adjusted for comorbid conditions. Groups of patients who died had higher rates of diabetes mellitus and heart failure. Age was not found to be associated with morbidity and mortality in other studies of gynecologic surgery, [11] POP surgery, [7] and gynecologic oncologic surgery. [10] The only prospective morbidity study included all major noncardiac surgical procedures in women aged 50 or over. [8] This study found age to be significantly associated with a greater incidence of cardiogenic pulmonary edema, myocardial infarction, ventricular arrhythmia, bacterial pneumonia, respiratory failure, and in-hospital mortality. Older patients were not found to be more likely than younger ones to experience neuropathy after dorsal lithotomy positioning. [6] A retrospective review of postoperative fever evaluations found that older age increases the likelihood that the chest x-ray would "be positive" (definition not given). [14]

In a retrospective analysis of 406 women undergoing elective vaginal surgery, cardiac morbidity was found to have occurred only among postmenopausal women. [12] The four congestive heart failures, one unstable angina, one unstable arrhythmia, and two deaths (apparently secondary to myocardial infarction) were not predicted by either the Goldman Cardiac Risk Index or the New York Heart Association functional classification of heart disease. Only hypertension and ischemic heart disease were found to be risk factors.

SUMMARY

Few studies have examined outcomes of gynecologic surgery in elderly women, and these have not evaluated typical geriatric complications. No studies have evaluated functional outcomes, and few have evaluated intermediate- or long-term quality-of-life changes. Mortality risks with gynecologic surgery are low and most commonly are due to cardiac or cancer complications.

Gyn 1 (Level B): **Prospective observational studies should be undertaken to discover the magnitude and severity of common geriatric perioperative complications of gynecologic surgery, eg, delirium, electrolyte imbalance, falls, deconditioning, urinary incontinence, functional loss, and discharge to rehabilitation or long-term-care facilities.**

Gyn 2 (Level B): **Observational studies are needed to establish the risk factors for geriatric perioperative complications of gynecologic surgery, eg, delirium, electrolyte imbalance, falls, deconditioning, urinary incontinence, functional loss, and discharge to rehabilitation or long-term-care facilities.**

Gyn 3 (Level B): **All gynecologic surgery studies that evaluate or describe outcomes, morbidity, or mortality should describe comorbidities, functional status, cognitive status, and estrogen status of elderly women participants.**

Gyn 4 (Level B): **The results from existing and future gynecologic surgery studies should be stratified by age, even when statistical power is low, to facilitate systematic reviews of gynecologic surgery outcomes.**

Gyn 5 (Level B): **Prospective observational studies are needed to compare the quality-of-life and functional outcomes of surgical and nonsurgical management of gynecologic conditions.**

Gyn 6 (Level A): **Randomized controlled trials are needed to determine which interventions in elderly women are effective in reducing geriatric surgical risks, eg, delirium, electrolyte imbalance, falls, deconditioning, urinary incontinence, functional loss, and discharge to rehabilitation or long-term-care facilities.**

Gyn 7 (Level A): **Randomized controlled trials are needed to determine whether pre- and postoperative local estrogen therapy improves surgical outcomes in a variety of gynecologic conditions.**

Gyn 8 (Level A): **Randomized controlled trials are needed to determine whether discontinuation of estrogen replacement therapy improves perioperative morbidity in elderly women.**

Gyn 9 (Level D): **Observational studies are needed to compare quality-of-life outcomes of different surgical techniques for gynecologic conditions, eg, urinary incontinence and pelvic organ prolapse.**

Gyn 10 (Level D): **Observational studies should be performed to determine patient and condition characteristics that are associated with improvement in quality of life after surgical treatment.**

Gyn 11 (Level D): **Guidelines for selecting candidates for gynecologic surgery from among older institutionalized populations on the basis of quality-of-life benefits should be prepared and validated.**

Gyn 12 (Level D): **As medical care changes and improves, descriptive observational studies should be performed to compare the risks of gynecologic surgery that are associated with age alone and those that are associated with comorbidities.**

UROGENITAL HEALTH

Gynecologists treat both anatomic and functional aspects of urogenital health and health maintenance. Certain well-known age-related changes are secondary to estrogen deficiency and are easily treated with estrogen replacement. However, age-related functional changes are heterogeneous, and many questions remain about their causes and therapy. We address the research in POP, vulvovaginal conditions, urinary incontinence, and sexual health.

PELVIC ORGAN PROLAPSE

The surgical and nonsurgical management of POP together constitute a substantial portion of gynecologic care for older women. The exact prevalence and natural history of POP are unknown. It is the most common reason for gynecologic surgery in women aged 65 and over. Surgical repair usually consists of full vaginal reconstruction. However, vaginal obliteration with the Le Fort colpocleisis is still a useful alternative to major surgery for some frail elderly women. There is also a resurgence in conservative therapy using pessaries, as the older population grows and the imperfection of long-term surgical results becomes more evident.

Quality of Data

Epidemiology. Data regarding the prevalence of POP requiring surgery are included in the section, above, on gynecologic surgery. Prevalence data for POP apart from surgical correction are few. One descriptive study using routine gynecologic care patients included 66 women aged 60 to 82. [15] One paper retrospectively reviewed admissions to a long-term-care facility. [16] Risk factors for POP that requires surgery were evaluated in a case-control study; [17] the risk factors for symptomatic pelvic floor dysfunction (including POP) were evaluated in a study using population-based cross-sectional interview data; [13] and risk factors for urinary incontinence or POP that requires surgery were assessed through a Kaiser Permanente database review. [4]

Complications. Hydronephrosis as a complication of POP has been reported in two retrospective case series. [18,19] No studies were found about other well-known complications, abrasions, or urinary retention due to a large cystocele.

Nonsurgical Management. We found no data on the natural history of POP. Articles about pessaries are based mostly on expert opinion, and some are case reports. One retrospective chart review reported indications, continuation, and complications. [20]

Surgical Management. A retrospective chart review evaluated age and voiding function following POP surgery. [21] One small prospective randomized study evaluated the effect of local estrogen prior to reconstructive vaginal surgery. [22] A case series compared the Le Fort procedure in medically compromised women to pelvic reconstruction in healthier women. [23] Some case series described major comorbidities, postoperative complications, and outcomes, [24,25] including one of POP repair under local anesthesia. [26] Several case series describing technique and results included younger and older women but rarely stratified them by age, and these studies are therefore not reviewed here.

Results

Epidemiology. In one study of older patients receiving routine gynecologic care, 50% to 60% were found to have stage II POP; stage III prolapse was present in 9% of the women aged 60 to 69 and 21% of the women aged 70 and over. [15] A review of long-term-care facility admissions found 25% of the women to have POP, 11% of which was beyond the introitus. [16] Age was found to be an independent risk factor for symptomatic pelvic floor dysfunction (including POP) in a large Australian household survey. [13] A Kaiser database study also found age to be an independent risk factor for pelvic floor surgery. [4] The effect of age was not evaluated in a case-control study of women aged 34 to 75. [17] Other risk factors that have been identified are parity, [4,13,17] body mass index, [4,13] and chronic lung disease or coughing. [4,13] Forceps delivery was found to be a risk factor in an epidemiologic survey, [13] but not a case-control study. [17] There was no difference in POP prevalence with a history of cesarean section or of nonoperative vaginal delivery, [13,17] once the number of vaginal deliveries was controlled for. [17] It must be noted that these studies evaluated the range of younger and older women. No studies evaluated the risk factors just for the older women.

Complications. In one study, 11% of 189 women undergoing POP surgery were found to have mild hydronephrosis and 4% had severe hydronephrosis. [18] Women with hydronephrosis were older (mean age 68 ± 10) than those without (mean age 61 ± 11). However, in multivariable logistic regression, only uterine (rather than anterior vaginal wall) prolapse was found to be statistically associated with hydronephrosis. Age was not associated. Among 323 POP surgical patients at the Cleveland Clinic who had preoperative imaging, 8% were found to have had hydronephrosis—4% mild, 3% moderate, and

1% severe. [19] Mean age was 75 in women with and 67 in women without hydronephrosis ($P < .001$). Uterine prolapse was more strongly associated than vaginal vault prolapse with hydronephrosis, even after adjusting for age and degree of prolapse. The two patients with renal insufficiency both had complete procidentia.

Nonsurgical Management. No studies compared types of pessaries. In a case series that preferentially placed Gellhorn pessaries, 96 of 101 women used a Gellhorn. [20] Of five women who could not retain a Gellhorn because of poor perineal support, four used a ring pessary and one a cube. Of 50 patients who continued pessary use 2 months to 5 years, 45 removed and reinserted the pessaries themselves. Forty percent discontinued pessary use because of inadequate symptom relief or inconvenience, but the authors did not further quantify this.

Surgical Management. A retrospective review of 23 women undergoing POP surgery did not find age to correlate with duration of catheterization (independently of estrogen status). [21] Among 43 women who underwent prolapse repair, preoperative vaginal estradiol, compared with placebo, was not found to influence the 3-year relapse rate, although bacteriuria was lower in the immediate postoperative period. [22] Twenty-one medically compromised women who underwent Le Fort procedures, mean age 82 years, and 42 women who had vaginal reconstruction, mean age 67, had a similar number of postoperative complications, including one cardiac arrhythmia and three urinary tract infections in each group. [23] Both groups had 90% to 95% long-term success. In a series of 33 women treated with colpocleises, mean age 78, postoperative complications included congestive heart failure (2) and pneumonia (1). [24] One woman required a second repair. Postoperative complications occurred in 29% of 38 women in another Le Fort procedure case series, including cardiac (11%), respiratory (5%), and urinary (13%) complications. [25] Local anesthesia was used successfully for vaginal POP repair in 20 women, mean age 80 years, including anterior and posterior colporrhaphy, enterocele repair, and Le Fort colpocleisis. [26] The only major complication was venous thrombosis. Pyometra followed a re-do Le Fort colpocleisis in a 92-year-old woman. [27]

Summary

Few data exist on the incidence of or risk factors for POP, with the exception of cases that undergo surgery. The benefit of estrogen prior to POP repair, if any, is unknown. Older age, parity, and operative vaginal delivery are risk factors for POP surgery. The risks of pregnancy alone, regardless of route of delivery, or of the number of vaginal deliveries are not clear. In women with POP, age may be a risk factor for the development of hydronephrosis, but uterine procidentia confers the most risk. Pessary management is virtually all by clinical experience, usually passed on by tradition or invented by individual physicians.

> *Gyn 13 (Level B)*: **Observational studies are needed to define long-term quality-of-life outcomes of nonoperative management of pelvic organ prolapse.**

> *Gyn 14 (Level B)*: **Observational studies are needed to define long-term quality-of-life outcomes of operative management of pelvic organ prolapse.**

Gyn 15 (Level B): Observational studies are needed to determine the patient factors, device factors, and management factors that are associated with successful long-term pessary use.

Gyn 16 (Level B): Pessaries (or other devices) should be developed for use in conservative management of pelvic organ prolapse in women with poor introital support and in whom currently available pessaries are not retained.

Gyn 17 (Level B): Basic science and clinical studies should be performed to delineate the pathophysiology of pelvic organ prolapse, particularly the way that genetic tissue factors confer risk.

Gyn 18 (Level B): Therapies to retard the progression of pelvic organ prolapse by targeting the pathophysiologic tissue factors should be developed.

Gyn 19 (Level B): Long-term observational studies are needed to determine the relative contributions of routes of delivery (cesarean section, operative vaginal, spontaneous vaginal) to the development of pelvic organ prolapse.

Gyn 20 (Level B): Observational studies are needed to determine the condition-specific functional impact of surgery for incontinence and pelvic organ prolapse in elderly women, including sexual function.

Gyn 21 (Level A): Long-term randomized controlled trials are needed to determine whether estrogen use, local or systemic, confers benefit or risk for the progression of pelvic organ prolapse.

Gyn 22 (Level A): Randomized controlled trials are needed to determine whether pre- and postoperative local estrogen therapy improves outcomes of pelvic organ prolapse surgery.

Gyn 23 (Level A): Long-term randomized controlled trials are needed to determine whether selective estrogen receptor modulator use confers benefit or risk for the progression of pelvic organ prolapse.

Gyn 24 (Level C): Randomized controlled trials should be performed to determine whether pessary use in early stages of pelvic organ prolapse retards progression.

Gyn 25 (Levels D, C): Long-term observational trials are needed to obtain indications as to whether pelvic floor muscle exercises retard the progression of pelvic organ prolapse; subsequently, these hypotheses need to be tested through randomized controlled trials.

Gyn 26 (Level D): Longitudinal observational studies are needed to define the natural history of untreated pelvic organ prolapse.

Gyn 27 (Level D): Observational studies are needed to determine the incidence of hydronephrosis in pelvic organ prolapse.

Gyn 28 (Level D): Observational studies are needed to determine modifiable risk factors for pelvic organ prolapse other than childbirth.

VULVOVAGINAL CONDITIONS

The nature of atrophic postmenopausal vulvovaginal changes is reasonably well established, but the contributions to these changes of aging, factors common in aging, and hypoestrinism are unclear. The pathophysiology of vaginal and, to a lesser extent, vulvar disorders is a unique combination of hormonal, dermatologic, microbiologic, structural supportive, environmental, neurologic, and psychologic factors. Vulvar pathophysiology is primarily dermatologic, with strong environmental influences and less well understood hormonal components.

The lower vagina, vulva, urethra, and bladder trigone have a common embryologic origin, the urogenital sinus, and are estrogen-responsive tissues. Dermatologic symptoms, vaginal discharge, dyspareunia, irritative voiding symptoms, and urinary tract infections may all be a consequence of prolonged hypoestrinism. Data regarding the prevalence of symptomatic vulvovaginal changes with aging are divergent and difficult to obtain without the inclusion of urologic symptoms such as dysuria, frequency, urgency, and urge incontinence.

Unclear factors associated with aging, hypoestrinism, or local environment increase vulvar susceptibility to dermatologic disorders, including lichen sclerosus, squamous hyperplasia, and neoplasia.

Quality of Studies

Relevant studies of urogenital symptoms include community-based observational surveys [28-32] and a case series of menopause clinic visits. [33] A meta-analysis summarized estrogen therapy trials, [34] an uncontrolled trial evaluated estrogen therapy, [35] and an observational study reported associations with sexual activity. [36] Vulvar cancer data are taken from a population-based study and case series. [37-39] Review articles and one randomized controlled trial are cited regarding vulvar dermatoses and neoplasia. [40-43]

Results

Two large surveys gathered data through personal interviews. [28,29] In one, urogenital symptoms were found to be prevalent in 30% of 3000 European women aged 55 to 75. [29] Eleven percent were found to have vaginal itch or burning, of whom 41% had a moderate problem and 17% a severe one. Of women aged 65 to 74, 9% reported having urinary frequency, 6% urinary incontinence, and 4% vaginal burning or itch. Of 2045 British women aged 55 to over 85 years interviewed in their homes, 49% reported having urogenital symptoms some time since menopause, and 31% within the past 2 years. [28] Vaginal itching occurred in 11%, vaginal dryness in 8%, dyspareunia in 2%, and irritative voiding symptoms in 16%. Only 27% were sexually active. Of 900 61-year-old Swedish questionnaire respondents, 38% reported vaginal dryness and dyspareunia, and 15% reported itch, discharge, and "smarting" pain. [32] Among 850 randomly selected postmenopausal Dutch women, 23% reported vaginal itching and 16% dyspareunia. [31] Clinically assessed vulvovaginal atrophy was evident in 34% of women evaluated in a menopause clinic. [33] Approximately 25% of the sexually active women had dyspareunia secondary to vulvovaginal pain.

A meta-analysis of 10 randomized controlled trials and 68 other relevant articles concerning older women, mean ages ranging from 54 to 72, showed that estrogen relieves urogenital atrophy symptoms, including vaginal dryness, itching, burning, and discharge; dyspareunia; urinary frequency; nocturia; urgency; dysuria; and recurrent urinary tract infections. [34] All administration routes were found to be effective. Intramuscular estrogen has been found to improve irritative voiding symptoms, as well as urge incontinence, in 84% to 94% of 24 postmenopausal women, mean age 70. [35] A cross-sectional analysis of women with a mean age of 57 found fewer symptoms and less vaginal atrophy in those who continued regular sexual activity through menopause than in those who did not. [36]

The incidence of vulvar dermatoses is unknown. [41,44] Lichen sclerosus may affect all age groups, but it seems to occur most commonly at times of low sex hormone output, in both the pediatric and postmenopausal ages. [44] Incidence is highest in the fifth and sixth decades in women. The incidence among dermatology referrals ranges from 1 in 300 to 1 in 1000, but the condition is more commonly seen by gynecologists who care for postmenopausal women. Squamous cell cancer occurs in 4% to 5% of known cases, but the contribution of lichen sclerosus to neoplasia is unknown. [44] Topical testosterone and progesterone are time-honored therapies, but their effectiveness may be no better than that of the carrier used without the steroid. [42] Topical petrolatum alone has been found to relieve symptoms in 75% of patients aged 35 to 83. [45] High- and medium-potency topical corticosteroids are the treatments of choice. [44]

The incidence of vulvar cancer rises sharply at age 60 until at least the ninth decade, reaching 0.02 to 0.03 in the ninth decade, [37,38] although melanoma may peak in the seventh decade. [39]

Summary

Most urogenital symptoms are related to hypoestrinism and are reversed with estrogen therapy. Symptoms are multifactorial, relating also to urinary tract dysfunction, microbial influences, dermatoses, and local environment. Aging-specific symptoms apart from endocrine failure are unclear. The incidence of vulvar cancer and non-neoplastic dermatoses rises with age. Susceptibility factors are poorly understood. The contributions of endocrine failure to these disorders are unknown.

Gyn 29 (Level B): **Quality-of-life instruments targeting vulvovaginal symptoms need to be developed and validated.**

Gyn 30 (Level B): **Clinical studies, including studies of young castrates, are needed to determine the relative contributions of hypoestrinism, local environment, and aging to vulvovaginal symptoms.**

Gyn 31 (Levels B, A): **Observational studies (and eventually randomized controlled trials) should be performed to determine what degree of quality-of-life improvement in frail older women can be attained by detection and treatment of vulvovaginal disorders.**

Gyn 32 (Level A): **Randomized controlled trials are needed to determine the impact of long-term local estrogen replacement therapy on the incidence and prevalence of urogenital symptoms.**

Gyn 33 (Level A): **Randomized controlled trials are needed to determine the relative contributions of local estrogen and vehicle to improved urogenital symptoms.**

Gyn 34 (Level D): **Basic science and clinical investigations are needed to learn more about the causes of lichen sclerosus.**

Gyn 35 (Level D): **Basic science and clinical investigations are needed to learn more about the age-related factors that increase susceptibility to vulvar cancer.**

Gyn 36 (Level D): **Observational studies should be performed to determine the profiles of susceptibility to vulvar cancer.**

Gyn 37 (Level C): **Randomized trials are needed to determine whether topical immune modulators (eg, imiquimod) reduce the incidence of vulvar cancer in vulnerable individuals.**

Gyn 38 (Level D): **Observational studies are needed to determine the prevalence of untreated vulvovaginal symptoms in frail and institutionalized populations.**

URINARY INCONTINENCE

Urinary incontinence in elderly persons is covered in the chapter on geriatric urology (see Chapter 10).

SEXUALITY

Two areas are of interest in older women's sexuality: sexual function and sexual dysfunction. Continued sexual activity into advanced age has been well documented. The fact that no diagnostic codes exist for female sexual dysfunction except psychologic disorders and dyspareunia bespeaks our remarkable ignorance, but medical knowledge of the pathophysiology of female sexual dysfunction is slowly expanding. The study of sexual dysfunction in elderly women is probably even more complex than that in younger women because of numerous relevant health and medication interactions, because of longer and more complex relationship issues, and because insufficient information is available about norms of physical response, as well as about the effects of androgens and estrogens (other than for urogenital atrophy).

Quality of Studies

Several questionnaires of varying scope and quality have been reported about sexual function and dysfunction in aging and are summarized in recent articles. [29,46–50] Demographic data are limited by convenience samples and low survey response rates. Community-based surveys have also been done. [46,50] One questionnaire was obtained before and after a three-part instructional program. [51] Masters and Johnson's 1966 work remains the definitive study of physiologic age-related changes in the sexual response cycle. [52] Most sexual dysfunction studies concern only the treatment of atrophic vaginitis. [47,50]

Results

Sexuality remains an important part of many older women's lives. One survey found that 30% of women aged 80 to 102 were sexually active, [53] as have other population–based studies. [29] Nonintercourse intimate activities increase in importance for men and maintain or increase in importance for women. [51] Many sexually "inactive" women continue to be interested in sexual relations and masturbation. [46,49,51] Advanced age is inversely associated with sexual activity in men but may not affect women when other factors, including partner status, are controlled for. [46] Heterosexual activity correlates with marital status [46,49] and is most often limited by lack of a partner or by male sexual dysfunction. [50,51] However, in one population survey, *satisfaction* with sexual activity or lack of activity was not found to correlate with marital status. [46] Age was associated with both activity and satisfaction in men but not in women. Specific medical conditions often but not invariably correlate with less activity or satisfaction, but overall health status is important uniformly. [46,47,49,50,54–56]

Age-related changes in the sexual response cycle, comparing pre- with postmenopausal women, include decreased skin flush, muscle tension, reaction time, secretions, vaginal lubrication and expansion, congestion, and number of contractions with orgasm. [52] Dyspareunia and decreased lubrication secondary to urogenital atrophy are the most common sexual dysfunction findings. [29,47,50,53,57] Urinary incontinence and POP also negatively impact sexual activity, [50] but not necessarily satisfaction. [58] However, little is known about specific disorders of desire, arousal, and orgasm in older women. Animal studies show that fibrosis of erectile tissue associated with cardiovascular disease may be linked with sexual arousal disorders in women, as has been found in men. [59,60] The sexual effects of a decline in androgens with age [61] or of hormone replacement therapy (HRT) [62] have not been evaluated in the geriatric age group.

Summary

Regular sexual activity of elderly women is often limited by lack of a partner. However, given the documented level of interest, it is likely that medicine could still make a positive impact on elderly women's sexual vitality and therefore on their sense of well-being. Research is sparse and needed in virtually every aspect of this field.

> *Gyn 39 (Level B)*: **Current investigations into the diverse causes of younger women's sexual dysfunction and its pathophysiology and management should be extended to include older women.**

> *Gyn 40 (Level B)*: **Observational studies are needed to determine the medication side effects that adversely affect specific aspects of sexual function in older women.**

> *Gyn 41 (Level B)*: **Observational studies are needed to define the adverse effects on older women's sexuality of specific medical conditions.**

> *Gyn 42 (Level B)*: **Dose-effect cohort studies of optimal dosage, frequency, and route of administration are needed to learn more about androgen replacement in elderly women.**

> *Gyn 43 (Level A)*: **Clinical trials are needed to determine the ability of androgen replacement in older women to enhance outcomes, including specific aspects of sexual function (eg, libido, orgasmic function).**

> *Gyn 44 (Level A)*: **Randomized controlled trials should be performed to determine whether oral estrogen replacement adversely affects**

sexual function in older women, presumably by decreasing free testosterone levels, and whether this is avoided by the use of transdermal estrogen.

Gyn 45 (Level D): **The emotional and physical components of the sexual response cycle in the older woman should be observed and defined in light of new and more sophisticated information about female sexuality.**

Gyn 46 (Level D): **Pilot studies should be performed to determine educational strategies for partners of cognitively impaired patients that enable them to deal with sexuality issues.**

Gyn 47 (Level C): **Clinical trials should be undertaken to improve the treatment of dyspareunia secondary to urogenital atrophy in women unable to use estrogen products.**

ROUTINE CARE OF THE WELL ELDERLY WOMAN

The benefits derived from routine gynecologic examination and subsequent care in both healthy and frail older women are unknown. Pelvic examination may prompt evaluation and treatment of several disorders, as well as provide an opportunity for cancer screening. However, little is known about the impact of gynecologic examination in specific populations, such as institutionalized, homebound, and frail older women. Does gynecologic evaluation lead to the detection and management of issues that impact quality of life that would otherwise be ignored or minimized by the community-dwelling patient? How can the additional costs to the primary care provider of routine gynecologic examination be adequately reimbursed? Essentially no studies answer these questions. This chapter summarizes the topics most reported in gynecologic care for the well older woman: cervical and breast cancer screening.

CERVICAL CANCER SCREENING

Cervical cancer screening with Papanicolaou (Pap) smears, initiated in 1943, has never been evaluated in a randomized controlled trial. However, the observational evidence is overwhelming that regular Pap smear screening reduces the incidence and mortality of invasive cervical cancer. The incidence of invasive cervical cancer is lower in women aged 65 and over, but mortality is higher, largely because stage at the time of diagnosis is more advanced. [63] Therefore, recommendations to discontinue screening in older age groups must be viewed with caution.

Quality of Studies

Epidemiology of Screening. Epidemiologic data regarding the prevalence of screening and of the incidence and prevalence of abnormalities in older women are obtained primarily from observational retrospective reviews of health databases, [64–71] cross-sectional and retrospective reviews, [70,72–79] and one prospective cohort study. [80] In addition, we found three screening intervention studies targeting or reporting on elderly women, [81–83] one prospective cohort study within a randomized controlled trial to determine the positive predictive value (PPV) of Pap smears, [84] and one prospective cohort study to evaluate the effect of Pap smears on mortality. [85] Two studies evaluate the influence of HRT on Pap smear abnormalities, one of them a prospective cohort nested in a randomized clinical trial of HRT and cardiovascular disease, [84] and one, a retrospective case analysis. [69]

Screening Improvement. One survey and a quasi-experimental study evaluated interventions to increase screening in elderly women. [81,82] Screening improvement trials with low-income women aged 40 and over were also found: [83] Mexican American and black women aged 40 to 70 years, [86] Cambodian women aged 50 years and over, [87] and black American women aged 40 and over. [88]

Screening Cost-effectiveness. The cost-effectiveness of screening for cervical cancer was calculated in a decision analysis applied to hypothetical 65-year-old women [89] and by using a retrospective chart review in an urban municipal hospital. [90]

Consensus Recommendations. The recommendations of national organizations for cervical cancer screening in older women are based primarily on expert opinion. [91–94]

Results

Epidemiology of Screening. Age was found to be inversely associated with having had a Pap smear in a retrospective database analysis, [71] a cross-sectional survey, [79] and a prospective cohort study. [80] However, in another study, of economically disadvantaged women aged 50 and over, age was not found to be a correlate of having had cervical cancer screening. [95] In this group, income and access to a telephone were strong correlates of cervical cancer screening. Low rates of screening may also occur more often in some ethnic minorities, as well as among women with less education and a lower socioeconomic status. [67,70,71,75–77,79,80] In an analysis of data from the Iowa Behavioral Risk Factor Surveillance System (BRFSS) and Iowa's Surveillance, Epidemiology, and End Results (SEER) study, barriers to screening were found to include rurality and limitations in activities of daily living. [96]

In a retrospective review of 96 abnormal Pap smears and their outcomes in women aged 55 and older, the prevalence of atypical cells of undetermined significance (ASCUS) was found to be 2%, lower than the 4% to 6% found in younger women. [69] The likelihood of pathology was also found to be lower: about 15% low-grade squamous intraepithelial lesion in the older women but 25% to 33% in the younger women. However, about 5% of ASCUS smears resulted in a diagnosis of cancer, including cervical, endometrial, and ovarian. An observational study of 1542 women aged 65 and over found a 1.5% prevalence of abnormal Pap smears. [64] Seventy-five percent of the women had not had regular Pap smear screening, and 25% had never been screened. Age, race, prior screening, and gynecologic symptoms failed to predict Pap smear abnormality. Two studies have found an association between HRT and abnormal (ASCUS) Pap smears. [69,84] These studies do not clarify whether a more active squamocolumnar junction due to hormonal influences places a woman at greater risk for true abnormalities or artifactual abnormalities, or whether a more accessible transition zone allows improved screening.

In a prospective cohort study nested within the Heart and Estrogen/progestin Replacement Study (HERS) randomized controlled trial, the incidence of new cytologic abnormalities within 2 years of a normal Pap smear was 23 per 1000 woman-years, with a PPV for dysplasia of 1%.[84] Centers for Disease Control and Prevention 1991–1998 data showed that the incidence of high-grade Pap smear abnormalities within 3 years of one normal Pap smear declined from 66 per 10,000 women aged 30 or younger to 10 per 10,000 women aged 65 or older.[97]

A review of cancer deaths in women in Australia aged 50 or over found that 70% could have been avoided by appropriate screening.[78] In the women aged 50 to 74, 67% had never been screened, and none of those aged 75 and over had had a Pap smear. A retrospective case analysis in 1989–1990 of 798 Scottish women with cervical intraepithelial neoplasia and cervical cancer found that the 26 aged 50 or over with microinvasive or invasive cancer had not been screened adequately.[72] Greater age was associated with a later stage at diagnosis of cancer [74,98] and a higher risk of death within 6 months of diagnosis [73] in cross-sectional epidemiologic studies using cancer registries. In women aged 21 to 96 years, each additional year of life conferred 3% increased odds of late-stage diagnosis.[74] Independent covariates were being unmarried and uninsured, but not race, education, income level, smoking status, medical comorbidity, or urban residence. In a Swedish population, the incidence of cervical cancer was only 3 per 100,000 among women aged 70 or over who had at least one normal Pap smear in the previous 10 years.[85]

Screening Improvement. Elderly black women improved their screening rates following a survey and when offered screening by a nurse practitioner.[81,82] Having lay health advisors interview low-income women was found to be effective "across age and insurance strata."[83] Other trials to improve screening rates included few elderly subjects.

Screening Cost-effectiveness. The cost per year of life saved in hypothetical 65-year-old women ranged from $2254 for triennial to $7345 for annual screening.[89] Triennial screening reduced cervical cancer mortality by 74%. It was calculated from a chart review that 100 Pap smears in low-income elderly women could save $5907 and 3.7 years of life.[90]

Consensus Recommendations. Consensus recommendations for frequency of Pap smears in older women vary from discontinuation after age 65 [94] to continued screening until age 70 [93,99] to no upper age limit.[91,92] The most commonly recommended screening interval is 3 years.

Posthysterectomy. Pap smears have little or no utility in women who have had a total hysterectomy (*corpus* and *cervix uteri*) for benign disease.[100,101] The American College of Obstetrics and Gynecology recommends "periodic" vaginal cuff Pap smears in women with any risk factors for cervical cancer or any endometrial, vaginal, or vulvar neoplasia.[91] Several factors speak for documenting at least one normal vaginal Pap smear in elderly women and possibly continuing "periodic" vaginal Pap smears:

- Most practitioners do not take a full past sexual history for older women.

- Data regarding the relevance of known risk factors (human papilloma virus, sexual practices) to vaginal intraepithelial neoplasia in older women are lacking.

- Data regarding the relevance of a remote operation for gynecologic cancer to vaginal Pap smears in elderly women are lacking.

■ Elderly women may not know why, and occasionally if, a hysterectomy was performed, and whether the hysterectomy was total (*corpus et cervix uteri*) or subtotal (*corpus uteri*).

Summary

Screening rates are low among women aged 65 or over, particularly those who are older, unmarried, and with poor medical financial coverage. In these women, the death rate from cervical cancer is much higher than in screened women, owing in large part to diagnosis at a more advanced stage. Extending the screening interval beyond 3 years leads to a greater incidence of abnormal Pap smears. Studies of Pap smear benefits have examined primarily disease incidence and mortality, rather than quality-of-life and functional issues, and thus have not included important outcomes relevant to geriatric care. Interventions to promote cervical cancer screening in elderly women are effective.

> *Gyn 48 (Level B)*: **Cost analysis should be performed to measure the comprehensive costs to the primary care provider of obtaining a Pap smear in an elderly woman and to compare these with current Medicare reimbursement.**

> *Gyn 49 (Level B)*: **As the baby boomers age, observational studies are needed to determine the cervical cancer incidence in a changing elderly population with different sexual risk factors and to compare this with previous incidence rates.**

> *Gyn 50 (Level B)*: **Observational studies are needed to delineate all factors associated with the increased mortality rate of cervical cancer among elderly women.**

> *Gyn 51 (Level A)*: **Clinical trials should be performed to determine whether strategies to improve cervical cancer screening in impoverished and minority elderly women result in decreased cervical cancer mortality, and which strategies are most cost-effective.**

> *Gyn 52 (Level D)*: **Observational studies should be performed to determine the relationship of well-established risk factors (eg, multiple sex partners, history of human papilloma virus, cervical dysplasia, smoking, medical or viral immune suppression) to the incidence of cervical or vaginal cancer in elderly women.**

> *Gyn 53 (Level D)*: **Observational studies should be performed to determine whether early detection of cervical neoplasia confers quality-of-life benefits on frail elderly women.**

BREAST CANCER SCREENING

Almost half of all breast cancers occur in women aged 65 and over. The average life expectancy of elderly women is usually underestimated. These facts imply that there is a substantial benefit to screening mammography for older women. However, few data exist to support or refute this presumption. Far fewer elderly than young women have been included in screening trials. Most studies use longevity as an outcome, rather than quality of life or burden of disease, which are of greater concern to older persons.

Quality of Studies

Only two randomized controlled trials of mammography, conducted in Sweden, included women to age 74 at entry. [102,103] Systematic reviews presented results from five Swedish trials, [104] seven randomized controlled trials and six case-control studies, [105] and thirteen randomized controlled trials with 7 to 9 years of follow-up. [106] Case-control studies from the Netherlands reported mammography benefit in women aged 65 and over. [107,108] Retrospective cohort and cross-sectional studies reported the impact of mammography on cancer incidence and stage at diagnosis in women aged 65 and over. [109–114] Studies have looked at the impact of age on the PPV, [108,110,111,115,116] recall rate, [110] cost-effectiveness, [117–119] and sensitivity among estrogen replacement therapy (ERT) users. [120] Retrospective database reviews have evaluated factors associated with screening prevalence. [96,121–125]

Results

Six of eight randomized controlled mammography trials demonstrated a 20% to 30% decline in mortality for women aged 50 to 70. [103] In 5 to 13 years, Swedish mammography trials demonstrated reduced mortality among women aged 50 to 69 (relative risk or RR 0.71), but no effect was seen in women aged 70 to 74. [104] The one trial including these older women was closed after only two screenings. A meta-analysis of seven randomized controlled trials including women to age 74 and six case-control studies including women to age 70 demonstrated that screening mammography reduces mortality (RR 0.70, 95% confidence interval or CI = 0.63 to 0.78 and RR 0.32, 95% CI = 0.28 to 0.38, respectively). [105] The true benefit may have been higher in the randomized controlled trials, which were confounded by low compliance rates in the treatment groups (50% to 80%) and prescreening in the control groups (20% to 30%). A meta-analysis of randomized controlled trials found lower mortality in screened women aged 50 to 74 years after 7 to 9 years of follow-up regardless of the number of mammographic views per screen, the screening interval, or the number of years of follow-up. [106] Case-control studies using one mammographic view every 2 years found lower mortality in women aged less than 65 years and 65 to 74 years (one with and one without statistical significance), but no demonstrable benefit in women aged 75 and over. [107,108] Retrospective cohort and cross-sectional studies have found among screened women aged 65 and over less metastatic disease and a lower stage at diagnosis. [109–114] One study in women aged 85 and over found that point estimates were similar but statistical significance was lost. [112]

The PPV of mammography increased with age in most, [110,111,115,116] but not all [108] studies. ERT has been found to have less negative impact on mammogram sensitivity in women aged 70 and older than in those who are younger. [120] Studies have found greatest cost-effectiveness in women with high bone mineral density (BMD) [117] and in women aged 50 to 79 [118] and 50 to 69. [119] Database reviews have shown costs (ie, Medicare copayment), functional activity limitations, advanced age, and rurality to be associated with less mammographic screening. [96,121–125]

Summary

Regular mammography benefits women to age 74 and probably to age 85, lowering breast cancer morbidity and mortality. Studies that have shown no statistical benefit in women aged 70 and over or 74 and over have evaluated only mortality. Studies looking at the burden of disease and stage at diagnosis have shown benefit to age 85 and perhaps beyond. Financial and functional barriers reduce screening.

> *Gyn 54 (Level B)*: **The results of existing and future mammography studies should be stratified by age, even when power is low, to facilitate systematic reviews of results in older women.**

> *Gyn 55 (Level B)*: **Observational studies are needed to determine what functional impairments and comorbid conditions are associated with a lack of mammography benefit.**

> *Gyn 56 (Level B)*: **Guidelines using functional impairment and comorbid condition measures for discontinuation of mammography should be developed and validated.**

> *Gyn 57 (Level A)*: **Randomized controlled trials are needed to determine the impact of mammography on the quality of life and burden of disease in older women.**

> *Gyn 58 (Level A)*: **Clinical trials are needed to determine whether strategies to improve mammography screening rates among impoverished and minority elderly women result in decreased breast cancer mortality or burden of disease, and which strategies are most cost-effective.**

> *Gyn 59 (Level D)*: **Observational studies should be performed to determine whether the increase in mammographic density that is related to hormone replacement therapy increases breast cancer mortality or burden of disease in older women.**

> *Gyn 60 (Level D)*: **The concurrence and variability of mammogram interpretations by different radiologists in elderly women should be observed and defined.**

ESTROGEN REPLACEMENT THERAPY

Estrogen is prescribed to elderly women as a preventive medication, not for menopausal symptoms. Because of the number of potential ERT candidates and the number of potentially affected organ systems, the decision to initiate or continue ERT is the greatest public health issue in geriatric gynecology. Although its prescription is within the purview of all primary care providers, as long as women have uteri that may bleed, gynecologists will play a substantial, and often the only, role in guiding and managing estrogen use. This summary addresses several of the topics most pertinent to elderly women. ERT and osteoporosis is addressed in the final section of this chapter.

ESTROGEN REPLACEMENT AND CARDIOVASCULAR DISEASE

Despite the huge body of literature published about the impact of ERT on cardiovascular disease, opinions about benefit and risks conflict in almost every therapeutic aspect. Even less is clear about the impact of ERT on cardiovascular disease in the elderly woman because data are sparse.

The research on estrogen, estrogen-progestin, and selective estrogen receptor modulator (SERM) therapy is reviewed. Except when estrogen alone is designated, the term *hormone replacement therapy* (HRT) will be used for both estrogen alone and estrogen plus progestin when studies either do not distinguish between the two or find little difference in main outcomes between them. SERMs have estrogenic effects in some organ systems (skeletal, cardiovascular) and antagonistic effects in other organs (breast, uterus). Currently available SERMs in the United States are tamoxifen, raloxifene, and toremifene. Toremifene is approved for the treatment of metastatic breast cancer. Data on potential preventive health benefits of this agent are inadequate and are not reviewed. Studies are cited that use cardiovascular disease, events, or mortality. Many additional studies can be found that report ERT, HRT, and SERM effects on cardiovascular risk factors.

Quality of Data

Estrogen. One systematic review of ERT and cardiovascular disease literature gave information specifically on older women. [126] Four randomized controlled trials, [127–130] ten prospective cohort studies, [126,131–139] three case-control studies, [140–142] and one cross–sectional study [143] were found. Four studies of carotid arterial disease that are relevant to elderly women were also found—one randomized clinical trial, [144] one cohort study, [145] one case–control study, [146] and one cross-sectional study. [147]

Estrogen Dosage. A recent Nurses' Health Study (NHS) report included 20,000 woman-years of conjugated equine estrogen (CEE) 0.3 mg per day, but ages were not reported. [131] One epidemiologic study of HRT and myocardial infarction stratified results by dose. [148]

Selective Estrogen Receptor Modulators. Four randomized controlled trials have evaluated tamoxifen use and cardiovascular endpoints. [149–152] No studies of raloxifene with cardiovascular outcomes have been published.

Results

Estrogen. In a 1991 systematic review of observational studies, [126] Stampfer and Colditz noted that two previous studies [139,153] found an apparent cardioprotective effect of estrogen across all ages, one found a stronger beneficial association in older women, [154] one found apparent benefit in women of all ages but more in younger women, [142] and one study with a mean age of 73 showed substantially less cardiovascular disease among HRT users. [138] Only an early observational publication from the Framingham trial found greater risk in older women taking HRT, [155] and these conclusions were later essentially retracted. [156] Four recent randomized controlled trials found no coronary heart disease benefit of HRT. Two were from the same 4-year trial, the HERS. [127,128] However, in the last 2 years of the trial, HRT was found to be associated with less coronary heart disease. The mean age of participants was 67, but no information specific to older women was given.

In a 3-year trial including 309 women, mean age 66 (range 42 to 80), HRT was not found to affect the progression of coronary atherosclerosis in women with established disease, even when stratified by age. [129] The Women's Health Initiative (WHI) enrolled women aged 50 to 79, mean age 63 at baseline, with over 8000 participants in each study arm. [130] The estrogen-progestin arm of the trial was stopped prematurely after an average of 5.2 years (range 3.5 to 8.5) because of an increase in a global risk index over that with placebo, which included small but statistically significant increases in nonfatal myocardial infarction, nonfatal stroke, pulmonary embolism, and deep-vein thrombosis. Age was not found to interact with HRT effects on any cardiovascular events (data not given). Results from the estrogen-only participants are still pending.

Most observational cohort studies have found lower coronary heart disease and improved survival in older (as well as younger) women taking HRT. The NHS has shown this in three trials, [131,133,134] which included women to age 75 at the 20-year follow-up, although most were under age 65. Current HRT users were found to have a coronary heart disease RR of 0.61 (95% CI = 0.52 to 0.71), but results were not stratified by age. An Iowa Women's Health Study 6-year follow-up (of women aged 55 to 69 years at entry) found current HRT users to have a 25% lower risk of death or coronary heart disease mortality, [135] with 50% risk reduction if use was longer than 5 years. [132] The Leisure World Cohort, mean initial age of 73 years, found a 20% lower all-cause mortality in ever-users than in never-users after 7.5 years of follow-up. [136] Current users had better health, but long duration of use was also found to be associated with benefit. However, in the NHS and the Iowa Women's Health Study, improved health was found to be associated only with current, not past, use. A Swedish cohort study found greater survival in older but not younger women who started HRT, probably because of preferential prescription only to healthy elderly women. [137] Another Swedish cohort study found a lower risk of myocardial infarction in women taking HRT. [157]

Two case-control studies and one cross-sectional analysis of older women found less coronary heart disease among HRT users. Kaiser Permanente patients on long-term HRT were found to have a 46% lower all-cause mortality, largely because there was less coronary heart disease. [140] A case-control study of women with a mean age of 65 found 65% less angiographically documented coronary arterial disease among HRT users. [142] The association was significant for women younger than 60 (P = .002) and aged 60 to 69 (P = .03), but not for those aged 70 and over (P= .5). A cross-sectional evaluation of women 65 to 100 years old, mean age 72, found a similar reduction in cardiovascular disease in HRT users both older and younger than 75 years. [143] In addition, an Italian case-control study found fewer nonfatal myocardial infarctions among women 60 years and older and younger than age 60 who had a late menopause. [141]

Three cross-sectional analyses and one randomized controlled trial evaluated ERT and carotid arterial disease. ERT use was found to be associated with a decrease in arterial wall thickness in older women. [145–147] In a randomized controlled trial of women aged 40 to 70 years, 4 months of ERT was found to be associated with increased carotid artery distensibility, but not significantly in the subgroup over the age of 59. [144]

Estrogen Dosage. The large cohort NHS observed that women using doses of ERT lower than CEE 0.625 mg per day obtain the same apparent cardioprotection as those using the standard strength, whereas those using higher estrogen dosages had less. [131,134] Furthermore, stroke risk tended to be less with lower dosages. However, results were not stratified by age, and the number of women in each therapy group is unknown. One observational study found that the reduction of risk for myocardial infarction with CEE 0.625 mg per day was not seen with the 0.3 mg dose, but these results were based on a small number of ERT users. [148]

Selective Estrogen Receptor Modulators. Two U.S. randomized controlled trials found a nonsignificant [150] or no [149] reduction in cardiovascular mortality with tamoxifen use. In contrast, European trials found a lower risk of fatal myocardial infarction [151,152] and hospitalization for cardiac disease. [158] Potential cardioprotective effects of raloxifene are currently being evaluated in the Raloxifene Use for The Heart (RUTH) trial. [159]

Summary

Conflicting results between high-quality large observational trials (showing benefit) and high-quality large randomized controlled trials (showing detriment) leave us in a quandary about the cardiovascular effects of hormone replacement. The discrepancies seem attributable either to crucial differences between the populations being studied, to the drugs being studied, or to a "healthy user effect" confounding observational trial outcomes even more than previously imagined. The randomized trials enrolled primarily older, overweight women who had not taken hormones for at least 5 to 10 years since menopause, gave them continuous estrogen plus progestin, and studied them for a short time relative to the postmenopausal life span. The observational trials studied primarily women who took hormones since menopause, at least half of whom took estrogen only, and whose average cardiovascular-related health measures (eg, weight, blood pressure, exercise) were better among hormone users than nonusers; greatest "benefit" was found with the longest use, although this was sometimes attenuated in advanced age. Interestingly, the most obvious cause of increased cardiovascular risk in the randomized trials could be attributed to a procoagulant effect of HRT, but the estrogen-only arm of the WHI was not discontinued prematurely, as would have been expected on the basis of thrombosis alone. Further study is necessary to understand hormone actions upon the cardiovascular system and to determine the patient characteristics that are associated with benefit and detriment.

At the current time, it is relatively contraindicated to start older postmenopausal women on ERT or HRT. However, the risks and benefits to those who have taken hormones since menopause are unclear. Results from the WHI to be completed in 2006 will guide the direction of current clinical care and future research. Although SERMs may improve cardiovascular risk profiles in older women, their effect on coronary heart disease and longevity in elderly women is unknown.

> **Gyn 61 (*Level B*): Basic science research, pilot studies, and observational trials are needed to determine which are the more sophisticated measures of potential cardiovascular benefits and risks associated with hormone replacement—C-reactive protein levels, homocysteine levels, activated protein C deficiency, intestinal calcium absorption.**

> **Gyn 62 (*Level A*): Placebo-controlled randomized trials, starting with women who have been on hormone replacement therapy for more than 5 years, are needed to determine whether continuation, lower-**

ing the dose, or discontinuation confers more cardiovascular benefit for older women.

Gyn 63 (Level A): **Randomized controlled trials should be performed to determine the effect in elderly women of selective estrogen receptor modulators on primary cardiovascular endpoints, such as myocardial infarction, cardiac death, pulmonary embolism, and stroke.**

Gyn 64 (Level A): **Randomized controlled trials should be performed to determine whether age modifies hormone effects on the cardiovascular system and cardiovascular risk factors (eg, platelet function, arterial distensibility, angiotensinogen levels, calcium absorption).**

Gyn 65 (Level B): **The results from existing and future studies of hormone replacement should be stratified by age, even when power is low, to facilitate systematic reviews.**

Gyn 66 (Level C): **Randomized controlled trials are needed to determine whether aspirin eliminates the thrombogenic effect of estrogen in elderly women.**

ESTROGEN REPLACEMENT THERAPY AND ALZHEIMER'S DISEASE

The age-specific incidence of Alzheimer's disease (AD) is higher for women than for men. [160] The effect of estrogen loss at menopause and of hormone replacement on the development of AD remains in question. Plausible biological theories and laboratory studies support a protective effect, but clinical studies have widely discrepant findings. Few risk factors for AD are known, with education being the only well-established modifiable one. Given the devastating nature of the disease and lack of other preventive strategies, hormone use or avoidance becomes an important individual and public health concern.

Quality of Data

Prevention. The biology of AD and potential neuroprotective mechanisms of estrogen have been well summarized in several reviews of AD and hormone therapy. [160–163] One randomized controlled trial of HRT for AD prevention has been published. [164] Large cohorts from which both prospective cohort and nested case-control studies were published include the Leisure World retirement community, [165,166] a longitudinal study of aging in Manhattan, [167] the Cardiovascular Health Study, [168] the Baltimore Longitudinal Study on Aging, [169] the Rancho Bernardo cohort, [170,171] the Duke Established Populations for Epidemiologic Studies of the Elderly, [172] the Italian Longitudinal Study on Aging, [173] the United Kingdom General Practice Research Database, [174] and the Cache County Study. [175] Preventive effects of endogenous estrogens were explored within the Study of Osteoporotic Fractures. [176] One cross-sectional study evaluated cognitive function and endogenous estrogens and androgens. [171] One longitudinal study compared cognitive ability over 2 years in older women taking no hormones, estrogen only, and estrogen-progestin. [177]

Treatment. Several clinical trials, including four with placebo control and randomization, have evaluated the effects of ERT in women with mild or moderate AD. [160,178–180] Many studies were small or used brief cognitive rating instruments. [160] All randomized controlled trials used oral CEE.

Results

Prevention. The Women's Health Initiative Memory Study randomized controlled trial showed worsening dementia with estrogen-progestin use for an average of 5 years (3 to 8) among women over age 65, 80% of whom had not taken hormones before. [164] AD specifically was increased with HRT, but at a slightly lower rate than for all-cause dementia. Among past users of estrogen alone, the increased risk of dementia was found not to be statistically significant. Too few women had used estrogen-progestin replacement prior to the study for meaningful comparison with the observational trials of long-term HRT use.

Observational data conflict regarding the protective effect of ERT or HRT use on AD. Apparent benefit was observed in large prospectively followed cohorts. [167,169,175] In a well-designed and -executed study of 1890 women and 1360 men over age 65 in Utah, incident dementia over a period of 3 years was found to be greater after age 80 among women. Women who had used hormones for more than 10 years (72% unopposed estrogen, mostly past use) were found to have the same AD incidence as men, whereas nonusers were found to have more than twice the risk. Women who used hormones less than 10 years had a greater risk of AD (not statistically significant), which essentially concurs with the randomized trial. [164] There was some suggestion that risk reduction with ERT or HRT is greater in women with two $\epsilon 4$ alleles ($P = .19$). [175] In contrast, one study found less cognitive decline with estrogen use in women negative for the APOE-$\epsilon 4$ allele, but not in $\epsilon 4$-positive women. [168] In a 2-year prospective study, cognitive performance was found to improve more for current unopposed estrogen users and less for estrogen-progestin users than for nonusers. [177] Another study found ERT use to be associated with less cognitive decline but not less impairment, but multivariate analyses did not confirm statistical significance. [172] Unexpectedly, higher serum estrone levels have been associated with worse performance on two cognitive tests, [176] but free estradiol with less decline. [181] Past, current, or no ERT use ever was not found to be associated with cognitive function in a large cohort. [170]

Retrospective case-control studies, [182–185] nested case-control studies, [165,166] and a cross–sectional study [173] have found less ERT use among demented women or less AD among ERT users. However, a large nested case-control study found similar odds ratios for AD among none ever, past, or current ERT users. [174] A case-control study based on pharmacy records found no association of ERT and AD. [186]

Treatment. Most treatment studies have found no benefit of ERT for AD, [160,178,179] the largest having 120 subjects. [180] One intriguing prospective cohort study within a randomized controlled trial found that ERT may enhance response to tacrine. [187] Some AD symptoms, such as naming, seem more amenable to improvement with ERT. [188]

Summary

Estrogen-progestin replacement therapy initiated in women who are several years postmenopausal increases the risk of dementia, including AD, with relatively short-term use. This does not entirely exclude the possibility of a neutral effect or benefit with long-term use, as found in some observational studies. It also does not exclude a potential benefit of estrogen alone, nor of HRT initiated at menopause. Discrepancies in study findings may relate to subgroups of women who respond favorably or adversely to hormones. These subgroups should be sought, to clarify the confusing clinical observations of postmenopausal hormone use. ERT has no proven benefit for women with established AD, but benefit in some individuals or synergism with cholinesterase inhibition is not excluded.

> *Gyn 67 (Level B)*: **Basic science research and animal studies are needed to determine the differential effects of estrogen and estrogen-progestin replacement on cognition.**

> *Gyn 68 (Level B)*: **Basic science research, animal studies, and observational studies are needed to determine which physiologic characteristics, if any, are associated with a benefit or detriment of long-term postmenopausal hormone use.**

> *Gyn 69 (Level B)*: **Basic science research is needed to reconcile and explain the discrepant findings of estrogen neuroprotection in the laboratory in comparison with cognitive detriment with estrogen-progestin in clinical experience.**

> *Gyn 70 (Level B)*: **Autopsy studies should be performed to determine the types of dementia most associated with postmenopausal hormone use.**

> *Gyn 71 (Level B)*: **Results from existing and future studies of hormone replacement and Alzheimer's disease should be stratified by age, even when power is low, to facilitate systematic reviews.**

> *Gyn 72 (Level A)*: **Randomized controlled trials of long-term postmenopausal hormone users are needed to determine whether discontinuation or continuation into the 70s, 80s, and 90s affects cognition.**

ESTROGEN REPLACEMENT THERAPY, MODIFIED ESTROGENS, AND CANCER

The incidence rates for both breast and colon cancer increase with advanced age, and they may be impacted by ERT or HRT. An abbreviated literature summary with issues pertinent to elderly women is summarized here. An increase in the incidence of endometrial cancer with the use of unopposed ERT is well understood and does not need comment.

Colon cancer is the leading cause of cancer mortality in women aged 85 and over. A protective influence of hormones was postulated by McMichael and Potter in 1980.[189] Given the vast number of observational studies that have looked at ERT and breast cancer, surprisingly little has been studied in elderly women.

Quality of Data

Colon Cancer. Approximately 40 studies have evaluated the association of ERT with colon cancer, including five meta-analyses,[190–193] and one randomized controlled trial with partial results.[130]

Breast Cancer. Despite the inclusion of many elderly women in breast cancer and ERT studies, few stratify results by age. The NHS provided data on a subset of women aged 60 to 64. [194] The Collaborative Group on Hormonal Factors in Breast Cancer summarized 51 studies from 21 countries and evaluated associations with age. [195] However, few older women were estrogen users. One large randomized controlled trial enrolled women to age 79. [130]

Selective Estrogen Receptor Modulators and Breast Cancer. The Multiple Outcomes of Raloxifene Evaluation (MORE) is a large randomized controlled trial that included women aged 31 to 80 and reported breast cancer results. [196] Eighty percent of the participants were aged 60 or over, mean age 67. The National Cancer Institute undertook a randomized controlled trial in 1990 to evaluate tamoxifen for the prevention of breast cancer in high-risk women. [149] Thirty percent of subjects were aged 60 and older, including 6% aged 70 and older.

Results

Colon Cancer. Of 35 observational studies reviewed, 23 suggested a protective effect of ERT on colon cancer, 11 were neutral, and 1 reported a negative impact. [190] Greater benefit is generally seen in studies published since 1990, [191] approximating an RR of 0.83 (95% CI = 0.66 to 1.04) in one meta-analysis. [189] The Leisure World cohort study of 7700 older women found 30% less colon cancer in current ERT users. [191] Risk reduction remained but lost statistical significance among past users. Other observational studies have also found current use but not longer duration to be beneficial. [192,193] A case-control study found a 65% ERT-related risk reduction, but the 23% reduction in those 70 and older was not statistically significant. [197] One third or more of subjects in the large randomized WHI were aged 65 or over. [130] Six fewer colon cancers per 10,000 women per year (statistically significant) occurred among estrogen-progestin users than with placebo after an average of 5 years (3.5 to 8.5). Age-specific risks were not evaluated.

Breast Cancer. In the NHS, breast cancer risk was found to be 70% higher in 60- to 64-year-old current ERT users who had been taking it at least 5 years. [194] A recent review of 51 epidemiologic studies, including 52,700 women with breast cancer, found a steady increase in risk among current ERT users of 1.023 for each year of hormone use. [195] RRs were 1.3 in women under age 60 and 1.40 in those aged 60 and over. However, the median age at breast cancer diagnosis was 60, and 92% of users stopped use prior to age 65, thus offering little information about the older woman. One third or more of subjects in the large randomized WHI were aged 65 or over. [130] Eight more breast cancers per 10,000 women per year (not statistically significant) occurred among estrogen-progestin users than among placebo users after an average of 5 years (3.5 to 8.5). No interactions with age were found.

Selective Estrogen Receptor Modulators and Breast Cancer. Raloxifene use for 3 years was associated with a 75% breast cancer risk reduction. [196] Estrogen-receptor-positive cancers were suppressed by 90%, but estrogen-receptor-negative cancers were not. Tamoxifen use for 4 years was found to reduce invasive breast cancer by 49% in 13,400 mostly younger women; this included a 55% reduction in those aged 60 and over. [149] No effect was seen on colon cancer.

Summary

Colon Cancer. Colon cancer is decreased among current HRT users, with concurrence of observational and randomized trial data. Although no study has shown statistical significance among women aged 65 and over, this is likely due to lack of data rather than a lack of effect. The effects of past use are unclear.

Breast Cancer. Long-term and current estrogen-progestin use slightly increases the risk of breast cancer, with concurrence of observational and randomized trial data. It is unclear whether age interacts with HRT. The effects of estrogen use alone are uncertain. Only observational data evaluate breast cancer mortality, which is not higher among HRT users. Still, relatively few data inform risks for the older woman. SERMs suppress, delay, or inhibit estrogen-receptor-positive breast cancers in young-elderly women, but study durations have been relatively short in relation to clinical breast cancer development (7 years).

> *Gyn 73 (Level B)*: **Cross-sectional or prospective cohort studies should be performed to determine the factors, whether breast cancer pathophysiology or other health factors, that are associated with the apparent lower mortality among women whose breast cancer is diagnosed during hormone replacement therapy use.**

> *Gyn 74 (Level B)*: **Observational studies are needed to determine what functional factors and comorbidities are associated with a lack of benefit of mammography or colon cancer screening, for the development of clinical guidelines.**

> *Gyn 75 (Level B)*: **The results from existing and future studies of estrogen, estrogen-progestin, and selective estrogen receptor modulator use should be stratified by age, even when power is low, to facilitate systematic reviews.**

> *Gyn 76 (Level A)*: **Randomized trials of continuous therapy since menopause are needed to determine the effects of estrogen and hormone replacement on breast and colon cancer incidence and mortality.**

> *Gyn 77 (Level A)*: **Randomized trials are needed to determine the effects of long-term use of selective estrogen receptor modulators on breast and colon cancer incidence and mortality.**

> *Gyn 78 (Level D)*: **Basic science and observational trials are needed to determine the mechanisms by which estrogen reduces colon cancer incidence.**

> *Gyn 79 (Level C)*: **Randomized trials are needed to determine whether estrogen or estrogen-progestin replacement after breast cancer treatment affects recurrence and mortality.**

OSTEOPOROSIS

Hormonal Therapies

The lifetime risk of osteoporotic fractures in a 50-year-old white woman has been estimated to be 30% to 40% in the United States, including a 15% to 18% risk for hip
fractures. [198] (See also Chapter 11, section on osteoporosis and falls.) In women aged 60
years and over, osteoporosis prevention or treatment has been the predominant reason for
initiation of ERT. [199] A lack of randomized data led to the Food and Drug Administration's
withdrawal of the indication of osteoporosis treatment for ERT, although it is still approved for prevention. Data from more recent research may reverse this. Some data are
also available for SERMs (raloxifene, tamoxifen). Studies on phytoestrogen effects in
elderly women have not been published.

Quality of Data

Estrogen. For a thorough discussion of studies pertinent to elderly women, the reader is
referred to reviews of this subject. [198,200–203] Cohort, case-control, and randomized controlled trials evaluate the effects of ERT on BMD and bone turnover in older
women. [200,202] Fracture data regarding elderly women are primarily from observational
studies. [204–212] Most earlier studies suffered from several design flaws, such as including
in the estrogen-user group women who had discontinued ERT use several years earlier. A
meta-analysis of fracture data in older women included published and unpublished reports
of all randomized clinical trials in the preceding decade. [203] The trials are well described
and five include young-old women [128,129,213–215] and two include middle-old
women. [180,216] A recent randomized controlled trial of HRT includes fracture data for
women aged 50 and over. [130]

Selective Estrogen Receptor Modulators. A large, well-conducted randomized controlled trial (MORE trial) reported the effect of raloxifene on BMD and fracture risk. [217] A
large, well-described cross-sectional case-control study of tamoxifen and fracture risk was
conducted in nursing-home residents aged 65 years and older. [218]

Results

Estrogen. Virtually all studies show improved BMD or bone turnover in the elderly
woman that was essentially equal to that in younger women. [200,202] However, fracture
benefit in older women is less clear. Studies generally show a reduction in risk that does
not achieve statistical significance. Pooled randomized controlled trial data of women
aged 60 and over showed a 21% hip fracture risk reduction ($P = .26$), and a 12% wrist
fracture risk reduction ($P = .63$). [203] These results do not prove a lack of ERT benefit,
because most randomized controlled trials were not designed with fracture as the primary
outcome, and the data regarding older women are heavily influenced by the large HERS
trial, [128] in which women with osteoporosis were systematically excluded, thereby limiting
the generalizability of the results. [219] Exclusion of the HERS trial (see above) led to a
more impressive fracture risk reduction of 38% ($P = .06$). In four observational studies it
is possible to distinguish between women who started HRT before and after age 60
years. [203,204,208,211,212] All show a large reduction in fractures among women starting before age 60 years, with three studies showing statistical significance. [208,211,212] However,

none found statistical significance among women who started after age 60. ERT was found to be most effective for hip fracture prevention among long-term and current ERT users aged 75 or over who started within 5 years of menopause. [211] One third or more of women in the randomized WHI were aged 65 or over. [130] Twenty-five percent to 35% fewer hip, vertebral, and other osteoporotic fractures occurred in the HRT group than in the placebo group. Age-specific rates were not given.

Low doses of ERT (0.3 mg esterified estrogen, 25 µg transdermal estrogen, 0.3 mg CEE) improved BMD in several studies, albeit less than standard doses. [202] One randomized controlled trial in 128 healthy white women aged 65 or over, mean age 73 ± 5 years, found an increase in BMD with low-dose ERT. [216] Fracture data are not available for low ERT doses.

Selective Estrogen Receptor Modulators. The MORE (raloxifene) trial included more than 7000 osteoporotic women aged 31 to 80 years, mean age 67. [217] Bone density was found to increase, but nonvertebral fractures were not significantly affected. Age was mentioned for only one outcome: the 50% reduction in vertebral fracture rate was the same "across all age groups." Tamoxifen was found to reduce fracture risk among nursing-home residents with 10 mg but not 20 mg daily. [218]

Summary

HRT reduces the risk of osteoporotic fractures, especially when started after menopause and used long term. The risk reduction when HRT is started in the 60s and 70s is not proven. Evidence points toward a modest (10% to 20%) effect. Low ERT doses help maintain BMD, but fracture benefit is unknown. SERMs are potentially an excellent alternative to ERT for osteoporosis. However, hip fracture data, particularly in middle-old and old-old women, are needed.

> *Gyn 80 (Level B)*: **Prospective cohort studies are needed to compare the quality-of-life outcomes of long-term estrogen, estrogen-progestin, selective estrogen receptor modulator, and bisphosphonate use.**

> *Gyn 81 (Level B)*: **Observational and pilot studies are needed to determine whether hormone replacement therapy and selective estrogen receptor modulators act synergistically with other fracture-prevention interventions, such as physical therapy for balance and strength.**

> *Gyn 82 (Levels B, A)*: **Observational and eventually randomized trials are needed to determine whether low-dose estrogen replacement therapy initiated at menopause reduces hip, vertebral, and other osteoporotic fractures in advanced age.**

> *Gyn 83 (Level B)*: **Results from existing and future studies of hormone replacement to prevent or treat osteoporosis need to be stratified by age, even when power is low, to facilitate systematic reviews.**

> *Gyn 84 (Level A)*: **Randomized trials are needed to determine the differences in overall quality of life with hormone replacement therapy, selective estrogen receptor modulators, and bisphosphonates.**

> *Gyn 85 (Level A)*: **A placebo-controlled randomized trial should be performed to determine whether bisphosphonates, hormone replacement therapy, or selective estrogen receptor modulators best reduce osteoporosis morbidity and mortality in frail and institutionalized elderly women, including data on overall cost, burden of care, and quality of life.**

> *Gyn 86 (Level A)*: **A randomized controlled trial should be performed to determine the fracture benefit of initiating selective estrogen receptor modulators after age 75 among both osteoporotic and osteopenic women.**

NONHORMONAL THERAPIES: CALCIUM AND VITAMIN D

The nonhormonal pharmacotherapeutics most relevant to osteoporosis in elderly women are nutritional supplementation (reviewed in this section) and bisphosphonates (reviewed in the next section). Other therapies (calcitonin, androgens, fluoride) have less demonstrated efficacy, are poorly studied in elderly women, or may even increase fracture risk.

The need for adequate calcium and vitamin D is well documented. Vitamin D promotes calcium absorption. Its benefit is largely lost within 2 years of discontinuation.[220]

Quality of Data

Randomized controlled trials of calcium and vitamin D and of combined therapy using fracture outcomes in older individuals have been reported. Large trials and moderate-sized trials have compared calcium plus vitamin D with placebo,[221–224] calcium with placebo,[225,226] vitamin D with calcium,[227] and vitamin D with placebo.[228] Several smaller trials have compared vitamin D with placebo, calcium, and other forms of vitamin D.[220] Dietary calcium and fracture associations were prospectively assessed in a large cohort.[229]

Results

Administration of vitamin D plus calcium was found to reduce hip, nonvertebral, and vertebral fractures in elderly women.[221–223] The Finnish study did not demonstrate fracture reduction, but power to do so and treatment duration were low.[224] Vitamin D alone was not found to reduce hip fractures in 2600 healthy and frail elderly women.[228] Calcium supplementation was found to lower the vertebral fracture rate in elderly women with baseline vertebral fractures, but not in those without.[225,226] Current calcium use was found to be associated with an increased hip-fracture risk in a large cohort, but this was presumed to be due to confounding by indication for supplements.[229]

Summary

Adequate intake of both vitamin D and calcium reduces fracture risk, and both are most important in those who are deficient or osteoporotic. Both together reduce vertebral and nonvertebral fractures in elderly women. Randomized data for the use of calcium alone are weak; data for vitamin D alone are slightly stronger, but still not certain.

> *Gyn 87 (Level D)*: **Observational trials and pilot studies are needed to determine the importance of factors in adolescence, such as milk**

and carbonated beverage consumption, on peak bone mass and bone matrix.

Gyn 88 (Level D): Observational studies are needed to define the costs and side effects associated with calcium and vitamin D supplementation.

Gyn 89 (Level C): Randomized trials are needed to determine the optimal time in a woman's life span to benefit from calcium supplementation.

Gyn 90 (Level C): Randomized trials should be performed to determine the best method of calcium supplementation to maximize absorption and minimize side effects.

Gyn 91 (Level C): Randomized trials are needed to determine the best form of vitamin D supplementation.

NONHORMONAL THERAPIES: BISPHOSPHONATES

Although the mechanism of action of bisphosphonates is incompletely understood, they have proven to be profoundly effective in the prevention and treatment of osteoporosis.

Quality of Studies

Bisphosphonates have undergone rigorous clinical efficacy trials, since their use for osteoporosis is a fairly new indication. Available data include randomized controlled trials in elderly women.

Alendronate. A meta-analysis including five randomized controlled trials published in 1994 and 1995 of alendronate use for at least 2 years reported data dichotomized at age 65.[230] Women aged 55 to 81 with and without existing vertebral fractures were studied in the Fracture Intervention Trial (FIT).[231–233]

Risedronate. The Vertebral Efficacy with Risedronate Therapy (VERT) trial reported approximately 1000 women, mean age 69, with low bone density and baseline vertebral fractures.[234]

Etidronate. Four etidronate randomized controlled trials with elderly women reported fracture data.[235–238]

Results

Alendronate. In the meta-analysis, the RRs for fracture ranged from 0.34 to 0.91, with the greatest risk reduction in those aged 65 and over.[230] In the FIT trial, women with a baseline vertebral fracture were found to have a reduced risk of subsequent vertebral or nonvertebral fracture.[231] Among women without a baseline vertebral fracture, only the risk for vertebral fracture was reduced. Results were consistent across age groups.[232] Among the women with baseline hip osteoporosis, the 36% reduction in clinical fractures was statistically significant, but no effect was demonstrable in women with higher baseline BMD.

Risedronate. Risedronate was found to reduce vertebral and nonvertebral fractures significantly in women with baseline osteoporosis, although in one report the nonvertebral fracture risk reduction was of borderline certainty ($P = .06$). [234,239] A trial of risedronate in 9000 severely osteoporotic women aged 70 or older (hip T score > 4.0) found a 30% decrease in hip fracture risk among those aged 70 to 79, but not significantly in women aged 80 and older ($P = .35$). [240]

Etidronate. In three of the four randomized controlled trials, mean ages 65 to 72 years, vertebral but not nonvertebral fractures were reduced. [235,236,238]

Summary

Bisphosphonates are well studied in elderly women and are effective. Alendronate decreases vertebral and nonvertebral fractures in osteoporotic women. A significant benefit in elderly women without osteoporosis is unlikely with therapy of short duration (> 4 years). Risedronate effectively lowers fracture rates in elderly osteoporotic women, although hip fracture benefit is less certain. Trials have included only osteoporotic women, so the preventive benefits of this agent are unknown. Etidronate is not first-line bisphosphonate therapy.

> *Gyn 92 (Level B)*: **Long-term observational studies are needed to obtain information about the efficacy, safety, and adverse effects of very long-term bisphosphonate use (30 to 40 years) for postmenopausal osteoporosis prevention and treatment.**

> *Gyn 93 (Level B)*: **Medications that selectively reduce bone resorption without limiting bone formation should be developed.**

> *Gyn 94 (Level B)*: **Medications that stimulate bone formation should be developed.**

> *Gyn 95 (Level A)*: **Randomized controlled trials are needed to determine the utility of bisphosphonates for osteoporosis benefit in healthy women.**

> *Gyn 96 (Level A)*: **Randomized controlled trials should be performed to determine the additive effects, if any, of hormonal and nonhormonal osteoporosis therapies.**

> *Gyn 97 (Level D)*: **Decision and cost-effectiveness analyses are needed to calculate whether health care dollars spent on medication, including evaluation and management of complications, would be better spent on physical and occupational therapy in frail elderly women.**

KEY RESEARCH QUESTIONS IN GERIATRIC GYNECOLOGY

Gyn KQ1: **How can the immediate and long-term functional impact of gynecologic surgery on older women be improved?**

Hypothesis-generating: Prospective or cross-sectional cohort studies are needed to give clues to the functional impact of gynecologic surgery on elderly women of differing functional status.

Hypothesis-testing studies are needed to define what preoperative, intraoperative, and postoperative interventions enhance functional recovery. Hypothesis-testing studies are needed to establish benefits and risks of estrogen replacement therapy preoperatively, both locally for incontinence and prolapse surgery, and systemically on the cardiovascular and hematologic systems (eg, thrombophilia).

Gyn KQ2: **How can normal urogenital function be maintained in aging and age-related conditions?**

Hypothesis-generating: Observational studies are needed to understand the epidemiology of urogenital disorders other than urinary incontinence, including vulvovaginal conditions, pelvic organ prolapse, and sexual dysfunction. Observational studies are needed to suggest preventive and therapeutic interventions (other than estrogen therapy) to minimize urinary incontinence, voiding dysfunction, pelvic organ prolapse, and vulvovaginitis. Hypothesis-generating studies are needed to find potential therapeutic interventions for sexual dysfunction in older women.

Hypothesis-testing studies are needed to determine the impact of estrogen replacement therapy on urogenital health. Hypothesis-testing studies are needed to evaluate the functional and quality-of-life benefits of currently available interventions for urinary incontinence and pelvic organ prolapse, including behavioral programs and pelvic floor reparative procedures. Hypothesis-testing studies are needed for the treatment of urinary incontinence in demented elderly women.

Gyn KQ3: **Which older women should be encouraged to initiate or continue estrogen replacement or other hormonal therapy?**

Hypothesis-generating: Observational studies are needed to sort out complex relationships among age, hormone replacement, and genetic and environmental predisposition to disease.

Hypothesis-testing studies are needed to establish the impact of selective estrogen receptor modulators and long-term (> 10 years) estrogen and estrogen-progestin replacement therapy on conditions that affect a large number of elderly women—cardiovascular disease, stroke, dementia, colon cancer, breast cancer, age-related macular degeneration, cataracts, poor dentition, arthritis, and osteoporosis. Sexual function issues should be included among the outcomes studied. Studies are needed to address the several hormone replacement therapeutic options, such as dose, route of administration, types and schedules of progestins, and the use of selective estrogen receptor modulators instead of estrogens and progestins. In all studies, the questions of continuation in old age should be addressed.

REFERENCES

1. Merrill RM. Prevalence corrected hysterectomy rates and probabilities in Utah. Ann Epidemiol 2001;11:127-135.
2. Wilcox LS, Koonin LM, Pokras R, et al. Hysterectomy in the United States, 1988-1990. Obstet Gynecol 1994;83:549-555.

3. Schofield MJ, Hennrikus DJ, Redman S, Sanson-Fisher RW. Prevalence and characteristics of women who have had a hysterectomy in a community survey. Aust N Z J Obstet Gynaecol 1991;31:153-158.

4. Olsen AL, Smith VJ, Bergstrom JO, et al. Epidemiology of surgically managed pelvic organ prolapse and urinary incontinence. Obstet Gynecol 1997;89:501-506.

5. Sultana CJ, Campbell JW, Pisanelli WS, et al. Morbidity and mortality of incontinence surgery in elderly women: an analysis of Medicare data. Am J Obstet Gynecol 1997;176:344-348.

6. Warner MA, Warner DO, Harper CM, et al. Lower extremity neuropathies associated with lithotomy positions. Anesthesiology 2000;93:938-942.

7. Panayiotis G, Ellenbogen A, Grunstein S. Major gynecologic surgical procedures in the aged. J Am Geriatr Soc 1978;26:459-462.

8. Polanczyk CA, Marcantonio E, Goldman L, et al. Impact of age on perioperative complications and length of stay in patients undergoing noncardiac surgery. Ann Intern Med 2001;134:637-643.

9. Virtanen HS, Makinen JI. Mortality after gynaecologic operations in Finland, 1986-1991. Br J Obstet Gynaecol 1995;102:54-57.

10. Nahhas WA, Brown M. Gynecologic surgery in the aged. J Reprod Med 1990;35:550-554.

11. Lambrou NC, Buller JL, Thompson JR, et al. Prevalence of perioperative complications among women undergoing reconstructive pelvic surgery. Am J Obstet Gynecol 2000;183:1355-1358; discussion 1359-1360.

12. Shackelford DP, Hoffman MK, Kramer PR, Jr., et al. Evaluation of preoperative cardiac risk index values in patients undergoing vaginal surgery. Am J Obstet Gynecol 1995;173:80-84.

13. MacLennan AH, Taylor AW, Wilson DH, Wilson D. The prevalence of pelvic floor disorders and their relationship to gender, age, parity and mode of delivery. BJOG 2000;107:1460-1470.

14. Fanning J, Neuhoff RA, Brewer JE, et al. Frequency and yield of postoperative fever evaluation. Infect Dis Obstet Gynecol 1998;6:252-255.

15. Swift SE. The distribution of pelvic organ support in a population of female subjects seen for routine gynecologic health care. Am J Obstet Gynecol 2000;183:277-285.

16. Quinlivan LG. The gynecological findings in elderly women. Geriatrics 1964;Sept:654-657.

17. Chiaffarino F, Chatenoud L, Dindelli M, et al. Reproductive factors, family history, occupation and risk of urogenital prolapse. Eur J Obstet Gynecol Reprod Biol 1999;82:63-67.

18. Gemer O, Bergman M, Segal S. Prevalence of hydronephrosis in patients with genital prolapse. Eur J Obstet Gynecol Reprod Biol 1999;86:11-13.

19. Beverly CM, Walters MD, Weber AM, et al. Prevalence of hydronephrosis in patients undergoing surgery for pelvic organ prolapse. Obstet Gynecol 1997;90:37-41.

20. Sulak PJ, Kuehl TJ, Shull BL. Vaginal pessaries and their use in pelvic relaxation. J Reprod Med 1993;38:919-923.

21. Theofrastous JP, Addison WA, Timmons MC. Voiding function following prolapse surgery. Impact of estrogen replacement. J Reprod Med 1996;41:881-884.

22. Mikkelsen AL, Felding C, Clausen HV. Clinical effects of preoperative oestradiol treatment before vaginal repair operation. A double-blind, randomized trial. Gynecol Obstet Invest 1995;40:125-128.

23. Denehy TR, Choe JY, Gregori CA, Breen JL. Modified Le Fort partial colpocleisis with Kelly urethral plication and posterior colpoperineoplasty in the medically compromised elderly: a comparison with vaginal hysterectomy, anterior colporrhaphy, and posterior colpoperineoplasty. Am J Obstet Gynecol 1995;173:1697-1701; discussion 1701-1692.

24. DeLancey JO, Morley GW. Total colpocleisis for vaginal eversion. Am J Obstet Gynecol 1997;176:1228-1232; discussion 1232-1235.

25. Ahranjani M, Nora E, Rezai P, Bujewski S. Neugebauer-Le Fort operation for vaginal prolapse. A review of 38 cases. J Reprod Med 1992;37:959-964.

26. Miklos JR, Sze EH, Karram MM. Vaginal correction of pelvic organ relaxation using local anesthesia. Obstet Gynecol 1995;86:922-924.

27. Kohli N, Sze E, Karram M. Pyometra following Le Fort colpocleisis. Int Urogynecol J Pelvic Floor Dysfunct 1996;7:264-266.

28. Barlow DH, Cardozo LD, Francis RM, et al. Urogenital ageing and its effect on sexual health in older British women. Br J Obstet Gynaecol 1997;104:87-91.

29. Barlow DH, Samsioe G, van Geelen JM. A study of European womens' experience of the problems of urogenital ageing and its management. Maturitas 1997;27:239-247.

30. Stenberg A, Heimer G, Ulmsten U. The prevalence of urogenital symptoms in postmenopausal women. Maturitas 1995;22 Suppl:S17-S20.

31. Rekers H, Drogendijk AC, Valkenburg HA, Riphagen F. The menopause, urinary incontinence and other symptoms of the genito-urinary tract. Maturitas 1992;15:101-111.

32. Iosif CS, Bekassy Z. Prevalence of genito-urinary symptoms in the late menopause. Acta Obstet Gynecol Scand 1984;63:257-260.

33. Versi E, Harvey MA, Cardozo L, et al. Urogenital prolapse and atrophy at menopause: a prevalence study. Int Urogynecol J Pelvic Floor Dysfunct 2001;12:107-110.

34. Cardozo L, Bachmann G, McClish D, et al. Meta-analysis of estrogen therapy in the management of urogenital atrophy in postmenopausal women: second report of the Hormones and Urogenital Therapy Committee. Obstet Gynecol 1998;92:722-727.

35. Ishigooka M, Hashimoto T, Tomaru M, et al. Effect of hormonal replacement therapy in postmenopausal women with chronic irritative voiding symptoms. Int Urogynecol J Pelvic Floor Dysfunct 1994;5:208-211.

36. Leiblum S, Bachmann G, Kemmann E, et al. Vaginal atrophy in the postmenopausal woman. The importance of sexual activity and hormones. JAMA 1983;249:2195-2198.

37. van der Velden J, van Lindert AC, Gimbrere CH, et al. Epidemiologic data on vulvar cancer: comparison of hospital with population-based data. Gynecol Oncol 1996;62:379-383.

38. Edwards CL, Balat O. Characteristics of patients with vulvar cancer: an analysis of 94 patients. Eur J Gynaecol Oncol 1996;17:351-353.

39. Raber G, Mempel V, Jackisch C, et al. Malignant melanoma of the vulva. Report of 89 patients. Cancer 1996;78:2353-2358.

40. Benign disorders of the vulva. In Beers MH, Berkow R (eds): The Merck Manual of Geriatrics, 3rd ed. Whitehouse Station, NJ: Merck Research Laboratories, 2000:1200-1201.

41. Elchalal U, Gilead L, Vardy DA, et al. Treatment of vulvar lichen sclerosus in the elderly: an update. Obstet Gynecol Surv 1995;50:155-162.

42. Lynch PJ, Edwards L. White patches and plaques. In Genital Dermatology. New York: Churchill Livingstone, 1994:149-162.

43. Wingate MB. Vulvar dystrophies in geriatric patients. Compr Ther 1986;12:39-42.

44. Powell JJ, Wojnarowska F. Lichen sclerosus. Lancet 1999;353:1777-1783.

45. Sideri M, Origoni M, Spinaci L, Ferrari A. Topical testosterone in the treatment of vulvar lichen sclerosus. Int J Gynaecol Obstet 1994;46:53-56.

46. Matthias RE, Lubben JE, Atchison KA, Schweitzer SO. Sexual activity and satisfaction among very old adults: results from a community-dwelling Medicare population survey. Gerontologist 1997;37:6-14.

47. Gentili A, Mulligan T. Sexual dysfunction in older adults. Clin Geriatr Med 1998;14:383-393.

48. Young M, Denny G, Young T, Luquis R. Sexual satisfaction among married women age 50 and older. Psychol Rep 2000;86:1107-1122.

49. Johnson BK. A correlational framework for understanding sexuality in women age 50 and older. Health Care Women Int 1998;19:553-564.

50. Gelfand MM. Sexuality among older women. J Womens Health Gend Based Med 2000;9 Suppl 1:S15-S20.

51. Wiley D, Bortz WM, 2nd. Sexuality and aging–usual and successful. J Gerontol A Biol Sci Med Sci 1996;51:M142-M146.

52. Masters WH, Johnson VE. Human Sexual Response. Boston, MA: Little, Brown, 1966.

53. Bretschneider JG, McCoy NL. Sexual interest and behavior in healthy 80- to 102-year-olds. Arch Sex Behav 1988;17:109-129.

54. Bortz WM, 2nd, Wallace DH. Physical fitness, aging, and sexuality. West J Med 1999;170:167-169.

55. Drory Y, Kravetz S, Weingarten M. Comparison of sexual activity of women and men after a first acute myocardial infarction. Am J Cardiol 2000;85:1283-1287.

56. Wright JG, Rudicel S, Feinstein AR. Ask patients what they want. Evaluation of individual complaints before total hip replacement. J Bone Joint Surg Br 1994;76:229-234.

57. Tobin JM, Harindra V. Attendance by older patients at a genitourinary medicine clinic. Sex Transm Infect 2001;77:289-291.

58. Barber MD, Visco AG, Wyman JF, et al. Sexual function in women with urinary incontinence and pelvic organ prolapse. Obstet Gynecol 2002;99:281-289.

59. Tarcan T, Park K, Goldstein I, et al. Histomorphometric analysis of age-related structural changes in human clitoral cavernosal tissue. J Urol 1999;161:940-944.

60. Park K, Goldstein I, Andry C, et al. Vasculogenic female sexual dysfunction: the hemodynamic basis for vaginal engorgement insufficiency and clitoral erectile insufficiency. Int J Impot Res 1997;9:27-37.

61. Kraemer RR, Synovitz LB, Gimpel T, et al. Effect of estrogen on serum DHEA in younger and older women and the relationship of DHEA to adiposity and gender. Metabolism 2001;50:488-493.

62. Slater CC, Zhang C, Hodis HN, et al. Comparison of estrogen and androgen levels after oral estrogen replacement therapy. J Reprod Med 2001;46:1052-1056.

63. Wright TC, Ferenczy A, Kurman RJ. Carcinoma and other tumors of the cervix. In Kurman RJ (ed): Blaustein's Pathology of the Female Genital Tract, 4th ed. New York: Springer-Verlag, 1994:279-326.

64. Mandelblatt J, Gopaul I, Wistreich M. Gynecological care of elderly women. Another look at Papanicolaou smear testing. JAMA 1986;256:367-371.

65. Fink DJ. Change in American Cancer Society Checkup Guidelines for detection of cervical cancer. CA Cancer J Clin 1988;38:127-128.

66. Mandelblatt JS, Hammond DB. Primary care of elderly women: is Pap smear screening necessary? Mt Sinai J Med 1985;52:284-290.

67. American Cancer Society. Cancer facts and figures, 1997. Racial and ethnic patterns. 1997.

68. Incidence of Pap test abnormalities within 3 years of a normal Pap test–United States, 1991-1998. MMWR Morb Mortal Wkly Rep 2000;49:1001-1003.

69. Rader AE, Rose PG, Rodriguez M, et al. Atypical squamous cells of undetermined significance in women over 55. Comparison with the general population and implications for management. Acta Cytol 1999;43:357-362.

70. Coughlin SS, Uhler RJ, Blackman DK. Breast and cervical cancer screening practices among American Indian and Alaska Native women in the United States, 1992-1997. Prev Med 1999;29:287-295.

71. Ruchlin HS. Prevalence and correlates of breast and cervical cancer screening among older women. Obstet Gynecol 1997;90:16-21.

72. van Wijngaarden WJ, Duncan ID. Rationale for stopping cervical screening in women over 50. BMJ 1993;306:967-971. [Erratum in BMJ 1993;306:1373].

73. Gatta G, Capocaccia R, Hakulinen T, et al. Variations in survival for invasive cervical cancer among European women, 1978-89. EUROCARE Working Group. Cancer Causes Control 1999;10:575-581.

74. Ferrante JM, Gonzalez EC, Roetzheim RG, et al. Clinical and demographic predictors of late-stage cervical cancer. Arch Fam Med 2000;9:439-445.
75. Ackermann SP, Brackbill RM, Bewerse BA, et al. Cancer screening behaviors among U.S. women: breast cancer, 1987-1989, and cervical cancer, 1988-1989. Morb Mortal Wkly Rep CDC Surveill Summ 1992;41:17-25.
76. Womeodu RJ, Bailey JE. Barriers to cancer screening. Med Clin North Am 1996;80:115-133.
77. Calle EE, Flanders WD, Thun MJ, Martin LM. Demographic predictors of mammography and Pap smear screening in US women. Am J Public Health 1993;83:53-60.
78. Mitchell H, Medley G, Higgins V. An audit of the women who died during 1994 from cancer of the cervix in Victoria, Australia. Aust N Z J Obstet Gynaecol 1996;36:73-76.
79. Mandelblatt J, Traxler M, Lakin P, et al. Mammography and Papanicolaou smear use by elderly poor black women. The Harlem Study Team. J Am Geriatr Soc 1992;40:1001-1007.
80. Ives DG, Lave JR, Traven ND, et al. Mammography and pap smear use by older rural women. Public Health Rep 1996;111:244-250.
81. Mandelblatt J, Traxler M, Lakin P, et al. Targeting breast and cervical cancer screening to elderly poor black women: who will participate? The Harlem Study Team. Prev Med 1993;22:20-33.
82. Mandelblatt J, Traxler M, Lakin P, et al. A nurse practitioner intervention to increase breast and cervical cancer screening for poor, elderly black women. The Harlem Study Team. J Gen Intern Med 1993;8:173-178.
83. Margolis KL, Lurie N, McGovern PG, et al. Increasing breast and cervical cancer screening in low-income women. J Gen Intern Med 1998;13:515-521.
84. Sawaya GF, Grady D, Kerlikowske K, et al. The positive predictive value of cervical smears in previously screened postmenopausal women: the Heart and Estrogen/progestin Replacement Study (HERS). Ann Intern Med 2000;133:942-950.
85. Stenkvist B, Bergstrom R, Eklund G, Fox CH. Papanicolaou smear screening and cervical cancer. What can you expect? JAMA 1984;252:1423-1426.
86. Suarez L, Nichols DC, Brady CA. Use of peer role models to increase Pap smear and mammogram screening in Mexican-American and black women. Am J Prev Med 1993;9:290-296.
87. Kelly AW, Fores Chacori M, Wollan PC, et al. A program to increase breast and cervical cancer screening for Cambodian women in a midwestern community. Mayo Clin Proc 1996;71:437-444.
88. Paskett ED, Phillips KC, Miller ME. Improving compliance among women with abnormal Papanicolaou smears. Obstet Gynecol 1995;86:353-359.
89. Fahs MC, Mandelblatt J, Schechter C, Muller C. Cost effectiveness of cervical cancer screening for the elderly. Ann Intern Med 1992;117:520-527.
90. Mandelblatt JS, Fahs MC. The cost-effectiveness of cervical cancer screening for low-income elderly women. JAMA 1988;259:2409-2413.
91. Committee on Gynecologic Practice. American College of Obstetricians and Gynecologists. ACOG committee opinion. Recommendations on frequency of Pap test screening. Number 152–March 1995. Int J Gynaecol Obstet 1995;49:210-211.
92. NIH Consensus Development Panel. National Institutes of Health Consensus Development Conference statement on cervical cancer. April 1-3, 1996. Gynecol Oncol 1997;66:351-361.
93. Miller AB, Anderson G, Brisson J, et al. Report of a national workshop on screening for cancer of the cervix. CMAJ 1991;145:1301-1325.
94. U.S. Preventive Services Task Force. Screening for cervical cancer. In Guide to Clinical Preventive Services, 2nd ed. Baltimore, MD: Williams and Wilkins, 1996:105-117.
95. Weinrich S, Coker AL, Weinrich M, et al. Predictors of Pap smear screening in socioeconomically disadvantaged elderly women. J Am Geriatr Soc 1995;43:267-270.

96. Schootman M, Fuortes LJ. Breast and cervical carcinoma: the correlation of activity limitations and rurality with screening, disease incidence, and mortality. Cancer 1999;86:1087-1094.

97. From the Centers for Disease Control and Prevention. Incidence of Pap test abnormalities within 3 years of a normal Pap test–United States, 1991-1998. JAMA 2000;284:2714-2715.

98. Chen F, Trapido EJ, Davis K. Differences in stage at presentation of breast and gynecologic cancers among whites, blacks, and Hispanics. Cancer 1994;73:2838-2842.

99. American Geriatrics Society Clinical Practice Committee. Screening for cervical carcinoma in older women. J Am Geriatr Soc 2001;49:655-657.

100. Pearce KF, Haefner HK, Sarwar SF, Nolan TE. Cytopathological findings on vaginal Papanicolaou smears after hysterectomy for benign gynecologic disease. N Engl J Med 1996;335:1559-1562.

101. Fox J, Remington P, Layde P, Klein G. The effect of hysterectomy on the risk of an abnormal screening Papanicolaou test result. Am J Obstet Gynecol 1999;180:1104-1109.

102. Tabar L, Fagerberg CJ, Gad A, et al. Reduction in mortality from breast cancer after mass screening with mammography. Randomised trial from the Breast Cancer Screening Working Group of the Swedish National Board of Health and Welfare. Lancet 1985;1:829-832.

103. Balducci L. Breast cancer in the older woman: recent advances. Ann Long Term Care 2001;9:37-44.

104. Nystrom L, Rutqvist LE, Wall S, et al. Breast cancer screening with mammography: overview of Swedish randomised trials. Lancet 1993;341:973-978.

105. Demissie K, Mills OF, Rhoads GG. Empirical comparison of the results of randomized controlled trials and case-control studies in evaluating the effectiveness of screening mammography. J Clin Epidemiol 1998;51:81-91.

106. Kerlikowske K, Grady D, Rubin SM, et al. Efficacy of screening mammography. A meta-analysis. JAMA 1995;273:149-154.

107. van Dijck JA, Holland R, Verbeek AL, et al. Efficacy of mammographic screening of the elderly: a case-referent study in the Nijmegen program in The Netherlands. J Natl Cancer Inst 1994;86:934-938.

108. van Dijck J, Verbeek A, Hendriks J, et al. Mammographic screening after the age of 65 years: early outcomes in the Nijmegen programme. Br J Cancer 1996;74:1838-1842.

109. Smith-Bindman R, Kerlikowske K, Gebretsadik T, Newman J. Is screening mammography effective in elderly women? Am J Med 2000;108:112-119.

110. Hunt KA, Rosen EL, Sickles EA. Outcome analysis for women undergoing annual versus biennial screening mammography: a review of 24,211 examinations. AJR Am J Roentgenol 1999;173:285-289.

111. Olivotto IA, Kan L, d'Yachkova Y, et al. Ten years of breast screening in the Screening Mammography Program of British Columbia, 1988-97. J Med Screen 2000;7:152-159.

112. McCarthy EP, Burns RB, Freund KM, et al. Mammography use, breast cancer stage at diagnosis, and survival among older women. J Am Geriatr Soc 2000;48:1226-1233.

113. Field LR, Wilson TE, Strawderman M, et al. Mammographic screening in women more than 64 years old: a comparison of 1- and 2-year intervals. AJR Am J Roentgenol 1998;170:961-965.

114. Gabriel H, Wilson TE, Helvie MA. Breast cancer in women 65-74 years old: earlier detection by mammographic screening. AJR Am J Roentgenol 1997;168:23-27.

115. Welch HG, Fisher ES. Diagnostic testing following screening mammography in the elderly. J Natl Cancer Inst 1998;90:1389-1392.

116. Kerlikowske K, Grady D, Barclay J, et al. Positive predictive value of screening mammography by age and family history of breast cancer. JAMA 1993;270:2444-2450.

117. Kerlikowske K, Salzmann P, Phillips KA, et al. Continuing screening mammography in women aged 70 to 79 years: impact on life expectancy and cost-effectiveness. JAMA 1999;282:2156-2163.

118. Lindfors KK, Rosenquist CJ. The cost-effectiveness of mammographic screening strategies. JAMA 1995;274:881-884.

119. Boer R, de Koning HJ, van Oortmarssen GJ, van der Maas PJ. In search of the best upper age limit for breast cancer screening. Eur J Cancer 1995;31A:2040-2043.

120. Kavanagh AM, Mitchell H, Giles GG. Hormone replacement therapy and accuracy of mammographic screening. Lancet 2000;355:270-274.

121. Kelaher M, Stellman JM. The impact of Medicare funding on the use of mammography among older women: implications for improving access to screening. Prev Med 2000;31:658-664.

122. Blustein J. Medicare coverage, supplemental insurance, and the use of mammography by older women. N Engl J Med 1995;332:1138-1143.

123. Carney PA, Goodrich ME, O'Mahony DM, et al. Mammography in New Hampshire: characteristics of the women and the exams they receive. J Community Health 2000;25:183-198.

124. Blustein J, Weiss LJ. The use of mammography by women aged 75 and older: factors related to health, functioning, and age. J Am Geriatr Soc 1998;46:941-946.

125. Rakowski W, Pearlman D, Rimer BK, Ehrich B. Correlates of mammography among women with low and high socioeconomic resources. Prev Med 1995;24:149-158.

126. Stampfer MJ, Colditz GA, Willett WC, et al. Postmenopausal estrogen therapy and cardiovascular disease. Ten-year follow-up from the nurses' health study. N Engl J Med 1991;325:756-762.

127. Shlipak MG, Simon JA, Vittinghoff E, et al. Estrogen and progestin, lipoprotein(a), and the risk of recurrent coronary heart disease events after menopause. JAMA 2000;283:1845-1852.

128. Hulley S, Grady D, Bush T, et al. Randomized trial of estrogen plus progestin for secondary prevention of coronary heart disease in postmenopausal women. Heart and Estrogen/progestin Replacement Study (HERS) Research Group. JAMA 1998;280:605-613.

129. Herrington DM, Reboussin DM, Brosnihan KB, et al. Effects of estrogen replacement on the progression of coronary-artery atherosclerosis. N Engl J Med 2000;343:522-529.

130. WHI Study Group. Risks and benefits of estrogen plus progestin in healthy postmenopausal women: principal results from the Women's Health Initiative randomized controlled trial. JAMA 2002;288:321-333.

131. Grodstein F, Manson JE, Colditz GA, et al. A prospective, observational study of postmenopausal hormone therapy and primary prevention of cardiovascular disease. Ann Intern Med 2000;133:933-941.

132. Sellers TA, Mink PJ, Cerhan JR, et al. The role of hormone replacement therapy in the risk for breast cancer and total mortality in women with a family history of breast cancer. Ann Intern Med 1997;127:973-980.

133. Grodstein F, Stampfer MJ, Colditz GA, et al. Postmenopausal hormone therapy and mortality. N Engl J Med 1997;336:1769-1775.

134. Grodstein F, Stampfer MJ, Manson JE, et al. Postmenopausal estrogen and progestin use and the risk of cardiovascular disease. N Engl J Med 1996;335:453-461.

135. Folsom AR, Mink PJ, Sellers TA, et al. Hormonal replacement therapy and morbidity and mortality in a prospective study of postmenopausal women. Am J Public Health 1995;85:1128-1132.

136. Henderson BE, Paganini-Hill A, Ross RK. Decreased mortality in users of estrogen replacement therapy. Arch Intern Med 1991;151:75-78.

137. Persson I, Adami HO, Bergstrom R, et al. Survival in women receiving hormone replacement therapy. A record-linkage study of a large population-based cohort. J Clin Epidemiol 1990;43:677-685.

138. Henderson BE, Paganini-Hill A, Ross RK. Estrogen replacement therapy and protection from acute myocardial infarction. Am J Obstet Gynecol 1988;159:312-317.

139. Bush TL, Barrett-Connor E, Cowan LD, et al. Cardiovascular mortality and noncontraceptive use of estrogen in women: results from the Lipid Research Clinics Program Follow-up Study. Circulation 1987;75:1102-1109.

140. Ettinger B, Friedman GD, Bush T, Quesenberry CP, Jr. Reduced mortality associated with long-term postmenopausal estrogen therapy. Obstet Gynecol 1996;87:6-12.

141. Fioretti F, Tavani A, Gallus S, et al. Menopause and risk of non-fatal acute myocardial infarction: an Italian case-control study and a review of the literature. Hum Reprod 2000;15:599-603.

142. Sullivan JM, Vander Zwaag R, Lemp GF, et al. Postmenopausal estrogen use and coronary atherosclerosis. Ann Intern Med 1988;108:358-363.

143. Manolio TA, Furberg CD, Shemanski L, et al. Associations of postmenopausal estrogen use with cardiovascular disease and its risk factors in older women. The CHS Collaborative Research Group. Circulation 1993;88:2163-2171.

144. Angerer P, Kothny W, Stork S, von Schacky C. Hormone replacement therapy and distensibility of carotid arteries in postmenopausal women: a randomized, controlled trial. J Am Coll Cardiol 2000;36:1789-1796.

145. Westendorp IC, Veld BA, Bots ML, et al. Hormone replacement therapy and intima-media thickness of the common carotid artery: the Rotterdam study. Stroke 1999;30:2562-2567.

146. Tremollieres FA, Cigagna F, Alquier C, et al. Effect of hormone replacement therapy on age-related increase in carotid artery intima-media thickness in postmenopausal women. Atherosclerosis 2000;153:81-88.

147. Jonas HA, Kronmal RA, Psaty BM, et al. Current estrogen-progestin and estrogen replacement therapy in elderly women: association with carotid atherosclerosis. CHS Collaborative Research Group. Cardiovascular Health Study. Ann Epidemiol 1996;6:314-323.

148. Hernandez Avila M, Walker AM, Jick H. Use of replacement estrogens and the risk of myocardial infarction. Epidemiology 1990;1:128-133.

149. Fisher B, Costantino JP, Wickerham DL, et al. Tamoxifen for prevention of breast cancer: report of the National Surgical Adjuvant Breast and Bowel Project P-1 Study. J Natl Cancer Inst 1998;90:1371-1388.

150. Costantino JP, Kuller LH, Ives DG, et al. Coronary heart disease mortality and adjuvant tamoxifen therapy. J Natl Cancer Inst 1997;89:776-782.

151. McDonald CC, Stewart HJ. Fatal myocardial infarction in the Scottish adjuvant tamoxifen trial. The Scottish Breast Cancer Committee. BMJ 1991;303:435-437.

152. McDonald CC, Alexander FE, Whyte BW, et al. Cardiac and vascular morbidity in women receiving adjuvant tamoxifen for breast cancer in a randomised trial. The Scottish Cancer Trials Breast Group. BMJ 1995;311:977-980.

153. Stampfer MJ, Willett WC, Colditz GA, et al. A prospective study of postmenopausal estrogen therapy and coronary heart disease. N Engl J Med 1985;313:1044-1049.

154. Gruchow HW, Anderson AJ, Barboriak JJ, Sobocinski KA. Postmenopausal use of estrogen and occlusion of coronary arteries. Am Heart J 1988;115:954-963.

155. Wilson PW, Garrison RJ, Castelli WP. Postmenopausal estrogen use, cigarette smoking, and cardiovascular morbidity in women over 50. The Framingham Study. N Engl J Med 1985;313:1038-1043.

156. Eaker ED, Castelli WP. Coronary heart disease and its risk factors among women in the Framingham Study. In Eaker E, Packard B, Wenger NK, et al (eds): Coronary Heart Disease in Women. New York: Haymarket Doyma, 1987:122-132.

157. Falkeborn M, Persson I, Adami HO, et al. The risk of acute myocardial infarction after oestrogen and oestrogen-progestogen replacement. Br J Obstet Gynaecol 1992;99:821-828.

158. Rutqvist LE, Mattsson A. Cardiac and thromboembolic morbidity among postmenopausal women with early-stage breast cancer in a randomized trial of adjuvant tamoxifen. The Stockholm Breast Cancer Study Group. J Natl Cancer Inst 1993;85:1398-1406.

159. Bush TL, Blumenthal R, Lobo R, Clarkson TB. SERMs and cardiovascular disease in women. How do these agents affect risk? Postgrad Med 2001;Spec No:17-24.

160. Birkhauser MH, Strnad J, Kampf C, Bahro M. Oestrogens and Alzheimer's disease. Int J Geriatr Psychiatry 2000;15:600-609.

161. Munoz DG, Feldman H. Causes of Alzheimer's disease. CMAJ 2000;162:65-72.

162. Monk D, Brodaty H. Use of estrogens for the prevention and treatment of Alzheimer's disease. Dement Geriatr Cogn Disord 2000;11:1-10.

163. Benson S. Hormone replacement therapy and Alzheimer's disease: an update on the issues. Health Care Women Int 1999;20:619-638.

164. Shumaker SA, Legault C, Thal L, et al. Estrogen plus progestin and the incidence of dementia and mild cognitive impairment in postmenopausal women: the Women's Health Initiative Memory Study: a randomized controlled trial. JAMA 2003;289:2651-2662.

165. Paganini-Hill A, Henderson VW. Estrogen deficiency and risk of Alzheimer's disease in women. Am J Epidemiol 1994;140:256-261.

166. Paganini-Hill A, Henderson VW. Estrogen replacement therapy and risk of Alzheimer disease. Arch Intern Med 1996;156:2213-2217.

167. Tang MX, Jacobs D, Stern Y, et al. Effect of oestrogen during menopause on risk and age at onset of Alzheimer's disease. Lancet 1996;348:429-432.

168. Yaffe K, Haan M, Byers A, et al. Estrogen use, APOE, and cognitive decline: evidence of gene-environment interaction. Neurology 2000;54:1949-1954.

169. Kawas C, Resnick S, Morrison A, et al. A prospective study of estrogen replacement therapy and the risk of developing Alzheimer's disease: the Baltimore Longitudinal Study of Aging. Neurology 1997;48:1517-1521.

170. Barrett-Connor E, Kritz-Silverstein D. Estrogen replacement therapy and cognitive function in older women. JAMA 1993;269:2637-2641.

171. Barrett-Connor E, Goodman-Gruen D. Cognitive function and endogenous sex hormones in older women. J Am Geriatr Soc 1999;47:1289-1293.

172. Fillenbaum GG, Hanlon JT, Landerman LR, Schmader KE. Impact of estrogen use on decline in cognitive function in a representative sample of older community-resident women. Am J Epidemiol 2001;153:137-144.

173. Baldereschi M, Di Carlo A, Lepore V, et al. Estrogen-replacement therapy and Alzheimer's disease in the Italian Longitudinal Study on Aging. Neurology 1998;50:996-1002.

174. Seshadri S, Zornberg GL, Derby LE, et al. Postmenopausal estrogen replacement therapy and the risk of Alzheimer disease. Arch Neurol 2001;58:435-440.

175. Zandi PP, Carlson MC, Plassman BL, et al. Hormone replacement therapy and incidence of Alzheimer disease in older women: the Cache County Study. JAMA 2002;288:2123-2129.

176. Yaffe K, Grady D, Pressman A, Cummings S. Serum estrogen levels, cognitive performance, and risk of cognitive decline in older community women. J Am Geriatr Soc 1998;46:816-821.

177. Rice MM, Graves AB, McCurry SM, et al. Postmenopausal estrogen and estrogen-progestin use and 2-year rate of cognitive change in a cohort of older Japanese American women: The Kame Project. Arch Intern Med 2000;160:1641-1649.

178. Henderson VW, Paganini-Hill A, Miller BL, et al. Estrogen for Alzheimer's disease in women: randomized, double-blind, placebo-controlled trial. Neurology 2000;54:295-301.

179. Wang PN, Liao SQ, Liu RS, et al. Effects of estrogen on cognition, mood, and cerebral blood flow in AD: a controlled study. Neurology 2000;54:2061-2066.

180. Mulnard RA, Cotman CW, Kawas C, et al. Estrogen replacement therapy for treatment of mild to moderate Alzheimer disease: a randomized controlled trial. Alzheimer's Disease Cooperative Study. JAMA 2000;283:1007-1015.

181. Yaffe K, Lui LY, Grady D, et al. Cognitive decline in women in relation to non-protein-bound oestradiol concentrations. Lancet 2000;356:708-712.

182. Waring SC, Rocca WA, Petersen RC, et al. Postmenopausal estrogen replacement therapy and risk of AD: a population-based study. Neurology 1999;52:965-970.

183. Harwood DG, Barker WW, Loewenstein DA, et al. A cross-ethnic analysis of risk factors for AD in white Hispanics and white non-Hispanics. Neurology 1999;52:551-556.

184. Henderson VW, Paganini-Hill A, Emanuel CK, et al. Estrogen replacement therapy in older women. Comparisons between Alzheimer's disease cases and nondemented control subjects. Arch Neurol 1994;51:896-900.

185. Mortel KF, Meyer JS. Lack of postmenopausal estrogen replacement therapy and the risk of dementia. J Neuropsychiatry Clin Neurosci 1995;7:334-337.

186. Brenner DE, Kukull WA, Stergachis A, et al. Postmenopausal estrogen replacement therapy and the risk of Alzheimer's disease: a population-based case-control study. Am J Epidemiol 1994;140:262-267.

187. Schneider LS, Farlow MR, Henderson VW, Pogoda JM. Effects of estrogen replacement therapy on response to tacrine in patients with Alzheimer's disease. Neurology 1996;46:1580-1584.

188. Henderson VW, Watt L, Buckwalter JG. Cognitive skills associated with estrogen replacement in women with Alzheimer's disease. Psychoneuroendocrinology 1996;21:421-430.

189. Hebert-Croteau N. A meta-analysis of hormone replacement therapy and colon cancer in women. Cancer Epidemiol Biomarkers Prev 1998;7:653-659.

190. Crandall CJ. Estrogen replacement therapy and colon cancer: a clinical review. J Womens Health Gend Based Med 1999;8:1155-1166.

191. Paganini-Hill A. Estrogen replacement therapy and colorectal cancer risk in elderly women. Dis Colon Rectum 1999;42:1300-1305.

192. Grodstein F, Newcomb PA, Stampfer MJ. Postmenopausal hormone therapy and the risk of colorectal cancer: a review and meta-analysis. Am J Med 1999;106:574-582.

193. Nanda K, Bastian LA, Hasselblad V, Simel DL. Hormone replacement therapy and the risk of colorectal cancer: a meta-analysis. Obstet Gynecol 1999;93:880-888.

194. Colditz GA, Hankinson SE, Hunter DJ, et al. The use of estrogens and progestins and the risk of breast cancer in postmenopausal women. N Engl J Med 1995;332:1589-1593.

195. Collaborative Group on Hormonal Factors in Breast Cancer. Breast cancer and hormone replacement therapy: collaborative reanalysis of data from 51 epidemiological studies of 52,705 women with breast cancer and 108,411 women without breast cancer. Lancet 1997;350:1047-1059.

196. Cummings SR, Eckert S, Krueger KA, et al. The effect of raloxifene on risk of breast cancer in postmenopausal women: results from the MORE randomized trial. Multiple Outcomes of Raloxifene Evaluation. JAMA 1999;281:2189-2197.

197. Newcomb PA, Storer BE. Postmenopausal hormone use and risk of large-bowel cancer. J Natl Cancer Inst 1995;87:1067-1071.

198. Kamel HK, Perry HM, 3rd, Morley JE. Hormone replacement therapy and fractures in older adults. J Am Geriatr Soc 2001;49:179-187.

199. Ettinger B, Pressman A, Silver P. Effect of age on reasons for initiation and discontinuation of hormone replacement therapy. Menopause 1999;6:282-289 [Erratum in Menopause 2000;7:135].

200. Miller KL. Hormone replacement therapy in the elderly. Clin Obstet Gynecol 1996;39:912-932.

201. Kenny AM, Prestwood KM. Osteoporosis: pathogenesis, diagnosis, and treatment in older adults. Rheum Dis Clin North Am 2000;26:569-591.

202. Doren M, Samsioe G. Prevention of postmenopausal osteoporosis with oestrogen replacement therapy and associated compounds: update on clinical trials since 1995. Hum Reprod Update 2000;6:419-426.

203. Torgerson DJ, Bell-Syer SE. Hormone replacement therapy and prevention of nonvertebral fractures: a meta-analysis of randomized trials. JAMA 2001;285:2891-2897.

204. Hutchinson TA, Polansky SM, Feinstein AR. Post-menopausal oestrogens protect against fractures of hip and distal radius. A case-control study. Lancet 1979;2:705-709.

205. Paganini-Hill A, Chao A, Ross RK, Henderson BE. Exercise and other factors in the prevention of hip fracture: the Leisure World study. Epidemiology 1991;2:16-25.

206. Ettinger B, Genant HK, Cann CE. Long-term estrogen replacement therapy prevents bone loss and fractures. Ann Intern Med 1985;102:319-324.

207. Kiel DP, Felson DT, Anderson JJ, et al. Hip fracture and the use of estrogens in postmenopausal women. The Framingham Study. N Engl J Med 1987;317:1169-1174.

208. Naessen T, Persson I, Adami HO, et al. Hormone replacement therapy and the risk for first hip fracture. A prospective, population-based cohort study. Ann Intern Med 1990;113:95-103.

209. Paganini-Hill A, Ross RK, Gerkins VR, et al. Menopausal estrogen therapy and hip fractures. Ann Intern Med 1981;95:28-31.

210. Kanis JA, Johnell O, Gullberg B, et al. Evidence for efficacy of drugs affecting bone metabolism in preventing hip fracture. BMJ 1992;305:1124-1128.

211. Cauley JA, Seeley DG, Ensrud K, et al. Estrogen replacement therapy and fractures in older women. Study of Osteoporotic Fractures Research Group. Ann Intern Med 1995;122:9-16.

212. Michaelsson K, Baron JA, Farahmand BY, et al. Hormone replacement therapy and risk of hip fracture: population based case-control study. The Swedish Hip Fracture Study Group. BMJ 1998;316:1858-1863.

213. Wimalawansa SJ. A four-year randomized controlled trial of hormone replacement and bisphosphonate, alone or in combination, in women with postmenopausal osteoporosis. Am J Med 1998;104:219-226.

214. Alexandersen P, Riis BJ, Christiansen C. Monofluorophosphate combined with hormone replacement therapy induces a synergistic effect on bone mass by dissociating bone formation and resorption in postmenopausal women: a randomized study. J Clin Endocrinol Metab 1999;84:3013-3020.

215. Orr-Walker BJ, Evans MC, Clearwater JM, et al. Effects of hormone replacement therapy on bone mineral density in postmenopausal women with primary hyperparathyroidism: four-year follow-up and comparison with healthy postmenopausal women. Arch Intern Med 2000;160:2161-2166.

216. Recker RR, Davies KM, Dowd RM, Heaney RP. The effect of low-dose continuous estrogen and progesterone therapy with calcium and vitamin D on bone in elderly women. A randomized, controlled trial. Ann Intern Med 1999;130:897-904.

217. Ettinger B, Black DM, Mitlak BH, et al. Reduction of vertebral fracture risk in postmenopausal women with osteoporosis treated with raloxifene: results from a 3-year randomized clinical trial. Multiple Outcomes of Raloxifene Evaluation (MORE) Investigators. JAMA 1999;282:637-645.

218. Breuer B, Wallenstein S, Anderson R. Effect of tamoxifen on bone fractures in older nursing home residents. J Am Geriatr Soc 1998;46:968-972.

219. Grady D, Cummings SR. Postmenopausal hormone therapy for prevention of fractures: how good is the evidence? JAMA 2001;285:2909-2910.

220. Gillespie WJ, Avenell A, Henry DA, et al. Vitamin D and vitamin D analogues for preventing fractures associated with involutional and post-menopausal osteoporosis. Cochrane Database Syst Rev 2001:CD000227.
221. Chapuy MC, Arlot ME, Duboeuf F, et al. Vitamin D3 and calcium to prevent hip fractures in the elderly women. N Engl J Med 1992;327:1637-1642.
222. Garay Lillo J, Parreno J, Gonzalez Y, Gonzalez JA. [Geminis: a prospective, multicentric, randomised study to evaluate the effect of tricalcium phosphate versus tricalcium phosphate plus 25(OH) vitamin D on the risk of fractures in older women]. Geriatrika 1997;13:24-28.
223. Dawson-Hughes B, Harris SS, Krall EA, Dallal GE. Effect of calcium and vitamin D supplementation on bone density in men and women 65 years of age or older. N Engl J Med 1997;337:670-676.
224. Inkovaara J, Gothoni G, Halttula R, et al. Calcium, vitamin D and anabolic steroid in treatment of aged bones: double-blind placebo-controlled long-term clinical trial. Age Ageing 1983;12:124-130.
225. Chevalley T, Rizzoli R, Nydegger V, et al. Effects of calcium supplements on femoral bone mineral density and vertebral fracture rate in vitamin-D-replete elderly patients. Osteoporos Int 1994;4:245-252.
226. Recker RR, Hinders S, Davies KM, et al. Correcting calcium nutritional deficiency prevents spine fractures in elderly women. J Bone Miner Res 1996;11:1961-1966.
227. Tilyard MW, Spears GF, Thomson J, Dovey S. Treatment of postmenopausal osteoporosis with calcitriol or calcium. N Engl J Med 1992;326:357-362.
228. Lips P, Graafmans WC, Ooms ME, et al. Vitamin D supplementation and fracture incidence in elderly persons: a randomized, placebo-controlled clinical trial. Ann Intern Med 1996;124:400-406.
229. Cumming RG, Cummings SR, Nevitt MC, et al. Calcium intake and fracture risk: results from the study of osteoporotic fractures. Am J Epidemiol 1997;145:926-934.
230. Liberman UA, Weiss SR, Broll J, et al. Effect of oral alendronate on bone mineral density and the incidence of fractures in postmenopausal osteoporosis. The Alendronate Phase III Osteoporosis Treatment Study Group. N Engl J Med 1995;333:1437-1443.
231. Black DM, Cummings SR, Karpf DB, et al. Randomised trial of effect of alendronate on risk of fracture in women with existing vertebral fractures. Fracture Intervention Trial Research Group. Lancet 1996;348:1535-1541.
232. Ensrud KE, Black DM, Palermo L, et al. Treatment with alendronate prevents fractures in women at highest risk: results from the Fracture Intervention Trial. Arch Intern Med 1997;157:2617-2624.
233. Cummings SR, Black DM, Thompson DE, et al. Effect of alendronate on risk of fracture in women with low bone density but without vertebral fractures: results from the Fracture Intervention Trial. JAMA 1998;280:2077-2082.
234. Harris ST, Watts NB, Genant HK, et al. Effects of risedronate treatment on vertebral and nonvertebral fractures in women with postmenopausal osteoporosis: a randomized controlled trial. Vertebral Efficacy With Risedronate Therapy (VERT) Study Group. JAMA 1999;282:1344-1352.
235. Harris ST, Watts NB, Jackson RD, et al. Four-year study of intermittent cyclic etidronate treatment of postmenopausal osteoporosis: three years of blinded therapy followed by one year of open therapy. Am J Med 1993;95:557-567.
236. Storm T, Kollerup G, Thamsborg G, et al. Five years of clinical experience with intermittent cyclical etidronate for postmenopausal osteoporosis. J Rheumatol 1996;23:1560-1564.
237. Montessori ML, Scheele WH, Netelenbos JC, et al. The use of etidronate and calcium versus calcium alone in the treatment of postmenopausal osteopenia: results of three years of treatment. Osteoporos Int 1997;7:52-58.

238. Lyritis GP, Tsakalakos N, Paspati I, et al. The effect of a modified etidronate cyclical regimen on postmenopausal osteoporosis: a four-year study. Clin Rheumatol 1997;16:354-360.
239. Reginster J, Minne HW, Sorensen OH, et al. Randomized trial of the effects of risedronate on vertebral fractures in women with established postmenopausal osteoporosis. Vertebral Efficacy with Risedronate Therapy (VERT) Study Group. Osteoporos Int 2000;11:83-91.
240. McClung MR. Bisphosphonates in osteoporosis: recent clinical experience. Expert Opin Pharmacother 2000;1:225-238.

10

GERIATRIC UROLOGY

Tomas L. Griebling, MD *

It is well recognized that the population of the United States is changing, as the proportion of older adults grows dramatically. Because disorders of the genitourinary system are particularly common in older adults, the specialty of urology will be significantly affected by these trends. Research is critically needed to provide data that will allow a better understanding of the unique nature of urologic disease in the older adult. This information will affect diagnostic and treatment interventions for older adults, particularly the role of urologic surgical therapy.

This chapter summarizes the available literature on the six conditions most commonly encountered in geriatric urology: urinary incontinence, urinary tract infections (UTIs), prostate disease and genitourinary malignancies, sexual dysfunction, stone disease, and renal transplantation. The goal of this review is to provide a framework for developing future research in geriatric urology.

METHODS

A comprehensive literature search was performed to identify literature relevant to geriatric urology. The search was conducted on the National Library of Medicine's PubMed database. The period covered was from 1985 to March 19, 2001. Older literature was included if it provided important historical or other unique information. Newer literature cited for some topics was added during manuscript revision, and results from searches for kidney and bladder neoplasms were also added. Several guidelines and consensus reviews regarding the evaluation and management of urinary incontinence, prostatic disease, and other genitourinary disorders provided pertinent information on the diagnosis and treatment of urologic conditions in older adults that was also extracted for this review.

The search was limited to the English language, human subjects, and an age delineation of 65 years and older. The following six topics were initially searched: prostate disease, renal transplantation, sexual dysfunction, stone disease, urinary incontinence, and urinary tract infections.

For the prostate, the search strategy combined terms for prostate radiology and surgery with terms for prostate diseases and procedures, age factors, postoperative care, outcomes, length of stay, functional status, and complications. This search resulted in 1519 references.

For renal transplantation, the search strategy combined the term *kidney transplantation* with the terms for age factors and postoperative course, along with the terms *reject, tissue donor, cadaveric donor,* and *patient selection.* This search resulted in 1530 references.

For sexual dysfunction, the search strategy used the terms *hormone replacement therapy, testosterone, aged, sexual dysfunctions, sex disorders, libido, penile erection,* and *impotence.* This search resulted in 1318 references.

For stone disease, the search strategy combined the terms *lithotripsy, urinary calculi, kidney calculi,* and *nephrostomy* with the terms for age factors, postoperative care, out-

---

* Assistant Professor of Urology, Assistant Scientist—Center on Aging, University of Kansas, Kansas City, KS.

comes, length of stay, functional status, and complications. This search resulted in 633 references.

For urinary incontinence, the terms used were *urinary incontinence, aged,* and *age factors* combined with *postoperative care, prognosis, outcome, length of stay, predict, forecast, recovery, functional status,* and *postoperative complications.* This search retrieved 1042 items.

For urinary tract infections, the search strategy was simply for the terms *urinary tract infections* and *aged.* It elicited 1132 references.

Analysis of titles and abstracts by the content expert resulted in the selection of the items used in this review.

SPECIFIC GENITOURINARY DISORDERS IN OLDER ADULTS

Although there has been a plethora of research related to the disorders commonly associated with aging and the genitourinary system, very little of this work has focused on the natural history, pathophysiology, or clinical outcomes in older adults. Clinical studies have commonly not been randomized; most lack long-term follow-up and do not separate outcomes for older adults from those for their younger counterparts. In addition, comparison of studies is complicated by a general lack of standardized operational terminology and validated, reproducible outcomes measures.

URINARY INCONTINENCE

Background and Epidemiology

The epidemiology of incontinence in the geriatric population has been closely examined. Urinary incontinence is a very common disorder among older adults; it is estimated that between 15% and 35% of community-dwelling adults in the United States aged 60 or over suffer from urinary incontinence. [1] The overall prevalence increases with age in both men and women. A recent survey of 10,458 community-dwelling men in Sweden revealed a linear relationship between the prevalence of urinary incontinence and age. [2] The overall prevalence of urinary incontinence was found to be 6.1% at 65 years, 9.6% at 75 years, 21.8% for those between 85 and 89, and 28.2% for those aged 90 years and over. A similar study in a cohort of 7949 older women with a mean age of 76.9 ± 5.0 years revealed that 41% reported urinary incontinence, with 14% suffering from daily incontinent episodes. [3] This latter study found the prevalence of urinary incontinence to be strongly associated with age, using multivariate regression analysis (odds ratio [OR] 1.3 per 5 years, 95% CI [confidence interval] 1.2 to 1.5). The authors also found that some common conditions associated with aging are strongly correlated with increased incontinence; these include prior hysterectomy, obesity, history of stroke, chronic obstructive pulmonary disease, diminished gait speed, and poor overall health. This finding supports prior studies that have also demonstrated the relationships between urinary incontinence and other chronic disorders associated with increasing age. [4]

Urinary incontinence can have significant negative impact on self-esteem and has been associated with increased rates of depression. [5,6] Incontinence also affects social aspects of quality of life and activities of daily living. [7,8] It may result in increased dependence on caregivers. Survey data suggest that at least 50% of homebound older adults suffer from urinary incontinence. [9] Those who are incontinent demonstrate significant impairments in social interaction. [10]

Incontinence has been identified as one of the major risk factors that in the United States leads to nursing-home admission, and this relationship has been extensively studied. Using data from the Longitudinal Study on Aging, Coward et al learned that incontinent people in less urbanized or populous areas are more at risk for nursing-home admission than are those in more populous areas. [11] A relative lack of community support services may explain this finding. Other geriatric syndromes that are associated with urinary incontinence can significantly increase the risk of functional dependence. In particular, cognitive impairment and gait abnormalities have been linked to increased rates of both isolated urinary incontinence and combined urinary and fecal incontinence. [12,13] Tinetti et al demonstrated a strong association between urinary incontinence and an increased risk of falls. [14] Seidel et al looked at the relationship between cognition and continence status in an attempt to predict discharge placement after inpatient rehabilitation. [15] They found that analysis of continence and cognitive status at the time of admission to rehabilitation services allows prediction of continence status at discharge that could impact placement decisions.

Even those who are continent at the time of admission to a nursing home have been shown to be at significantly increased risk for the development of urinary incontinence. The estimated incidence of new-onset urinary incontinence in nursing-home residents is approximately 27% per year. [16] However, age itself has not been identified as a risk factor. In a review of 434 nursing-home residents, Palmer et al identified incontinent episodes or poor behavioral adjustment within 2 weeks of admission, male gender, dementia, or impaired mobility within 2 months as significant risk factors for chronic incontinence in nursing-home residents. [17]

Although urinary incontinence is certainly more prevalent among older adults, it should not be considered a normal or inevitable part of aging. A variety of diagnostic and therapeutic techniques have been developed to address this condition; many have shown great promise for improving or eliminating incontinence even in very elderly persons. In addition, there is an increased awareness of the role of preventive therapies. [18]

Types of Urinary Incontinence

Although urinary incontinence has been operationally defined in a variety of ways, the central feature is considered to be the involuntary loss of urine. This may be either acute or chronic. Urinary incontinence that is acute in onset is often transient and is typically caused by nonurologic factors such as fecal impaction, delirium, or polypharmacy. Correction of the underlying problem often leads to resolution of the urinary incontinence.

There are a variety of forms of chronic urinary incontinence, including stress incontinence, urge incontinence, overflow incontinence, and functional incontinence. Mixed patterns are very common. Determining the type of urinary incontinence an individual has is critically important because type influences the choice and success of a given therapy. Surgical therapies are commonly used to treat stress incontinence and selected patients with urge incontinence.

Stress incontinence is caused by a decrease in outlet resistance at the level of the bladder neck. Leakage occurs when the pressure in the bladder exceeds the outlet closure pressure. Patients describe episodes of incontinence with activities that increase intra-abdominal pressure, such as coughing, sneezing, or laughing. This may be caused by either urethral hypermobility or intrinsic sphincter deficiency. Research has suggested that apoptosis of the rhabdosphincter cells may be one of the primary causes of sphincteric dysfunction in older adults. [19,20]

Urge incontinence is typically caused by overactivity of the detrusor muscles in the bladder wall. Abnormal contractions during bladder filling lead to a sensation of urgency, and if strong enough, these contractions may cause urinary leakage. Urge incontinence is often associated with neurologic disorders, such as prior stroke.

Overflow incontinence is caused by an inability to completely empty the bladder with each voiding attempt. This is often caused by poor detrusor contractility and may be associated with chronic conditions such as diabetes mellitus and some neurologic disorders. Patients typically describe constant dribbling incontinence caused by leakage from the full bladder. Sensation is often diminished, and patients may not sense an elevated postvoid residual volume.

A unique form of incontinence in the elderly population is detrusor hyperactivity with impaired contractility. [21] This is essentially a combination of urge and overflow incontinence. In these cases, the bladder demonstrates abnormal contractions with filling but diminished contractile function during the voiding effort. It is particularly common in frail elderly persons.

Functional incontinence refers to loss of independent urinary control caused by other functional limitations, such as diminished mobility or cognition. Common causes of mobility limitations include arthritis and gait disturbances. Urinary incontinence seen in people with dementia is often functional in origin.

Nocturia is another very common complaint in older adults and is often associated with functional incontinence. Nocturia can have significant physical and psychosocial impacts, including a higher risk of falls and sleep deprivation. The pathophysiology of nocturia in older adults is still not completely understood.

Diagnostic Evaluation

The evaluation of the patient with urinary incontinence must begin with a detailed history and physical examination. This provides the most valuable information for diagnosis and therapeutic planning. However, a variety of other techniques have been developed, ranging from validated survey instruments to predictive algorithms and sophisticated urodynamic tests. Although these tools are widely employed in the evaluation of the incontinent patient, few studies have examined their utility specifically for the older adult. [22,23]

A large number of both self- and interviewer-administered survey instruments have been designed to assess types and degrees of urinary incontinence. However, there is no clear consensus about which instruments are best or should be used particularly in the geriatric population. One study demonstrated that brief questionnaires may be inaccurate and tend to correlate poorly with urodynamic findings in older adults. [24]

The role of formal urodynamic tests and video imaging studies in the evaluation of geriatric urinary incontinence remains controversial. The World Health Organization convened worldwide consensus conferences on urinary incontinence in 1998 and 2001. A committee focused on geriatric incontinence met at each of these conferences to review and discuss issues related to the evaluation and management of incontinence in older adults. The committee concluded that, although urodynamic studies are generally not required as part of a routine evaluation, they may be particularly important in evaluating geriatric patients being considered for anti-incontinence surgery.[25] These studies can help to differentiate stress, urge, and overflow incontinence, which can affect surgical decisions. Other authors concur with this recommendation for formal urodynamic evaluation prior to development of surgical plans.[26,27] Diokno et al examined the utility of urodynamics in a community-based sample of 167 women aged 60 years and older.[28] In this sample, 26.9% were 70 to 79 years old and 7.2% were 80 years or older. The researchers found that provocative stress tests, including cough and the Valsalva maneuver, significantly distinguish continent from incontinent persons and differentiate between stress and other forms of urinary incontinence. The overall sensitivity and specificity were 39.5% and 98.5%, respectively. Similarly, Wagg et al used urodynamics to identify age-related differences in bladder neck and urethral capacity in older women, including a loss of external sphincter function associated with stress incontinence.[29] Fluoroscopic video imaging is often used with multichannel urodynamics and may enhance interpretation of results. A study of a group of 69 elderly women (mean age of 72.5 years) revealed voiding cystourethrography to be useful for identifying factors associated with urge incontinence seen on urodynamics.[30]

Treatment

Biobehavioral Therapies. A variety of biobehavioral therapies have been developed to address urinary incontinence, including bladder retraining, pelvic floor muscle exercises, and prompted or assisted voiding routines. These conservative therapies are usually recommended as first-line treatment options, particularly for geriatric patients.[25,31] Although they have been shown to be effective in general, few have been studied in elderly persons.[32] In addition, interpretation and generalization is often difficult because many studies include a heterogeneous population with various forms of urinary incontinence.[31]

Wyman et al performed a randomized clinical trial comparing bladder training with scheduled toileting, pelvic floor muscle exercises, and a combination of the two techniques; their subjects were 204 women with a mean age of 61 ± 10 years who were suffering from stress or urge incontinence, or both.[33] After a 12-week intervention program, the group using the combined treatments was found to have significantly fewer incontinent episodes than did groups using either technique alone. However, at 3-month follow-up, there was no significant difference between groups, suggesting that enrollment in a structured intervention program may be more important than the exact protocol. In a single-arm trial, Publicover and Bear examined the utility of scheduled voiding with weekly clinician counseling.[34] In a group of 19 women aged 64 to 88 years (mean age 75.2), they found that behavioral intervention significantly reduces the number of urinary incontinent episodes during treatment and at 6-month follow-up. The causes and types of incontinence were not defined in this study.

Prompted voiding techniques have also been developed and used successfully with nursing-home residents.[35] Ouslander et al demonstrated an overall response rate of 41% in a cohort of 191 elderly incontinent nursing-home residents (mean age 84.5 years) who underwent a prompted toilet training program.[36] These researchers found that the overall wet percentage went from 26.7% to 6.4% and was sustained at 9.6% after 9 weeks.

Several studies have examined the differences between drug and behavioral therapies. In a randomized controlled trial comparing pelvic floor exercises with biofeedback to anticholinergic medications for treatment of urge incontinence, Burgio et al demonstrated superior results for the behavioral therapy. [37] In this study, 197 women were randomized to behavioral therapy, anticholinergic medication, or placebo. Subjects were 55 to 92 years old (mean age 67.7 ± 7.5 years). Behavioral therapy was found to result in an 80.7% reduction in urge incontinent symptoms; anticholinergics, in only a 68.5% reduction; and placebo, in 39.4% (all, $P < .05$). In a subsequent modified crossover trial, the same researchers found that, in a cohort of 35 women aged 55 to 91 years (mean 69.3 ± 7.9), the combination of oxybutynin and pelvic floor exercises supplemented with biofeedback is successful in reducing urge incontinent episodes by 84.3% to 88.5%. [38] In comparison, women on medication or behavioral therapy alone demonstrated improvements of 57.5% to 72.7%. Szonyi et al found similar results in a randomized, double-blind, controlled trial with 57 elderly subjects aged 72 to 98 years (mean 82.2 ± 6.06). [39] The overall efficacy of the combination of oxybutynin and behavioral therapy was found to be superior to that of placebo or of either medical or behavioral therapy alone.

Pharmacotherapy. Pharmacotherapy has been widely used to treat urinary incontinence, particularly for the treatment of urge incontinence. The most commonly used medications for urge incontinence are anticholinergics; examples are oxybutynin and tolterodine. Both have shown efficacy in older adults, but their use can be associated with significant side effects, including dry mouth, constipation, blurred vision, and confusion. Newer drugs currently in development are more uroselective and may have fewer systemic side effects in older adults.

Few pharmacologic agents are available for the treatment of stress incontinence. Phenylpropanolamine was used in the past to treat some patients with mild stress urinary incontinence. However, the U.S. Food and Drug Administration recently removed this drug from the market because of an associated increased risk of stroke. At this time, the only medication that shows some efficacy in the treatment of stress incontinence is topical vaginal estrogen. Published results are somewhat controversial, and there is a large amount of conflicting data. Data on geriatric cohorts is extremely limited, and many studies are confounded by heterogeneous subject demographics, outcomes measurements, and diagnostic criteria. However, a meta-analysis by Fantl et al did present supportive evidence that estrogen replacement subjectively improves urinary incontinence symptoms in postmenopausal women. [40]

Complementary Therapy. To date, there have been almost no studies examining the role of complementary therapies in the treatment of urinary incontinence in elderly persons. However, interest in such treatments is likely to increase. One uncontrolled pilot study examined the outcomes of acupuncture in a group of 15 elderly women with urge or mixed urinary incontinence that was refractory to other behavioral or medical therapies. [41] Mean age was 76.4 years (range 66 to 82). All subjects underwent 12 acupuncture treatments over a 6-week period. Twelve of the 15 women (80%) considered themselves significantly improved at 3-month follow-up.

Surgery. Surgical therapy has long been a mainstay of treatment, particularly for stress urinary incontinence. It is widely used in treating younger women, but there is some hesitation to choose surgery for older women. Most agree that the first line of treatment for stress incontinence in older women, particularly those who are frail, should be conservative therapy. [25] Although there is a plethora of data on the indications, efficacy, and potential complications of a wide variety of surgical procedures for the treatment of stress urinary incontinence, very little research has focused on the geriatric patient. Most published studies include a wide range of patients, and it is often difficult to extract results specific to older adults. Research in this field is also hampered by a lack of standardized diagnostic criteria, terminology, and outcomes measures. In addition, there is a dearth of well-designed randomized trials that directly compare the various forms of surgery such as bladder neck injection of bulking agents, retropubic or transvaginal bladder neck suspensions, or pubovaginal sling procedures. Many studies have short-term follow-up of 1 or 2 years, and they often lack information regarding specific reporting intervals. A number of leading professional organizations, including the American Urological Association, the International Continence Society, and the World Health Organization, have identified these limitations in the available research and have made recommendations to improve the quality of future studies. [25,42,43]

The risks of morbidity and mortality for geriatric patients undergoing anti-incontinence surgery are similar to those of other major surgical procedures. In a review of 66,478 Medicare patients, Sultana et al found the overall postoperative surgical mortality to be 0.3% at 30 days, 0.5% at 60 days, and 0.6% at 90 days. [44] The mean and median patient age in this cohort was 71 years. The risk of significant postoperative morbidity and mortality was found to increase linearly with age. In the group aged 75 to 84 years, the mortality rates were 0.5%, 0.7%, and 0.9% at 30, 60, and 90 days, respectively. In the cohort of those 85 years and older, the postoperative mortality rates were 1.6%, 2.0%, and 2.3%, respectively. Median length of hospital stay and readmission rates were also somewhat higher in this older cohort. However, in a multivariate analysis age was not identified as an independent risk factor for morbidity or mortality. The authors concluded that anti-incontinence surgery can be done safely in all age groups, and that the associated comorbidities in very elderly persons are likely more significant contributors to postoperative morbidity and mortality than is age itself.

Injection therapy represents an effective, minimally invasive surgical treatment for stress urinary incontinence caused by intrinsic sphincter deficiency. The procedure can be performed under local or general anesthesia. A bulking agent is injected into the submucosal space at the level of the bladder neck with the use of cystoscopic guidance. Although a variety of materials have been used for the injections, the most widely used material is glutaraldehyde cross-linked collagen. The material acts to increase outlet pressure at the bladder neck. Overall success is approximately 80% in women and 15% in men. Many patients need repeat injections over time to maintain continence. Most studies include a diverse range of patient ages, but the treatment appears to be effective in older women. One study examining the response to collagen injection in elderly women reported a 77% cure rate at 2 years of follow-up (mean age 76 years, range 62 to 90). [45] The procedure is minimally invasive and repeatable, which makes it attractive for use in older adults. Most studies have found that age does not correlate with outcomes for injection therapy. [46–48]

Open surgical procedures for female stress incontinence include bladder neck suspensions or pubovaginal slings. The suspension procedures may be performed via either a transvaginal or retropubic approach. Several studies have examined the utility of these procedures in elderly women. Nitti et al retrospectively examined the results of the Raz transvaginal suspension procedure in 92 women aged 65 to 87 years (mean 72 years).[49] At a mean of 17 months of follow-up, the overall success rates were 100% for those with mild incontinence, 93% for those with moderate incontinence, and 65% for those with severe incontinence. The researchers compared these results with those from a cohort of 141 patients younger than 65 years. Overall, they found similar continence and complication rates in the two groups. They concluded that this procedure can be done safely and effectively for patients regardless of age.

Pubovaginal sling procedures are being used in increasing numbers for the treatment of female stress urinary incontinence. In contrast to suspension procedures, which place sutures in the periurethral tissues and suspend the urethra to decrease its hypermobility or angulation, sling procedures place a supportive graft underneath the urethra. The procedure has been shown to be effective for stress incontinence caused by either urethral hypermobility or intrinsic sphincter deficiency. Carr et al looked at the results of pubovaginal sling in a retrospective cohort of 19 elderly women (median age 72 years, range 70 to 82).[50] The researchers compared their results with those in a group of 77 women with a median age of 60 years (range 26 to 69). The overall morbidity and success rates of the sling procedure were equivalent in the two groups. Stress incontinence had been resolved in 100% of the older women and 97% of the younger women at a mean follow-up of 22 months. No patients developed significant urinary retention, and the rate of postoperative urinary urgency was 10% in both groups. The researchers concluded that pubovaginal sling cystourethropexy is a safe and effective surgical option for both older and younger women.

Tension-free vaginal tape is a new procedure that uses a synthetic mesh for the suburethral sling. To date there have been limited studies on its use, and follow-up is quite short. However, the short-term data do demonstrate good continence outcomes even in elderly patients.[51] Longer term follow-up in a larger sample will be necessary, as synthetic materials are prone to increased rates of urethral erosion and infection.

Needed Research in Urinary Incontinence

Future studies need to include standardized operational definitions for urinary incontinence, a clear separation of the types of incontinence included in the study population, and requirements for patient inclusion and exclusion.

Although a number of survey instruments are currently used to evaluate patients with incontinence, few have been developed or validated for use in older adults. In the area of diagnostic evaluation, there is a need to better define the role of formal urodynamic testing, including videourodynamics in the assessment of older patients with urinary incontinence. This is particularly important for those considered as surgical candidates.

Urinary incontinence and pelvic organ prolapse often coexist in older women. Additional research on the diagnosis and management of prolapse in older women is needed, particularly to help define the role of surgical therapy in this population.

Several sets of clinical guidelines have been developed for the evaluation and management of urinary incontinence. Formal outcomes research is needed to identify the utility of these guidelines in both institutionalized and community-dwelling older adults.

Although there has been some research examining the association between urinary incontinence and other chronic health conditions in older adults, more work is needed to better understand these complex interactions. Examination of the relationship between urinary incontinence and other functional impairments, such as cognitive and physical limitations, will be particularly important. Urinary incontinence is commonly associated with chronic neurologic conditions, such as stroke, Parkinson's disease, multiple sclerosis, and Alzheimer's disease. The urologic implications of these disorders, particularly for rehabilitation outcomes, are still relatively poorly understood. In addition, there is a need for additional work on the urologic outcomes in geriatric patients with spinal cord injuries.

Research on behavioral techniques and pharmacotherapy for urinary incontinence must include older adult subjects. Ideally, these treatments should be analyzed for evidence of age-related effects. Studies should also include a variety of subjects, including community-dwelling older adults and people residing in assisted-living and long-term-care environments.

Studies regarding surgical therapy for urinary incontinence should examine outcomes, including potential complications in older adults. Although short-term studies are necessary to begin this work, long-term data will be required to fully evaluate the risks and benefits of anti-incontinence surgeries in older patients. Ideally, this would include 5- to 10-year follow-up with both subjective and objective outcomes measures. Standard surgical techniques, such as injection of bulking agents at the bladder neck, bladder neck suspension procedures, pubovaginal sling cystourethropexy, and artificial urinary sphincter placement, need to be examined in older patient populations in a prospective fashion, with an appropriate length of follow-up.

New anti-incontinence surgical techniques are being developed for both men and women. Many of these procedures are minimally invasive, and they have the potential to offer good clinical outcomes with less surgical risk. However, they need to be studied in comparison with currently accepted procedures. Prospective randomized trials that include older adults in a subgroup analysis would be the ideal. Innovative surgical techniques for urge incontinence such as sacral nerve stimulator implantation also need to be studied in a prospective fashion in this patient population.

Quality of life and cost must be considered in the evaluation and treatment of urinary incontinence in older adults. These types of studies help to define clinical needs from a social standpoint. Ultimately, this information helps to shape decisions about health care policy and reimbursement.

> *Urol 1 (Level B)*: **Studies are needed on the pathophysiology of nocturia, which occurs in a wide variety of conditions, including heart failure, renal failure, vascular insufficiency, sleep disorders, prostate enlargement, and polyuria of various causes.**

> *Urol 2 (Level B)*: **Studies are needed to establish the validity of new and existing survey instruments to assess the types and degrees of urinary incontinence in older adults.**

> *Urol 3 (Level B)*: **Systematic prospective cohort or case-control studies are needed to determine whether urodynamic and imaging techniques are associated with better outcomes in urinary incontinence in older patients.**

> *Urol 4 (Level A)*: **Depending on the results of studies of the impact of urodynamic and imaging techniques on outcomes (Urol 3), the ef-**

fect of particular urodynamic or imaging studies on the accuracy of diagnosis and outcomes of treatment should be assessed in randomized controlled trials.

Urol 5 (Level A): **Further randomized controlled trials are needed to test the efficacy and safety of both new and established anticholinergic drugs for the management of urinary incontinence in older adults.**

Urol 6 (Level A): **Randomized controlled trials with large numbers of subjects will be required to determine whether acupuncture or other complementary therapies have a significant beneficial effect in treating urge or mixed urinary incontinence in older patients.**

Urol 7 (Level A): **The bladder neck suspension and sling procedures have been proven effective in older women studied an average of 17 months after surgery. Prospective cohort studies with longer-term follow-up periods are needed to determine whether these procedures have sustained longevity.**

Urol 8 (Level B): **Prospective cohort studies are needed to explore the factors that identify which elderly patients will do better with early surgical intervention than with more conservative treatment options.**

Urol 9 (Level A): **Performing randomized controlled trials to extend the studies of factors that identify appropriate candidates for early surgery for incontinence could lead to the development and validation of predictive models useful for guiding treatment decisions for various types of urinary incontinence in older patients (see also Key Research Questions in Geriatric Urology, end of chapter).**

URINARY TRACT INFECTIONS

UTIs and asymptomatic bacteruria are common in older adults, particularly those in long-term-care settings. Although there is consensus that symptomatic infections should be treated with antibiotics, the implications of recurrent infections and asymptomatic bacteruria on long-term morbidity and mortality outcomes are more controversial. In a prospective cohort study of 1491 women, Abrutyn et al did not find UTI to be a risk factor for mortality. [52] In contrast, they did find age and poor self-reported health status to be significant predictors of mortality. However, a previous longitudinal cohort study of 1148 men and women reported by Nordenstam et al did demonstrate a significant increase in 5-year mortality for men with bacteruria. [53] The similar finding in women disappeared when those with indwelling catheters were excluded from the analysis. In contrast, Nicolle et al reported no significant survival difference between men with and without asymptomatic bacteruria. [54]

Bacteruria has been shown to be a transient phenomenon in older adults. Monane et al performed a prospective observational study on 61 women. [55] Subjects included both community-dwelling persons and long-term-care residents. The researchers found asymptomatic bacteruria to be present in 20% of all urine samples and in one third of all subjects over 6 months of follow-up. Variation was seen on a month-by-month basis, with frequent spontaneous alterations in positive and negative specimens.

These data support the consensus that asymptomatic bacteruria in the older adult does not usually warrant initiation of antibiotic therapy. In a randomized trial of antibiotic treatment for 50 institutionalized elderly women (mean age 83.4 ± 8.8 years) with asymptomatic bacteruria, Nicolle et al found no short-term benefits to be associated with therapy. However, they did identify increased long-term risks, including reinfection with resistant organisms.[56] Similarly, Ouslander et al found that treating asymptomatic bacteruria in institutionalized elderly women does not improve rates of chronic urinary incontinence.[57]

Bacteruria is also commonly associated with chronic indwelling catheter use and typically does not require treatment. However, UTIs associated with short-term catheterization of less than 2 weeks in older adults should be addressed. In a prospective randomized controlled trial, Harding et al examined the role of antibiotic therapy in a group of 119 women with catheter-acquired UTIs[58] and found that infections resolve spontaneously more often in younger women than in those aged 65 years or older (89% versus 62%; $P < .001$). They also found that single-dose antibiotic therapy is generally effective, although more so in the younger women.

Raz et al examined the risk factors associated with recurrent UTI in a case-control study of 149 postmenopausal women referred for evaluation and treatment of UTIs.[59] Compared with the 53 age-matched control subjects, the case subjects tended to have at least one of three common urologic conditions believed to predispose them to infection: urinary incontinence (41% versus 9%, $P < .001$), cystocele (19% versus 0%, $P < .001$), and elevated postvoid residual urine volume (28% versus 2%, $P < .001$). Age was not identified as a significant risk factor in this study.

Two studies have shown the prevalence of UTI in hip fracture patients to be approximately 23% to 25%.[60,61] Catheterization was not found to be a significant risk factor. However, female gender, prior history of UTIs, poor general medical health, and delay in operative treatment of the fracture were found to be predictors of UTI. The identification and treatment of UTIs in this patient population are also important to help prevent potential infection of implanted orthopedic prostheses.

Vaginal estrogen replacement has long been a mainstay of therapy for the prevention of recurrent UTIs in postmenopausal women.[62] Many patients find cream-based preparations messy and uncomfortable. A recent randomized open, parallel study by Eriksen revealed good response to an estrogen-impregnated vaginal device (Estring).[63] Its use has not been studied in a geriatric population; however, improved satisfaction could lead to increased adherence by older patients.

Cranberry juice and other cranberry preparations have long been used as prophylactic treatments for recurrent UTIs. It is hypothesized that cranberries contain compounds that prevent bacterial adhesion to the urothelium. Studies support the prophylactic use of cranberry products, particularly in institutionalized older adults.[64] Avorn et al performed a randomized, double-blind, placebo-controlled trial with 153 older women (mean age 78.5 years).[65] Consumption of 300 mL of cranberry juice each day was found to reduce the odds of clinically significant bacteriuria ($\geq 10^5$ organisms) with associated pyuria to 42% of that seen in the control subjects ($P = .004$). In another study, Kontiokari et al compared consumption of cranberry-lingonberry juice, *Lactobacillus GG*, and placebo in a group of 150 women previously diagnosed with acute *Escherichia coli* UTIs.[66] They found a 20% reduction in the absolute risk of recurrent UTI (defined as a urine culture with $\geq 10^5$

colony-forming units of bacteria) for the women who drank the juice in comparison with the control group (P = .023, 95% CI = 3% to 36%). The recurrence rate for those who consumed *Lactobacillus* did not differ from that of the control group in this series.

Most research on UTIs in older adults has examined patient risk factors and the bacteriology associated with infection. Studies are often confusing because they lack detailed information on what constitutes an infection. The definition of asymptomatic bacteriuria is especially a problem. Future research studies must clearly state the inclusion and exclusion criteria used for subject selection.

Clinical drug studies of new antibiotic agents need to consider the unique needs of older adults. They must include issues of safety, efficacy, and tolerability in this patient population. Special attention must be paid to drug-drug interactions and the issue of polypharmacy. Studies on the epidemiology of infection are needed, particularly with regard to development of resistant pathogens. Research on prophylaxis should include specific analysis of indications and outcomes in older adults.

> *Urol 10 (Level B)*: **Additional research is needed to clarify the operational definitions of urinary tract infection and of asymptomatic bacteruria.**

> *Urol 11 (Level B)*: **The natural history and potential risks of urinary tract infection or asymptomatic bacteruria and forms of preventive therapy warrant further study (see Key Research Questions in Geriatric Urology, end of chapter).**

> *Urol 12 (Level A)*: **Research on new antibiotic agents for the treatment of urinary tract infection should include randomized controlled trials specifically designed to assess the safety and efficacy of these drugs in geriatric patient populations.**

PROSTATE DISEASES

Prostate disorders are common in men of all ages, although the incidence and prevalence increase with age. The most common disorders include prostatitis and chronic pelvic pain, benign prostatic hyperplasia (BPH), and prostate cancer. This review focuses on BPH and prostate cancer. Although a variety of treatment options now exist for both of these disorders, emphasis herein is placed on surgical therapy in the older adult.

Benign Prostatic Hyperplasia

BPH is caused by a proliferation of the stromal components of the prostate, typically beginning after age 40 and leading to functional obstructive changes. The development of lower urinary tract voiding symptoms in men appears to be related to this hyperplastic aging process. In a cross-sectional analysis of 1557 men (mean age 51.3 years, range 40 to 96), Haidinger et al found that increasing age is an independent risk factor for onset of symptoms. [67] Other studies have supported this finding but suggest that age does not influence the outcome of subsequent surgery for BPH. [68] Interestingly, symptoms such as urinary urgency and frequency have also been found to be correlated with increasing age in women, but outlet obstruction is uncommon. In a prospective cohort analysis of 2280 men followed for almost 25 years, the development of obstructive voiding symptoms such as urgency, frequency, hesitancy, decreased force and caliber of urinary stream, and nocturia was found to be highly predictive of the need for prostate surgery, and the risk varies significantly by age. [69] These authors found that men aged 62 to 68 years are more likely than their younger counterparts to require surgery.

Over the past 15 years there has been a general shift from surgical to medical therapy as the preferred initial treatment for most patients with BPH. The development of safe, clinically effective pharmacologic agents, including α_1-adrenoceptor antagonists such as doxazosin, terazosin, and tamsulosin, and 5-α-reductase inhibitors such as finasteride, has led to a decline in rates of surgery for BPH. [70–72] Breslin et al reviewed a series of 1822 BPH patients in a single private practice between July 1, 1987 and June 30, 1991 and determined that the rate of surgery dropped from 28% in the first year of the study to 8% in the last year. [73] This matches the timing of the increased acceptance and use of pharmacotherapy for the treatment of BPH. In a review of the Medicare database, Holtgrewe identified a 30% decline in surgery for BPH despite an increase in the number of older men enrolled in the program. [74]

Phytotherapy has recently gained popularity as a medical treatment option for BPH. Several compounds have been used, including *Pygeum africanum*, *Hypoxis rooperi*, and *Serenoa repens*. There have been few randomized controlled trials of these types of agents, and research is complicated by the lack of standardization in the preparation of most of these compounds. A recent meta-analysis by Wilt et al examined data from 18 trials involving 2939 men. [75] They found an improvement in obstructive urinary symptoms with many different phytotherapy preparations. However, most studies have limited follow-up of less than 1 year, and none targeted geriatric patients. [76]

Despite the increase in the use of pharmacotherapy for the treatment of BPH, some patients ultimately require surgical intervention. Several studies support the fact that surgical therapy for BPH, such as transurethral resection of the prostate (TURP), is generally well tolerated even by elderly patients. A study by Concato et al revealed that, after adjusting for age and severity of comorbidity, there is no difference in 5-year mortality between older men undergoing TURP and those undergoing open surgery. [77] Ibrahim et al also showed that there is no increase in morbidity or mortality with advancing patient age for men undergoing surgery for BPH. [78] Improvements in surgical technique have decreased operative times and the associated risks, such as hyponatremia due to absorption of large volumes of irrigation fluid used in surgery. [79] In a retrospective analysis of 229 men between the ages of 80 and 97, Ilkjaer et al found that overall outcomes from TURP are excellent. [80] In this study, the perioperative mortality rate was 2%, and complications such as UTI or bleeding occurred in 21%. These data match historical control data on younger subjects. [79] In long-term follow-up (range 6 to 16 years), the overall satisfaction rate was excellent, at 86%. In a separate retrospective population-based study of 621 men undergoing TURP for treatment of BPH, Pientka et al found that age is not a risk factor for perioperative morbidity or mortality. [81] This was found to be true for both those with and without significant underlying comorbidities.

Alterations in sexual function have been reported after TURP for treatment of BPH. However, age may also influence these clinical outcomes. In an analysis of postprostatectomy sexual adjustment in 72 men aged 50 to 79 years (mean age 65 years), Libman et al found age to be a significant risk factor for postoperative erectile dysfunction. [82]

A wide variety of minimally invasive surgical therapies for the treatment of BPH have been developed over the past 20 years. Examples include microwave thermotherapy, laser tissue ablation, high-intensity focused ultrasound, tissue electrovaporization, placement of intraprostatic stents, and transurethral needle ablation. These types of therapy offer several potential advantages for older adults, including decreased blood loss, fluid absorption, and anesthetic requirements. However, most studies on these types of therapies lack long-term follow-up, and none have focused on geriatric patients. In outcome analyses, none of these treatments matched the level of results obtained with TURP, currently considered the gold standard surgical option. [83–85]

Prostate Cancer

Age has clearly been identified as a risk factor for the development of prostate cancer. Early detection is possible in most cases by the use of a combination of serum prostate-specific antigen (PSA) testing and digital rectal examination. The American Cancer Society currently recommends annual screening examination using the combination of PSA and digital rectal examination for men aged 50 and over who have a life expectancy of at least 10 years. [86] Men in high-risk groups, including black Americans and those with a first-degree relative with prostate cancer, should begin screening at 40 to 45 years of age.

Using data from the Baltimore Longitudinal Study of Aging, Carter et al have reported that biennial testing in older men may provide similar results in terms of cancer detection at a significant cost savings. [87] The age at which annual prostate cancer screening may be suspended is much more controversial. Most urologists agree that patients need an estimated 10-year life expectancy to justify definitive therapy for localized prostate cancer, such as radical prostatectomy or radiation therapy. The median current life expectancy for men in the United States who have reached age 65 is estimated to be approximately 82 years. Therefore, one could argue to continue screening with annual PSA and rectal examination into the mid-70s for many men. However, this has not been adequately examined. It is currently recommended that the risks and benefits of screening and the possible need for treatment be discussed with elderly men prior to making decisions about screening. [88,89]

PSA levels appear to correlate directly with increasing age, and some authors have argued for the use of age-adjusted normal ranges for interpretation of results. [90] However, other authors disagree. In a study of 773 men, Catalona et al found that age-specific PSA cutoffs enhance specificity but lack appropriate sensitivity. [91] They found that 20% to 60% of cancer in men aged 60 and over would have been missed with the use of age-specific PSA norms.

Age may also influence the choice of treatments for prostate cancer. Many urologic surgeons are reluctant to perform radical prostatectomy on patients aged 70 years and over. However, recent literature suggests that projected life expectancy may be a more useful diagnostic criterion for surgical selection than patient age alone. [92] However, the best methods to establish projected life expectancy have not been definitively established. It has been shown that surgical therapy is generally well tolerated by elderly men if they are carefully selected and screened for comorbid disease. [93,94] However, this must be balanced with data that identify increased age at the time of diagnosis as a strong predictor of a decreased probability of surgically curable prostate cancer. [95]

Age also appears to affect patient choices about treatment options. In a study using a convenience sample of 163 men seen at an urban Veterans Affairs Medical Center, Mazur and Merz found that patients were willing to trade off complications from surgery for increased potential cancer survival. [96] Mean patient age was 65.2 years (range 35 to 84). Overall, 62% of the patients were willing to accept a 100% chance of postoperative urinary incontinence and 83% were willing to accept a 100% chance of erectile dysfunction for better 5-year survival. Age influences the results; older subjects are less willing to accept complications for increased survival. In a similar trial, these authors also reported that older patients are more willing to accept expectant management than radical surgery. [97] These results were found to be influenced by age within the context of pre-existing urologic conditions. Subjects with current urinary dribbling or incontinence or sexual dysfunction were found to be much more likely to prefer expectant management over surgery.

Outcomes and complications may differ with patient age. Kerr and Zincke reported a significantly higher rate of postoperative urinary incontinence in elderly men after radical prostatectomy. [98] They compared outcomes from 191 men aged 55 years or younger at the time of surgery with 51 men who were aged 75 years or older. In this retrospective cohort analysis, 16% of the elderly patients but only 3% of the younger patients reported significant urinary incontinence ($P = .001$). A large population-based study of Medicare claims data for 101,604 men revealed that there is an increase in 30-day mortality after radical prostatectomy that is associated with age ($< 0.5\%$ for men aged 65 to 69 years, and approximately 1% for men aged 75 years and older). [99]

Disease-free survival may also be influenced by patient age at the time of surgery. In a retrospective study of 489 consecutive men treated with radical prostatectomy, Öbek et al reported that age may be an independent prognostic factor for the risk of biochemical recurrence. [100] At a mean follow-up of 25.4 months, 12% of those 70 years or younger but 25% of older men were found to demonstrate rising PSA levels ($P = .01$). The researchers also found that younger age is associated with a longer time to recurrence ($P < .02$).

The effects of surgical intervention for localized prostate cancer on general and disease-specific quality of life can be substantial. In a cross-sectional analysis of 528 managed-care enrollees, Litwin et al found significant impairment in health-related quality of life for men who underwent radical prostatectomy. [101] This was found to occur even after adjusting for age and pre-existing urinary and sexual dysfunction. Stanford et al reported similar results in a population-based longitudinal cohort of 1291 men who underwent radical prostatectomy with 24-month follow-up. [102] Patients aged 65 to 74 years constituted 40.9% of subjects, and 2.8% were between ages 75 and 79. Urinary and sexual dysfunction side effects were found to be more common in the older men and to lead to a decrease in quality of life.

Changes in quality of life have also been reported in men with metastatic prostate cancer. Hormonal manipulation with either surgical or medical androgen ablation is commonly used in the treatment of these men. Litwin et al reported that there is no significant difference in health-related quality of life in elderly men (mean age 71.2 to 75.4 years) treated with orchiectomy and those receiving pharmacologic agents for androgen ablation. [103] Survival data have historically been equivalent between these treatment options.

The biology of prostate cancer has recently attracted a great deal of research attention. The role of androgens in the growth and spread of prostate cancer has been extensively examined. Prostate cancer is unique in that it is typically a very slow-growing tumor. Adequate follow-up of at least 5 to 10 years or more will be required to provide adequate interpretation of results for most prostate cancer studies.

Needed Research in Prostate Disease

Although there has been a large amount of research on prostate diseases, including both BPH and prostate cancer, relatively few studies have targeted geriatric patients. The greatest advances have come in the understanding of the pathophysiology of prostate disorders and the relationship to the normal aging process. Currently, there is a strong focus on the molecular biology of prostate disease and possible preventive therapies. Studies of new technology, such as gene therapy for BPH and prostate cancer, should include prospective research with older men.

Pharmacotherapy for BPH has certainly changed the initial approach to this disorder for most patients. As new, more uroselective products are developed for the treatment of BPH, they must be tested for safety and efficacy in older men. Phytotherapy is becoming quite popular, and additional research is needed to better understand the pharmacologic mechanisms of these products. Randomized placebo-controlled trials will be needed to establish outcomes data, particularly for older adults.

Research has established the safety and efficacy of TURP surgical therapy for BPH, even in quite elderly men. Research on new, less invasive surgical techniques needs to examine clinical outcomes, including complications, in older men. Results must be compared with the current gold standard, TURP, and studies should ideally be randomized. Future research on both surgical and nonsurgical therapies for BPH must also include an analysis of cost and the impact on health-related quality of life.

The optimal treatments for localized and metastatic prostate cancer in elderly men remain controversial. The biological nature of prostate cancer is unique in that it is generally a slow-growing tumor. Therefore, it will be critical that future clinical research studies include adequate long-term follow-up of at least 5 to 10 years.

A large amount of research has focused on the role of screening for prostate cancer by the use of PSA testing and rectal examination. It is now widely accepted that patients should have a projected life expectancy of at least 10 years to be considered for definitive treatment of localized prostate cancer with either radical prostatectomy or radiation therapy. Most research on life expectancy is population based. However, in order to use this 10-year clinical criterion, we need to develop better models for prediction of life expectancy for individuals. There is also no clear consensus regarding when routine screening in older men may be discontinued. Studies to identify the risks and benefits of continued screening, including potential costs and complications from screening and treatment, will be needed to answer this question. Decision-analysis models that include patients' desires regarding evaluation and treatment may be helpful in this regard.

The role of hormone therapy in the management of metastatic prostate cancer has been extensively examined. However, there are still conflicting data on its utility, especially in elderly men. Future studies on this topic will need to include information about health-related quality of life, which may be significantly altered with hormonal therapy. The use of hormone replacement in older men is still poorly understood. Testosterone replacement therapy may have significant impacts with regard to emotional health, libido and sexual function, and prevention of osteoporosis and other orthopedic disorders.

Urol 13 (Level A): **Randomized controlled trials in elderly men are needed to compare phytotherapies with placebo or with established medical therapies for benign prostatic hyperplasia.**

Urol 14 (Level A): **Randomized trials in elderly men are needed to compare minimally invasive surgical therapies for benign prostatic hyperplasia with the gold standard procedure, transurethral resection of the prostate.**

Urol 15 (Level A): **Randomized controlled trials are needed to compare outcomes of early transurethral resection of the prostate with outcomes of initial medical therapy followed by subsequent transurethral resection of the prostate when clinically necessary.**

Urol 16 (Level B): **Prospective cohort studies and decision-analysis models are needed to identify the characteristics that predispose an older patient with benign prostatic hyperplasia to benefit from early transurethral resection of the prostate (see Key Research Questions in Geriatric Urology, end of chapter).**

Urol 17 (Level B): **Because screening for prostate cancer is so widespread, it may be very difficult to design a randomized controlled trial comparing prostate-specific antigen screening with rectal examination alone, using risks, benefits, and costs as outcome measures. Therefore, the decision as to when to stop routine screening for prostate cancer in elderly men may depend on prospective cohort studies.**

Urol 18 (Level A): **Because there is so much uncertainty regarding the best treatment plan for localized or locally metastatic prostate cancer, it is justified and indeed necessary to design randomized clinical trials in large populations of elderly men, with subgroup analyses, to examine the effects of clinical characteristics on treatment decisions.**

OTHER GENITOURINARY MALIGNANCIES

Bladder cancer and renal malignancies, including both renal cell carcinomas and transitional cell carcinomas of the upper urinary tract, are more common in older than in younger adults. However, the natural history, pathophysiology, and long-term treatment outcomes of these disorders have not been extensively studied in older adults.

Transitional cell carcinoma is the most common malignant tumor of the urinary bladder in the United States. Superficial tumors are usually treated by endoscopic resection. However, the overall recurrence rate is up to 70%, and long-term surveillance is recommended to identify recurrent disease. Adjuvant intravesical chemotherapy or immunotherapy with Bacillus-Calmette-Guerin is commonly used to treat recurrences. In contrast, the standard treatment for muscle-invasive bladder cancer is radical cystectomy and urinary diversion. This major surgery may be associated with significant risk of perioperative morbidity and mortality. Research has shown that radical cystectomy with urinary diversion can be safely performed in elderly patients; however, the long-term outcomes have not been assessed. [104–107] In particular, the effects of such major surgery on activities of daily living, instrumental activities of daily living, and overall rehabilitation status in older adults have not been clearly identified. The efficacy of less invasive forms of surgical therapy, including partial cystectomy or aggressive endoscopic resection with adjuvant radiation or chemotherapy, has not been studied in older adults.

Renal and adrenal malignancies, particularly small, incidentally detected tumors, are also more common in older adults. However, the natural history of these types of tumors, particularly in elderly patients, needs additional study.[108] Renal and adrenal tumors are often chemo- and radioresistant. Traditional surgical therapies for these types of tumors include radical nephrectomy, nephroureterectomy, or adrenalectomy. Newer, less invasive techniques such as laparoscopic surgery, cryotherapy, and nephron-sparing surgery have been used in older adults and may offer the promise of reduced morbidity.[109]

Additional research regarding the natural history and pathophysiology of both bladder and renal cancer is needed. In particular, the most appropriate diagnostic and treatment modalities for management of the small, incidental renal or adrenal mass need to be better defined. Outcome analyses for new, minimally invasive treatment options will be particularly valuable.

> **Urol 19 (Level A)**: **Randomized clinical trials are needed to determine the overall safety and long-term efficacy of less invasive therapy for bladder and renal malignancies in older adults, comparing these with the standard procedures (radical cystectomy and radical nephrectomy).**

> **Urol 20 (Level A)**: **Predictive outcomes models to identify who would most benefit from the various forms of therapy for bladder and renal malignancies need to be developed and validated (see Key Research Questions in Geriatric Urology, end of chapter).**

SEXUAL DYSFUNCTION

Sexual dysfunction occurs in both men and women, and the overall prevalence of these disorders increases with age. However, like other genitourinary complaints, sexual dysfunction should not be accepted as a normal part of aging. Recent research has examined this issue in an attempt to sort out differences resulting from the physiology of aging and from other causes.

Male Sexual Dysfunction

The prevalence of sexual complaints increases with age. Panser et al conducted a population-based cross-sectional study of 2115 men and found that, in comparison with men aged 40 to 49 years, older men (70 to 79 years) are more worried about their overall sexual function (24.9% versus 46.6%) and report that they experienced worse actual performance over the past year.[110] The older men also have rated higher levels of dissatisfaction, decreased libido, and impaired erectile function. However, in a multivariate analysis, age itself was not found to be an independent predictor of the results. On the basis of survey results from a convenience sample of 1680 men in different geographic locations, Jønler et al confirmed that the prevalence of erectile dysfunction increases with age.[111] In an analysis of data from the Massachusetts Male Aging Study, Johannes et al reported the crude incidence rate for erectile dysfunction to be 25.9 cases per 1000 man-years (95%

CI = 22.5 to 29.9). [112] The incidence increases significantly with increasing age, with 12.4, 29.8, and 46.4 cases per 1000 man-years for men in their 40s, 50s, and 60s, respectively. They also found that other risk factors for erectile dysfunction include lower education as well as comorbid disease, such as diabetes mellitus, heart disease, and hypertension.

Diabetes and use of hydrogen-blocker medications for the treatment of gastric acidity and reflux were found to be significant risk factors for erectile dysfunction (relative risk [RR] for both, 2.3) in a cross-sectional survey study of older men by Helgason et al. [113] They also identified prostate cancer as a significant risk factor (RR 1.9). However, they did not conclude that age itself is a risk factor. Despite these increases in the prevalence of sexual dysfunction, older men remain interested in sexual function and activity. [114] A similar trend has been documented in a small convenience survey of older men residing in long-term-care facilities. [115] Sexual dysfunction in older adults has been associated with a decreased quality of life and mental health impairment, including depression. [116–118]

Several multidimensional assessment instruments have been developed to identify the levels of sexual dysfunction and their impact on disease-specific quality of life. [119–121] These survey instruments have been well designed and appear to have appropriate reliability and validity when used with elderly persons.

Female Sexual Dysfunction

An instrument to evaluate female sexual dysfunction has been developed and validated. [122] Very little is known about the psychosocial and physiologic aspects of female sexual dysfunction. Interest is growing both in the scientific community and the lay public. Several studies have documented that sexual dysfunction in women increases with age, but the causes of these changes are still poorly understood. [123,124] A survey of 964 women in a primary care practice revealed that 98.8% expressed at least one sexual concern. [125] Mean patient age in this study was 45.4 ± 16.8 years, with a range of 18 to 87 years. (See also Chapter 9, section on sexuality.)

Influence of Comorbid Disease

Several studies have presented early data to suggest that most sexual dysfunction in older adults is related to the effects of other chronic comorbid diseases rather than normal aging alone. [126] The most common associated disorders include hypertension, diabetes mellitus, atherosclerosis, and other diseases of the cardiovascular system. [127–131] Associated changes in penile vasculature lead to impairment of penile blood flow and subsequent erectile dysfunction. Sexual dysfunction related to impaired penile blood flow is also a side effect of many antihypertensive medications, particularly those containing β-blockers.

Chronic pain is associated with an increased rate of sexual dysfunction and may be associated with the concomitant increase in depressive symptoms in chronic pain patients. [132] Similarly, patients with end-stage renal disease on peritoneal dialysis display increased rates of sexual dysfunction, depression, and impaired quality of life. [133] Gastrointestinal and urinary diversion surgeries are common in older adults for treatment of bladder and bowel cancers. Ostomy patients typically report poorer quality of life and limitations in sexual function than do patients without a stoma. [134–136] These changes are often caused by impaired body image and lack of knowledge about techniques to improve sexual function despite these handicaps.

Studies of the relationship between sleep apnea and sexual dysfunction have provided conflicting data. Karacan and Karatas examined 22 men with sleep apnea (mean age 54, range 27 to 73) and found that erectile function improved in one third of the men with use of continuous positive airway pressure. [137] However, Schiavi et al did not find sleep apnea to be a significant risk for erectile dysfunction in a similar cohort of 70 men aged 45 to 75 years. [138]

Neurologic disorders are very common in older adults, and in retrospective cohort studies several have been associated with impaired sexual function. Stroke appears to be a cause of significant sexual dysfunction in both men and women. [139] Right hemispheric stroke appears to cause greater impairments than left hemispheric stroke. [140] It must also be remembered that any sexual dysfunction will affect both the individual patient and his or her partner(s). [141] Parkinson's disease is also associated with sexual dysfunction. In a cohort study of 50 subjects (mean age 67.3 years) with evidence of autonomic nervous system dysfunction, Koller et al found a 70% rate of sexual impairment. [142]

Dementing illnesses such as Alzheimer's disease can significantly impair the sexual function of both patients and partners. [143] Inappropriate sexual behaviors are common in this patient population, occurring in approximately 15% of affected individuals. [144] Clinical management of these associated behavior disorders can be difficult and may lead to requirements for placement in long-term care. Anecdotal information suggests that antiandrogens, estrogen, gonadotropin-releasing hormone analogues, selective serotonin-reuptake inhibitors, and cimetidine may be helpful. [145,146] Additional randomized placebo-controlled trials will be necessary to identify the utility of these types of pharmacotherapies in older adults with inappropriate sexual behaviors associated with cognitive impairment.

Treatment of Sexual Dysfunction

Over the past decade, the variety of options for the treatment of sexual dysfunction, particularly erectile dysfunction, has increased dramatically. Clinical evaluation has been simplified, and invasive testing is usually deferred in favor of empiric, goal-directed therapy. The introduction of sildenafil citrate (Viagra) has revolutionized the clinical management of erectile dysfunction. Although studies have shown general clinical efficacy, research stratified by age is still lacking. [147,148] Trials for the use of sildenafil citrate in women are in progress. Early data suggest that it may improve sexual function in younger women (< 65 years). [149] The widespread acceptance of oral therapy for sexual dysfunction has led to a decreased use of other forms of treatment, including intracavernosal injection therapy, vacuum erection devices, and penile prosthesis.

Needed Research in Sexual Dysfunction

Research on sexual function and dysfunction in older adults has focused primarily on basic physiology and pathophysiology. The general associations between chronic disorders such as diabetes mellitus and vascular disease have been identified, but more work will be needed to examine these complex relationships. The development of new diagnostic and therapeutic options must include prospective analysis of utility in older adults. Potential side effects of therapy must be carefully examined. For example, currently used oral medications have potential interactions with other drugs that may lead to cardiovascular complications. Critical outcomes analysis in older persons will be needed to determine safety and efficacy of new products.

The physiology of sexual function and dysfunction in older women is very poorly understood. Research is critically needed to better understand this basic biology in order to develop effective treatment modalities. Cost and quality-of-life research is also needed regarding sexuality in both older men and women.

> *Urol 21 (Level B)*: **Most of the studies that examine the relationship between sexual dysfunction and comorbid conditions are small retrospective reviews or case series, and they typically do not focus on elderly subjects. Larger, well-designed prospective cohort studies will be necessary to confirm these associations in older adult populations (see Key Research Questions in Geriatric Urology, end of chapter).**

> *Urol 22 (Level B)*: **Time series (before-and-after) studies may be sufficient to assess the effect of sildenafil on sexual function of women aged 65 to 74, 75 to 84, and 86 years and older.**

> *Urol 23 (Level B)*: **Time series (before-and-after) studies may be sufficient to assess the effect of sildenafil on sexual function of men aged 65 to 74, 75 to 84, and 86 years and older.**

> *Urol 24 (Level B)*: **Prospective clinical series are needed to examine the use of intracavernosal injections, vacuum erection devices, and penile prostheses by men who are nonresponsive to sildenafil or are ineligible to use it.**

STONE DISEASE

Urinary tract stone disease is one of the most common disorders treated by the urologist. It is estimated that approximately one in every five individuals will experience an episode of urolithiasis at some point in life. The risk factors and symptoms associated with the development and passage of urinary stones are the same in older and younger persons. Swallowing difficulties and fear of increased incontinence are common in older adults and may cause decreased fluid intake, which can increase the propensity for stone production.

Very few studies have examined the surgical management of stone disease in geriatric patients. Extracorporeal shock-wave lithotripsy (ESWL) has become a popular form of effective, minimally invasive therapy, especially for stones in the renal collecting system and upper ureter. Kramolowsky et al reviewed the utility of ESWL as a function of age. [150] They examined a cohort of 789 consecutive patients undergoing ESWL for treatment of stones in the upper urinary tract. Of these patients, 96 (12%) were aged 70 or over, with a mean age of 75 (range 70 to 93). A total of 905 treatment procedures were performed, of which 107 procedures were in the older group. No significant differences were identified between the groups with regard to treatment-related complications, length of postoperative hospitalization, or clinical efficacy. The need to perform secondary procedures to render patients stone-free was similar in the groups (12.5% older, 13% younger).

Newer forms of minimally invasive surgical therapy for stone disease have revolutionized the care of patients with urolithiasis. Surgical procedures include retrograde ureteroscopic stone extraction and percutaneous nephrostolithotomy. Many of these procedures also use lithotripsy technology such as ultrasound, electrohydraulic shock-wave therapy, and holmium laser energy.

Although it is estimated that stone disease occurs in older adults with the same incidence as younger people, there has been almost no research on the evaluation and management of this disorder in adults aged 65 and over. Studies are needed to define the role of formal metabolic evaluation and medical management in these patients. Established and evolving surgical technologies need to be examined in older adults with regard to utility, safety, and clinical efficacy. Many of these newer techniques are minimally invasive and may offer potential benefits for older adults that are significantly better than those of more invasive procedures. Cost and health-related quality of life must also be considered in studies on diagnosis and treatment of urolithiasis.

> *Urol 25 (Level B)*: **Cohort studies are needed to evaluate the safety and clinical efficacy of minimally invasive surgical techniques in older adults with stone disease.**

RENAL TRANSPLANTATION

End-stage renal disease (ESRD) is a common clinical problem with a variety of causes, and the prevalence increases with increasing age. Although chronic peritoneal or hemodialysis is effective therapy for ESRD, renal transplant is often the preferred form of therapy because of better survival and overall and disease-specific quality of life. [151] The incidence rates for ESRD have more than doubled for most age groups over the past decade. [152] In fact, the incidence for those aged 75 and over has increased by a factor of 2.4 times. In 1996 in the United States, 73,000 new ESRD cases were identified, and 46% of these patients were aged 65 years or over. [153] ESRD has important implications for overall quality of life. Beusterien et al reported significant impairment in essentially all quality-of-life domains, with ESRD patients scoring lower than those with congestive heart failure or clinical depression. [154] In an analysis of Medicare claims data for almost 43,000 transplants, Whiting et al demonstrated a significant cost savings for transplant over chronic dialysis even when quality of life was not figured into the cost-equation models. [155]

The role of renal transplantation in older adults with ESRD has long been a source of controversy, particularly in terms of the ethical and cost implications. Becker et al pointed out that the debate focuses both on whether older adults should undergo transplant, and whether kidneys from older donors should be used for older recipients, given a theoretically shorter graft life span. [156] They concluded that physiologic function is more important than age in the determination of suitability for transplant. A number of studies have examined the utility of renal transplant in older adults. Recent research has focused on the use of kidney grafts taken from older adults as donors for both older and younger recipients.

The Older Adult as Donor

Studies on data from the United Network for Organ Sharing have suggested that overall graft survival from donors aged 55 and over is approximately 10% lower than for grafts from younger donors. However, results depend largely on how graft survival is defined.

Many studies combine perioperative deaths with other causes of graft loss. Other research examines outcomes more critically, using biochemical parameters.

Shimmura et al examined predonation creatinine clearance for living related donors and found no significant differences in graft survival that are based on this parameter. [157] Hayashi et al suggested that graft survival from living related older donors is most likely due to the fact that no preservation or significant cold ischemia time is required for these transplants. [158] They also pointed out that follow-up in the living related older donor (age > 66) revealed no significant changes in postoperative serum creatinine in comparison with younger historical controls. In a retrospective cohort analysis of extreme-age donors (< 10 or > 60 years old), Ferraresso et al reported actuarial graft survival at 1 and 4 years of 90% and 87% in kidneys from older living related donors. These figures are statistically equivalent to historical controls. [159]

There is continued controversy over whether older kidney grafts should be used exclusively for older recipients. In a retrospective cohort study using biochemical parameters, Vianello et al found that grafts from persons of "high donor age" (50 to 66 years) had lower survival than did grafts from younger persons. [160] They concluded that when kidneys from donors aged 50 years and over are used, they should probably be given to recipients with an estimated life expectancy of no more than 10 to 15 years. However, a more recent retrospective analysis of 509 transplants challenges this conclusion. [161] These investigators compared results stratified by both donor and recipient age. This study was unique in that it considered age as a continuous rather than a categorical variable. They found that the age of both the donor and recipient independently influences the overall graft survival rates when results are censored for deaths. They found no interaction between these variables, which suggests that trying to match the ages of donors and recipients may not be necessary.

Chronic organ rejection does not appear to differ on the basis of the age of the graft donor. In a retrospective cohort analysis comparing graft survival from 112 older living related donors (55 to 81 years) with that from 87 younger donors (< 45 years), Kumar et al found no difference in overall graft survival between the groups. [162] In addition, they found no difference in graft function, using biochemical parameters, including serum creatinine or glomerular filtration rate. However, they did identify a significantly higher rate of acute graft rejection in kidneys obtained from the older donors.

Although the quality of transplanted kidneys is very important, a recent prospective multicenter case-control study by Remuzzi et al suggested that volume of functioning nephrons in the transplant may be of equal significance. [163] In this analysis of grafts from older (≥ 60 years) cadaveric donors, they found that en bloc transplant of both kidneys of "marginal quality" yields better clinical results than transplant of a single, more "ideal" older kidney.

The Older Adult as Recipient

Although it has been well documented that older adults can successfully undergo kidney transplantation for renal replacement therapy, statistics on graft survival usually show lower success in older adults than in younger recipients. However, the method used to define graft loss is important for analysis and interpretation. Most studies include perioperative deaths as a graft loss. However, in a retrospective cohort analysis comparing 206 recipients aged 60 years or over with 1640 younger recipients, Doyle et al found no significant differences in graft survival when death is censored as a cause of graft loss. [164] In fact, graft loss in older adults appears to be due more to perioperative mortality than to other factors. [165]

The primary risk factor for perioperative mortality in older renal transplant recipients appears to be concomitant cardiopulmonary disease. In a small retrospective analysis of 26 kidney recipients aged 60 years or over, Schulak et al found that both overall patient and graft actuarial survivals are influenced by the presence of cardiovascular comorbidity. [166] Low-risk patients had 1- and 3-year graft and patient survival rates of 91% and 84%, respectively, but high-risk patients had survival rates of 67% and 58%. Their findings are supported by data reported by Tesi et al in an analysis of 1222 consecutive transplants. [167] They found that underlying cardiovascular disease was the leading cause of death in both older and younger recipients.

The presence of underlying cardiovascular disease certainly influences patient selection for transplant. In a sociodemographic cohort analysis of 4118 subjects started on dialysis between 1986 and 1987, Gaylin et al found cardiovascular disease to be the most predictive parameter of who received a transplant. [168] This suggests that potential recipients are being well screened to help maximize clinical outcomes.

There are data to suggest that the immunosuppression requirements for older graft recipients are lower than for younger patients. [169] This likely reflects the fact that overall immune response tends to decrease with the normal aging process. Soran et al found in a cohort of 230 older (> 60 years) recipients that the administration of tacrolimus, a relatively new immunosuppressive agent, results in overall graft survival rates for repeat transplants equal to that of first transplants. [170]

Needed Research in Renal Transplantation

There has been a large amount of research on renal transplantation for the management of ESRD in older adults. Most of this work has focused on the use of kidneys from older donors for younger recipients. More recent studies have examined the ability to perform transplants in older recipients. As surgical techniques for renal harvest and transplant improve, these methods will need to be studied in older adult populations. Laparoscopic donor nephrectomy for living related kidney donors has recently gained widespread attention as a minimally invasive technique. As transplant surgeons continue to push the age limits for donation, this technique will need to be examined in older adults.

Our understanding of immunosuppression has improved dramatically over the past several years. As new immunosuppressive agents are developed, their safety and efficacy will need to be studied in older adults who may now be eligible for transplant. In addition, the impact of various forms of renal replacement therapy (chronic dialysis versus transplantation) on health-related quality of life in older adults should be addressed.

> *Urol 26 (Level B)*: **The role of renal transplantation in older adults has grown recently, with the expansion of both donor and recipient age limits and other clinical criteria. Research is needed to clarify the unique needs of geriatric transplant patients, particularly with regard to immunosuppression and clinical outcomes. The effect of age of the kidney donor, age of the recipient, methods and degrees of immunosuppression, and the presence of concomitant disease need to be evaluated in prospective cohort studies.**

KEY RESEARCH QUESTIONS IN GERIATRIC UROLOGY

Urol KQ1: **Research is needed to better define the pathophysiology and natural history of the most common genitourinary disorders affecting older adults. These include but are not limited to urinary incontinence, urinary tract infection, prostate diseases, urologic malignancies, sexual dysfunction, stone disease, and renal failure and transplantation.**

Hypothesis-generating: Basic science and clinical studies are recommended to examine these issues, particularly the impact of common comorbid illnesses that may influence genitourinary health, for example, diabetes mellitus, hypertension, and chronic neurologic conditions. Large-scale cohort studies, well-designed case-control studies, and community-based research techniques are needed to develop this baseline knowledge.

Hypothesis-testing research that is based on this improved understanding of genitourinary disorders in older adults should then be conducted. Randomized therapeutic trials with appropriate operational definitions and adequate longitudinal follow-up should be developed to identify the most effective surgical and nonsurgical treatment options for each of these conditions.

Urol KQ2: **Research is needed to develop and validate predictive models to identify appropriate candidates for early surgical or other more active therapies for urologic disorders versus appropriate candidates for an initial trial of more conservative treatment options.**

Hypothesis-generating research: For most urologic conditions that affect older adults, a range of treatment options are available, including conservative nonsurgical therapies, biobehavioral treatments, pharmacotherapy, or surgical interventions. There is a perceived general tendency to favor initial trials of conservative therapy in older adults. Research is needed to determine whether delay in treatment may make subsequent surgical intervention more difficult or less successful. Conversely, it is possible that a planned course of preoperative nonsurgical therapy may potentially improve subsequent surgical outcomes. In addition, models to determine what preoperative evaluation techniques best influence outcomes should be developed. For example, which patient undergoing treatment for urinary incontinence would most benefit from formal urodynamic evaluation? Ideally, these models should be created on the basis of findings from randomized controlled clinical trials of diagnostic evaluations and treatments outlined in Urol KQ1, above.

Hypothesis-testing research to determine the validity and reliability of these predictive models will then be required. This will involve prospective cohort studies and clinical trials of these models.

Urol KQ3: **Research is needed to analyze the longitudinal outcomes of various urologic therapies, including potential risks, benefits, and costs.**

Hypothesis-generating research: The genitourinary disorders that affect older adults are diverse, and each presents unique diagnostic dilemmas and treatment challenges. Large-scale, prospective cohort studies and randomized controlled clinical trials will be needed to identify the impact of the information gained from work on Urol KQ1 and Urol KQ2. Emphasis should be placed on risks and benefits associated with health-related quality of life, improvement or preservation of functional capacity, and costs. The development of cooperative databases from multiple clinical centers will help to facilitate this type of outcomes research.

Hypothesis-testing research using randomized controlled trials will subsequently be required to demonstrate the clinical utility and longevity of these therapies. It will be critically important for these studies to be designed with a sufficient follow-up interval to document the durability of outcomes.

REFERENCES

1. Burgio KL, Matthews KA, Engel BT. Prevalence, incidence and correlates of urinary incontinence in healthy, middle-aged women. J Urol 1991;146:1255-1259.
2. Malmsten UG, Milsom I, Molander U, Norlen LJ. Urinary incontinence and lower urinary tract symptoms: an epidemiological study of men aged 45 to 99 years. J Urol 1997;158:1733-1737.
3. Brown JS, Seeley DG, Fong J, et al. Urinary incontinence in older women: who is at risk? Study of Osteoporotic Fractures Research Group. Obstet Gynecol 1996;87:715-721.
4. Diokno AC, Brock BM, Herzog AR, Bromberg J. Medical correlates of urinary incontinence in the elderly. Urology 1990;36:129-138.
5. Johnson TM, Kincade JE, Bernard SL, et al. The association of urinary incontinence with poor self-rated health. J Am Geriatr Soc 1998;46:693-699.
6. Dugan E, Cohen SJ, Bland DR, et al. The association of depressive symptoms and urinary incontinence among older adults. J Am Geriatr Soc 2000;48:413-416.
7. Grimby A, Milsom I, Molander U, et al. The influence of urinary incontinence on the quality of life of elderly women. Age Ageing 1993;22:82-89.
8. Wyman JF, Harkins SW, Fantl JA. Psychosocial impact of urinary incontinence in the community-dwelling population. J Am Geriatr Soc 1990;38:282-288.
9. Noelker LS. Incontinence in elderly cared for by family. Gerontologist 1987;27:194-200.
10. Breakwell SL, Walker SN. Differences in physical health, social interaction, and personal adjustment between continent and incontinent homebound aged women. J Community Health Nurs 1988;5:19-31.
11. Coward RT, Horne C, Peek CW. Predicting nursing home admissions among incontinent older adults: a comparison of residential differences across six years. Gerontologist 1995;35:732-743.
12. Jirovec MM, Wells TJ. Urinary incontinence in nursing home residents with dementia: the mobility-cognition paradigm. Appl Nurs Res 1990;3:112-117.
13. Chiang L, Ouslander J, Schnelle J, Reuben DB. Dually incontinent nursing home residents: clinical characteristics and treatment differences. J Am Geriatr Soc 2000;48:673-676.

14. Tinetti ME, Inouye SK, Gill TM, Doucette JT. Shared risk factors for falls, incontinence, and functional dependence: unifying the approach to geriatric syndromes. JAMA 1995;273: 1348-1353.
15. Seidel GK, Millis SR, Lichtenberg PA, Dijkers M. Predicting bowel and bladder continence from cognitive status in geriatric rehabilitation patients. Arch Phys Med Rehabil 1994;75: 590-593.
16. Ouslander JG, Kane RL, Abrass IB. Urinary incontinence in elderly nursing home patients. JAMA 1982;248:1194-1198.
17. Palmer MH, German PS, Ouslander JG. Risk factors for urinary incontinence one year after nursing home admission. Res Nurs Health 1991;14:405-412.
18. Fonda D, Resnick NM, Kirschner-Hermanns R. Prevention of urinary incontinence in older people. Br J Urol 1998;82 Suppl 1:5-10.
19. Strasser H, Tiefenthaler M, Steinlechner M, et al. Urinary incontinence in the elderly and age-dependent apoptosis of rhabdosphincter cells. Lancet 1999;354:918-919.
20. Strasser H, Tiefenthaler M, Steinlechner M, et al. Age dependent apoptosis and loss of rhabdosphincter cells. J Urol 2000;164:1781-1785.
21. Resnick NM, Yalla SV. Detrusor hyperactivity with impaired contractile function: an unrecognized but common cause of incontinence in elderly patients. JAMA 1987;257:3076-3081.
22. DuBeau CE, Resnick NM. Evaluation of the causes and severity of geriatric incontinence: a critical appraisal. Urol Clin North Am 1991;18:243-256.
23. Weiss BD. Diagnostic evaluation of urinary incontinence in geriatric patients. Am Fam Physician 1998;57:2675-2684, 2688-2690.
24. Kirschner-Hermanns R, Scherr PA, Branch LG, et al. Accuracy of survey questions for geriatric urinary incontinence. J Urol 1998;159:1903-1908.
25. Fonda D, Benvenuti F, Castleden M, et al. Management of incontinence in older people. In Abrams P, Khoury S, Wein A (eds): Incontinence: 1st International Consultation on Incontinence. Plymouth, United Kingdom: World Health Organization (WHO) and International Union Against Cancer (UICC), 1998:731-773.
26. O'Donnell PD. Special considerations in elderly individuals with urinary incontinence. Urology 1998;51:20-23.
27. Galloway NT. Surgical treatment of urinary incontinence in geriatric women. Am J Med Sci 1997;314:268-272.
28. Diokno AC, Normolle DP, Brown MB, Herzog AR. Urodynamic tests for female geriatric urinary incontinence. Urology 1990;36:431-439.
29. Wagg AS, Lieu PK, Ding YY, Malone-Lee JG. A urodynamic analysis of age associated changes in urethral function in women with lower urinary tract symptoms. J Urol 1996;156:1984-1988.
30. Fielding JR, Lee JH, Dubeau CE, et al. Voiding cystourethrography findings in elderly women with urge incontinence. J Urol 2000;163:1216-1218.
31. Fantl JA, Newman DK, Colling J, et al. Managing Acute and Chronic Urinary Incontinence. Clinical Practice Guideline. Quick Reference Guide for Clinicians, No. 2. 1996 Update. Rockville, MD: U.S. Department of Health and Human Services. Public Health Service, Agency for Health Care Policy and Research, 1996. AHCPR Publication No. 96-0682.
32. Hadley EC. Bladder training and related therapies for urinary incontinence in older people. JAMA 1986;256:372-379.
33. Wyman JF, Fantl JA, McClish DK, Bump RC. Comparative efficacy of behavioral interventions in the management of female urinary incontinence. Continence Program for Women Research Group. Am J Obstet Gynecol 1998;179:999-1007.
34. Publicover C, Bear M. The effect of bladder training on urinary incontinence in community-dwelling older women. J Wound Ostomy Continence Nurs 1997;24:319-324.

35. Lyons SS, Specht JKP. Research-based protocol: prompted voiding for persons with urinary incontinence. Iowa City, IA: The University of Iowa Gerontological Nursing Interventions Research Center, Research Development and Dissemination Core, 1999.

36. Ouslander JG, Schnelle JF, Uman G, et al. Predictors of successful prompted voiding among incontinent nursing home residents. JAMA 1995;273:1366-1370.

37. Burgio KL, Locher JL, Goode PS, et al. Behavioral vs drug treatment for urge urinary incontinence in older women: a randomized controlled trial. JAMA 1998;280:1995-2000.

38. Burgio KL, Locher JL, Goode PS. Combined behavioral and drug therapy for urge incontinence in older women. J Am Geriatr Soc 2000;48:370-374.

39. Szonyi G, Collas DM, Ding YY, Malone-Lee JG. Oxybutynin with bladder retraining for detrusor instability in elderly people: a randomized controlled trial. Age Ageing 1995;24:287-291.

40. Fantl JA, Cardozo L, McClish DK. Estrogen therapy in the management of urinary incontinence in postmenopausal women: a meta-analysis. First report of the Hormones and Urogenital Therapy Committee. Obstet Gynecol 1994;83:12-18.

41. Bergstrom K, Carlsson CP, Lindholm C, Widengren R. Improvement of urge- and mixed-type incontinence after acupuncture treatment among elderly women–a pilot study. J Auton Nerv Syst 2000;79:173-180.

42. American Urological Association Female Stress Urinary Incontinence Clinical Guidelines Panel. Report on the surgical management of female stress urinary incontinence. American Urological Association, 1997.

43. Stohrer M, Goepel M, Kondo A, et al. The standardization of terminology in neurogenic lower urinary tract dysfunction: with suggestions for diagnostic procedures. International Continence Society Standardization Committee. Neurourol Urodyn 1999;18:139-158.

44. Sultana CJ, Campbell JW, Pisanelli WS, et al. Morbidity and mortality of incontinence surgery in elderly women: an analysis of Medicare data. Am J Obstet Gynecol 1997;176:344-348.

45. Khullar V, Cardozo LD, Abbott D, Anders K. GAX collagen in the treatment of urinary incontinence in elderly women: a two year follow up. Br J Obstet Gynaecol 1997;104:96-99.

46. Stanton SL, Monga AK. Incontinence in elderly women: is periurethral collagen an advance? Br J Obstet Gynaecol 1997;104:154-157.

47. Winters JC, Chiverton A, Scarpero HM, Prats LJ. Collagen injection therapy in elderly women: long-term results and patient satisfaction. Urology 2000;55:856-861.

48. Faerber GJ. Endoscopic collagen injection therapy in elderly women with type I stress urinary incontinence. J Urol 1996;155:512-514.

49. Nitti VW, Bregg KJ, Sussman EM, Raz S. The Raz bladder neck suspension in patients 65 years old and older. J Urol 1993;149:802-807.

50. Carr LK, Walsh PJ, Abraham VE, Webster GD. Favorable outcome of pubovaginal slings for geriatric women with stress incontinence. J Urol 1997;157:125-128.

51. Migliari R, De Angelis M, Madeddu G, Verdacchi T. Tension-free vaginal mesh repair for anterior vaginal wall prolapse. Eur Urol 2000;38:151-155.

52. Abrutyn E, Mossey J, Berlin JA, et al. Does asymptomatic bacteriuria predict mortality and does antimicrobial treatment reduce mortality in elderly ambulatory women? Ann Intern Med 1994;120:827-833.

53. Nordenstam GR, Brandberg CA, Oden AS, et al. Bacteriuria and mortality in an elderly population. N Engl J Med 1986;314:1152-1156.

54. Nicolle LE, Henderson E, Bjornson J, et al. The association of bacteriuria with resident characteristics and survival in elderly institutionalized men. Ann Intern Med 1987;106:682-686.

55. Monane M, Gurwitz JH, Lipsitz LA, et al. Epidemiologic and diagnostic aspects of bacteriuria: a longitudinal study in older women. J Am Geriatr Soc 1995;43:618-622.

56. Nicolle LE, Mayhew WJ, Bryan L. Prospective randomized comparison of therapy and no therapy for asymptomatic bacteriuria in institutionalized elderly women. Am J Med 1987;83:27-33.

57. Ouslander JG, Schapira M, Schnelle JF, et al. Does eradicating bacteriuria affect the severity of chronic urinary incontinence in nursing home residents? Ann Intern Med 1995;122:749-754.

58. Harding GK, Nicolle LE, Ronald AR, et al. How long should catheter-acquired urinary tract infection in women be treated? A randomized controlled study. Ann Intern Med 1991;114:713-719.

59. Raz R, Gennesin Y, Wasser J, et al. Recurrent urinary tract infections in postmenopausal women. Clin Infect Dis 2000;30:152-156.

60. Hedstrom M, Grondal L, Ahl T. Urinary tract infection in patients with hip fractures. Injury 1999;30:341-343.

61. Johnstone DJ, Morgan NH, Wilkinson MC, Chissell HR. Urinary tract infection and hip fracture. Injury 1995;26:89-91.

62. Griebling TL, Nygaard IE. The role of estrogen replacement therapy in the management of urinary incontinence and urinary tract infection in postmenopausal women. Endocrinol Metab Clin North Am 1997;26:347-360.

63. Eriksen B. A randomized, open, parallel-group study on the preventive effect of an estradiol-releasing vaginal ring (Estring) on recurrent urinary tract infections in postmenopausal women. Am J Obstet Gynecol 1999;180:1072-1079.

64. Dignam R, Ahmed M, Denman S, et al. The effect of cranberry juice on UTI rates in a long term care facility [abstract]. J Am Geriatr Soc 1997;45:S53.

65. Avorn J, Monane M, Gurwitz JH, et al. Reduction of bacteriuria and pyuria after ingestion of cranberry juice. JAMA 1994;271:751-754.

66. Kontiokari T, Sundqvist K, Nuutinen M, et al. Randomised trial of cranberry-lingonberry juice and Lactobacillus GG drink for the prevention of urinary tract infections in women. BMJ 2001;322:1571.

67. Haidinger G, Temml C, Schatzl G, et al. Risk factors for lower urinary tract symptoms in elderly men. For the Prostate Study Group of the Austrian Society of Urology. Eur Urol 2000;37:413-420.

68. Krogh J, Jensen JS, Iversen HG, Andersen JT. Age as a prognostic variable in patients undergoing transurethral prostatectomy. Scand J Urol Nephrol 1993;27:225-229.

69. Epstein RS, Lydick E, deLabry L, Vokonas PS. Age-related differences in risk factors for prostatectomy for benign prostatic hyperplasia: the VA Normative Aging Study. Urology 1991;38:9-12.

70. Cooper KL, McKiernan JM, Kaplan SA. Alpha-adrenoceptor antagonists in the treatment of benign prostatic hyperplasia. Drugs 1999;57:9-17.

71. Medina JJ, Parra RO, Moore RG. Benign prostatic hyperplasia (the aging prostate). Med Clin North Am 1999;83:1213-1229.

72. Lee M, Sharifi R. Benign prostatic hyperplasia: diagnosis and treatment guideline. Ann Pharmacother 1997;31:481-486.

73. Breslin DS, Muecke EC, Reckler JM, Fracchia JA. Changing trends in the management of prostatic disease in a single private practice: a 5-year followup. J Urol 1993;150:347-350.

74. Holtgrewe HL. Economic issues and the management of benign prostatic hyperplasia. Urology 1995;46:23-25.

75. Wilt TJ, Ishani A, Rutks I, MacDonald R. Phytotherapy for benign prostatic hyperplasia. Public Health Nutr 2000;3:459-472.

76. Lowe FC, Ku JC. Phytotherapy in treatment of benign prostatic hyperplasia: a critical review. Urology 1996;48:12-20.

77. Concato J, Horwitz RI, Feinstein AR, et al. Problems of comorbidity in mortality after prostatectomy. JAMA 1992;267:1077-1082.

78. Ibrahim AI, el-Malik E, Ghali AM, et al. Effect of age, comorbidity and type of surgery on perioperative complications and mortality of prostatectomy. Br J Urol 1995;76:341-345.

79. Mebust WK, Holtgrewe HL, Cockett AT, Peters PC. Transurethral prostatectomy: immediate and postoperative complications. A cooperative study of 13 participating institutions evaluating 3,885 patients. J Urol 1989;141:243-247.

80. Ilkjaer LB, Lund L, Nielsen KT. Outcome of transurethral prostatectomy in men over 80 years. Scand J Urol Nephrol 1998;32:270-272.

81. Pientka L, van Loghem J, Hahn E, et al. Comorbidities and perioperative complications among patients with surgically treated benign prostatic hyperplasia. Urology 1991;38:43-48.

82. Libman E, Fichten CS, Creti L, et al. Transurethral prostatectomy: differential effects of age category and presurgery sexual functioning on postprostatectomy sexual adjustment. J Behav Med 1989;12:469-485.

83. Tubaro A, Vicentini C, Renzetti R, Miano L. Invasive and minimally invasive treatment modalities for lower urinary tract symptoms: what are the relevant differences in randomised controlled trials? Eur Urol 2000;38 Suppl 1:7-17.

84. Djavan B, Marberger M. Minimally invasive procedures as an alternative to medical management for lower urinary tract symptoms of benign prostatic hyperplasia. Curr Opin Urol 2001;11:1-7.

85. Djavan B, Madersbacher S, Klingler HC, et al. Outcome analysis of minimally invasive treatments for benign prostatic hyperplasia. Tech Urol 1999;5:12-20.

86. Smith RA, von Eschenbach AC, Wender R, et al. American Cancer Society guidelines for the early detection of cancer: update of early detection guidelines for prostate, colorectal, and endometrial cancers. Also: update 2001–testing for early lung cancer detection. CA Cancer J Clin 2001;51:38-75; quiz 77-80.

87. Carter HB, Epstein JI, Chan DW, et al. Recommended prostate-specific antigen testing intervals for the detection of curable prostate cancer. JAMA 1997;277:1456-1460.

88. American College of Physicians. Screening for prostate cancer. Ann Intern Med 1997;126:480-484.

89. American Urological Association Prostate Cancer Clinical Guidelines Panel. Report on the management of clinically localized prostate cancer. Baltimore, MD: American Urological Association, 1995.

90. Uygur MC, Erol D, Cetinkaya M, et al. The correlation between prostate-specific antigen and age. Analysis of prostate-specific antigen values from 4,846 Turkish men with symptomatic benign prostatic hyperplasia. Eur Urol 1997;32:416-419.

91. Catalona WJ, Southwick PC, Slawin KM, et al. Comparison of percent free PSA, PSA density, and age-specific PSA cutoffs for prostate cancer detection and staging. Urology 2000;56:255-260.

92. Corral DA, Bahnson RR. Survival of men with clinically localized prostate cancer detected in the eighth decade of life. J Urol 1994;151:1326-1329.

93. Middleton AW. Radical prostatectomy for carcinoma in men more than 69 years old. J Urol 1987;138:1185-1188.

94. Post PN, Kil PJ, Hendrikx AJ, et al. Comorbidity in patients with prostate cancer and its relevance to treatment choice. BJU Int 1999;84:652-656.

95. Carter HB, Epstein JI, Partin AW. Influence of age and prostate-specific antigen on the chance of curable prostate cancer among men with nonpalpable disease. Urology 1999;53:126-130.

96. Mazur DJ, Merz JF. Older patients' willingness to trade off urologic adverse outcomes for a better chance at five-year survival in the clinical setting of prostate cancer. J Am Geriatr Soc 1995;43:979-984.

97. Mazur DJ, Merz JF. How older patients' treatment preferences are influenced by disclosures about therapeutic uncertainty: surgery versus expectant management for localized prostate cancer. J Am Geriatr Soc 1996;44:934-937.

98. Kerr LA, Zincke H. Radical retropubic prostatectomy for prostate cancer in the elderly and the young: complications and prognosis. Eur Urol 1994;25:305-311; discussion 311-302.

99. Lu-Yao GL, Albertsen P, Warren J, Yao SL. Effect of age and surgical approach on complications and short-term mortality after radical prostatectomy–a population-based study. Urology 1999;54:301-307.

100. Obek C, Lai S, Sadek S, et al. Age as a prognostic factor for disease recurrence after radical prostatectomy. Urology 1999;54:533-538.

101. Litwin MS, Hays RD, Fink A, et al. Quality-of-life outcomes in men treated for localized prostate cancer. JAMA 1995;273:129-135.

102. Stanford JL, Feng Z, Hamilton AS, et al. Urinary and sexual function after radical prostatectomy for clinically localized prostate cancer: the Prostate Cancer Outcomes Study. JAMA 2000;283:354-360.

103. Litwin MS, Shpall AI, Dorey F, Nguyen TH. Quality-of-life outcomes in long-term survivors of advanced prostate cancer. Am J Clin Oncol 1998;21:327-332.

104. Rosario DJ, Becker M, Anderson JB. The changing pattern of mortality and morbidity from radical cystectomy. BJU Int 2000;85:427-430.

105. Game X, Soulie M, Seguin P, et al. Radical cystectomy in patients older than 75 years: assessment of morbidity and mortality. Eur Urol 2001;39:525-529.

106. Soulie M, Straub M, Game X, et al. A multicenter study of the morbidity of radical cystectomy in select elderly patients with bladder cancer. J Urol 2002;167:1325-1328.

107. Saika T, Suyama B, Murata T, et al. Orthotopic neobladder reconstruction in elderly bladder cancer patients. Int J Urol 2001;8:533-538.

108. Doherty JG, Rufer A, Bartholomew P, Beaumont DM. The presentation, treatment and outcome of renal cell carcinoma in old age. Age Ageing 1999;28:359-362.

109. Hsu TH, Gill IS, Fazeli-Matin S, et al. Radical nephrectomy and nephroureterectomy in the octogenarian and nonagenarian: comparison of laparoscopic and open approaches. Urology 1999;53:1121-1125.

110. Panser LA, Rhodes T, Girman CJ, et al. Sexual function of men ages 40 to 79 years: the Olmsted County Study of Urinary Symptoms and Health Status Among Men. J Am Geriatr Soc 1995;43:1107-1111.

111. Jønler M, Moon T, Brannan W, et al. The effect of age, ethnicity and geographical location on impotence and quality of life. Br J Urol 1995;75:651-655.

112. Johannes CB, Araujo AB, Feldman HA, et al. Incidence of erectile dysfunction in men 40 to 69 years old: longitudinal results from the Massachusetts male aging study. J Urol 2000;163:460-463.

113. Helgason AR, Adolfsson J, Dickman P, et al. Factors associated with waning sexual function among elderly men and prostate cancer patients. J Urol 1997;158:155-159.

114. Mulligan T, Moss CR. Sexuality and aging in male veterans: a cross-sectional study of interest, ability, and activity. Arch Sex Behav 1991;20:17-25.

115. Mulligan T, Palguta RF. Sexual interest, activity, and satisfaction among male nursing home residents. Arch Sex Behav 1991;20:199-204.

116. Araujo AB, Johannes CB, Feldman HA, et al. Relation between psychosocial risk factors and incident erectile dysfunction: prospective results from the Massachusetts Male Aging Study. Am J Epidemiol 2000;152:533-541.

117. Araujo AB, Durante R, Feldman HA, et al. The relationship between depressive symptoms and male erectile dysfunction: cross-sectional results from the Massachusetts Male Aging Study. Psychosom Med 1998;60:458-465.

118. Helgason AR, Adolfsson J, Dickman P, et al. Sexual desire, erection, orgasm and ejaculatory functions and their importance to elderly Swedish men: a population-based study. Age Ageing 1996;25:285-291.

119. Rosen RC, Riley A, Wagner G, et al. The International Index of Erectile Function (IIEF): a multidimensional scale for assessment of erectile dysfunction. Urology 1997;49:822-830.

120. Cappelleri JC, Siegel RL, Osterloh IH, Rosen RC. Relationship between patient self-assessment of erectile function and the erectile function domain of the international index of erectile function. Urology 2000;56:477-481.

121. Glick HA, McCarron TJ, Althof SE, et al. Construction of scales for the Center for Marital and Sexual Health (CMASH) Sexual Functioning Questionnaire. J Sex Marital Ther 1997;23:103-117.

122. Rosen R, Brown C, Heiman J, et al. The Female Sexual Function Index (FSFI): a multidimensional self-report instrument for the assessment of female sexual function. J Sex Marital Ther 2000;26:191-208.

123. Purifoy FE, Grodsky A, Giambra LM. The relationship of sexual daydreaming to sexual activity, sexual drive, and sexual attitudes for women across the life-span. Arch Sex Behav 1992;21:369-385.

124. Berman JR, Berman L, Goldstein I. Female sexual dysfunction: incidence, pathophysiology, evaluation, and treatment options. Urology 1999;54:385-391.

125. Nusbaum MR, Gamble G, Skinner B, Heiman J. The high prevalence of sexual concerns among women seeking routine gynecological care. J Fam Pract 2000;49:229-232.

126. Mulligan T, Retchin SM, Chinchilli VM, Bettinger CB. The role of aging and chronic disease in sexual dysfunction. J Am Geriatr Soc 1988;36:520-524.

127. Wespes E. Erectile dysfunction in the ageing man. Curr Opin Urol 2000;10:625-628.

128. Jensen J, Lendorf A, Stimpel H, et al. The prevalence and etiology of impotence in 101 male hypertensive outpatients. Am J Hypertens 1999;12:271-275.

129. Schachter M. Erectile dysfunction and lipid disorders. Curr Med Res Opin 2000;16 Suppl 1:s9-s12.

130. Jaffe A, Chen Y, Kisch ES, et al. Erectile dysfunction in hypertensive subjects: assessment of potential determinants. Hypertension 1996;28:859-862.

131. Ledda A. Diabetes, hypertension and erectile dysfunction. Curr Med Res Opin 2000;16 Suppl 1:s17-s20.

132. Monga TN, Tan G, Ostermann HJ, et al. Sexuality and sexual adjustment of patients with chronic pain. Disabil Rehabil 1998;20:317-329.

133. Steele TE, Wuerth D, Finkelstein S, et al. Sexual experience of the chronic peritoneal dialysis patient. J Am Soc Nephrol 1996;7:1165-1168.

134. Nordstrom GM, Nyman CR. Male and female sexual function and activity following ileal conduit urinary diversion. Br J Urol 1992;70:33-39.

135. Bjerre BD, Johansen C, Steven K. Sexological problems after cystectomy: bladder substitution compared with ileal conduit diversion. A questionnaire study of male patients. Scand J Urol Nephrol 1998;32:187-193.

136. Bjerre BD, Johansen C, Steven K. A questionnaire study of sexological problems following urinary diversion in the female patient. Scand J Urol Nephrol 1997;31:155-160.

137. Karacan I, Karatas M. Erectile dysfunction in sleep apnea and response to CPAP. J Sex Marital Ther 1995;21:239-247.

138. Schiavi RC, Mandeli J, Schreiner-Engel P, Chambers A. Aging, sleep disorders, and male sexual function. Biol Psychiatry 1991;30:15-24.

139. Monga TN, Lawson JS, Inglis J. Sexual dysfunction in stroke patients. Arch Phys Med Rehabil 1986;67:19-22.

140. Coslett HB, Heilman KM. Male sexual function. Impairment after right hemisphere stroke. Arch Neurol 1986;43:1036-1039.

141. Korpelainen JT, Nieminen P, Myllyla VV. Sexual functioning among stroke patients and their spouses. Stroke 1999;30:715-719.

142. Koller WC, Vetere-Overfield B, Williamson A, et al. Sexual dysfunction in Parkinson's disease. Clin Neuropharmacol 1990;13:461-463.

143. Litz BT, Zeiss AM, Davies HD. Sexual concerns of male spouses of female Alzheimer's disease patients. Gerontologist 1990;30:113-116.

144. Tsai SJ, Hwang JP, Yang CH, et al. Inappropriate sexual behaviors in dementia: a preliminary report. Alzheimer Dis Assoc Disord 1999;13:60-62.

145. Levitsky AM, Owens NJ. Pharmacologic treatment of hypersexuality and paraphilias in nursing home residents. J Am Geriatr Soc 1999;47:231-234.

146. Wiseman SV, McAuley JW, Freidenberg GR, Freidenberg DL. Hypersexuality in patients with dementia: possible response to cimetidine. Neurology 2000;54:2024.

147. Rosas SE, Wasserstein A, Kobrin S, Feldman HI. Preliminary observations of sildenafil treatment for erectile dysfunction in dialysis patients. Am J Kidney Dis 2001;37:134-137.

148. Dinsmore WW, Hodges M, Hargreaves C, et al. Sildenafil citrate (Viagra) in erectile dysfunction: near normalization in men with broad-spectrum erectile dysfunction compared with age-matched healthy control subjects. Urology 1999;53:800-805.

149. Kaplan SA, Reis RB, Kohn IJ, et al. Safety and efficacy of sildenafil in postmenopausal women with sexual dysfunction. Urology 1999;53:481-486.

150. Kramolowsky EV, Quinlan SM, Loening SA. Extracorporeal shock wave lithotripsy for the treatment of urinary calculi in the elderly. J Am Geriatr Soc 1987;35:251-254.

151. Schaubel D, Desmeules M, Mao Y, et al. Survival experience among elderly end-stage renal disease patients: a controlled comparison of transplantation and dialysis. Transplantation 1995;60:1389-1394.

152. Wolfe RA, Held PJ, Hulbert-Shearon TE, et al. A critical examination of trends in outcomes over the last decade. Am J Kidney Dis 1998;32:S9-S15.

153. Wolfe RA, Port FK, Webb RL, et al. II. Incidence and prevalence of ESRD. United States Renal Data System 1998 Annual Data Report. Am J Kidney Dis 1998;32:S38-S49.

154. Beusterien KM, Nissenson AR, Port FK, et al. The effects of recombinant human erythropoietin on functional health and well-being in chronic dialysis patients. J Am Soc Nephrol 1996;7:763-773.

155. Whiting JF, Woodward RS, Zavala EY, et al. Economic cost of expanded criteria donors in cadaveric renal transplantation: analysis of Medicare payments. Transplantation 2000;70:755-760.

156. Becker BN, Ismail N, Becker YT, et al. Renal transplantation in the older end stage renal disease patient. Semin Nephrol 1996;16:353-362.

157. Shimmura H, Tanabe K, Ishikawa N, et al. Influence of donor renal reserve on the long-term results of living kidney transplantation from elderly donors. Transplant Proc 1999;31:2874-2876.

158. Hayashi T, Koga S, Higashi Y, et al. Living-related renal transplantation from elderly donors (older than 66 years of age). Transplant Proc 1995;27:984-985.

159. Ferraresso M, Berardinelli L, Bellapi A, Vegeto A. Long-term function and survival rates of kidneys from extreme-age donors in the cyclosporine era. Transplant Proc 1998;30:2274-2275.

160. Vianello A, Mastrosimone S, Calconi G, et al. Influence of donor age on cadaver kidney graft function and survival: univariate and multivariate analyses. Nephron 1993;65:541-548.

161. Roodnat JI, Zietse R, Mulder PG, et al. The impact of donor age on renal graft survival. Transplant Proc 2000;32:136-138.

162. Kumar A, Verma BS, Srivastava A, et al. Long-term followup of elderly donors in a live related renal transplant program. J Urol 2000;163:1654-1658.
163. Remuzzi G, Grinyo J, Ruggenenti P, et al. Early experience with dual kidney transplantation in adults using expanded donor criteria. Double Kidney Transplant Group (DKG). J Am Soc Nephrol 1999;10:2591-2598.
164. Doyle SE, Matas AJ, Gillingham K, Rosenberg ME. Predicting clinical outcome in the elderly renal transplant recipient. Kidney Int 2000;57:2144-2150.
165. Phillips AO, Bewick M, Snowden SA, et al. The influence of recipient and donor age on the outcome of renal transplantation. Clin Nephrol 1993;40:352-354.
166. Schulak JA, Mayes JT, Johnston KH, Hricik DE. Kidney transplantation in patients aged sixty years and older. Surgery 1990;108:726-731; discussion 731-723.
167. Tesi RJ, Elkhammas EA, Davies EA, et al. Renal transplantation in older people. Lancet 1994;343:461-464.
168. Gaylin DS, Held PJ, Port FK, et al. The impact of comorbid and sociodemographic factors on access to renal transplantation. JAMA 1993;269:603-608.
169. Ismail N, Hakim RM, Helderman JH. Renal replacement therapies in the elderly: Part II. Renal transplantation. Am J Kidney Dis 1994;23:1-15.
170. Soran A, Basar H, Shapiro R, et al. Renal retransplantation in elderly recipients under tacrolimus-based immunosuppression. Transplant Proc 2000;32:663-664.

11

GERIATRIC ORTHOPEDICS

Susan Day, MD*

By the year 2020 about 20% of the population, or an estimated 60 million people, will be aged 65 years or over. Increasing age leads to increasing vulnerability in the musculoskeletal system through injury and disease. Approximately 80% of those older persons will have musculoskeletal complaints.

Significant osteoarthritis of the hip or knee will be reported by 40% to 60% of older persons. Disabling osteoarthritis of the weight-bearing joints commonly leads to joint replacement surgery, which was performed an average of 648,000 times annually from 1993 to 1995. [1] In 1996, 74% of the total knee replacements and 68% of the total hip replacements were performed on patients aged 65 and older. [1] As the number of elders in the population increases, so will the need for joint replacement surgery. Joint arthroplasty is expected to increase by at least 80% by 2030. [1]

Age-related changes in bone and soft tissue are commonly associated with disabling fractures. In the first 5 years following menopause, women lose up to 25% of their bone mass. In the United States, osteoporosis affects approximately 20 million persons, and every year 1.3 million fractures are attributed to this condition. Muscle strength decreases on average by about one third after age 60, which can lead to difficulty maintaining balance and predispose a person to falls. By the age of 90, one third of women and one sixth of men will experience a hip fracture. About two thirds of those who fracture a hip do not return to their prefracture level of functioning. The cost of treating all osteoporotic fractures was estimated to be $13.8 billion in 1995 and is expected to double in the next 50 years. Most of this cost can be attributed to the treatment and postoperative care of hip fractures. [1]

Thus, it is vital at this time to evaluate the agenda for research on orthopedic management of geriatric patients. We approached this task by surveying the orthopedic literature to assess the status of knowledge and the quality of research on which present practice is based. By detecting areas where research has been lacking or of poor quality, or where results have been inconsistent or controversial, we have identified research studies that are urgently needed.

METHODS

The searches were conducted on the National Library of Medicine's PubMed database in March 2001. Eleven topics were searched: demographics, arthritis, and fractures; impact of musculoskeletal conditions on overall function; joint replacement; rotator cuff and surgery; spinal stenosis and surgery; fracture care, in general; hip fracture care; wrist fracture care; spine fracture care; proximal humerus fracture care; and amputation surgery.

For epidemiology, the search strategy was to combine terms for aged, arthritis epidemiology, and fractures epidemiology with terms for demography, male or female, social class, and ethnic groups. This search yielded 1129 references.

* Clinical Instructor, Michigan State University; Grand Rapids Orthopaedics Residency Program, Grand Rapids, MI.

For overall function, the search strategy combined terms for aged, musculoskeletal diseases, or fractures with terms for function, recovery of function, and activities of daily living (ADLs). This search uncovered 1656 references.

On joint replacement, the search combined terms for aged and arthroplasty, replacement, and statistics and numeric data with terms for utilization, cohort studies, physicians' practice patterns, incidence, indicators, postoperative complications, treatment outcome, risk factors, follow-up studies, recovery, predict, prognosis, functional status, indication, complications, etiology, forecast, or length of stay. This search yielded 1272 references.

The search strategy for rotator cuff surgery was identical except *rotator cuff surgery* was substituted for *arthroplasty, replacement*. This search generated 110 references.

When *spinal stenosis surgery* was substituted, the search yielded 235 references.

For fracture care, the search strategy was to add terms for aged, fractures, osteoporosis, and risk factors and then merge them with terms for treatment and fracture fixation or complications, bone transplantation, bone substitutes, or casts. This search produced 1592 references.

For the care of hip fractures, the search strategy was long and complex. It is available from the author. The number of items retrieved was 2449.

The search strategy for wrist fractures was simpler: it used terms for aged and fractures and wrist injuries and excluded several terms that had been used in the general fracture care search (see above). This search found 153 references.

The search strategy for spine fractures used terms for aged and fractures and spinal fractures, and it excluded a host of terms used in the searches above. It retrieved 764 titles.

The search strategy for proximal humerus fractures was exactly the same, except for substituting *shoulder* for *spinal*. It led to 140 references.

Finally, the search strategy for amputations included terms for aged, amputation, and energy metabolism, combined with terms for wound healing, prostheses, implants, rehabilitation, or utilization. This search yielded 272 references.

NORMAL MUSCULOSKELETAL AGING AND THE AGING ATHLETE

A comprehensive review of the literature did not find any studies identifying normal ranges of motion of the extremities in older persons. No articles were found addressing the treatment of the otherwise healthy elderly patient who sustains a sports-related musculoskeletal injury. It is not currently known whether treatments recommended for younger patients with musculoskeletal injuries are applicable in part or at all to the older patient with a similar problem.

To prepare for the care of an increasingly active and vigorous older population, research is needed to define normative and incidence data.

> ***Ortho 1 (Level B)*: Observational studies are needed to define the normal range of motion of the extremities in older people without musculoskeletal disease. Such studies should also examine the range of motion necessary for activities of daily living and instrumental activities of daily living.**

Ortho 2 (Level D): Observational studies of older athletes are needed to define the incidence and nature of sports-related injuries in older athletes and to examine the utility of arthroscopy in the treatment of knee and shoulder injuries.

FACTORS THAT INFLUENCE POSTOPERATIVE OUTCOME

Age alone does not appear to be a prognostic factor for outcome following orthopedic surgical procedures. Pre-existing medical condition, however, plays a significant role in postoperative outcome; medical comorbidities influence physiologic reserve, postoperative complications, and capacity for rehabilitation. Many patients require treatment of a medical condition prior to elective joint replacement surgery. [2]

Following hip fracture, host factors, not injury severity, are the primary determinants of long-term survival. [3] One-year mortality following hip fracture can be predicted on admission by the number of medical conditions: with no other medical conditions, mortality is 0%; with one or two, mortality is 14%; with three or more, the mortality is 24%. [4]

Malnutrition is common in older patients. The incidence of malnutrition among orthopedic patients is thought to be 20%. Many studies have shown that weight loss in older persons is a major predictor of mortality. In addition, poor nutrition can lead to weakness, fatigue, and decreased muscle mass, muscle strength, and bone mineral density. Poor nutrition is, therefore, a risk factor for poor outcome following surgery because of wound-healing complications, delayed recovery, and increased infection rate. Low preoperative serum albumin has been correlated with decreased postfracture quality of life [5] and increased postfracture mortality rate. [6]

On the other hand, good nutrition is associated with decreased fracture risk. In a cohort study of women aged 55 to 69 who were assessed with a food frequency questionnaire and followed up 2 to 3 years later, a reduced risk of hip fracture was shown in those with increased dietary protein consumption. [7] (See also Chapter 13, section on preoperative nutrition.)

The outcome of elderly patients who have undergone surgery for hip fracture [8–11] and joint arthroplasty [12] improves with dietary supplementation. Older patients with a hip fracture demonstrate an increase in serum insulin-like growth factor 1 (IGF-1) in response to increased dietary protein. [10,13] IGF-1, which normally decreases in the aging process, may be responsible for the improvement seen in bone quality and outcome following fracture. It may be difficult, however, to improve nutrition in those hospitalized with a hip fracture. Many hospitalized elderly patients receive inadequate calories during their hospital stay. [14] Even if adequate calories are provided in the postoperative period, the nutritional status of malnourished patients does not improve. [15]

Pre- and perioperative medical conditions and nutrition clearly influence long-term outcome; interventions to influence those outcomes are critical and should be examined.

Ortho 3 (Level B): Observational and case-control studies are needed to determine the elements of preoperative evaluation and treatment that are associated with reduction in mortality in older orthopedic surgery patients.

Ortho 4 (Level B): **Case-control studies are needed to compare the incidence of malnutrition among older hip fracture patients to that in the general population of older adults. Databases examining risk factors for hip fracture should be expanded (when possible) to include detailed nutritional measures.**

Ortho 5 (Level B, A): **Observational studies using multivariate regression analysis are needed to identify which nutritional deficiencies (eg, calcium, protein) appear to be predictive of bad outcomes following hip surgery in older patients. Randomized controlled trials based on these findings are then needed to determine the type and duration of nutritional supplementation that would most effectively improve surgical outcome and fracture healing.**

DEGENERATIVE JOINT DISEASE

Osteoarthritis (OA, degenerative joint disease) is the most common articular disease among those aged 65 and older. It commonly leads to decreased function and loss of independence. Although the joints of the hand are the most commonly affected, they are less likely than the knee or hip to be symptomatic.

Clinically, OA is diagnosed by pain that worsens with activity and lessens with rest. Joints may feel as though they are locking or giving way. Older adults with OA demonstrate decreased flexibility [16] and decreased quadriceps strength. [17] Impairment in mobility often leads to difficulty with ADLs. Painful ambulation and disturbances in gait, as are commonly seen in arthritic joints, may predispose an older person to falling. [18] A self-reported history of arthritis and painful or limited motion is predictive of recurrent nonsyncopal falls by older adults. [19] There are many other factors that contribute to falling, including lower-extremity muscle weakness; deficits in balance; impaired visual, proprioceptive, and cognitive function; sedative medications; and comorbid medical conditions. The contribution of a single factor such as hip or knee OA to falling is difficult to estimate and should be a topic of further research. [20]

Pharmacologic management of OA usually begins with acetaminophen, the recommended analgesic for symptomatic OA in adults. In cases where acetaminophen at full dosage (3000 to 4000 mg per day) does not control symptoms, nonsteroidal anti-inflammatory drugs (NSAIDs) may be used. These medications exert their anti-inflammatory and analgesic effects by inhibition of prostaglandin synthesis via inactivation of the COX enzymes. Reduction of prostaglandin synthesis can have a negative impact on the kidneys and stomach, leading to renal impairment and gastric ulceration. These agents are also associated with sodium retention that can lead to hypertension or edema. Elderly patients taking NSAIDs are particularly vulnerable to these side effects; 20% to 30% of all hospitalizations and deaths due to peptic ulcer disease in this age group are attributable to NSAID therapy. [21]

Selective COX-2 inhibitors, celecoxib and rofecoxib, have been studied in patients with OA. Celecoxib has been found to be more effective than placebo and comparable in efficacy with naproxen in patients with hip or knee OA, and rofecoxib has been shown to be comparable to ibuprofen and diclofenac in patients with hip or knee OA. [21] Endoscopic studies have demonstrated a lower incidence of gastroduodenal ulcers than with conventional NSAID therapy and comparable to that of placebo. [21]

Local treatments include topical capsaicin and methylsalicylate creams as adjunctive agents. Intra-articular injections of cortisone may be effective when there are effusions or local inflammatory signs. [22]

Intra-articular injections of hyaluronate and hylan are now often being used for the treatment of symptomatic knee osteoarthrosis. A randomized controlled clinical trial of three (hylan) or five (hyaluronate) weekly intra-articular injections showed that they provided sustained pain relief and improved function, at least as effectively as continuous treatment with NSAIDs, with fewer side effects. [23,24] It is not currently known how this substance exerts its therapeutic effect.

Exercise benefits elderly persons, improving symptoms in those with arthritis and preventing hip fracture by increasing bone density [25] and muscle strength [26] and thereby decreasing falling. [27] Other studies have shown that resistance training in older adults increases muscle mass [28] and improves neural coordination and strength. [29]

OA is a common and morbid problem in later life, and painful arthritis of the hip or knee is a risk factor for falls. Further research is needed to define the importance of OA of the knee or hip as an independent risk factor for falls and to examine the risks and benefits of surgical and nonsurgical therapies on risk reduction.

SURGICAL TREATMENT OF DEGENERATIVE JOINT DISEASE

Older patients may be more vulnerable to joint disease because of age-related changes in the musculoskeletal system. The surgical management of joint disease consists largely of joint replacement. Joint replacement surgery can significantly improve patients' health and well-being. An outcome study found that following hip or knee replacement, those patients who were 75 years of age and older had improved their preoperative scores on the Medical Outcomes Study 36-item Short Form Health Survey (SF-36), becoming similar to population norms for this age group. [30] A review of 99 consecutive elective hip and knee arthroplasties in patients aged 80 years and older found significantly improved postoperative knee and hip scores with no increased complication rate when they were compared with a younger, otherwise matched control group. [31] Postoperative outcome has been demonstrated to be predominantly dependent on preoperative function, [32] and not age. Surgical management of joint disease can improve physical function, which could positively influence comorbidities, improve strength and balance, and reduce the rate of injurious falls.

DEGENERATIVE DISEASE OF THE HIP

Surgical treatment of osteoarthritis of the hip in the older patient is limited to total joint arthroplasty. Advanced age alone does not appear to be a contraindication to joint reconstruction. Poor outcomes appear to be related to comorbidities rather than age. The best outcomes for total hip arthroplasty have, however, been shown in those younger than 75. [33] Total hip replacement in patients aged 80 and older results in more complications than in younger patients, including increased rates of dislocation and femoral fractures. [34] However, total hip replacement improves pain and physical activity [35] and increases independence and function. [36]

Fixation of the components in total hip arthroplasty is a topic of considerable debate. A cementless acetabular component is most commonly used. Concern about the increased cost of porous coated implants and the ability for bony ingrowth in the older patient have generally led to the use of a cemented femoral stem in the older patient. However, Konstantoulakis et al reviewed hip arthroplasties in patients aged 65 and older and found that uncemented hip arthroplasties in this age group showed no signs of subsidence or osteolysis after 4 years of follow-up. [37] An autopsy study by Lester et al of cementless femoral components, with an average time in situ of 22 months, in patients with an average age of 87 years found that the implants were well fixed and stable. [38] It would seem from the literature that age has no bearing on the success of different fixation methods, cement versus bony ingrowth. Cost, however, may be a significant issue.

Wear debris may lead to implant loosening. The atrophy of bone and muscle may also be a contributing factor in implant loosening. However, pelvic osteolysis, which can result from polyethylene wear debris, was not found in patients older than 70 years followed for a minimum of 5 years. [39] The influence of age on cellular response to wear debris has not been studied. Aging affects cell number and most likely affects cellular response. This is potentially an interesting area of study.

When implants become loose, they often become painful, necessitating revision surgery. Revision hip surgery in patients over age 75 has been found to improve function and relieve pain, although the complication rate (death 13.3% and dislocation 20%) was higher than in patients younger than 75. [40]

The incidence of dislocation of total hip components is 1% to 2%. The most common causes of recurrent dislocation, reported in a study conducted by Joshi et al, are component malposition (58%) and failure of the abductor mechanism (42%). [41] Ekelund et al found a higher dislocation rate for total hip replacements performed for complications from proximal femoral fractures. [42] Treatment may consist of revision surgery or repair of the abductor mechanism, if possible. Revision of a total hip replacement to bipolar arthroplasty (large head with no acetabular component) has been shown to be helpful as a salvage treatment for instability of the hip. [43]

Hip disease is a problem that limits the quality of life and functional independence of older persons. Advances will depend on studies to address areas of uncertainty in treatment, such as optimal techniques for fixation, outcomes after hip revision, the effect of age on wear debris, and prevention of periprosthetic fracture.

DEGENERATIVE DISEASE OF THE KNEE

Surgical options for the arthritic knee include arthroscopy and arthroplasty. Arthroscopic debridement of the arthritic knee has been shown to improve function, decrease pain, and decrease need for total joint replacement. [44] However, patients with angular malalignment of the knee do poorly following arthroscopic debridement, [45,46] and this is a more significant factor than age in outcome. [46] Results of a recent randomized controlled clinical trial have shown no difference in outcome between placebo and arthroscopic debridement and arthroscopic lavage of osteoarthritic knees. [47]

End-stage osteoarthritis of the knee is generally treated with total knee arthroplasty that reliably provides significant and persistent relief of pain and improved physical function. Age does not appear to have a negative impact on patient outcomes. [48] Patients over the age of 80 followed for 12 months after total knee replacement demonstrated improved pain, emotional reaction, sleep, and physical mobility. [49] Those older than 85 had significant improvement in pain and function after total knee replacement, although most still required the use of a cane for walking outdoors. [50,51] Successful knee replacement surgery has been demonstrated in patients 90 and older. Although no surgical complications occurred in this age group, there were several nonsurgical complications, including confusion, urinary retention, atrial fibrillation, atrial flutter, gallstone retention, and gastrointestinal bleeding. [52]

All total knee components are generally cemented, especially in elderly patients. Cemented, all-polyethylene tibial components have been recommended for patients older than 75 because the component is less expensive, [53] and studies have shown a high rate of survivorship without the need for revision surgery and without symptomatic loosening. [54] In recent years, patellar resurfacing has been controversial. Studies have shown, however, that patellar resurfacing results in better stair-climbing ability and improved overall function. [55]

Interestingly, after total knee arthroplasty, bone mineral density of the proximal femur improves. [56] This increase in bone density may be related to an increase in loading of the proximal femur as a result of improved mobility. This improvement in bone density could prevent or lessen the likelihood of an injurious fall.

Arthroscopy of osteoarthritic knees has been shown to be unsuccessful in the management of symptoms. The role of knee arthroscopy in the older patient with knee pain is unclear. Although the potential benefits of knee replacement are clear, there remain several unanswered issues: patient selection for various procedures, issues of optimal hardware, and the outcomes related to gait and balance.

DEGENERATIVE DISEASE OF THE SHOULDER

Degenerative disease of the shoulder is fairly common. Out of 100 randomly chosen people aged 65 and older, 34% were found to have significant shoulder pain and 30% had disability related to decreased shoulder movement. [57] Rotator cuff disease is the major cause of shoulder disability. The degenerative change in the rotator cuff that occurs as a result of overuse can lead to a tear with minimal trauma. Large tears in the rotator cuff are more common in the older population. [58] Tears of the rotator cuff may result in the loss of the primary stabilizers of the glenohumeral joint, leading to articular wear and arthritis.

Treatment of rotator cuff disease generally begins with rotator cuff strengthening exercises and anti-inflammatory medication. In a review of 124 patients with rotator cuff tears treated conservatively, those with well-preserved motion and strength did well with nonoperative treatment, in contrast to those with limited motion and strength on first evaluation. [59] Patients who experience significant sleep loss due to shoulder pain are unlikely to be satisfied with nonoperative treatment. [60]

Rotator cuff repair is usually associated with an acromioplasty and occasionally a distal clavicle resection. Surgery is often performed in an open manner through a standard approach, with the deltoid removed from the acromion and distal clavicle. In general, the larger the rotator cuff tear, the poorer the results. [58,61] A follow-up study nearly 7 years after open rotator cuff repair in 72 patients found that age was not a factor in functional outcome. [61] Retrospective reviews of 92 patients aged 62 and older [62] and 69 patients aged 70 and older [63] found, with standardized scoring, improved function, decreased pain, and satisfactory results more than 2 years following open rotator cuff repair.

Rehabilitation after rotator cuff surgery is important. The greatest improvement in strength occurs in the first 6 months after surgery, but strength continues to improve 12 months after surgery [64] and can ultimately equal that of the nonoperative shoulder. [65]

Symptomatic, failed repairs of massive rotator cuff tears can be managed with muscle transfer as a salvage procedure. The latissimus dorsi [66] or central quadriceps tendon can be used as a free tendon graft. Harvest of the central quadriceps tendon in elderly patients was found to be associated with significant reduction in knee reliability and function. [67]

Significant degenerative change of the glenohumeral joint is initially treated with anti-inflammatory medication and function-maintaining exercise. Surgical management may consist of total shoulder arthroplasty, hemiarthroplasty, or bipolar hemiarthroplasty.

Shoulder arthroplasty is commonly performed for end-stage glenohumeral arthritis. Total shoulder arthroplasty involves resurfacing of the glenoid in addition to replacement of the humeral head. The indications for resurfacing the glenoid have not been clearly defined, but generally resurfacing is reserved for cases with an intact rotator cuff. Total shoulder arthroplasty demonstrated significantly greater pain relief and improved internal rotation than that achieved with hemiarthroplasty. [68] Hemiarthroplasty is often utilized to eliminate the problem of glenoid loosening, which can occur in total shoulder arthroplasty as a result of proximal humeral migration due to a torn rotator cuff. Improvement in function and comfort has been demonstrated following hemiarthroplasty performed in patients with massive rotator cuff tearing. [69,70] Bipolar hemiarthroplasty is also used to treat glenohumeral arthritis associated with rotator cuff tearing. It has been theorized that the oversized humeral head would increase the stability of the joint, increase the abductor lever arm, and power and prevent impingement of the tuberosities. Concerns have been raised regarding the potential for overstuffing the glenohumeral joint and the generation of polyethylene wear debris. A review of the literature did not find any reports comparing bipolar hemiarthroplasty with standard hemiarthroplasty in the rotator cuff–deficient shoulder.

Although shoulder disease is common and disabling, much remains to be learned on its optimal surgical management. Changes in the aging shoulder and in potential tissue donor sites will likely influence possible surgical approaches. The goals for improved function from total knee arthroplasty are readily identified, but range and function goals for the shoulder may be more subtle.

COMPLICATIONS OF JOINT REPLACEMENT SURGERY

Thromboembolism

Venous thromboembolism occurs in 40% to 70% of patients who undergo hip or knee replacement without postoperative thromboprophylaxis. Patients who have total knee arthroplasty are 3.2 times more likely than patients who have total hip arthroplasty to develop deep-vein thrombosis (DVT). [71] Patients aged 65 and older who have had total hip arthroplasty and who have an increased body mass index have an increased risk of rehospitalization for thromboembolic events. [72]

With thromboprophylaxis, the incidence of DVT is 15% in those having hip replacement and 30% in those with knee replacements. [73] The risk for thromboembolism continues for at least 1 month postoperatively, [74] with the rate of proximal DVT 2.4% at 1 week after surgery and increasing to 8.2% at 1 month after surgery. [75] The risk of fatal pulmonary embolism after total knee arthroplasty without thromboprophylaxis is 0.4%. [76]

Those with hip fractures demonstrate a high rate of DVT, and, if surgery is delayed more than 48 hours, 62% of patients have venographic evidence of DVT. [77] Autopsies performed on patients with surgically treated hip fractures demonstrate that the incidence of fatal pulmonary embolism is between 0.37% and 3.3%. [78]

A variety of medications and mechanisms have been proposed to decrease the rate of thromboembolism. The safest and most efficacious method of prophylaxis remains controversial. Mechanical modalities include external pneumatic compression sleeves and foot pumps. These work by decreasing stasis in the gastroc-soleus complex, by improving venous return, and also by increasing fibrinolysis. They are placed on the patient prior to and worn throughout surgery. It is recommended that the sleeves be discontinued when the patient is more ambulatory. Pneumatic compression has been shown to be effective after total hip arthroplasty only in patients with body mass index (weight in kg / height in meters ^{2}) of less than 25. [72] The arteriovenous impulse system has been shown to be effective in reducing thromboembolic events after hemiarthroplasty of the hip [79] and comparable to enoxaparin in preventing DVT following total hip replacement. [80]

Aspirin has long been used for thromboprophylaxis. In the Pulmonary Embolism Prevention (PEP) trial, [81] 17,444 randomized patients undergoing surgery for hip fracture or elective arthroplasty received 160 mg of aspirin daily for 35 days after surgery. The study concluded that this regimen reduced pulmonary embolism 43% and symptomatic DVT 29%. In this study, thromboembolic events were not recorded if they were not symptomatic. With this protocol there was no significant increase in bleeding complications. Aspirin has been shown to effective for thromboprophylaxis in doses of 160 mg [81] and 375 mg. [79]

Warfarin has been shown to be protective against DVT after total hip and knee arthroplasty. The goal is to keep the INR between 2 and 3. Warfarin used in combination with pneumatic compression results in a prevalence of DVT of 5% and a prevalence of bleeding complications of 0.9%. [82] A meta-analysis of thromboembolic prophylaxis following elective total hip arthroplasty [83] found that warfarin and pneumatic compression were the best prophylactic agents in terms of safety and efficacy. Sensitivity to anticoagulant effects is enhanced by age 80 years or greater, hip fracture fixation, and weight greater than 180 pounds. [84]

Enoxaparin, a low-molecular-weight heparin (LMWH), is commonly used for thromboprophylaxis. In elderly patients with hip fracture, a 40 mg once daily dose of enoxaparin was found to be effective in prevention of DVT without major bleeding complications. [85] The rate of thromboembolic event during and after prophylaxis with enoxaparin has been reported to be 2% and the rate of major hemorrhage 2.9%. [73] Bleeding complications are reported by 23.7% of individuals over the age of 65 receiving enoxaparin but by only 16.5% of control persons; [86] the result is a lower hemoglobin level and a higher transfusion rate in the enoxaparin group. The complication rate was lower if the first dose of enoxaparin was given more than 10 hours postoperatively. A meta-analysis revealed that LMWH may be more protective against thromboembolism following total joint arthroplasty but that there was a slightly greater risk of clinically important bleeding. [87] A study of 263 patients who had undergone total knee arthroplasty found an 11.3% incidence of bleeding complications in those patients using enoxaparin but only a 4.6% incidence in patients using warfarin, with no significant difference in the rate of DVT between the groups. [88] The bleeding complications reported with the LMWHs may be attributed to the fact that these medications are cleared by renal excretion. Patients with decreased renal function may develop accumulation of the drug and hemorrhagic problems. [89]

There are several effective therapies for the prevention of thromboembolism in older patients who have undergone hip and knee procedures. Most of these are associated with some risk of bleeding and some residual risk of thromboembolism. The optimal regimen for older patients and for specific procedures remains to be determined. For further discussion of thromboembolism and surgery, see Chapter 13.

Periprosthetic Fracture

Periprosthetic femur fractures have been estimated to occur in 2.5% of patients following total hip arthroplasty. [90] The cause is usually loosening of the implant due to osteoporosis [91] or osteolysis secondary to wear debris. [92] The incidence of these fractures is likely to increase the longer the implant is in place. Treatment can consist of plate fixation if the implant is stable or stem revision with or without cerclage wiring and bone strut grafts if the initial stem is loose. [93–95]

Fracture around a total knee arthroplasty generally occurs around the femoral component. Treatment may consist of open reduction and internal fixation [96] or intramedullary rodding, [97] that is, placing the rod in the intercondylar notch, between the medial and lateral femoral condyles of the femoral component. If the fracture is comminuted, treatment is difficult. Tani et al have described intramedullary fibular grafting as a means for reconstructing large segmental defects. [98]

Risk factors for periprosthetic fractures resemble those for osteoporotic fracture (old age or poor bone quality). Development of and risk for these fractures are also likely influenced by the site (hip or knee) and possibly by the nature of fixation for the device (cemented or noncemented). Further research is needed to understand causes and to design and test preventive strategies.

Infection

Infection of a joint after total hip or knee arthroplasty may be the result of hematogenous seeding. Treatment is generally removal of the implant and placement of a block of cement that has been mixed with antibiotics to act as a cement spacer. A relatively new technique is to cement total joint components loosely in place with antibiotic-impregnated cement as an "articulating" spacer. Treatment with debridement and retention of joint components and antibiotic therapy is usually successful if the infection is caught within 2 weeks of symptoms. [99] The success of these techniques in the older patient has not been established.

> *Ortho 6 (Level B)*: **Basic studies are needed to determine the mechanism of action of hylan and hyaluronate injections in providing long-term pain relief from knee arthritis. Additional clinical studies are needed to examine the long-term effect on cartilage in older persons during repeated courses of treatment.**

Ortho 7 (Level A): A randomized clinical trial is needed to examine if hylan and hyaluronate injections delay or reduce the likelihood of total knee arthroplasty in elderly patients.

Ortho 8 (Level B): Existing databases should be examined (or expanded) in an effort to determine the independent contribution that hip or knee osteoarthritis holds as a risk factor for falls by older people.

Ortho 9 (Level B): Databases examining the effects of joint replacement surgery should assess baseline and postoperative rates of falling to determine the effects of replacement on falls risk in older persons.

Ortho 10 (Level B): Further laboratory and clinical studies of COX-2 inhibitors should examine the effects of these agents in older persons on fracture healing, tissue healing (eg, after rotator cuff injury), and on bony ingrowth (into joint replacements).

Ortho 11 (Level B): Case-control studies should examine the surgical and functional outcome in older patients for various methods of fixation and various surgical approaches in total hip replacement. Such studies should examine the outcomes for cementless components in osteoporotic bone.

Ortho 12 (Levels B, A): Observational studies are needed to define the outcome of revision hip surgery in elderly patients. Careful reporting of factors associated with outcome would help define future level A studies to further define the optimal approach to this problem.

Ortho 13 (Level D): Basic laboratory studies are needed to define the influence of age on the cellular response to wear debris.

Ortho 14 (Level B): Observational studies are needed to define the type of hip procedure (cemented or uncemented) that is associated with the lower incidence of periprosthetic fractures in elderly patients. Additional observational studies are needed to generate information on the outcomes of various treatments for periprosthetic fractures in preparation for hypothesis-testing studies.

Ortho 15 (Level B): Observational studies are needed to define the subpopulation of older patients who might respond to arthroscopy or meniscectomy.

Ortho 16 (Level B): Observational studies are needed to identify older patients at risk for less than optimal outcome after total knee arthroplasty, for example, those with peripheral vascular disease or neuropathy.

Ortho 17 (Level B): Additional observational studies focused on patients aged 85 years and over who undergo total knee arthroplasty are needed to identify risk factors for postoperative morbidity and to begin to define interventional strategies to reduce that risk.

Ortho 18 (Level D): Case-control studies are needed to determine whether metal-backed or all-polyethylene tibial components should be used in arthroplasty for elderly patients and whether there are indications for each.

Ortho 19 (Level B): Observational studies of older patients undergoing treatment for comminuted distal femur fractures are needed to examine the possible utility of total knee arthroplasty as a reconstructive procedure in this setting.

Ortho 20 (Level B): Observational studies are needed to further define those benefits of total knee arthroplasty (eg, increased range of motion, increased strength, decreased pain), which serve to improve gait and balance. Ultimately, such studies may begin to determine whether or not total knee arthroplasty helps to reduce the risk of hip fracture.

Ortho 21 (Level B): Case-control or focused cohort studies are needed to compare functional outcomes in older people with shoulder disease who do not undergo surgery with those who undergo rotator cuff surgery, hemiarthroplasty, or total shoulder replacement. Key outcomes for comparison include improved function and decreased pain. Such studies should address how the desired outcomes may change with age, from those aged 65 to 75 years to those aged 90 years and over.

Ortho 22 (Level A): Randomized controlled clinical trials are needed of the various preventive regimens (alone or in combination) to identify the safest and most effective treatment strategy for preventing thromboembolism after joint replacement surgery in older patients. Such studies should also address how long deep-vein thrombosis prophylaxis should continue in elderly patients who have had recent total joint replacements or hip fracture.

Ortho 23 (Level B): Further retrospective studies are needed to examine risk factors beyond age and poor bone quality for periprosthetic fractures. Case-control studies could possibly suggest protective factors, such as the nature of the implant (cemented or uncemented) and the use of antiresorptive therapies.

Ortho 24 (Level A): Randomized controlled trials are needed to determine with certainty whether specific prostheses or antiresorptive therapies would be effective at minimizing the risk of periprosthetic fracture.

Ortho 25 (Level B): Observational studies and subgroup analyses are needed to determine if features of periprosthetic infections are different in elderly patients and to examine differences in outcome for elderly patients when specific established or emerging approaches are used.

DEGENERATIVE SPINE DISEASE

Degenerative disease of the spine (spondylosis) includes spondylolisthesis, which is characterized by the forward displacement of one vertebral body on another, disc herniation or degeneration, facet joint degeneration, osteophytes, foraminal stenosis, and radiculopathy. Degenerative spondylosis and radiculopathy may occur in the cervical or lumbar spine. These conditions are usually managed conservatively.

Surgical intervention is reserved for those with progressive neurologic deficit or severe functional incapacitation. Surgical decompression in cervical spondylotic myelopathy is usually anterior decompression and fusion in patients with three or fewer levels or in patients with kyphosis; a posterior decompression is used for those with more extensive disease.[100] Elderly patients can benefit from decompression;[101–103] however, incomplete recovery is more likely in patients older than 70, and outcome has been found to be related more to the clinical picture and the duration of the symptoms than to age.[103]

Surgical treatment of lumbar spinal stenosis generally consists of decompressive laminectomy plus fusion with or without instrumentation. Patients aged 65 and older have outcomes that are as good as those for younger patients.[104] The complication rate may be higher for patients aged 75 and older[105] and has been reported to be 6%[106] to 10%.[107] After 4 years of follow-up, patients aged 60 years and over who had surgical treatment for spinal stenosis were found to have better outcomes than those who had nonsurgical treatment.[108] In a meta-analysis, patients suffering from degenerative spinal stenosis for up to 8 years were found to have responded best to decompression without fusion, whereas those with symptoms of 15 years or more had better results with decompression and fusion with instrumentation.[109] These studies suggest that earlier intervention is more successful, possibly because of better overall health and functional reserve and fewer medical comorbidities in younger patients. This is supported by the finding that the most powerful predictor of a good outcome was the patient's report of good or excellent health before surgery.[110] Shorter duration of symptoms may be associated with less nerve degeneration and atrophy. This is supported by the results of a study that revealed that the outcome following surgically treated lumbar spinal stenosis was better when there was a shorter preoperative duration of symptoms.[111] A 10-year follow-up study found that more than half of the patients evaluated their postsurgical results as excellent or good.[112]

Stenosis can recur within a few years following decompression, and the rate of recurrence has been reported to be from 18% to 27%.[111,113,114] This may be attributed to vertebral levels that had unrecognized stenosis and were, therefore, not decompressed or stabilized in the initial surgery. Bone regrowth has also been demonstrated following decompression.[115] Bone regrowth may be associated with postoperative spinal instability.[116]

Fusion with instrumentation is associated with a better outcome than fusion without instrumentation if there is instability after surgical decompression.[117] Instrumentation in an osteoporotic spine can, however, be difficult. Larger screws can be used in the pedicle, but these can cause the pedicle to fracture. The pedicle can fracture if the screw diameter is greater than 70% of the outer diameter of the pedicle in cases were bone mineral density is low.[118]

Patients with osteoporosis have less bone to harvest for fusion, and the bone is commonly of poor structural quality. A decreased number of osteoprogenitor cells in the autogenous bone graft often necessitates supplemental material to encourage osteoinduction and osteoconduction.

Advanced age does not appear to preclude benefit from cervical-spine decompressive surgery, although recovery of neurologic function may be less complete in older than in younger patients. Available studies suggest that a longer duration of symptoms prior to surgery reduces the eventual degree of recovery. Benefit is also seen from lumbar surgery, although at the risk of higher complication rates. Osteoporosis makes surgery more difficult and reduces the quality of bone harvested for grafts. These issues raise several significant research problems.

> ***Ortho 26 (Level B)***: **Observational studies are needed to examine the impact of aging on bone fusion or fracture healing and to begin examining strategies to augment the bone healing response after fusion or fracture. Candidate strategies include growth factors.**

> ***Ortho 27 (Level B)***: **Case-control or focused cohort studies are needed to refine understanding of which patients benefit (in terms of symptom control and function) most from spinal decompression versus conservative management. Important covariates include duration of symptoms and degree of neurologic deficits and perhaps the degree of osteoporosis. Such studies should attempt to clarify when elderly patients should be referred for spinal decompression in order to experience maximum benefit.**

DEGENERATIVE DISEASE OF THE FOOT AND ANKLE

There is a high incidence of foot problems in the elderly age group. If older persons are to remain ambulatory, foot care is essential. Foot deformity resulting from aging or degenerative disease can lead to gait and balance disturbance. A comprehensive review of the literature found very few articles addressing foot-related issues in the elderly population.

Shoe wear is an important factor in maintaining balance. A randomized controlled trial of twenty-five patients to evaluate balance while barefoot and in different types of shoe wear determined that bare feet and walking shoes maximize balance and that high heels create a balance hazard. [119] (See also Chapter 13, section on falls prevention.)

Onychomycosis is a common problem affecting 2% to 13% of all persons. Treatment is oral antifungal agents. The efficacy and side effects of these medications in elderly patients have not been well established. A review of the literature did not find any articles pertaining exclusively to the elderly age group.

Posterior tibial tendon insufficiency and hallux valgus often lead to severe deformity of the foot. Treatment can range from conservative care with shoe wear modifications and orthotics to extensive reconstruction and fusion. A review of the literature, however, found no articles evaluating reconstruction in the older patient.

Fractures of the ankle are relatively common. Of all ankle fractures, 20% to 30% occur in elderly persons. [120] A study comparing operatively treated and nonoperatively treated ankle fractures in patients aged 65 and over found better outcomes in the nonoperatively treated group. [120]

The treatment of ankle arthritis is either fusion or total ankle arthroplasty. The results of ankle fusion can deteriorate over time as a result of transverse tarsal or subtalar degenerative joint disease. Elderly patients are thought to be good candidates for total joint replacement because degenerative changes in other areas of the foot are most likely and because older patients may be less active than younger ones. A review of the literature found no articles dealing with this procedure exclusively in the elderly patient.

Relatively little is known about the effect of foot and ankle problems on gait and balance in older people, even though these would appear to be important outcomes when assessing the utility of surgery for such disorders in this population. Research needs to define indications for surgery and orthotics in the treatment of disorders of the foot and ankle in the older person.

> *Ortho 28 (Level B)*: **Observational studies examining how foot and ankle deformity influence gait and balance in the older person are needed. Those deformities that are associated with significant gait problems should be the focus of research on surgical and nonsurgical approaches to these conditions. Appropriate outcome measures (eg, healing, gait improvement) from specific techniques of foot and ankle reconstruction need to be defined. In addition, more study is needed to identify characteristics of footwear that maximize balance.**

> *Ortho 29 (Level C)*: **Controlled trials are needed to identify safe and effective treatment for fungal disease of the foot.**

BONE INSUFFICIENCY AND FALLS

Bone loss is commonly associated with aging. Significant bone loss, which results in skeletal fragility, is termed *osteoporosis*. (See also Chapter 9, section on Osteoporosis.) Osteoporosis is a major health problem, affecting 10 million people in the United States. Another 18 million are at risk for developing the disease. [121] Low bone mineral density predicts fracture risk but cannot identify individuals who will have a fracture. Therefore, an understanding of the factors that result in a fall and the subsequent fracture is essential. At least 30% of individuals fall at least once in their life. Only 5% of falls result in fracture. Most fractures occur in the home. [122] The nature of the fall determines the type of fracture, and bone density and factors that increase or attenuate the force determine whether a fracture will occur. [123] A prospective case-control study demonstrated that a fall to the side, decreased bone density in the hip, and impaired mobility were all-important risk factors for hip fracture. [124] Neuromuscular and visual impairments, as well as femoral neck bone mineral density, are significant and independent predictors of hip fracture in elderly mobile women. [125–127] Balance is a prerequisite for mobility and ADL function [128] and is affected by medical comorbidities. Herndon et al reported on chronic medical conditions in patients aged 65 and older, finding that a self-reported history of anemia or stroke increased risk of a fall. [129] A comprehensive review of risk factors for falls summarizes 11 separate risk factors and reviews studies that demonstrate that the greater the number of risk factors, the greater the likelihood of falls. [130] This report also summarizes the strategies that have, in controlled trials, been shown to reduce the incidence of falls, although none has been sufficiently powered to demonstrate a reduction in fractures. (See also Chapter 13, section on falls prevention.)

Nursing-home residents are at particular risk for injurious falls. Institutionalized fallers have low serum 25-hydroxyvitamin D and high serum parathyroid hormone levels. [131] Minimal trauma fractures are common, usually with no clear precipitating factors other than severely impaired mobility. [132] Extreme weight loss and poor health have been shown to increase the risk of hip fracture. [133,134]

With aging, decreased muscle strength and impaired coordination are common, which results in an increased likelihood of falling and a decreased ability to break the fall. Physical activity throughout life has been found to reduce the risk of falling. [135–138] Fractures of the hip, wrist, and spine are a significant cause of morbidity and mortality among elderly persons. The cost of treating these fractures is $14 billion annually, and this is expected to increase to $60 billion by the year 2020. [1]

Fractures occur in osteoporotic bone, but osteoporosis per se does not predict who will fracture. Falls are the result of cumulative risk factors, and there is good evidence for strategies that reduce falls in community-dwelling older persons who have fallen. Whether those same strategies reduce fractures has not been determined (sample size inadequately powered). Risk factors for minimal-trauma fractures are being developed, although intervention studies have not been undertaken. Studies are generally lacking on the best surgical approaches, such as using joint replacement for fractures that occur close to a joint and using techniques or materials that provide the best fixation in osteopenic bone.

> *Ortho 30 (Level A)*: **Adequately powered randomized clinical trials are needed to determine if falls-prevention strategies for older persons will translate into fracture reduction for treated patients.**

> *Ortho 31 (Level A)*: **Cohort studies or randomized controlled trials are needed to compare the functional recovery of patients whose fractures occur close to a joint and who are treated with either total joint replacement or standard care.**

> *Ortho 32 (Level B)*: **Methodologic studies are needed to describe outcomes with various approaches to fixation in osteopenic bone.**

FRACTURES OF THE HIP

The number of elderly persons with hip fractures will double to 2.6 million by the year 2025. [139] The lifetime risk of hip fracture is 11.1% for men and 22.7% for women. [140] Almost half of all hip fractures occur in patients aged 80 or over. An estimated 18% to 28% of older hip fracture patients die within 1 year of their fracture. [140]

There are many determinants of hip fractures. The two main factors are falls and decreased bone density. Increased fracture risk has been demonstrated with lifestyle factors, such as weight loss or low body weight, [133,134,141–143] decreased physical activity, [143,144] increased tobacco use, [145,146] and poor socioeconomic status. [147] Increased fracture risk has also been found to be associated with medical comorbidities such as stroke, [148] end-stage renal disease, [149,150] and visual impairment. [151]

There has been considerable debate as to which came first, the fall or the fracture. Most studies report that the fall precedes the fracture. In fact, over 90% of all fractures are the result of falling [152–156] Hip fractures typically result from falls that result in direct impact on the hip, typically a fall to the side. External hip protectors have been found to prevent hip fractures. [157,158] A controlled study [159] and a randomized controlled clinical trial [160] found the rate of hip fracture to be significantly lower when hip protectors are worn. However, one study found only 44% adherence in wearing the device. [159] Reasons cited for not wearing the protector included skin irritation and being bedridden. (See also Chapter 13, section on falls prevention.)

For all but the very sick, operative treatment of hip fractures is recommended. Mortality rates following nonoperative treatment for hip fractures has been found to be high. [161] The timing of surgery following hip fracture is critical. The sooner the better, but medical stabilization before surgery is required. Once the patient is medically stable, surgery is recommended, if possible within 24 hours. Operative delay more than 2 calendar days has been found to be associated with higher mortality within 1 year in patients who were independent, cognitively intact ,and able to walk prior to fracture. [162] There is a significant increase in mortality in those patients whose surgery is delayed more than 24 hours. [163,164] The choice of regional or general anesthesia does not influence outcome. [165]

Fractures of the hip include intertrochanteric fractures and femoral neck fractures. There may be some differences in the patients that sustain each type of fracture. In a prospective study of elderly patients admitted for hip fracture, patients with intertrochanteric fractures were found to be slightly older and sicker and to have longer hospital stays; they were less likely at 2 months postfracture to have recovered ADLs than were patients with a femoral neck fracture. [166] Recovery at 1 year following hip fracture did not differ between fracture types. Patients with an intertrochanteric hip fracture had higher mortality rates at 2 and 6 months after fracture than did those with a femoral neck fracture.

The basic principle of treating hip fractures is secure fracture fixation to promote healing and early mobilization. Intertrochanteric hip fractures are generally treated by open reduction and internal fixation. A sliding hip screw–plate construct (compression hip screw) or a cephalomedullary nail (gamma nail) may be used for treatment. Although there has been shown to be less femoral shortening with the gamma nail, [167] no difference between the two treatments with respect to functional recovery has been found. [168] An increased complication rate has been shown with the gamma nail. [168] The gamma nail may, however, be a more versatile implant, useful in treating a variety of fracture patterns. [169] As there is currently no literature to suggest that use of this device improves outcome in routine intertrochanteric hip fractures, the sliding hip screw is thought to be the implant of choice for treating intertrochanteric hip fractures. For peritrochanteric fractures or fractures with subtrochanteric extension, the gamma nail is superior in stability and decreases operative blood loss, [170–172] and complications can be minimized by attention to surgical technique. [173]

Hemiarthroplasty has been proposed for treating unstable intertrochanteric hip fractures in debilitated elderly patients. [174,175] Hemiarthroplasty can also be used to salvage an intertrochanteric hip fracture that has had a failure of internal fixation. [176]

Femoral neck fractures may be fixed with internal fixation if nondisplaced. However, Hudson et al found higher revision and mortality rates in patients who had internal fixation than in those who had hemiarthroplasty for femoral neck fracture. [177] Internal fixation for femoral neck fracture has been associated with greater readmission and reoperation than hemiarthroplasty, without improvement in function. [178] In a review of 312 community-dwelling ambulatory patients admitted for femoral neck fracture, the choice of hemiarthroplasty or internal fixation also was found to have no impact on recovery of physical ADLs or instrumental ADLs. [179]

Hemiarthroplasty is performed when femoral neck fractures are displaced or the quality of the bone is poor. Cement may be used as a grout to improve stem fixation. There is no difference between the use of a bipolar or unipolar hemiarthroplasty for the treatment of femoral neck fractures. [180–182] Furthermore, the bipolar prosthesis has been shown to have increased polyethylene wear because of impingement of the metal shell notching the femoral component. [183] Patients with cemented implants have been found to have a higher perioperative mortality than those in which no cement was used. [184] However, in a randomized prospective trial comparing cemented and uncemented bipolar hemiarthroplasties in 53 patients with femoral neck fracture, the patients with cemented stems were found to fare better with less pain and need for fewer walking aids than did those with uncemented stems, and there was no difference in complications. [185]

Total hip arthroplasty may also be used to treat femoral neck fractures. Better outcome following femoral neck fracture has been reported with total hip arthroplasty than with hemiarthroplasty [186] or with internal fixation. [187,188] Revision rates have been shown to be lower for total hip arthroplasty (2.2%) than for cemented hemiarthroplasty (7.9%) and uncemented hemiarthroplasty (13%). [189] An increased rate of operative complications (17%), [190] dislocations (12%), [188] and implant loosening [191] has been shown if total hip arthroplasty is performed for femoral neck fractures than if the replacement is done for osteoarthritis.

Immediate postoperative weight bearing to tolerance following hip fracture fixation has not been shown to result in hardware failure or loss of fixation. [192]

Delirium is a common problem following operative treatment of hip fractures. Stromberg et al in a randomized clinical trial found a 13% incidence of delirium postoperatively in patients with hip fractures. [193] Postoperative delirium is more likely to occur in patients aged 80 and older, those with prefracture cognitive impairment, and ADL functional impairment or high medical comorbidity; if the delirium persists more than 1 month following hip fracture, there is poor functional recovery. [194] Following hip fracture, patients with dementia, delirium, or depression are more likely to remain in the hospital longer. [195] For further discussion of delirium in surgical patients, see the chapter on cross-cutting issues (Chapter 13).

Bone mineral density decreases in the operative side following femoral neck fracture. [196] A decline in bone mineral density has also been demonstrated in the contralateral hip in the year following hip fracture. [197,198] Bone mineral density does, however, increase in the following 5 years, in most cases replacing the loss from the first year. Those patients who do not regain bone density in the contralateral hip are at risk for a second hip fracture. [199] Patients with a history of hip fracture have a greater risk for developing another hip fracture. A review of orthopedists and internists found that neither specialty adequately addresses the prevention of a second hip fracture. [200]

The primary determinants of long-term survival following hip fracture are host factors and not injury severity. [3] The mortality following hip fracture has been found to be predictable on admission by the number of medical conditions: with no other diagnosis, mortality is 0%; with one or two, mortality is 14%; and with three or more, the mortality is 24%. [4] Following a hip fracture, medically ill and functionally impaired patients demonstrate an immediate increase in mortality, but those with no comorbidities and few impairments have a gradual increase in mortality that continues for 5 years postfracture. [201] Increased mortality has also been demonstrated in those with mental impairment [195,202] and decreased postoperative ambulatory level. [203] Age at the time of fracture is also predictive of mortality. [204] The 1-year mortality of nonagenarians is 46% [205] and of centenarians is 56%. [206] Men in general appear to have a higher mortality rate after hip fracture than women. [204,207] Poor et al attributed this to interaction of the fracture with serious underlying medical conditions. [208]

Following hip fracture, there is a dramatic decline in physical function at 2 years that is independent of the effects of increasing age, pre-existing medical conditions, and disabilities. [209] Prefracture mobility is the most significant factor in predicting continued ability to live at home. [210] By 1 year, only 41% of hip fracture patients are back to their prefracture ambulatory ability, 40% of those ambulating require assistive devices, 12% go from community ambulation to household ambulation, and 8% become nonfunctional ambulators. [211] Patients aged 85 and older who live independently and alone before a fracture are at high risk for nonrecovery of ADLs and instrumental ADLs. Recovery of ADLs occurs in only 73%, and only 48% recover instrumental ADLs. [212] The chance that a patient with a hip fracture will make any further recovery after 4 months is minimal, and that recovery is directly influenced by increasing age, coexisting diseases, and complications. [213] Only 17% of institutionalized elderly patients regain their overall functional ability, and only 13% return to their pre-injury ambulatory status.

Hip fracture is a disorder of late life and one that is too often associated with substantial long-term disability. Although surgical techniques have progressed and pre- and perioperative care have improved, long-term outcomes have failed to keep pace. Surgical advances include improved devices for fixation, better understanding of the importance of timing (best if in the first 24 hours), and weight bearing as tolerated for most repairs. Further advances can be expected as other key issues are addressed: whether or not cement should be used with hemiarthroplasty; comparisons of available techniques for repair of intertrochanteric fracture to identify the optimal approach; and techniques or interventions to reduce hardware failure. Reducing 1- and 2-year mortality and improving long-term functional outcomes for patients is a more daunting task and will likely require approaches to reduce perioperative delirium, to improve continuity between care settings (hospital, rehabilitation setting, and home), to optimally manage medical comorbidities (including osteoporosis), and to provide effective (perhaps extended) rehabilitation and nutritional support services.

Ortho 33 (Level B): **Observational studies are needed to examine the effect of shortening of the fractured limb on gait and balance.**

Ortho 34 (Level B): **Observational studies are needed to learn whether modalities such as electrical stimulation or ultrasound can speed the fracture healing response in the older patient and therefore decrease fracture collapse or hardware failure.**

Ortho 35 (Level B): **Methodologic studies are needed to identify elderly patients with hip fracture who are at high risk for operative intervention and postoperative complications and to devise clinical pathways for their care. Database analyses of the pre-hospital,** in-hospital, and rehabilitation periods of elderly orthopedic patients should be performed to identify clinical management strategies that result in decreased morbidity and improved functional recovery.

Ortho 36 (Level A): Controlled trials are needed to compare outcomes using cement and noncemented hardware for hemiarthroplasty. Additional controlled trials are needed to compare techniques for repair of intertrochanteric hip fractures.

Ortho 37 (Level B): Current clinical databases should be expanded to include long-term and functional outcomes of older orthopedic surgical patients recovering from hip fracture.

FRACTURES OF THE WRIST

Wrist fractures are a common consequence of osteoporosis. Wrist fractures are more likely to occur in women with low bone mineral density who are healthy and active and have good neuromuscular function, when they put out the hand to break the fall. [214] As common as distal radius fractures are in the elderly age group, there is a paucity of research regarding treatment and outcome. The expert consensus seems to be that most of these fractures do well in the elderly patient, regardless of treatment. However, this assumption has not been well studied. Fractures may require either closed manipulation and immobilization or surgical treatment.

Older patients with low levels of activity have been found to be satisfied with wrist fractures treated nonoperatively; 88% are able to return to their prefracture activities. [215] Up to 30 degrees of dorsal angulation and 5 mm of radial shortening have been found to be acceptable in elderly patients. [216]

More active individuals may be candidates for operative stabilization. Surgical treatment may consist of closed reduction and pinning, open reduction and pinning, open reduction and internal fixation with plate and screws, or external fixation alone or in combination with wiring or plating. Percutaneous pinning is simple and has been shown to give results superior to those of manipulation and casting alone. [217] If the fracture is extensively comminuted, however, reduction may be lost.

Plate fixation [218,219] is advantageous because it may be used in combination with bone grafting to restore structural integrity, and plate fixation allows for earlier motion. Plates are commonly placed on the dorsal aspect of the wrist and as a result can interfere with extensor tendon activity.

External fixation is commonly used to address the concern of radial shortening and comminution. This procedure uses an external device that applies pins proximally and distally to the fracture and applies traction to keep the fracture out to length. Bone grafting of the fracture site is commonly carried out to supplement the fixation. [220] Unfortunately, because the fracture is at the end of the bone, the external fixator needs to span the wrist joint, which can result in wrist stiffness. Also, because the distal pins are placed in the metacarpal and this bone is small, fractures can result. Frame loosening can occur as a result of placement of the pins in osteoporotic bone. Bone graft or bone substitute is commonly used for filling in the void after an impacted fracture is brought back out to length. Options for bone void filler include autograft, allograft, and bone void fillers. Autograft is often not a good choice for the elderly patient, as the number of mesenchymal cells in the host bone may be limited. In addition, because many of these patients are osteoporotic, the structural integrity of the graft material is not adequate. Allograft bone is commonly used instead. Additionally, there are many bone substitutes. An injectable, remodellable bone cement has been developed, but its use for elderly patients has not been studied. However, Sanchez-Sotelo et al have shown it to provide good results in comparison with conservative treatment. [221]

Outcome 10 years following distal radius fracture was shown by Warwick et al to be satisfactory. [222] Radial shortening and finger stiffness were found to be related to less satisfactory outcomes.

Wrist fracture is common in older women, and although it is not well studied, most patients appear to have a good outcome. However, for those fractures requiring operative intervention, issues regarding osteoporosis and whether autograft or allograft is better require further study.

> *Ortho 38 (Level B)*: **Observational studies are needed to compare operative with nonoperative management to suggest which method is better with regard to outcome (time to union and function) following wrist fracture in the older patient.**

> *Ortho 39 (Level D)*: **Descriptive studies are needed to determine the range of motion and strength of the wrist necessary for good activities of daily living function in older persons.**

> *Ortho 40 (Level D)*: **Case series describing outcomes with various fixation methods are needed to suggest the best fixation method for wrist fractures in older patients.**

> *Ortho 41 (Level C)*: **Controlled trials of various graft materials are needed to determine the best graft material to supplement wrist fracture internal fixation in older patients.**

FRACTURES OF THE SPINE

Osteoporotic vertebral compression fractures are very common, affecting 25% of women aged 70 years and older and 40% of women aged 80 and older. [223] Vertebral fractures are associated with significant performance impairments in physical, functional, and psychosocial domains [224] and increased risk of mortality [225] and hospitalization. [226]

Vertebral fractures typically occur in the lumbar and thoracic region and result in loss of normal alignment of the spine. Kyphosis can cause severely deformed posture, which commonly leads to a reduction in pulmonary capacity [227] and decreased physical mobility. [228,229] These fractures typically result from very minimal trauma, such as sneezing, lifting, bending, or coughing. Conservative treatment is generally indicated. Rest, physical therapy, and occasionally bracing are used for treatment. Nasal calcitonin has been reported to have an analgesic effect when used following compression fractures. [230]

In situations where there are persistent neurologic symptoms, surgical treatment may be indicated. Lee and Yip evaluated 497 patients with compression fractures and found a 2% incidence of spinal cord compression. [231] Treatment consisted of anterior decompression and iliac crest bone graft. The authors found incomplete recovery, but in general the results were satisfactory. Vertebroplasty is a relatively new technique involving percutaneous administration, under fluoroscopic guidance, of polymethylmethacrylate into the vertebral body. Improvement in symptoms following treatment has been reported by up to 90% of patients. [232,233] Of those with compression fractures due to metastatic disease, only half of those treated with vertebroplasty report good relief of symptoms. [233]

Complications of vertebroplasty have been reported in 6% of cases. Cortet et al found no adverse effect from the procedure, and at 6 months, no vertebral fracture had occurred. [234] With open or surgically controlled placement of the polymethylmethacrylate under fluoroscopic guidance, the potential risk of chemical, compressive, or thermal effects of cement leakage on the neural structures is eliminated. [235] Fracture adjacent to vertebrae augmented with cement has been shown as a late complication. [236]

Vertebral fractures are common and often cause severe acute and chronic pain. Surgical therapy is reserved for those with neurologic deficits. Vertebroplasty is a relatively new and promising therapy for the pain of fracture, but much remains to be learned about its indications, the timing of the procedure, and its benefits and complications.

> *Ortho 42 (Level A)*: **Randomized controlled trials are needed to compare vertebroplasty with current usual care (no treatment) in older patients. The studies should compare indications (acute and or chronic pain) for vertebroplasty, complications, benefits, and long-term effects of each approach, and they should also examine the effects on adjacent vertebrae (eg, fracture, deformity) following vertebroplasty.**

FRACTURES OF THE PROXIMAL HUMERUS

The proximal humerus commonly fractures when there is a fall directly onto the shoulder by persons whose bone quality is poor. The proximal humerus may fracture into two, three, or four parts. Treatment includes a sling with range of motion started when the patient is comfortable, internal fixation, or humeral head replacement. Nonoperative treatment of three- and four-part proximal humerus fractures has shown good results. In a 10-year follow-up of nonoperatively treated three- and four-part proximal humerus fractures, despite poor reduction and decreased range of motion, most patients were satisfied with their outcome. [237] A randomized controlled trial demonstrated that patients treated with open reduction with internal fixation had no better outcome than did patients treated nonoperatively. [238] The complication rate was higher in the operatively treated patients.

Operative treatment of proximal humerus fractures is considered when the reduction is poor. The indications for open reduction and internal fixation have generally been limited to two- and three-part fractures and some types of four-part fractures if the bone quality is adequate. Plate fixation and indirect reduction have been associated with a low rate of avascular necrosis and nonunion. [239] The valgus-impacted four-part proximal humerus fracture has been treated with open reduction and internal fixation; 74% of those treated were satisfied with their result. [240] Complications of open reduction and internal fixation include nonunion, malunion, subacromial impingement, and adhesive capsulitis.

Hemiarthroplasty has been the mainstay of treatment for significantly displaced three- and four-part proximal humerus fractures in older patients. Better results are seen if the decision to perform hemiarthroplasty is made early after the fracture. [241] After hemiarthroplasty performed for three- and four-part proximal humerus fractures, several authors have noted in their patients decreased range of motion but good pain relief. [242–244] Others have found their patients to have decreased range of motion and continued pain. [245,246] Complications of hemiarthroplasty include infection, nerve injury, intraoperative fractures, instability, and tuberosity nonunion.

The results of operative repair for three- and four-part proximal humeral fracture are conflicting. Results for nonoperatively treated patients are probably not worse than those undergoing surgical repair, yet there are substantial limitations in shoulder range and functional abilities. Substantial additional study is needed on this topic.

> *Ortho 43 (Level B)*: **Observational studies are needed to more clearly define what constitutes a good outcome following a proximal humerus fracture in the older patient.**

> *Ortho 44 (Level A)*: **Controlled studies are needed to compare operative with nonoperative repair of proximal humerus fractures in older patients.**

> *Ortho 45 (Level A)*: **Controlled studies are needed to compare various operative repairs for proximal humerus fractures in older patients.**

KEY RESEARCH QUESTIONS IN GERIATRIC ORTHOPEDICS

The morbidity related to musculoskeletal disorders in the elderly patient is significant. Degenerative joint disease and fractures of the spine and extremities have a tremendous impact on function, especially in the oldest individuals. Research is needed in many areas, particularly in ways to decrease the amount of fall-related trauma, to improve implant fixation in osteoporotic bone, to enhance fracture healing in the aged patient, and to optimize outcomes following fracture. Outcome studies should be performed to evaluate treatment, but what defines a successful outcome in this age group remains to be established.

Ortho KQ1: How can implant fixation in osteoporotic bone be improved?

Hypothesis-generating research studies should focus on the technical aspects of specific fixation techniques (eg, cemented, noncemented implants) and postoperative care (eg, antiresorptive agents, calcium, vitamin D, exercise). Database analyses and observational studies of specific implants currently used in operations on elderly patients should elucidate risk factors (eg, degree of osteoporosis) and technical contributions to implant fixation. Further hypothesis-generating research should focus on the development of widely acceptable measures and timeframes for healing and fixation to be used as benchmarks in the evaluation of elderly patients after implant fixation.

Hypothesis-testing research may start with cohort studies to compare fixation rates according to implant type. Multivariate analyses for such studies may clarify the role of device characteristics versus the presence of specific diseases in predicting successful fixation in older patients. Finally, randomized trials of specific implants alone or in combination with specific therapies to treat the underlying bone disease may be required.

Ortho KQ2: **How can fracture healing in the aged person be enhanced?**

Hypothesis-generating research should include studies to identify risk factors for poor healing and the effects on healing of commonly prescribed therapies for osteoporosis. Basic research needs to examine growth factors and other modalities that may enhance healing for future clinical trials. Further hypothesis-generating research should focus on the development of widely acceptable measures and timeframes for healing to be used as benchmarks in the evaluation of elderly patients after fracture.

Hypothesis-testing research may include randomized trials of specific therapies to enhance fracture healing. Cohort studies should compare healing rates under different strategies for fracture management. Multivariate analyses from such studies may clarify the role of patient-level characteristics versus the management of specific fractures in predicting optimal healing in older patients.

Ortho KQ3: **How can the outcomes after fracture be optimized in elderly patients?**

Hypothesis-generating research should include methodologic studies to identify high-risk elderly patients and devise clinical pathways for their care. Database analyses of the pre-hospital, in-hospital, and rehabilitation periods of elderly orthopedic patients should be performed to identify clinical management strategies that result in decreased morbidity and improved functional recovery. Hypothesis-generating research should also include the expansion of current clinical databases to include long-term and functional outcomes of older orthopedic surgical patients. Observational studies and database analysis should focus on refinement of risk factors for poor outcome in surgically versus nonsurgically treated elderly patients (eg, for humerus, wrist, vertebral fractures) and describe outcomes in various settings (eg, acute rehabilitation, skilled nursing facility, home) and with various approaches (eg, organized fracture service, weight bearing as tolerated after hip repair) used to manage specific high-priority fractures (eg, hip).

Hypothesis-testing research studies to address this question would be aimed at defining the benefits of specific interventions in older patients. Randomized trials of elderly patients treated for specific fractures (eg, vertebrae, wrist, humerus) are needed to clarify the role of operative therapy in improving function and quality of life. Case-control or randomized studies of clinical pathways to elucidate the benefit of pathways in obtaining better functional outcomes and reducing in-hospital adverse events and optimizing long-term recovery are needed. The aim of these studies would also be to identify treatment strategies that reduce the incidence of perioperative complications, wound-related problems, and deep-vein thrombosis, which are especially prevalent in older orthopedic patients.

REFERENCES

1. Praemer A, Furner S, Rice DP. Musculoskeletal Conditions in the United States, 2nd ed. Rosemont, IL: American Academy of Orthopaedic Surgeons, 1999.
2. Clelland C, Worland RL, Jessup DE, East D. Preoperative medical evaluation in patients having joint replacement surgery: added benefits. South Med J 1996;89:958-960.

3. van der Sluis CK, Timmer HW, Eisma WH, ten Duis HJ. Outcome in elderly injured patients: injury severity versus host factors. Injury 1997;28:588-592.

4. Svensson O, Stromberg L, Ohlen G, Lindgren U. Prediction of the outcome after hip fracture in elderly patients. J Bone Joint Surg Br 1996;78:115-118.

5. Ponzer S, Tidermark J, Brismar K, et al. Nutritional status, insulin-like growth factor-1 and quality of life in elderly women with hip fractures. Clin Nutr 1999;18:241-246.

6. Burness R, Horne G, Purdie G. Albumin levels and mortality in patients with hip fractures. N Z Med J 1996;109:56-57.

7. Munger RG, Cerhan JR, Chiu BC. Prospective study of dietary protein intake and risk of hip fracture in postmenopausal women. Am J Clin Nutr 1999;69:147-152.

8. Tkatch L, Rapin CH, Rizzoli R, et al. Benefits of oral protein supplementation in elderly patients with fracture of the proximal femur. J Am Coll Nutr 1992;11:519-525.

9. Sullivan DH, Nelson CL, Bopp MM, et al. Nightly enteral nutrition support of elderly hip fracture patients: a phase I trial. J Am Coll Nutr 1998;17:155-161.

10. Schurch MA, Rizzoli R, Slosman D, et al. Protein supplements increase serum insulin-like growth factor-I levels and attenuate proximal femur bone loss in patients with recent hip fracture: a randomized, double-blind, placebo-controlled trial. Ann Intern Med 1998;128: 801-809.

11. Koval KJ, Maurer SG, Su ET, et al. The effects of nutritional status on outcome after hip fracture. J Orthop Trauma 1999;13:164-169.

12. Lavernia CJ, Sierra RJ, Baerga L. Nutritional parameters and short term outcome in arthroplasty. J Am Coll Nutr 1999;18:274-278.

13. Bonjour JP, Schurch MA, Rizzoli R. Nutritional aspects of hip fractures. Bone 1996;18:139S-144S.

14. Sullivan DH, Sun S, Walls RC. Protein-energy undernutrition among elderly hospitalized patients: a prospective study. JAMA 1999;281:2013-2019.

15. Paillaud E, Bories PN, Le Parco JC, Campillo B. Nutritional status and energy expenditure in elderly patients with recent hip fracture during a 2-month follow-up. Br J Nutr 2000;83:97-103.

16. Messier SP, Loeser RF, Hoover JL, et al. Osteoarthritis of the knee: effects on gait, strength, and flexibility. Arch Phys Med Rehabil 1992;73:29-36.

17. Slemenda C, Heilman DK, Brandt KD, et al. Reduced quadriceps strength relative to body weight: a risk factor for knee osteoarthritis in women? Arthritis Rheum 1998;41:1951-1959.

18. Sudarsky L. Geriatrics: gait disorders in the elderly. N Engl J Med 1990;322:1441-1446.

19. King MB, Tinetti ME. Falls in community-dwelling older persons. J Am Geriatr Soc 1995;43:1146-1154.

20. Ling SM, Bathon JM. Osteoarthritis in older adults. J Am Geriatr Soc 1998;46:216-225.

21. American College of Rheumatology Subcommittee on Osteoarthritis Guidelines. Recommendations for the medical management of osteoarthritis of the hip and knee: 2000 update. Arthritis Rheum 2000;43:1905-1915.

22. Hochberg MC, Altman RD, Brandt KD, et al. Guidelines for the medical management of osteoarthritis. Part I. Osteoarthritis of the hip. American College of Rheumatology. Arthritis Rheum 1995;38:1535-1540.

23. Adams ME, Atkinson MH, Lussier AJ, et al. The role of viscosupplementation with hylan G-F 20 (Synvisc) in the treatment of osteoarthritis of the knee: a Canadian multicenter trial comparing hylan G-F 20 alone, hylan G-F 20 with non-steroidal anti-inflammatory drugs (NSAIDs) and NSAIDs alone. Osteoarthritis Cartilage 1995;3:213-225.

24. Altman RD, Moskowitz R. Intraarticular sodium hyaluronate (Hyalgan) in the treatment of patients with osteoarthritis of the knee: a randomized clinical trial. Hyalgan Study Group. J Rheumatol 1998;25:2203-2212.

25. Nelson ME, Fiatarone MA, Morganti CM, et al. Effects of high-intensity strength training on multiple risk factors for osteoporotic fractures: a randomized controlled trial. JAMA 1994;272:1909-1914.

26. Butler RN, Davis R, Lewis CB, et al. Physical fitness: benefits of exercise for the older patient. 2. Geriatrics 1998;53:46, 49-52, 61-42.

27. Province MA, Hadley EC, Hornbrook MC, et al. The effects of exercise on falls in elderly patients: a preplanned meta-analysis of the FICSIT Trials. Frailty and Injuries: Cooperative Studies of Intervention Techniques. JAMA 1995;273:1341-1347.

28. Evans WJ. Exercise, nutrition, and aging. Clin Geriatr Med 1995;11:725-734.

29. Tseng BS, Marsh DR, Hamilton MT, Booth FW. Strength and aerobic training attenuate muscle wasting and improve resistance to the development of disability with aging. J Gerontol A Biol Sci Med Sci 1995;50 Spec No:M113-M119.

30. March LM, Cross MJ, Lapsley H, et al. Outcomes after hip or knee replacement surgery for osteoarthritis: a prospective cohort study comparing patients' quality of life before and after surgery with age-related population norms. Med J Aust 1999;171:235-238.

31. Brander VA, Malhotra S, Jet J, et al. Outcome of hip and knee arthroplasty in persons aged 80 years and older. Clin Orthop 1997;Dec:67-78.

32. Fortin PR, Clarke AE, Joseph L, et al. Outcomes of total hip and knee replacement: preoperative functional status predicts outcomes at six months after surgery. Arthritis Rheum 1999;42:1722-1728.

33. Young NL, Cheah D, Waddell JP, Wright JG. Patient characteristics that affect the outcome of total hip arthroplasty: a review. Can J Surg 1998;41:188-195.

34. Newington DP, Bannister GC, Fordyce M. Primary total hip replacement in patients over 80 years of age. J Bone Joint Surg Br 1990;72:450-452.

35. Brodie LJ, Sloman RM. Changes in health status of elderly patients following hip replacement surgery. J Gerontol Nurs 1998;24:5-12.

36. Boettcher WG. Total hip arthroplasties in the elderly: morbidity, mortality, and cost effectiveness. Clin Orthop 1992;Jan:30-34.

37. Konstantoulakis C, Anastopoulos G, Papaeliou A, et al. Uncemented total hip arthroplasty in the elderly. Int Orthop 1999;23:334-336.

38. Lester DK, Campbell P, Ehya A, Rude RK. Assessment of press-fit hip femoral components retrieved at autopsy. Orthopedics 1998;21:27-33.

39. Maloney WJ, Galante JO, Anderson M, et al. Fixation, polyethylene wear, and pelvic osteolysis in primary total hip replacement. Clin Orthop 1999;Dec:157-164.

40. Radcliffe GS, Tomichan MC, Andrews M, Stone MH. Revision hip surgery in the elderly: is it worthwhile? J Arthroplasty 1999;14:38-44.

41. Joshi A, Lee CM, Markovic L, et al. Prognosis of dislocation after total hip arthroplasty. J Arthroplasty 1998;13:17-21.

42. Ekelund A, Rydell N, Nilsson OS. Total hip arthroplasty in patients 80 years of age and older. Clin Orthop 1992;Aug:101-106.

43. Parvizi J, Morrey BF. Bipolar hip arthroplasty as a salvage treatment for instability of the hip. J Bone Joint Surg Am 2000;82-A:1132-1139.

44. McGinley BJ, Cushner FD, Scott WN. Debridement arthroscopy: 10-year followup. Clin Orthop 1999;Oct:190-194.

45. Salisbury RB, Nottage WM, Gardner V. The effect of alignment on results in arthroscopic debridement of the degenerative knee. Clin Orthop 1985;Sep:268-272.

46. Harwin SF. Arthroscopic debridement for osteoarthritis of the knee: predictors of patient satisfaction. Arthroscopy 1999;15:142-146.

47. Moseley JB, O'Malley K, Petersen NJ, et al. A controlled trial of arthroscopic surgery for osteoarthritis of the knee. N Engl J Med 2002;347:81-88.

48. Hawker G, Wright J, Coyte P, et al. Health-related quality of life after knee replacement. J Bone Joint Surg Am 1998;80:163-173.

49. Birdsall PD, Hayes JH, Cleary R, et al. Health outcome after total knee replacement in the very elderly. J Bone Joint Surg Br 1999;81:660-662.

50. Dickstein R, Heffes Y, Shabtai EI, Markowitz E. Total knee arthroplasty in the elderly: patients' self-appraisal 6 and 12 months postoperatively. Gerontology 1998;44:204-210.

51. Laskin RS. Total knee replacement in patients older than 85 years. Clin Orthop 1999;Oct:43-49.

52. Belmar CJ, Barth P, Lonner JH, Lotke PA. Total knee arthroplasty in patients 90 years of age and older. J Arthroplasty 1999;14:911-914.

53. Gioe TJ, Bowman KR. A randomized comparison of all-polyethylene and metal-backed tibial components. Clin Orthop 2000;Nov:108-115.

54. Pagnano MW, Levy BA, Berry DJ. Cemented all polyethylene tibial components in patients age 75 years and older. Clin Orthop 1999;Oct:73-80.

55. Schroeder-Boersch H, Scheller G, Fischer J, Jani L. Advantages of patellar resurfacing in total knee arthroplasty. Two-year results of a prospective randomized study. Arch Orthop Trauma Surg 1998;117:73-78.

56. Ishii Y, Yagisawa K, Ikezawa Y. Changes in bone mineral density of the proximal femur after total knee arthroplasty. J Arthroplasty 2000;15:519-522.

57. Chakravarty KK, Webley M. Disorders of the shoulder: an often unrecognised cause of disability in elderly people. BMJ 1990;300:848-849.

58. Hattrup SJ. Rotator cuff repair: relevance of patient age. J Shoulder Elbow Surg 1995;4:95-100.

59. Itoi E, Tabata S. Conservative treatment of rotator cuff tears. Clin Orthop 1992;Feb:165-173.

60. Hawkins RH, Dunlop R. Nonoperative treatment of rotator cuff tears. Clin Orthop 1995;Dec:178-188.

61. Motycka T, Kriegleder B, Landsiedl F. Results of open repair of the rotator cuff–a long-term review of 79 shoulders. Arch Orthop Trauma Surg 2001;121:148-151.

62. Grondel RJ, Savoie FH, 3rd, Field LD. Rotator cuff repairs in patients 62 years of age or older. J Shoulder Elbow Surg 2001;10:97-99.

63. Worland RL, Arredondo J, Angles F, Lopez-Jimenez F. Repair of massive rotator cuff tears in patients older than 70 years. J Shoulder Elbow Surg 1999;8:26-30.

64. Rokito AS, Zuckerman JD, Gallagher MA, Cuomo F. Strength after surgical repair of the rotator cuff. J Shoulder Elbow Surg 1996;5:12-17.

65. Hartsell HD. Postsurgical shoulder strength in the older patient. J Orthop Sports Phys Ther 1993;18:667-672.

66. Miniaci A, MacLeod M. Transfer of the latissimus dorsi muscle after failed repair of a massive tear of the rotator cuff: a two to five-year review. J Bone Joint Surg Am 1999;81:1120-1127.

67. Comley AS, Krishnan J. Donor site morbidity after quadriceps tendon harvest for rotator cuff repair. Aust N Z J Surg 1999;69:808-810.

68. Gartsman GM, Roddey TS, Hammerman SM. Shoulder arthroplasty with or without resurfacing of the glenoid in patients who have osteoarthritis. J Bone Joint Surg Am 2000;82:26-34.

69. Worland RL, Jessup DE, Arredondo J, Warburton KJ. Bipolar shoulder arthroplasty for rotator cuff arthropathy. J Shoulder Elbow Surg 1997;6:512-515.

70. Zuckerman JD, Scott AJ, Gallagher MA. Hemiarthroplasty for cuff tear arthropathy. J Shoulder Elbow Surg 2000;9:169-172.

71. Fujita S, Hirota S, Oda T, et al. Deep venous thrombosis after total hip or total knee arthroplasty in patients in Japan. Clin Orthop 2000;Jun:168-174.

72. White RH, Gettner S, Newman JM, et al. Predictors of rehospitalization for symptomatic venous thromboembolism after total hip arthroplasty. N Engl J Med 2000;343:1758-1764.

73. Leclerc JR, Gent M, Hirsh J, et al. The incidence of symptomatic venous thromboembolism during and after prophylaxis with enoxaparin: a multi-institutional cohort study of patients who underwent hip or knee arthroplasty. Canadian Collaborative Group. Arch Intern Med 1998;158:873-878.

74. Dahl OE, Gudmundsen TE, Haukeland L. Late occurring clinical deep vein thrombosis in joint-operated patients. Acta Orthop Scand 2000;71:47-50.

75. Caprini JA, Arcelus JI, Motykie G, et al. The influence of oral anticoagulation therapy on deep vein thrombosis rates four weeks after total hip replacement. J Vasc Surg 1999;30:813-820.

76. Ansari S, Warwick D, Ackroyd CE, Newman JH. Incidence of fatal pulmonary embolism after 1,390 knee arthroplasties without routine prophylactic anticoagulation, except in high-risk cases. J Arthroplasty 1997;12:599-602.

77. Zahn HR, Skinner JA, Porteous MJ. The preoperative prevalence of deep vein thrombosis in patients with femoral neck fractures and delayed operation. Injury 1999;30:605-607.

78. Bergqvist D, Fredin H. Pulmonary embolism and mortality in patients with fractured hips–a prospective consecutive series. Eur J Surg 1991;157:571-574.

79. Kennedy JG, Soffe KE, Rogers BW, et al. Deep vein thrombosis prophylaxis in hip fractures: a comparison of the arteriovenous impulse system and aspirin. J Trauma 2000;48:268-272.

80. Warwick D, Harrison J, Glew D, et al. Comparison of the use of a foot pump with the use of low-molecular-weight heparin for the prevention of deep-vein thrombosis after total hip replacement: a prospective, randomized trial. J Bone Joint Surg Am 1998;80:1158-1166.

81. Prevention of pulmonary embolism and deep vein thrombosis with low dose aspirin: Pulmonary Embolism Prevention (PEP) trial. Lancet 2000;355:1295-1302.

82. Woolson ST, Robinson RK, Khan NQ, et al. Deep venous thrombosis prophylaxis for knee replacement: warfarin and pneumatic compression. Am J Orthop 1998;27:299-304.

83. Freedman KB, Brookenthal KR, Fitzgerald RH, Jr., et al. A meta-analysis of thromboembolic prophylaxis following elective total hip arthroplasty. J Bone Joint Surg Am 2000;82-A:929-938.

84. Messieh M, Huang Z, Johnson LJ, Jobin S. Warfarin responses in total joint and hip fracture patients. J Arthroplasty 1999;14:724-729.

85. Barsotti J, Gruel Y, Rosset P, et al. Comparative double-blind study of two dosage regimens of low-molecular weight heparin in elderly patients with a fracture of the neck of the femur. J Orthop Trauma 1990;4:371-375.

86. Shaieb MD, Watson BN, Atkinson RE. Bleeding complications with enoxaparin for deep venous thrombosis prophylaxis. J Arthroplasty 1999;14:432-438.

87. Imperiale TF, Speroff T. A meta-analysis of methods to prevent venous thromboembolism following total hip replacement. JAMA 1994;271:1780-1785.

88. Stern SH, Wixson RL, O'Connor D. Evaluation of the safety and efficacy of enoxaparin and warfarin for prevention of deep vein thrombosis after total knee arthroplasty. J Arthroplasty 2000;15:153-158.

89. Fairweather RB. When should low-molecular-weight heparin be monitored? CAP Today 1999;13:48-50.

90. Kyle RF, Crickard GE, 3rd. Periprosthetic fractures associated with total hip arthroplasty. Orthopedics 1998;21:982-984.

91. Wu CC, Au MK, Wu SS, Lin LC. Risk factors for postoperative femoral fracture in cementless hip arthroplasty. J Formos Med Assoc 1999;98:190-194.

92. Younger AS, Dunwoody I, Duncan CP. Periprosthetic hip and knee fractures: the scope of the problem. Instr Course Lect 1998;47:251-256.

93. Jukkala-Partio K, Partio EK, Solovieva S, et al. Treatment of periprosthetic fractures in association with total hip arthroplasty–a retrospective comparison between revision stem and plate fixation. Ann Chir Gynaecol 1998;87:229-235.

94. Siegmeth A, Menth-Chiari WA, Wozasek GE, Vecsei V. Femur fractures in patients with hip arthroplasty: indications for revision arthroplasty. J South Orthop Assoc 1998;7:251-258.

95. Incavo SJ, Beard DM, Pupparo F, et al. One-stage revision of periprosthetic fractures around loose cemented total hip arthroplasty. Am J Orthop 1998;27:35-41.

96. Weber D, Peter RE. Distal femoral fractures after knee arthroplasty. Int Orthop 1999;23: 236-239.

97. Weber D, Pomeroy DL, Schaper LA, et al. Supracondylar nailing of distal periprosthetic femoral fractures. Int Orthop 2000;24:33-35.

98. Tani Y, Inoue K, Kaneko H, et al. Intramedullary fibular graft for supracondylar fracture of the femur following total knee arthroplasty. Arch Orthop Trauma Surg 1998;117:103-104.

99. Crockarell JR, Hanssen AD, Osmon DR, Morrey BF. Treatment of infection with debridement and retention of the components following hip arthroplasty. J Bone Joint Surg Am 1998;80:1306-1313.

100. Orr RD, Zdeblick TA. Cervical spondylotic myelopathy: approaches to surgical treatment. Clin Orthop 1999;Feb:58-66.

101. Taylor J, Johnston RA, Caird FI. Surgical treatment of cervical spondylotic myelopathy in elderly patients. Age Ageing 1991;20:407-412.

102. Kohno K, Kumon Y, Oka Y, et al. Evaluation of prognostic factors following expansive laminoplasty for cervical spinal stenotic myelopathy. Surg Neurol 1997;48:237-245.

103. Tanaka J, Seki N, Tokimura F, et al. Operative results of canal-expansive laminoplasty for cervical spondylotic myelopathy in elderly patients. Spine 1999;24:2308-2312.

104. Sanderson PL, Wood PL. Surgery for lumbar spinal stenosis in old people. J Bone Joint Surg Br 1993;75:393-397.

105. Deyo RA, Cherkin DC, Loeser JD, et al. Morbidity and mortality in association with operations on the lumbar spine: the influence of age, diagnosis, and procedure. J Bone Joint Surg Am 1992;74:536-543.

106. Kalbarczyk A, Lukes A, Seiler RW. Surgical treatment of lumbar spinal stenosis in the elderly. Acta Neurochir (Wien) 1998;140:637-641.

107. Vitaz TW, Raque GH, Shields CB, Glassman SD. Surgical treatment of lumbar spinal stenosis in patients older than 75 years of age. J Neurosurg 1999;91:181-185.

108. Atlas SJ, Keller RB, Robson D, et al. Surgical and nonsurgical management of lumbar spinal stenosis: four-year outcomes from the Maine lumbar spine study. Spine 2000;25:556-562.

109. Niggemeyer O, Strauss JM, Schulitz KP. Comparison of surgical procedures for degenerative lumbar spinal stenosis: a meta-analysis of the literature from 1975 to 1995. Eur Spine J 1997;6:423-429.

110. Katz JN, Stucki G, Lipson SJ, et al. Predictors of surgical outcome in degenerative lumbar spinal stenosis. Spine 1999;24:2229-2233.

111. Jonsson B, Annertz M, Sjoberg C, Stromqvist B. A prospective and consecutive study of surgically treated lumbar spinal stenosis: Part I: Clinical features related to radiographic findings. Spine 1997;22:2932-2937.

112. Iguchi T, Kurihara A, Nakayama J, et al. Minimum 10-year outcome of decompressive laminectomy for degenerative lumbar spinal stenosis. Spine 2000;25:1754-1759.
113. Katz JN, Lipson SJ, Chang LC, et al. Seven- to 10-year outcome of decompressive surgery for degenerative lumbar spinal stenosis. Spine 1996;21:92-98.
114. Caputy AJ, Luessenhop AJ. Long-term evaluation of decompressive surgery for degenerative lumbar stenosis. J Neurosurg 1992;77:669-676.
115. Postacchini F, Cinotti G. Bone regrowth after surgical decompression for lumbar spinal stenosis. J Bone Joint Surg Br 1992;74:862-869.
116. Guigui P, Barre E, Benoist M, Deburge A. Radiologic and computed tomography image evaluation of bone regrowth after wide surgical decompression for lumbar stenosis. Spine 1999;24:281-288; discussion 288-289.
117. Yone K, Sakou T, Kawauchi Y, et al. Indication of fusion for lumbar spinal stenosis in elderly patients and its significance. Spine 1996;21:242-248.
118. Hirano T, Hasegawa K, Washio T, et al. Fracture risk during pedicle screw insertion in osteoporotic spine. J Spinal Disord 1998;11:493-497.
119. Lord SR, Bashford GM. Shoe characteristics and balance in older women. J Am Geriatr Soc 1996;44:429-433.
120. Salai M, Dudkiewicz I, Novikov I, et al. The epidemic of ankle fractures in the elderly–is surgical treatment warranted? Arch Orthop Trauma Surg 2000;120:511-513.
121. NIH Consensus Development Panel of Osteoporosis Prevention, Diagnosis and Therapy. Osteoporosis prevention, diagnosis, and therapy. JAMA 2001;285:785-795.
122. Aharonoff GB, Dennis MG, Elshinawy A, et al. Circumstances of falls causing hip fractures in the elderly. Clin Orthop 1998;Mar:10-14.
123. Nevitt MC, Cummings SR. Type of fall and risk of hip and wrist fractures: the study of osteoporotic fractures. The Study of Osteoporotic Fractures Research Group. J Am Geriatr Soc 1993;41:1226-1234.
124. Greenspan SL, Myers ER, Kiel DP, et al. Fall direction, bone mineral density, and function: risk factors for hip fracture in frail nursing home elderly. Am J Med 1998;104:539-545.
125. Dargent-Molina P, Hays M, Breart G. Sensory impairments and physical disability in aged women living at home. Int J Epidemiol 1996;25:621-629.
126. Ivers RQ, Cumming RG, Mitchell P, Attebo K. Visual impairment and falls in older adults: the Blue Mountains Eye Study. J Am Geriatr Soc 1998;46:58-64.
127. Klein BE, Klein R, Lee KE, Cruickshanks KJ. Performance-based and self-assessed measures of visual function as related to history of falls, hip fractures, and measured gait time. The Beaver Dam Eye Study. Ophthalmology 1998;105:160-164.
128. Era P, Avlund K, Jokela J, et al. Postural balance and self-reported functional ability in 75-year-old men and women: a cross-national comparative study. J Am Geriatr Soc 1997;45:21-29.
129. Herndon JG, Helmick CG, Sattin RW, et al. Chronic medical conditions and risk of fall injury events at home in older adults. J Am Geriatr Soc 1997;45:739-743.
130. American Geriatrics Society, British Geriatrics Society, and American Academy of Orthopaedic Surgeons Panel on Falls Prevention. Guideline for the prevention of falls in older persons. J Am Geriatr Soc 2001;49:664-672.
131. Stein MS, Wark JD, Scherer SC, et al. Falls relate to vitamin D and parathyroid hormone in an Australian nursing home and hostel. J Am Geriatr Soc 1999;47:1195-1201.
132. Kane RS, Burns EA, Goodwin JS. Minimal trauma fractures in older nursing home residents: the interaction of functional status, trauma, and site of fracture. J Am Geriatr Soc 1995;43:156-159.
133. Langlois JA, Visser M, Davidovic LS, et al. Hip fracture risk in older white men is associated with change in body weight from age 50 years to old age. Arch Intern Med 1998;158:990-996.

134. Meyer HE, Tverdal A, Selmer R. Weight variability, weight change and the incidence of hip fracture: a prospective study of 39,000 middle-aged Norwegians. Osteoporos Int 1998;8: 373-378.

135. Grisso JA. Prevention of falls in patients with osteoporosis. Rev Rhum Engl Ed 1997;64:75S-77S.

136. Graafmans WC, Ooms ME, Hofstee HM, et al. Falls in the elderly: a prospective study of risk factors and risk profiles. Am J Epidemiol 1996;143:1129-1136.

137. Tinetti ME, Speechley M, Ginter SF. Risk factors for falls among elderly persons living in the community. N Engl J Med 1988;319:1701-1707.

138. Sorock GS, Labiner DM. Peripheral neuromuscular dysfunction and falls in an elderly cohort. Am J Epidemiol 1992;136:584-591.

139. Gullberg B, Johnell O, Kanis JA. World-wide projections for hip fracture. Osteoporos Int 1997;7:407-413.

140. Oden A, Dawson A, Dere W, et al. Lifetime risk of hip fractures is underestimated. Osteoporos Int 1998;8:599-603.

141. Ensrud KE, Cauley J, Lipschutz R, Cummings SR. Weight change and fractures in older women. Study of Osteoporotic Fractures Research Group. Arch Intern Med 1997;157:857-863.

142. Farahmand BY, Michaelsson K, Baron JA, et al. Body size and hip fracture risk. Swedish Hip Fracture Study Group. Epidemiology 2000;11:214-219.

143. Farahmand BY, Persson PG, Michaelsson K, et al. Physical activity and hip fracture: a population-based case-control study. Swedish Hip Fracture Study Group. Int J Epidemiol 2000;29:308-314.

144. Gregg EW, Pereira MA, Caspersen CJ. Physical activity, falls, and fractures among older adults: a review of the epidemiologic evidence. J Am Geriatr Soc 2000;48:883-893.

145. Hoidrup S, Prescott E, Sorensen TI, et al. Tobacco smoking and risk of hip fracture in men and women. Int J Epidemiol 2000;29:253-259.

146. Stewart A, Calder LD, Torgerson DJ, et al. Prevalence of hip fracture risk factors in women aged 70 years and over. Qjm 2000;93:677-680.

147. Bacon WE, Hadden WC. Occurrence of hip fractures and socioeconomic position. J Aging Health 2000;12:193-203.

148. Ramnemark A, Nilsson M, Borssen B, Gustafson Y. Stroke, a major and increasing risk factor for femoral neck fracture. Stroke 2000;31:1572-1577.

149. Alem AM, Sherrard DJ, Gillen DL, et al. Increased risk of hip fracture among patients with end-stage renal disease. Kidney Int 2000;58:396-399.

150. Coco M, Rush H. Increased incidence of hip fractures in dialysis patients with low serum parathyroid hormone. Am J Kidney Dis 2000;36:1115-1121.

151. Ivers RQ, Norton R, Cumming RG, et al. Visual impairment and risk of hip fracture. Am J Epidemiol 2000;152:633-639.

152. Hayes WC, Myers ER, Morris JN, et al. Impact near the hip dominates fracture risk in elderly nursing home residents who fall. Calcif Tissue Int 1993;52:192-198.

153. Cummings SR, Nevitt MC. A hypothesis: the causes of hip fractures. J Gerontol 1989;44:M107-M111.

154. Cumming RG, Klineberg RJ. Fall frequency and characteristics and the risk of hip fractures. J Am Geriatr Soc 1994;42:774-778.

155. Lauritzen JB. Hip fractures: incidence, risk factors, energy absorption, and prevention. Bone 1996;18:65S-75S.

156. Parkkari J, Kannus P, Palvanen M, et al. Majority of hip fractures occur as a result of a fall and impact on the greater trochanter of the femur: a prospective controlled hip fracture study with 206 consecutive patients. Calcif Tissue Int 1999;65:183-187.

157. Lauritzen JB, Petersen MM, Lund B. Effect of external hip protectors on hip fractures. Lancet 1993;341:11-13.
158. Lauritzen JB. Hip fractures. Epidemiology, risk factors, falls, energy absorption, hip protectors, and prevention. Dan Med Bull 1997;44:155-168.
159. Ekman A, Mallmin H, Michaelsson K, Ljunghall S. External hip protectors to prevent osteoporotic hip fractures. Lancet 1997;350:563-564.
160. Kannus P, Parkkari J, Niemi S, et al. Prevention of hip fracture in elderly people with use of a hip protector. N Engl J Med 2000;343:1506-1513.
161. Lyon LJ, Nevins MA. Nonoperative management as primary therapy. J Am Geriatr Soc 1987;35:77-78.
162. Zuckerman JD, Skovron ML, Koval KJ, et al. Postoperative complications and mortality associated with operative delay in older patients who have a fracture of the hip. J Bone Joint Surg Am 1995;77:1551-1556.
163. Beringer TR, Crawford VL, Brown JG. Audit of surgical delay in relationship to outcome after proximal femoral fracture. Ulster Med J 1996;65:32-38.
164. Hamlet WP, Lieberman JR, Freedman EL, et al. Influence of health status and the timing of surgery on mortality in hip fracture patients. Am J Orthop 1997;26:621-627.
165. Koval KJ, Aharonoff GB, Rosenberg AD, et al. Hip fracture in the elderly: the effect of anesthetic technique. Orthopedics 1999;22:31-34.
166. Fox KM, Magaziner J, Hebel JR, et al. Intertrochanteric versus femoral neck hip fractures: differential characteristics, treatment, and sequelae. J Gerontol A Biol Sci Med Sci 1999;54:M635-M640.
167. Bess RJ, Jolly SA. Comparison of compression hip screw and gamma nail for treatment of peritrochanteric fractures. J South Orthop Assoc 1997;6:173-179.
168. Baumgaertner MR, Curtin SL, Lindskog DM. Intramedullary versus extramedullary fixation for the treatment of intertrochanteric hip fractures. Clin Orthop 1998;Mar:87-94.
169. Chevalley F, Gamba D. Gamma nailing of pertrochanteric and subtrochanteric fractures: clinical results of a series of 63 consecutive cases. J Orthop Trauma 1997;11:412-415.
170. Di Fiore M, Giacomello A, Vigano E, Zanoni A, Jr. The gamma nail and the compression-sliding plate in the treatment of pertrochanteric fractures: anesthesiologic aspects. Chir Organi Mov 1993;78:59-62.
171. Park SR, Kang JS, Kim HS, et al. Treatment of intertrochanteric fracture with the Gamma AP locking nail or by a compression hip screw—a randomised prospective trial. Int Orthop 1998;22:157-160.
172. Habernek H, Wallner T, Aschauer E, Schmid L. Comparison of ender nails, dynamic hip screws, and Gamma nails in the treatment of peritrochanteric femoral fractures. Orthopedics 2000;23:121-127.
173. Lyddon DW, Jr. The prevention of complications with the Gamma Locking Nail. Am J Orthop 1996;25:357-363.
174. Vahl AC, Dunki Jacobs PB, Patka P, Haarman HJ. Hemiarthroplasty in elderly, debilitated patients with an unstable femoral fracture in the trochanteric region. Acta Orthop Belg 1994;60:274-279.
175. Chan KC, Gill GS. Cemented hemiarthroplasties for elderly patients with intertrochanteric fractures. Clin Orthop 2000;Feb:206-215.
176. Stoffelen D, Haentjens P, Reynders P, et al. Hip arthroplasty for failed internal fixation of intertrochanteric and subtrochanteric fractures in the elderly patient. Acta Orthop Belg 1994;60:135-139.
177. Hudson JI, Kenzora JE, Hebel JR, et al. Eight-year outcome associated with clinical options in the management of femoral neck fractures. Clin Orthop 1998;Mar:59-66.

178. Parker MJ, Pryor GA. Internal fixation or arthroplasty for displaced cervical hip fractures in the elderly: a randomised controlled trial of 208 patients. Acta Orthop Scand 2000;71:440-446.

179. Young Y, Brant L, German P, et al. A longitudinal examination of functional recovery among older people with subcapital hip fractures. J Am Geriatr Soc 1997;45:288-294.

180. Wathne RA, Koval KJ, Aharonoff GB, et al. Modular unipolar versus bipolar prosthesis: a prospective evaluation of functional outcome after femoral neck fracture. J Orthop Trauma 1995;9:298-302.

181. Cornell CN, Levine D, O'Doherty J, Lyden J. Unipolar versus bipolar hemiarthroplasty for the treatment of femoral neck fractures in the elderly. Clin Orthop 1998;Mar:67-71.

182. Calder SJ, Anderson GH, Jagger C, et al. Unipolar or bipolar prosthesis for displaced intracapsular hip fracture in octogenarians: a randomised prospective study. J Bone Joint Surg Br 1996;78:391-394.

183. Incavo SJ, Ninomiya J, Howe JG, Mayor MB. Failure of the polyethylene liner leading to notching of the femoral component in bipolar prostheses. Orthop Rev 1993;22:728-732.

184. Lennox IA, McLauchlan J. Comparing the mortality and morbidity of cemented and uncemented hemiarthroplasties. Injury 1993;24:185-186.

185. Emery RJ, Broughton NS, Desai K, et al. Bipolar hemiarthroplasty for subcapital fracture of the femoral neck. A prospective randomised trial of cemented Thompson and uncemented Moore stems. J Bone Joint Surg Br 1991;73:322-324.

186. Squires B, Bannister G. Displaced intracapsular neck of femur fractures in mobile independent patients: total hip replacement or hemiarthroplasty? Injury 1999;30:345-348.

187. Neander G, Adolphson P, von Sivers K, et al. Bone and muscle mass after femoral neck fracture: a controlled quantitative computed tomography study of osteosynthesis versus primary total hip arthroplasty. Arch Orthop Trauma Surg 1997;116:470-474.

188. Johansson T, Jacobsson SA, Ivarsson I, et al. Internal fixation versus total hip arthroplasty in the treatment of displaced femoral neck fractures: a prospective randomized study of 100 hips. Acta Orthop Scand 2000;71:597-602.

189. Gebhard JS, Amstutz HC, Zinar DM, Dorey FJ. A comparison of total hip arthroplasty and hemiarthroplasty for treatment of acute fracture of the femoral neck. Clin Orthop 1992;Sep:123-131.

190. Lee BP, Berry DJ, Harmsen WS, Sim FH. Total hip arthroplasty for the treatment of an acute fracture of the femoral neck: long-term results. J Bone Joint Surg Am 1998;80:70-75.

191. Broos PL. Prosthetic replacement in the management of unstable femoral neck fractures in the elderly: analysis of the mechanical complications noted in 778 fractures. Acta Chir Belg 1999;99:190-194.

192. Koval KJ, Sala DA, Kummer FJ, Zuckerman JD. Postoperative weight-bearing after a fracture of the femoral neck or an intertrochanteric fracture. J Bone Joint Surg Am 1998;80:352-356.

193. Stromberg L, Ohlen G, Nordin C, et al. Postoperative mental impairment in hip fracture patients: a randomized study of reorientation measures in 223 patients. Acta Orthop Scand 1999;70:250-255.

194. Marcantonio ER, Flacker JM, Michaels M, Resnick NM. Delirium is independently associated with poor functional recovery after hip fracture. J Am Geriatr Soc 2000;48:618-624.

195. Holmes J, House A. Psychiatric illness predicts poor outcome after surgery for hip fracture: a prospective cohort study. Psychol Med 2000;30:921-929.

196. Neander G, Adolphson P, Hedstrom M, et al. Decrease in bone mineral density and muscle mass after femoral neck fracture: a quantitative computed tomography study in 25 patients. Acta Orthop Scand 1997;68:451-455.

197. Zerahn B, Olsen C, Stephensen S, et al. Bone loss after hip fracture is correlated to the postoperative degree of mobilisation. Arch Orthop Trauma Surg 1998;117:453-456.

198. Dirschl DR, Henderson RC, Oakley WC. Accelerated bone mineral loss following a hip fracture: a prospective longitudinal study. Bone 1997;21:79-82.

199. Dirschl DR, Piedrahita L, Henderson RC. Bone mineral density 6 years after a hip fracture: a prospective, longitudinal study. Bone 2000;26:95-98.

200. Kamel HK, Hussain MS, Tariq S, et al. Failure to diagnose and treat osteoporosis in elderly patients hospitalized with hip fracture. Am J Med 2000;109:326-328.

201. Magaziner J, Lydick E, Hawkes W, et al. Excess mortality attributable to hip fracture in white women aged 70 years and older. Am J Public Health 1997;87:1630-1636.

202. van Dortmont LM, Douw CM, van Breukelen AM, et al. Outcome after hemi-arthroplasty for displaced intracapsular femoral neck fracture related to mental state. Injury 2000;31:327-331.

203. Imura K, Ishii Y, Yagisawa K, Matsueda M. Postoperative ambulatory level after hip fracture in the elderly predicts survival rate. Arch Orthop Trauma Surg 2000;120:369-371.

204. Schroder HM, Erlandsen M. Age and sex as determinants of mortality after hip fracture: 3,895 patients followed for 2.5-18.5 years. J Orthop Trauma 1993;7:525-531.

205. Jennings AG, de Boer P. Should we operate on nonagenarians with hip fractures? Injury 1999;30:169-172.

206. Forster MC, Calthorpe D. Mortality following surgery for proximal femoral fractures in centenarians. Injury 2000;31:537-539.

207. Diamond TH, Thornley SW, Sekel R, Smerdely P. Hip fracture in elderly men: prognostic factors and outcomes. Med J Aust 1997;167:412-415.

208. Poor G, Atkinson EJ, O'Fallon WM, Melton LJ, 3rd. Determinants of reduced survival following hip fractures in men. Clin Orthop 1995;Oct:260-265.

209. Norton R, Butler M, Robinson E, et al. Declines in physical functioning attributable to hip fracture among older people: a follow-up study of case-control participants. Disabil Rehabil 2000;22:345-351.

210. Parker MJ, Palmer CR. Prediction of rehabilitation after hip fracture. Age Ageing 1995;24:96-98.

211. Koval KJ, Skovron ML, Aharonoff GB, et al. Ambulatory ability after hip fracture: a prospective study in geriatric patients. Clin Orthop 1995;Jan:150-159.

212. Koval KJ, Skovron ML, Aharonoff GB, Zuckerman JD. Predictors of functional recovery after hip fracture in the elderly. Clin Orthop 1998;Mar:22-28.

213. Koot VC, Peeters PH, de Jong JR, et al. Functional results after treatment of hip fracture: a multicentre, prospective study in 215 patients. Eur J Surg 2000;166:480-485.

214. Kelsey JL, Browner WS, Seeley DG, et al. Risk factors for fractures of the distal forearm and proximal humerus. The Study of Osteoporotic Fractures Research Group. Am J Epidemiol 1992;135:477-489.

215. Young BT, Rayan GM. Outcome following nonoperative treatment of displaced distal radius fractures in low-demand patients older than 60 years. J Hand Surg [Am] 2000;25:19-28.

216. Kelly AJ, Warwick D, Crichlow TP, Bannister GC. Is manipulation of moderately displaced Colles' fracture worthwhile? A prospective randomized trial. Injury 1997;28:283-287.

217. Board T, Kocialkowski A, Andrew G. Does Kapandji wiring help in older patients? A retrospective comparative review of displaced intra-articular distal radial fractures in patients over 55 years. Injury 1999;30:663-669.

218. Rikli DA, Regazzoni P. Fractures of the distal end of the radius treated by internal fixation and early function: a preliminary report of 20 cases. J Bone Joint Surg Br 1996;78:588-592.

219. Ring D, Jupiter JB, Brennwald J, et al. Prospective multicenter trial of a plate for dorsal fixation of distal radius fractures. J Hand Surg [Am] 1997;22:777-784.

220. Herrera M, Chapman CB, Roh M, et al. Treatment of unstable distal radius fractures with cancellous allograft and external fixation. J Hand Surg [Am] 1999;24:1269-1278.

221. Sanchez-Sotelo J, Munuera L, Madero R. Treatment of fractures of the distal radius with a remodellable bone cement: a prospective, randomised study using Norian SRS. J Bone Joint Surg Br 2000;82:856-863.

222. Warwick D, Prothero D, Field J, Bannister G. Radiological measurement of radial shortening in Colles' fracture. J Hand Surg [Br] 1993;18:50-52.

223. Lyles KW. Management of patients with vertebral compression fractures. Pharmacotherapy 1999;19:21S-24S.

224. Lyles KW, Gold DT, Shipp KM, et al. Association of osteoporotic vertebral compression fractures with impaired functional status. Am J Med 1993;94:595-601.

225. Kado DM, Browner WS, Palermo L, et al. Vertebral fractures and mortality in older women: a prospective study. Study of Osteoporotic Fractures Research Group. Arch Intern Med 1999;159:1215-1220.

226. Ensrud KE, Thompson DE, Cauley JA, et al. Prevalent vertebral deformities predict mortality and hospitalization in older women with low bone mass. Fracture Intervention Trial Research Group. J Am Geriatr Soc 2000;48:241-249.

227. Schlaich C, Minne HW, Bruckner T, et al. Reduced pulmonary function in patients with spinal osteoporotic fractures. Osteoporos Int 1998;8:261-267.

228. Ryan SD, Fried LP. The impact of kyphosis on daily functioning. J Am Geriatr Soc 1997;45:1479-1486.

229. Cortet B, Houvenagel E, Puisieux F, et al. Spinal curvatures and quality of life in women with vertebral fractures secondary to osteoporosis. Spine 1999;24:1921-1925.

230. Lyritis GP, Paspati I, Karachalios T, et al. Pain relief from nasal salmon calcitonin in osteoporotic vertebral crush fractures: a double blind, placebo-controlled clinical study. Acta Orthop Scand Suppl 1997;275:112-114.

231. Lee YL, Yip KM. The osteoporotic spine. Clin Orthop 1996;Feb:91-97.

232. Jensen ME, Evans AJ, Mathis JM, et al. Percutaneous polymethylmethacrylate vertebroplasty in the treatment of osteoporotic vertebral body compression fractures: technical aspects. AJNR Am J Neuroradiol 1997;18:1897-1904.

233. Barr JD, Barr MS, Lemley TJ, McCann RM. Percutaneous vertebroplasty for pain relief and spinal stabilization. Spine 2000;25:923-928.

234. Cortet B, Cotten A, Boutry N, et al. Percutaneous vertebroplasty in the treatment of osteoporotic vertebral compression fractures: an open prospective study. J Rheumatol 1999;26:2222-2228.

235. Wenger M, Markwalder TM. Surgically controlled, transpedicular methyl methacrylate vertebroplasty with fluoroscopic guidance. Acta Neurochir (Wien) 1999;141:625-631.

236. Grados F, Depriester C, Cayrolle G, et al. Long-term observations of vertebral osteoporotic fractures treated by percutaneous vertebroplasty. Rheumatology (Oxford) 2000;39:1410-1414.

237. Zyto K. Non-operative treatment of comminuted fractures of the proximal humerus in elderly patients. Injury 1998;29:349-352.

238. Zyto K, Ahrengart L, Sperber A, Tornkvist H. Treatment of displaced proximal humeral fractures in elderly patients. J Bone Joint Surg Br 1997;79:412-417.

239. Hessmann M, Baumgaertel F, Gehling H, et al. Plate fixation of proximal humeral fractures with indirect reduction: surgical technique and results utilizing three shoulder scores. Injury 1999;30:453-462.

240. Jakob RP, Miniaci A, Anson PS, et al. Four-part valgus impacted fractures of the proximal humerus. J Bone Joint Surg Br 1991;73:295-298.

241. Bosch U, Skutek M, Fremerey RW, Tscherne H. Outcome after primary and secondary hemiarthroplasty in elderly patients with fractures of the proximal humerus. J Shoulder Elbow Surg 1998;7:479-484.

242. Hawkins RJ, Switlyk P. Acute prosthetic replacement for severe fractures of the proximal humerus. Clin Orthop 1993;Apr:156-160.
243. Goldman RT, Koval KJ, Cuomo F, et al. Functional outcome after humeral head replacement for acute three- and four-part proximal humeral fractures. J Shoulder Elbow Surg 1995;4:81-86.
244. Wretenberg P, Ekelund A. Acute hemiarthroplasty after proximal humerus fracture in old patients: a retrospective evaluation of 18 patients followed for 2-7 years. Acta Orthop Scand 1997;68:121-123.
245. Zyto K, Wallace WA, Frostick SP, Preston BJ. Outcome after hemiarthroplasty for three- and four-part fractures of the proximal humerus. J Shoulder Elbow Surg 1998;7:85-89.
246. Movin T, Sjoden GO, Ahrengart L. Poor function after shoulder replacement in fracture patients: a retrospective evaluation of 29 patients followed for 2-12 years. Acta Orthop Scand 1998;69:392-396.

12

GERIATRIC REHABILITATION

Helen Hoenig, MD, MPH; Hilary C. Siebens, MD*

Rehabilitation focuses on the functional outcomes of pathologic processes and uses a variety of therapeutic interventions to restore function. Geriatric rehabilitation differs from rehabilitation in younger persons in that many older patients suffer from multiple conditions that interact to produce disability. [1] Hence, an understanding of the disablement process is critical to rehabilitation of older persons. [2] This chapter reviews the current understanding of the way disability occurs, the use of rehabilitation to treat disability, and the gaps in research in this area.

METHODS

The basic search was conducted on the National Library of Medicine's PubMed database. The period covered was from 1980 through March 28, 2001. This search combined the terms *rehabilitation, recovery of function,* or *rehabilitation nursing* with terms for the following five conditions or topics: arthritis or arthroplasty; equilibrium, posture, gait, falls, or fractures; cerebrovascular disorders; exercise or physical fitness; and amputees. This search generated 5967 references.

The authors later added terms for physical therapy, occupational therapy, activities of daily living, self-help devices, and durable medical equipment. They also added a search on CINAHL (Cumulative Index to Nursing and Allied Health Literature), focusing on *wheelchair, walker, cane,* and *assistive technology.* Finally, in making the final selection for this project, they reviewed pertinent rehabilitation texts and their references, as well as references cited in some of the papers derived from the search.

THEORETICAL UNDERPINNINGS FOR GERIATRIC REHABILITATION

Rehabilitation is a comparatively new field of medicine, the development of which has occurred primarily because of successes in other areas of medicine. Historically, people did not survive acute illness, so rehabilitation was moot. Because coping with old age, chronic illness, and disability are relatively novel, rehabilitation does not have the long experience available to other areas of medicine. Thus, theoretical constructs for treatment of disability and rehabilitation are, comparatively speaking, less developed. For this reason, the field of rehabilitation is less ready for definitive randomized trials than are other areas of geriatric medicine. In many respects, rehabilitation research is analogous to can-

* Hoenig: Associate Professor of Medicine, Division of Geriatrics, Department of Medicine, Center for the Study of Aging and Human Development, Duke University Medical Center; Chief, Physical Medicine and Rehabilitation Service, Durham VA Medical Center, Durham, NC. Siebens: Professor of Clinical Medicine, Professor of Clinical Physical Medicine and Rehabilitation, University of California, Irvine, College of Medicine, Irvine, CA.

Acknowledgment: We gratefully acknowledge Michael O'Grady, MD, for systematically reviewing and summarizing the literature on exercise and sarcopenia.

cer research. The condition (disability or cancer) often is multicausal, with causal factors occurring over a lifetime, and multimodal treatment often is required. Successes in cancer research have occurred through a combination of epidemiologic research, followed by basic science research, followed by multiphasic human studies with considerable coordination among clinical care providers. Similar efforts are needed in rehabilitation, although currently the field lacks the cohesiveness seen in cancer research. The research priorities for rehabilitation recommended herein reflect the need for further epidemiologic and theoretical work.

Disability is a complex behavior with biologic causes (eg, deconditioning, age-related changes, illness), as well as social and economic causes. There are several theoretical frameworks for the causation of disability that tie together the traditional biomedical and biopsychosocial models of illness. The conceptual framework for disability most commonly used in rehabilitation medicine is the one adopted by the World Health Organization, which portrays the progression of disease to disability and handicap as a stepwise process. [3] Geriatric medicine in the United States more often uses a model originally espoused by Nagi and refined by Verbrugge, Jette, and others. [4,5] Recent revisions by the World Health Organization focus on the use of empowering terminology (eg, using the term *social participation* instead of *handicap*) and on the role of personal and environmental contextual factors. [6]

The ongoing empirical work testing these models is research of substantial importance to geriatrics in general and geriatric rehabilitation specifically. It is vital to the future of geriatric rehabilitation to determine how the trajectory of disability differs for different diseases and combinations of diseases. In addition, we need to better understand the extent and ways in which the disablement process is modified by social and environmental factors, as well as by aging per se and health care. Examples of applications to geriatric rehabilitation research are briefly reviewed herein.

One key question is whether disability represents the "final common pathway" or if the disablement process is unique for each person. The concept of the final common pathway is based on the premise that different diseases lead to common expressions of disability or frailty. [7] For example, lower-extremity impairment, upper-extremity impairment, visual or hearing impairment, and affective disorders all predict functional dependence—someone with three impairments has a 60% likelihood of developing disability in the next year, whereas the likelihood among persons with no impairments is 7%. [8] Data show that in many older adults there appears to be an orderly progression of disability, with self-care activities that are dependent on lower-extremity function (eg, mobility) being lost before those that are dependent on upper-extremity function (eg, self-feeding). [9] One consequence of the final common pathway thesis is the assumption that rehabilitation treatment could be directed to the disability irrespective of the underlying causal pathway. The clinical result might be screening for functional impairment via self-reported questionnaire with direct referral to physical therapy (PT) or occupational therapy (OT), and without evaluation by a physician to determine the reason why the patient has impaired function. Since many physicians have little training in evaluating the underlying causes of disability, [10] there is substantial appeal to this approach.

There is increasing evidence that disability does not necessarily progress in a uniform manner and that differences in the acquisition and progression of disability may be important. Guralnik et al showed that stroke, hip fracture, and cancer, but not heart attack, are associated with the rapid development of severe mobility disability or "catastrophic disability." [11] They found that the incidence of catastrophic versus a more slowly progressive pattern of developing disability varies with age. People aged 85 or over with multiple medical conditions are more likely to have progressive rather than catastrophic disability. The pattern of disability acquisition, in turn, was found to be associated with mortality outcomes. For some conditions causing catastrophic disability, the timing of exercise or other rehabilitative interventions may be important. For example, there is some evidence that early surgery and early, intensive rehabilitation may improve outcomes after hip fracture over those seen with delayed surgery and rehabilitation. [12,13] In addition, there is evidence that diseases interact in unique ways. Some diseases appear to have multiplicative effects in producing disability; examples are the combination of osteoarthritis and heart disease, or hip fracture and cerebrovascular accident. [14]

A key factor both in the clinical treatment of patients and in planning a research agenda is remembering that the impact of disability at the individual and at societal levels must be distinguished. We readily appreciate that at the individual level some diseases are highly disabling (eg, spinal cord injury), but that other diseases are less disabling (eg, osteoarthritis). For example, in a representative sample of noninstitutionalized older Americans, a history of stroke was found to be associated with a twofold greater likelihood of disability and persons with arthritis were found to have a 1.5-fold greater likelihood of disability than do persons without these diseases. [15] In developing a research agenda, one wants to target the conditions of greatest importance both at the individual level and at the societal level. Societal impact is determined by the amount of disability produced by the condition in an individual and the prevalence of the disease in the population. Although there is substantial epidemiologic data on the prevalence and incidence of disability in the older population, [16] there is little information on the disabling impact of specific diseases at the societal level. A study by Verbrugge and Patrick illustrates the kind of information that is needed; they found that among men aged 70 or over, arthritis ranks as the number 1 cause of activity limitation, whereas cerebrovascular disease ranks as number 7. [17] This is because, as illustrated by the previously mentioned representative sample of noninstitutionalized older Americans, although arthritis produces less disability than stroke in any given individual, it occurs much more commonly than stroke (53% versus 5%). [15]

Better information on which diseases and conditions, alone and in combination, produce what kinds of disability could lead to the development of rehabilitative treatments that more precisely target the underlying mechanisms producing disability, thus improving the efficacy of rehabilitation. For example, exercise has been viewed as something of a panacea for functional deficits in the older population. However, a review by Keysor and Jette shows that relatively few exercise interventions have resulted in improved functional skills, even though improvements occur at the organ system level (eg, increased strength). [18] Keysor and Jette attribute these findings to an oversimplified theoretical rationale for exercise effects on severity of disability. They found that two of the five studies that showed improvement in functional outcomes targeted persons with chronic arthritis. Functional disability due to arthritis may respond better to exercise than do other causes of functional disability (eg, spinal stenosis).

A number of studies have shown that psychologic and social factors are associated with disability. These are particularly important factors for disability outcomes over time. For example, although correlations as high as 80% have been reported between measures of motor impairment and functional disability in persons recovering from acute spinal cord injury, [19] the correlations are lower among persons with chronic spinal cord injury. [20] Moreover, even though the extent and type of physical limitations bear a relationship to self-perceptions of disability, the relationship is not uniform. Only 70% of those reporting major mobility limitations and 80% of those using a wheelchair were found to perceive themselves as having a disability. [21] Increasingly, we are appreciating the influence of mental state on outcomes for a variety of diseases. Coexisting depression can adversely affect functional outcomes; stroke patients who are depressed, for example, have poorer functional outcomes. [22] Financial supports enable people to pay for personal assistance or equipment that in turn increases independence. Most insurance policies now cover the more basic types of adaptive equipment, but it can be difficult to obtain reimbursement for anything other than a standard wheelchair or commode. For instance, few insurance policies cover motorized scooters. Similarly, the physical environment is a key factor influencing functional outcomes among people with physical impairments. The Americans with Disabilities Act was enacted with this in mind. Someone who must use a wheelchair for mobility will be able to carry out activities in and outside the home only if the environment is wheelchair accessible. However, few studies have examined the role of these factors in the care of the older patient and how they may differ uniquely with age.

In addition, we need to understand the impact of disability from the perspective of the family and caregiver. The psychologic and financial burdens families face when patients survive with severe chronic disabilities are huge; these burdens are a source of significant anger at the health care system, and unmet needs may be common. [23,24] However, little is known about the effects of different types of caregiving on patients' outcomes from surgical and rehabilitation treatments. Some work suggests that, in the setting of chronic disease, training family and friends in methods of assisting patients and identifying family goals improves patient outcomes and prevents caregiver burnout. [25–28]

We need to understand better the ways people cope with disability over time (eg, avoiding the activity, using personal assistance, using assistive technology), the trade-offs between differing coping strategies, and if these vary for specific diseases and conditions. For example, is a wheelchair as beneficial for someone with the inability to walk because of cardiopulmonary disease as it is for someone who is unable to walk because of paraplegia or arthritis? Other key areas for further investigation include patient, family, and societal attitudes (eg, the influence of self-efficacy and sick-role perceptions on outcomes, induced disability with provision of personal assistance) and the costs and benefits of various types of assistive technology and enhanced environmental access (eg, the costs and benefits of using the principles of universal design both in the home and in public places, ie, deliberately designing products and environment to be usable by people of diverse abilities).

Giacomini discusses the merits and hazards of clinical research that attempts to draw on both qualitative and quantitative research traditions. [29] On one hand, she argues persuasively that qualitative findings may lose integrity when reduced and operationalized as quantitative variables. On the other hand, she points out that the two research traditions address essentially different questions about the world, so their findings tend to complement rather than compete as contributions to knowledge. Rehabilitation research in particular needs to support the development of methodology to better adapt and incorporate work from these two traditional research approaches. Disability is the product of both social and physical (biomedical) phenomena; therefore, rehabilitation research must draw from methodology developed to study both.

Empirical data are needed to better elucidate the disablement process and its treatment, but conceptual and theoretical models are needed as well. Such models help to put existing data into context, establishing directions for future research and facilitating rigorous research methodology. To a substantial extent, rehabilitation research has been characterized by inadequate theorization, scientifically poor methodology, and inadequate descriptions of the studied services. [30,31] In a review of rehabilitation research, Johnston et al noted that most studies identify the inputs (ie, patient characteristics) and the outputs (eg, functional outcomes), but that what happened in rehabilitation usually is defined vaguely. [32]

Several researchers have attempted to provide theoretical models for differing aspects of rehabilitation. For example, Strasser and Falconer focused on the rehabilitation team, and Kramer examined the patient perspective. [33,34] Other investigators have tried to apply to rehabilitation research existing models for the disablement process and the health services research model of structure, process, and outcomes. [35–37] Hoenig et al applied the standard health services research framework of structure, process, and outcome to published stroke rehabilitation research in a comprehensive review of the literature to identify gaps in the research and then used their findings to develop and validate a model for the structure of rehabilitation care (Figure 1). [38,39] This model is used to organize sections of this chapter on the components of rehabilitation treatment. However, this work serves only as a beginning; considerable additional work is needed. Multiple studies will be needed over the next decade. Some elements of a rehabilitation taxonomy will apply across conditions and rehabilitation disciplines; other elements will need to be specific to the condition being treated. The development of a uniform terminology for use across all rehabilitation studies is essential for the progress of rehabilitation research.

> *Rehab 1 (Level B)*: **The first step required, in support of all other recommended research efforts, is to develop uniform terminology, so that multisite research consortia can be formed to allow faster progress, as was done in the field of cancer research over the past 50 years.**

> *Rehab 2 (Levels B, A)*: **Hypothesis-testing research is needed to determine the costs and benefits of treatment that is targeted generically at the disability versus treatment that addresses the underlying diseases and impairments.**

> *Rehab 3 (Level B)*: **If it is important to individualize treatment on the basis of underlying cause (see Rehab 2), then additional research will be needed to identify the most efficient diagnostic methods to distinguish among causes of disability, with an eye to identifying characteristics that may affect treatment planning and outcomes. For example, a sudden acute event may need condition-specific treatment, whereas a slow decline in function may be amenable to treatment at the level of disability.**

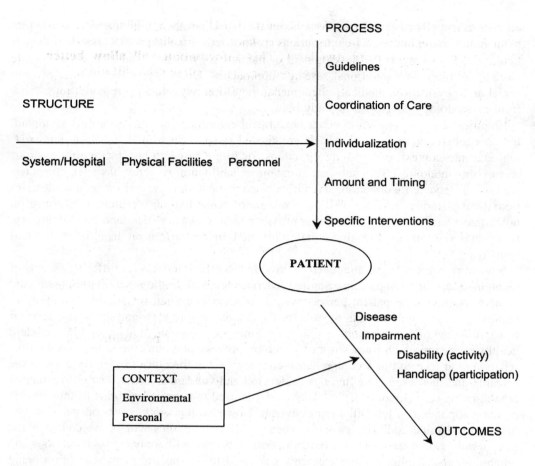

Figure 12.1—The structure, process, outcome rehabilitation model. (Based on Duncan PW, Hoenig H, Hamilton B, Samsa G. Characterizing medical rehabilitation interventions. In: Fuhrer MJ, ed.: Assessing Medical Rehabilitation Practices: The Promise of Outcomes Research. Baltimore: Brookes Publishing Co., 1997:307-17; and Hoenig H, Horner R, Duncan PW, et al. New horizons in stroke rehabilitation research. J Rehab Res Dev 1999; 36[1]:19-31.)

> ***Rehab 4 (Level B)***: **Mechanistic studies are needed on the physiologic processes underlying geriatric disability and on the potential effect of the biology of aging on response to rehabilitation, particularly for sarcopenia and recovery from acute illness.**
>
> ***Rehab 5 (Levels B, A)***: **Hypothesis-generating research followed by hypothesis-testing research is needed to better define the point in the disablement process when treatment is optimally instituted and whether or not optimal timing differs according to the disablement process (catastrophic versus progressive) or the underlying condition.**
>
> ***Rehab 6 (Level B)***: **A longitudinal, nationally representative cohort study is needed to define the disabling impact of different diseases**

and conditions at the societal level, stratified by age group and major categories of interest to geriatrics (eg, nursing-home residents versus community dwellers). This information will allow better prioritization of research endeavors in geriatric rehabilitation.

Rehab 7 (Level B): Observational and cohort studies are needed to identify the key social and environmental risk factors for current disability or progression into disability for the older patient, and the influence of these factors on rehabilitation outcomes.

Rehab 8 (Level B): Cross-sectional studies and longitudinal cohort studies of the relations between caregiving and outcomes are needed.

Rehab 9 (Level B): Adequate investigation of such factors as coping strategies, attitudes, and the cost versus the benefits of assistive technology and improved access will require both qualitative and quantitative research, and considerable work is needed to develop methods for combining the results of both these research traditions.

Rehab 10 (Levels B, A): Research is needed to articulate a clear theory or model of rehabilitation treatment that can then be tested.

Rehab 11 (Level B): Research is needed to delineate the components of the rehabilitation "black box" (eg, the dosage of rehabilitation).

COMPONENTS OF REHABILITATION

STRUCTURE OF CARE

Settings

In 1997 the Commission on Accreditation of Rehabilitation Facilities defined three levels of inpatient medical rehabilitation (rehabilitation units in acute care or rehabilitation hospitals, and two levels of nursing-home rehabilitation), as well as outpatient and home health rehabilitation. [40] Although regulatory standards have changed since then, much of the research on the effect of various care settings on rehabilitation outcomes has been based on this traditional classification. The relationship of rehabilitation outcomes to setting for care has been most thoroughly studied for stroke rehabilitation, where better outcomes have been shown consistently for patients treated in specialized stroke units. [41] Similarly, treatment in geriatric evaluation units has been shown to improve outcomes over usual care. [42,43] What is unclear is why rehabilitation outcomes vary across settings. Since costs of care can vary markedly across settings, [44] this is a question of some interest. For example, Duncan et al showed that compliance with guidelines of the Agency for Health Care Policy and Research for stroke rehabilitation varies among postacute-care settings, and that better compliance is associated with better 6-month outcomes for stroke patients. [45]

Reimbursement has been and continues to be an important factor affecting the use of rehabilitation. [45–48] Reimbursement for rehabilitation is in flux, with the emergence and more recent decline of health maintenance organizations and the use of prospective payment for inpatient rehabilitation in the near future.

Providers

There are many different kinds of rehabilitation providers. Qualifications vary according to years of education (eg, master's degree for a physical therapist versus an associate degree for a PT assistant), training in unique therapeutic techniques (eg, occupational therapist versus physical therapist), and licensure (eg, unlicensed PT aide versus licensed PT assistant). In addition, state requirements for licensure and the privileges conferred with licensure vary considerably. In some states, physical therapists are allowed to treat patients without physician referral (open access); in others, physician referral is required. The effects of these regulatory differences are unknown. Though many third-party payers require physician referral irrespective of state regulations, such regulatory differences might have important effects on the utilization of PT, on the amount and kind of physician supervision provided to patients receiving PT, and on patient outcomes.

The differences in training among rehabilitation providers are believed to account for the distinct attributes of each type of provider; however, in reality very little is known about the relative merits of the different types of rehabilitation providers. Moreover, there can be considerable overlap in the services rendered by the different providers. The use of multiple different providers in rehabilitation is based on the belief that the resultant group interaction offers significant benefits to patients (eg, the combined treatment of functional mobility by OT, PT, and nursing may act to reinforce newly learned techniques). However, even though the comprehensive treatment team has been the foundation of rehabilitation, evidence of its effectiveness has been meager. [49] Indeed, we even lack data on how commonly multiple providers are involved in rehabilitative treatment. The use of a single type of provider may be common for the treatment of musculoskeletal disorders or postoperative care with orthopedic surgery, and the importance of team approach to successful rehabilitation of those conditions may be no more than a myth.

The benefits of a team approach have been studied for several conditions common in the older population, with inconclusive results for any of the conditions studied. For example, one meta-analysis of stroke studies did not show a significant difference in effect according to provider type (ie, PT versus OT). [50] Yet another meta-analysis showed that more successful stroke units are characterized by coordinated multidisciplinary rehabilitation, the use of education and training programs, and specialization of medical and surgical staff. [41] Among patients with rheumatoid arthritis, one randomized trial showed that team care predicts better overall health at 1 year than does usual care, as measured by the Sickness Impact Profile, but another randomized trial found just the opposite, with no differences between groups receiving team care and usual care. [51,52] With regard to geriatric rehabilitation specifically, Weiland et al examined Veterans Affairs geriatric units and found them to be a fairly diverse group, falling into two categories: standard (56% of geriatric units) and nonstandard (44% of geriatric units). Standard units were found to have better outcomes and, among other qualities, were characterized by the use of specifically assigned physicians, nurses, and social workers. [53]

The paucity of objective information about the benefits of using specific types of rehabilitation providers is remarkable in light of the high costs of rehabilitation and the potential for savings with the use of paraprofessionals. For example, in North Carolina salaries in 1994 for PT assistants ranged from $18,000 to $37,000, and salaries for physical therapists ranged from $34,000 to $80,000. [54]

Equipment

Most of the research data on rehabilitation equipment pertains to equipment used to provide physical modalities of one sort or another or for specific types of exercise (see the next section). However, studies of stroke rehabilitation show that the availability of rehabilitation equipment (eg, onsite apartment designed for use by people with physical disability) may be associated with better functional outcomes. [55,56]

PROCESS OF CARE: INTERVENTIONS

Interventions used in geriatric rehabilitation include exercise, adaptive techniques (modifications of the way an activity is performed), assistive technology (eg, canes, walkers, wheelchairs), physical modalities (eg, heat, cold, ultrasound), and orthotic (braces, splints) and prosthetic (artificial limbs) devices. [57] These are first briefly summarized, and then a more detailed review of the two most commonly used interventions, exercise and assistive technology, is provided.

Exercise programs are used to increase general flexibility, muscular strength, and aerobic endurance, but exercises may be used for more specific purposes (eg, preserving bone density, reducing joint pain, increasing coordination after a stroke). Different types of exercises have varying levels of data supporting their efficacy for specific conditions.

Adaptive techniques involve modifying a task so that it can be performed despite physical limitations. Adaptive techniques often are combined with assistive technology. The use of adaptive techniques and assistive technology enables the person to interact more favorably with the environment. For example, the use of a cane can make walking easier and safer. Although assistive devices can be purchased without the involvement of a rehabilitation provider, rehabilitation specialists often make recommendations about which devices will be most helpful in improving function and facilitating independence.

Physical modalities use physical processes to treat the patient; examples are ultrasound, diathermy, transcutaneous electrical nerve stimulation, whirlpool, massage, and the application of heat or cold. Research data on the efficacy of many physical modalities is limited. [58–60]

Orthotic devices are externally applied devices that act to support the musculoskeletal system. Examples are inserts or specially adapted shoes for arthritic problems of the feet, splinting and padding for overuse syndromes such as carpal tunnel syndrome, and braces to support an unstable or weak joint, such as an ankle-foot orthosis used after a stroke. Prosthetics are devices that act to substitute or replace a missing body part; examples are a prosthetic eye or prosthetic limb. Individual orthotic and prosthetic devices have been studied in some detail, but we need systematic research and a systematic review of the effectiveness of commonly used orthotics and prosthetics.

Benefits and Types of Exercise

There is substantial evidence that regular physical activity has a number of health benefits. For example, greater physical activity is associated with a twofold increase in the likelihood of dying without disability. [61] Given that physical activity is good, the question arises whether some kinds of physical activity are better than others. Each type of exercise appears to have unique benefits. Exercise can be classified in five categories: resistance, aerobic (endurance), balance, flexibility, and functionally based. Within each category there are various subtypes, depending on how the exercise is delivered (eg, water based or weight bearing, isotonic or isokinetic), the rate at which the difficulty of the exercise is increased, and the frequency of exercise. This chapter provides an overview of the research on the use of the five categories of exercise to treat older patients but does not review research on the subtypes.

Resistance Exercise

Strength training has been a focus of considerable research in geriatrics. This is due, in part, to the strong evidence that muscle mass declines with age. [62,63] Work has been done to characterize the underlying physiology behind the change in muscle mass, but the cause of age-related decline in muscle mass, or *sarcopenia*, remains elusive. Factors that have been explored include loss of spinal alpha motor neurons causing denervation atrophy, loss of specific types of muscle fibers, increased vulnerability to contraction-induced muscle injury, incomplete tissue repair, disuse muscle atrophy, malnutrition, and reduced trophic factor release (eg, testosterone).

Much of the interest in resistive exercise has been generated because, not only are there age-related changes in muscle strength, but resistive exercise has been shown to improve a number of physiologic parameters of great importance to the older person, including insulin sensitivity, bone mineral density, aerobic capacity, and muscle strength. In addition, a variety of epidemiologic studies have related muscle strength to functional outcomes. For example, Gibbs et al showed that low baseline quadriceps strength predicts decline in walking speed 2 and 4 years later, [64] and others have shown that slower walking speed predicts dependence in self-care. [65] Thus, a logical chain of evidence in support of resistance exercise for the older population is apparent. Since muscle mass and function decline with aging, and resistance exercise can increase leg strength, and leg strength is associated with gait speed, and gait speed is associated with disability, many geriatricians have expected that resistance exercise would improve functional outcomes. Indeed, many basic activities of daily living (ADLs) are more dependent on gross motor strength than on aerobic capacity.

A review by Keysor and Jette showed that relatively few exercise interventions have improved functional skills, even though improvements occur at the organ system level (eg, increased strength). [18] The most consistent positive effects from exercise were found to be in strength, aerobic capacity, flexibility, and walking and standing balance, with over half of studies that examined these outcomes showing benefit. However, of the exercise studies that examined ADLs or overall disability, few showed benefit. For example, 14 of 21 studies that examined gait speed as an outcome showed a beneficial effect from exercise, but only 5 of 14 studies that examined ADLs showed a beneficial effect. A number of factors may account for these findings. It may be that functional benefits become apparent with greater improvements in strength. Investigators have examined combination interventions (eg, nutritional support plus resistive exercise), hoping to increase the benefits of resistance exercise in the older population, but none have shown added benefits over resistance exercise alone. [66,67] The lack of functional benefit from resistive exercise alone also may be because other factors besides muscle strength are determinants of functional performance. For example, leg strength explains only 25% to 30% of 6-minute walk distances. [68,69] Another factor that may account for the lack of functional benefit may be the specificity of exercise training; there is some evidence that the effect of resistive exercise on muscle function may quite specific, [70,71] such that resistive exercise performed at one speed may improve performance at that speed but not at another speed. In turn, this might mean that function would be improved the most in those tasks performed at similar speeds to the exercise training itself. Studies are examining functionally based resistive exercise in the hope of helping patients generalize to specific functional tasks the gains in muscle strength achieved with resistive exercise (see below, the section on functionally based exercise).

Aerobic (Endurance) Exercise

Much of the research on aerobic exercise has focused on younger adults. Even so, there is a substantial body of research on the effects of aerobic exercise on the older adult. Most studies show that aerobic exercise can improve aerobic capacity. For example, Keysor and Jette report that 70% of studies of aerobic conditioning exercise in older adults showed improvements in aerobic capacity, but that the effect of aerobic exercise on body composition is less consistent. [18] Green and Crouse report in their meta-analysis that exercise training significantly improves maximum oxygen consumption in older people, with the magnitude being slightly less than that seen in younger people and inversely related to the individual's age. [72] Studies of aerobic exercise for specific conditions commonly seen in older adults have shown beneficial effects. For example, a meta-analysis showed that aerobic exercise significantly reduces systolic blood pressure in older adults. [73] Weight-bearing exercise for prevention of bone loss in postmenopausal women, walking for treatment of intermittent claudication, and exercise-based rehabilitation for coronary heart disease are additional examples. [74–76] However, it must be noted that a recent review of randomized trials of treatment for coronary heart disease found a bias toward younger adults, and few studies examined age-specific efficacy. [77] With regard to functional outcomes, a review found that longitudinal studies consistently show that long-term physical activity is related to postponement of disability in older adults, but that randomized trials of aerobic training do not necessarily support the results of longitudinal studies. [78] The reasons for this are unclear. However, much of the physiologic benefit of aerobic exercise is the prevention of or reduction in the severity of diseases whose end-organ effects cause disability (eg, stroke in uncontrolled hypertension), so older people who already suffer disability may experience less benefit.

Balance Exercise

Exercises can be designed to deliberately stress the systems involved in balance, including the musculoskeletal system and the vestibular system. When used to stress the vestibular system, these have been termed *habituation exercises*, and they appear to have efficacy in the treatment of benign positional vertigo. [79] Various types of exercise interventions, including Tai Chi, have been used to treat persons at risk for falls, with apparent benefit. [80–82] Balance exercise appears to be most effective when it is used as a part of a comprehensive or multifaceted approach; [83] the use of exercise to treat falls is discussed in detail (see the section on falls, below). Though we have made substantial progress in our understanding of balance exercise, its role in relation to other kinds of exercise needs additional study (see Rehab 18, below).

Flexibility Exercise

In a 1999 review of flexibility training, Krivickas pointed out that researchers have largely ignored flexibility training. [84] Most people, including professionals, believe that flexibility is beneficial; however, the belief is based on remarkably few data. Correlations have been observed between flexibility deficits and specific types of injuries, but all of these studies were in adolescents or young adults. Despite the fact that many disease processes common among elderly people can adversely affect flexibility (eg, stroke, arthritis), there are few studies in the older population of the effect on outcomes of a loss of range of motion or of the efficacy of exercise interventions to restore flexibility. One study found a relationship in older persons between decreased hip and ankle range of motion and a history of falls. [85] Another study compared flexibility exercise alone with flexibility exercise plus resistance training in older men and found that range of motion increases with the flexibility exercise alone but does not increase when resistance training is included, which suggests that resistance training may act to decrease flexibility. [86] With this exception, studies of flexibility have included the flexibility exercise as one component of a multifaceted exercise intervention. Research is needed to identify the unique contribution of flexibility exercise relative to other types of exercise (see Rehab 18, below).

Functionally Based Exercise

Functionally based exercises may be particularly beneficial for older persons. Functionally based exercise has been studied among disabled older patients in assisted-living centers and in demented patients in nursing homes, and as a type of stroke rehabilitation termed *massed activity* or *constraint therapy*. There is some evidence that the effects of exercise may be quite specific, with the greatest effect occurring with muscle function similar to that of the exercise itself. [70,71] This produces a dilemma, since a primary goal of exercise for the older person is to improve functional performance across diverse activities. The use of functionally based exercise may offer a solution to this problem.

Task-specific resistive exercise has been used successfully to improve the endurance during and rapidity of rising from sitting to standing by persons with mobility disability who live in congregate housing facilities. [87] Task-specific training involves training in tasks that are components of an act, for example, of rising from a supine to a sitting position on the side of the bed (which involves, first, rolling to one side, then moving the legs over the side of the bed, and finally pushing up to a seated position). As needed, partial assistance is provided or weights are added (eg, with a weighted vest) to ensure that task difficulty is sufficiently but not overly challenging.

In the nursing-home setting, functionally based exercises have been incorporated into daily routines. Examples include having the patient perform an extra sit-to-stand with each transfer or using graded steps that require the patient to independently perform an ever-increasing portion of ADLs. One of the benefits of functionally based exercises is that they appear to be effective even for demented patients. For example, in a randomized trial, Schnelle et al showed that an exercise program integrated into the daily nursing care of demented nursing-home patients results in improved endurance during ADLs. [88] However, this type of intervention appears to require increased nursing staff time. Rogers et al showed that patients undergoing skills training take, on average, twice as long to complete a given self-care task than do those in usual care. However, they require nearly 50% less physical assistance with self-care, and disruptive behavior declines by more than 50%. [89]

Recently Morris et al used a quasi-experimental design to compare the impact of nurses trained to elicit greater patient participation during daily care activities with a resistance and aerobic exercise program and with a control group. Both the exercise and the nursing rehabilitation groups were found to have better functional outcomes than the usual care group. However, the nursing rehabilitation group showed a trend ($P = .07$) for greater response than the exercise group. [90]

Massed activity (repetitive exercise activities for up to 8 hours per day), often used in conjunction with constraint therapy wherein the unaffected limb is constrained, is a new form of treatment for stroke patients that may have substantial efficacy for both acute and chronic stroke. [91] The activities include both functional activities and specific exercises to develop components of movement needed for functional activities. There is some evidence that this therapeutic approach may be effective not only for motor deficits but for aphasia as well. [92]

As with other types of exercise reviewed, a pressing need is to compare the efficacy of functionally based exercise with other types of exercise for various conditions and patient populations (see Rehab 18, below).

Comparisons of Types of Exercise

Few studies have compared the relative merits of differing forms of exercise for the same condition. Ettinger et al carried out a randomized trial of resistance exercise, aerobic exercise, and health education for knee osteoarthritis and found that they are both more effective than health education alone, but not significantly different from one another. [93] The study by Morris et al described in the preceding section was also a comparative study. [90] A meta-analysis of the Frailties and Injuries: Cooperative Studies of Intervention Techniques trials showed that the adjusted fall incidence ratio for treatment arms that included general exercise was 0.90 and for those that included balance was 0.83. [80] A somewhat different result may be seen in a study by Wolfson et al that showed that balance and strength training have different outcomes. [82] Specifically, their randomized study showed that balance training improves balance measures and strength training improves strength, and that there is no interaction between the two types of training.

Adaptive Techniques and Assistive Technology

Increasingly, assistive technology is being used to cope with disability. [94] In 1995, requests for durable medical equipment amounted to $6.27 million, 25.7% more than in 1994. [95] Although the majority of assistive device users are aged 65 or over, recent increases in the use of most devices far exceed the increase in population, even after accounting for age. From 1980 to 1994, the U.S. population increased by 19.1%; however, the age-adjusted use of leg braces increased by 52.1%, canes by 37.0%, walkers by 70.1%, and wheelchairs by 82.6%. [96] The increased popularity of assistive technology is due in part to the remarkable improvements in assistive technology design, both in functionality and in appearance. For example, design options for wheelchairs have exploded in the past two decades; wheelchairs are now lighter and many are motorized, and the ability to customize the wheelchair itself to the physical dimensions of the rider is improved. [97,98]

Despite the growing use of assistive technology, remarkably little information from research about its use in general and even less on its use by older persons is available. This lack is particularly striking when it is compared with the considerable body of work in geriatrics on the use of formal and informal support, another commonly used method for coping with disability. Nonetheless, assistive technology offers great potential benefit for the older population. Epidemiologic data and one randomized trial show that assistive technology may decrease task difficulty, decrease hours of personal assistance, and decrease costs for institutional care. [99–101]

However, most studies of assistive technology have examined either the functionality of the equipment at a basic engineering level or technology utilization in general, examining overall use rather than use that is specific to the device or the activity. [102] Studies of assistive technology usage show that many disabled people lack potentially helpful devices, many of the devices that are provided are not used, and problems with device utility are common. [103–106] For example, one investigator found that up to half of the mobility aids owned by older persons are in disrepair or ill-fitting, and many devices are not used at all. [107] Some disuse may be due to improved health or changes in personal preferences. Two studies found that the primary reason cited by patients for discarding aids is improved health. [108,109] In addition, there appear to be gender differences in use of technology. [104] However, the provision process itself also appears to be a problem. For example, one study of older wheelchair users showed that they commonly obtain wheelchairs without professional assistance, but that those who do this are more likely to report problems with the wheelchair. [103] Problems with acquisition of assistive technology reported by O'Day and Corcoran include lack of funds to purchase the most suitable equipment, fraud and abuse by providers, and denials of needed equipment by third-party payers. [110] It is noteworthy that one study that examined an improved process for provision of bath aids reported that it resulted in higher device utilization and greater patient safety during bathing. [111] However, the functionality of wheelchairs in nursing homes, where more assistance might be available, is equally if not more filled with problems. [112] Key rehabilitation investigators are calling now for an investment in research to assess the outcomes of assistive technology. [113]

OUTCOMES OF CARE

Considerable work has been done on measuring functional outcomes in geriatric rehabilitation. Several excellent texts are available that review the current state of the field; one example is *Measuring Health* by McDowell and Newell. [114] Two major gaps persist in outcome measures: one concerns the most distal of functional outcomes, social participation (eg, community mobility) and quality of life, and the other concerns the use of outcome measures for specific types of interventions (eg, assistive technology) for specific conditions. Future research in all areas of rehabilitation will need to compare outcome measures across studies and across conditions, to allow attainment of consensus on which measures are most useful in what circumstances.

> *Rehab 12 (Levels B, A)*: **Hypothesis-generating research followed by hypothesis-testing research is needed to identify the critical factors responsible for the more optimal outcomes seen in some settings.**

> *Rehab 13 (Levels B, A)*: **Hypothesis-generating research followed by hypothesis-testing research is needed to examine the effect of changes in Medicare reimbursement on access to rehabilitation and the quality of rehabilitative care.**

Rehab 14 (Level A): **Randomized trials are needed to investigate the trade-offs of using less costly paraprofessionals to provide rehabilitation treatment, of using streamlined teams, and of using diverse strategies for team coordination and communication.**

Rehab 15 (Levels B, A): **Observational studies followed by randomized trials are needed to identify which conditions are best treated with a team approach (eg, disability resulting from multiple medical problems or a condition like stroke that causes multiple physical impairments) versus which conditions are treated equally well by a single provider (eg, disability due to a single condition causing a limited physical impairment, like osteoarthritis of the knee).**

Rehab 16 (Level A): **Randomized controlled trials are needed to examine whether specific kinds of resistive exercise, modes of exercise delivery, and combinations of treatments (eg, psychosocial intervention plus exercise intervention) might enhance functional outcomes for older persons, and which functional outcomes are affected to the greatest extent.**

Rehab 17 (Level A): **Randomized trials are needed on the health, functional, and quality-of-life benefits of aerobic exercise in older persons who are already disabled. The study population should be homogeneous with regard to amount and type of disability, and methodologic consideration should be given to how to deal with underlying medical conditions in the population and the differences they might produce in response to exercise. The outcome measures should be clearly specified; they might include physiologic parameters such as blood pressure, body composition, oxygen-carrying capacity, measures of physical function such as 6-minute walk distance, self-reported difficulty with activities of daily living, and measures of health-related quality of life like the Medical Outcomes Study 36-item Short Form 36 (SF 36).**

Rehab 18 (Levels B, A): **Hypothesis-generating research (eg, databases, cohort studies, case series) followed by hypothesis-testing research is needed to examine the benefits of differing types of exercise for specific conditions.**

Rehab 19 (Levels B, A): **Observational and cohort studies are greatly needed to identify effect size for key outcomes, which devices are promising enough to merit later comparative clinical trials, and what long-term follow-up shows among older people using assistive devices. These should be followed by randomized trials of the most promising devices.**

REHABILITATION FOR SPECIFIC CONDITIONS

There are important age-related differences in rehabilitation for nearly every condition treated with rehabilitation, primarily because of the high prevalence of multiple comorbid conditions in the older population and age-related changes in physiology of a variety of organ systems that impact physical function. One study showed that medical comorbidity scores higher than 5 on the Cumulative Illness Rating Scale predicts greater length of stay and less gain in functional status, and 60% of geriatric patients receiving rehabilitation have scores of 6 or more.[115] Greater lengths of stay and lower functional outcomes have been reported for older patients for most conditions in which this has been examined. For example, among patients with spinal cord injury, it was found that length of stay is 58 days and the gain in score on the Functional Independence Measure is 27.8 among patients aged 60 and over, but the length of stay is 43 days and the gain on the Functional Independence Measure is 38.2 among patients aged 18 to 39.[116] Unfortunately, age-specific differences in outcomes have not been examined for all conditions treated with rehabilitation. For example, a National Institutes of Health consensus statement on rehabilitation of persons with traumatic brain injury states that little attention has been paid to the needs of high-risk age groups (eg, elderly persons), and it recommends research to examine the consequences and effects of rehabilitation after traumatic brain injury in elderly persons.[117] In addition, data are lacking on the disabling impact of specific medical conditions in the older population as a whole or for particular subsets (eg, nursing-home patients). Given the lack of empirical data to guide the selection of conditions to cover, the conditions reviewed herein were selected on the basis of prevalence in the older population along with likely utility and importance of rehabilitation to condition-specific outcomes. No doubt, important conditions are not included in this review.

ARTHRITIC AND RELATED MUSCULOSKELETAL PROBLEMS

Rehabilitation interventions are used widely to treat arthritic conditions. Research into their effectiveness is of great importance, and rehabilitation treatment of arthritic conditions is an active area of research. However, an important caveat in reviewing the literature and an important priority for research on rehabilitative treatment of arthritic conditions is to specify the underlying pathophysiology and the joint being studied. Otherwise, important findings may be overlooked. For example, two recent reviews of exercise for osteoarthritis showed conflicting results. Although differing methods may account for the discrepancies, another possibility is that the less conclusive analysis included studies of both the hip and the knee whereas the more conclusive study examined the knee alone.[59,118] From an anatomic point of view, it is likely that exercise is not as effective for a deep ball-and-socket joint like the hip as it is for a more mobile joint like the knee, where the muscles and tendons provide considerable support to the joint, and exercises that strengthen the muscles therefore are likely to affect the biomechanical function of the joint. Thus, a review that combines studies of the two joints might come up with inconclusive results, not because of the ineffectiveness of the intervention but rather because of the effectiveness differential.

Similarly, it might make sense at first glance to review painful musculoskeletal conditions of a given joint as a general group. However, there likely are important differences in response to therapy, depending on the underlying cause of the musculoskeletal disorder. Consider, for example, osteoporosis and osteoarthritis of the spine, with spinal stenosis as the specific example of the latter. Spinal stenosis is a consequence of bony hypertrophy and narrowing of the central neural canal. There is little reason to believe that exercise would reduce bony hypertrophy; if anything, just the opposite would result. Moreover, it is difficult to envision how alterations in the strength or mechanics of the paraspinous muscles would affect the central canal. On the other hand, the underlying pathophysiology of osteoporosis likely would be affected beneficially by weight-bearing exercise; moreover, pain from the flexion deformities seen after compression fractures in spinal osteoporosis might well respond to flexibility and strengthening exercises for the paraspinous muscles. Indeed, one recent review of exercise for low back pain distinguished among major disease categories and found important differences in outcomes. [119]

A number of studies of exercise, assistive technology, and orthotics show that these can be effective strategies to reduce disability due to diverse musculoskeletal disorders, although the specific type and amount of exercise and the most useful devices and orthotics depend on the specific joints affected and the underlying disorder(s).

We lack comparisons of home-based versus clinic-based exercise for arthritic conditions. What is the difference in short- and long-term efficacy of exercise therapy for osteoarthritis of the knee from a one-time PT evaluation with recommendations for home exercise versus PT in the clinic three times weekly for 3 to 4 weeks? Does the amount and kind of patient education when prescribing a mobility aid affect outcomes? Which patients prescribed a cane would benefit from seeing a physical therapist for gait training, and which patients need no more assistance than that available from untrained staff at a local medical supply store?

STROKE

Post-stroke rehabilitation can be provided in a rehabilitation hospital, a subacute rehabilitation unit, a skilled nursing facility, or via home health or on an outpatient basis. Guidelines published in 1995 by the Agency for Health Care Policy and Research (renamed: Agency for Healthcare Research and Quality) as well as guidelines published in 2003 by the Veterans Health Administration suggest that choice of rehabilitation setting be dictated by the severity of the patient's impairment, the availability of family and social support, and the patient's or family's preferences [120,121] The research evidence on settings for stroke rehabilitation and use of massed activity to treat stroke-related deficits are discussed above, in the section on interventions.

Studies have shown surprising plasticity in the adult brain. [122] Currently, investigators are studying not only massed activity but also combinations of exercise and pharmacologic treatment (eg, sympathomimetics) in an attempt to enhance the responsiveness of the brain to interventions designed to facilitate motor recovery via neuronal plasticity. [123] This research has not targeted the older population per se, but since strokes are common in the older population, the work is pertinent to geriatric rehabilitation. Investigation into interventions to mold and enhance neural plasticity is a very exciting area of research in stroke rehabilitation, and work in this area that focuses on older persons will be needed.

A number of comorbid conditions can have important effects on stroke outcomes. Kelly-Hayes and Paige provide a review of psychosocial factors important to stroke recovery. [124] For example, depression is common after stroke and is associated with poor functional outcomes, and treatment of stroke-related depression may improve cognitive function post-stroke. [125,126] Stroke patients with dysphagia are at risk for malnutrition, which can adversely affect functional outcomes. [127] One study showed that early nutritional support in these patients reduces mortality. [128] Malnutrition may also adversely affect functional recovery by reducing endurance, interfering with rebuilding muscle strength, and increasing the risk of pressure ulcers and infectious complications.

CARDIAC DISEASE

The federal guidelines for cardiac rehabilitation note that elderly patients are referred for cardiac rehabilitation less frequently than younger persons, but that they likely would benefit from exercise-based cardiac rehabilitation. [129] However, there is little hard evidence of this because most cardiology clinical research has not specifically examined the older population. [77] In addition, the effect of comorbid cardiopulmonary disease on rehabilitation outcomes for other conditions needs further study in light of data suggesting that, for example, cardiac disease in combination with arthritis produces more disability that either condition alone. [11] We have good evidence that there are important age-related changes in cardiac function, [130] and cardiac disease is common in the older population.

HIP FRACTURE

The goals of hip fracture rehabilitation are to restore functional ambulation and independent self-care; however, many people have substantial decline in physical function after hip fracture despite surgery and rehabilitation. Several studies have shown that high-intensity postoperative PT may prevent postoperative complications and promote better functional outcomes. [13,131,132] However, a review suggests that definitive proof of the merits of early, high-intensity PT after acute hip fracture is lacking. [12] A prospective case series of nearly 600 patients aged 65 and over with hip fracture who were allowed full weight bearing showed that, after 1 year or more, 5.3% of those treated by internal fixation suffer loss of fixation or nonunion and 0.6% of those treated with hemiarthroplasty require revision. [133] However, a Cochrane Review concludes that there is insufficient evidence to determine the effects of early weight bearing after the internal fixation of an intracapsular proximal femoral fracture. [134] The merits of postoperative ambulation restrictions like "partial weight bearing" or "touch-down weight bearing" need further study, as older adults may have difficulty comprehending these instructions if they have cognitive deficits or postoperative delirium, and such restrictions in turn may interfere with optimal postoperative PT.

AMPUTATION

Amputation in older persons usually occurs in the setting of severe peripheral vascular disease, often in association with longstanding diabetes mellitus, sometimes complicated by hypertension or tobacco abuse. Comorbid disease, including cardiopulmonary disease, stroke, retinopathy, and prior amputation, are common and may affect the functional outcome (as does the level of amputation). Premorbid functional limitations and comorbid conditions must be considered both preoperatively in determining the level of amputation and the ability to tolerate repeated surgery, and postoperatively in determining the goals for rehabilitation. There are recent advances in design of artificial limbs that increase biomechanical efficiency, but at considerable financial cost. Andrews, as well as Cutson and Bongiorni, provide recent reviews of rehabilitation for the older amputee. [135,136] The cost-benefit trade-offs for older patients differ markedly from those seen with younger persons, for whom amputation usually is traumatic but the cardiovascular and musculoskeletal systems are otherwise intact.

DECONDITIONING, SARCOPENIA, AND FRAILTY

Deconditioning occurs with a decrease in activity level for whatever reason, and typically it includes loss of strength, loss of flexibility, and metabolic and hemodynamic abnormalities (eg, calcium wasting, orthostatic hypotension).[137] Deconditioning may occur with disuse because of pain, incoordination, or any other cause of decreased physical activity. A common cause of deconditioning is enforced immobility as a consequence of acute illness or hospitalization. Early mobilization during hospitalization and regular participation in exercise during hospitalization and after discharge are thought to be the most helpful interventions to prevent and treat deconditioning. However, evidence for the efficacy of exercise among acutely ill older patients is just beginning to appear.[138,139]

Deconditioning is thought to be one of the factors underlying the sarcopenia and frailty sometimes found with aging. Treatment of sarcopenia and related frailty is an active area of research in geriatrics. Research on deconditioning, sarcopenia, and frailty is highly pertinent to geriatric rehabilitation in that exercise, alone or in combination with other treatments (eg, growth hormone, nutritional support), is being used as a treatment for sarcopenia; moreover, deconditioning, sarcopenia, and frailty can adversely affect rehabilitation outcomes. The evidence on exercise interventions is reviewed in the intervention section of this chapter. However, some evidence supports the concept that sarcopenia is a complex condition due to the interaction of multiple factors, both hormonal and environmental.[140,141] The efficacy of rehabilitation treatment for sarcopenia likely will be enhanced as the complex physiologic abnormalities underlying this condition are better understood.

FALLS

"Falls" is a diagnosis not often mentioned in connection with rehabilitation, but rehabilitation interventions are among those often used to prevent falls. The most commonly used rehabilitation interventions in falls prevention programs are various types of exercise and home assessment with environmental modification. A review of randomized trials of falls prevention interventions identified 23 studies that included exercise, 9 studies of home assessment and surveillance, 1 study of hip protectors, and no studies of footwear.[142] The authors concluded that the majority of exercise studies suggest a decrease in falling, with balance training appearing to be the most effective exercise intervention, and they concluded that the majority of home assessment studies showed benefit as well. A Cochrane review of 18 falls prevention trials and one planned meta-analysis concludes that the evidence does not support the effect of exercise alone in establishing protection against falls, but that the evidence does support the use of exercise as one of multiple interventions specifically targeting identified risk factors in individual patients.[143] An editorial by Tinetti[144] identifies two research needs on falls: Research that focuses intently on single interventions (as opposed to the multifocal interventions previously tested) to better establish the potency of each intervention and to establish its utility for subgroups of patients, and research that would enable implementation in clinical practice of the results of this research. The American Geriatrics Society, the British Geriatrics Society, and the American Academy of Orthopaedic Surgeons recently issued a research agenda for falls and identified the following priorities: cost-effectiveness studies of falls-prevention strategies; examination of risk stratification to identify persons most at risk and persons who would benefit the most; treatment interventions for specific subgroups of patients, including hospitalized patients and those with cognitive impairment; identification of the most effective elements of exercise programs (eg, types of exercise, duration, frequency); identification of patient groups most likely to benefit from home safety assessment; and examination of the merits of mobility aids for falls prevention. [145]

For further discussion of falls prevention, see Chapter 13 on cross-cutting issues.

PAIN

Acute, chronic, and acute-on-chronic pain problems are common in older patients. This is not surprising, given the prevalence of musculoskeletal problems and malignancies in this age group. Unfortunately, pain may be under-recognized in older patients, especially those with cognitive disorders. [146] Currently, the management of pain in older patients includes the use of medications, injections, exercise, physical modalities like heat or cold, behavioral approaches, assistive devices, and orthotics. [146,147] However, we know little about which interventions are most effective.

For further discussion of pain management, see Chapter 2, Geriatric Anesthesia.

> *Rehab 20 (Level B)*: **Epidemiologic and observational studies of older patients with specific disabling conditions are needed in order to identify risk factors and to select key outcomes for measurement in future clinical trials.**

> *Rehab 21 (Levels B, A)*: **Observational and cohort studies are needed to define the efficacy and safety of specific types of exercise, assistive devices, and orthotics for arthritic and musculoskeletal conditions. These studies could lead later to controlled trials comparing the most promising interventions.**

> *Rehab 22 (Levels B, A)*: **Observational and cohort studies are needed in the rehabilitation of musculoskeletal conditions to obtain preliminary data on the effects of the location of the physical therapy, the level of expertise of therapists needed, and how much is accomplished by education of elderly patients. This could lead eventually to controlled trials assessing these variables.**

> *Rehab 23 (Levels B, A)*: **Hypothesis-generating research followed by hypothesis-testing research is needed to identify the key components facilitating better outcomes that are seen in some settings and to identify ways to optimize treatment and outcomes among elderly patients unable to tolerate therapy in a stroke unit or rehabilitation hospital.**

> *Rehab 24 (Level A)*: **Randomized controlled trials of exercise-based cardiac rehabilitation, as a function of age and comorbid conditions, would be very valuable and are urgently needed.**

> *Rehab 25 (Level A)*: **Randomized controlled trials are needed to test the efficacy and safety for elderly patients of early, high-intensity physical therapy following hip fracture surgery and of postoperative restrictions on ambulation.**

Rehab 26 (Levels B, A): Observational and cohort studies should be performed to compare the costs and benefits of using newer prostheses in younger and older persons; factors found to be associated with better outcomes for older persons should then be tested in controlled trials.

Rehab 27 (Levels B, A): Basic laboratory research is needed to determine the factors that cause sarcopenia or that interact to cause it in older persons. Findings from this research should then be used in clinical trials of interventions to prevent or treat sarcopenia.

Rehab 28 (Level A): Randomized trials are needed to examine the merits of specific falls-prevention interventions (eg, types or duration or frequency of exercise, mobility aids, home safety interventions) and for specific subgroups of elderly patients (eg, cognitively impaired, hospitalized) and to examine the cost-effectiveness of various falls-prevention strategies.

Rehab 29 (Levels B, A): Observational and cohort studies are needed to clarify the natural history of pain syndromes, identify risk factors, and describe the effects of treatment approaches. Ultimately, the most promising approaches should be identified and tested in controlled trials.

KEY RESEARCH QUESTIONS IN GERIATRIC REHABILITATION

Rehab KQ1: What is the process in elderly persons underlying the development of disability and the factors influencing the disablement process?

Hypothesis-generating research: A nationally representative longitudinal study is needed to address two related research questions. First, what is the disability impact for older adults of specific diseases, both at the individual level and at the population level? For a variety of conditions, we have individual-level data on the amount of associated disability and population-level data on their incidence and prevalence, but we lack population-level data on the resultant disability. Second, how does the disablement process differ in older adults, what factors modify the disablement process, and do these vary across conditions? This latter investigation should examine the processes underlying catastrophic or acute-onset disability versus progressive disability. Existing longitudinal studies should be assessed to see if they could be adapted for these purposes. In addition, mechanistic studies are needed on the physiologic processes underlying geriatric disability and the potential effect of the biology of aging on response of older adults to rehabilitation.

Hypothesis-testing research pertinent to the disablement process in older adults is described under Rehab KQ2 and Rehab KQ3.

Rehab KQ2: **What are the costs and benefits of targeting treatment at differing aspects of the disablement process in elderly persons?**

Hypothesis-generating research: There is considerable diversity in the approaches used to treat common physical impairments and disabilities in the older population (eg, arthritic knee pain is treated with nonsteroidal medication, herbal preparations, injectable medications, narcotics, liniment, heat, canes, braces, exercise, and joint replacement). Observational studies are needed to identify current treatment patterns for various physical impairments and functional disabilities in the older population. The population(s) studied should be representative of disabled older persons, including nursing-home residents, persons with cognitive impairment, and community-dwelling older persons. Outcomes measured should include quality of care, costs, and function. Registries, administrative data, patient and provider surveys, and medical records could be used.

Hypothesis-testing research is needed to determine the costs and benefits of treatment targeted at the disability versus treatment targeted at the underlying disease or impairment. Rehabilitative interventions can be directed at the disability itself (eg, dependence on a wheelchair) or at underlying impairments (eg, muscle weakness). Evaluation to specify the underlying process can be time consuming and expensive, and some diagnostic tests have the potential for adverse effects. The merits of focusing on treatment of the disability may vary with the patient population and the underlying process. Randomized trials are needed, with careful definition of the populations and disabilities studied. Results of hypothesis-generating studies for both this key question and Rehab KQ1 should be used to identify the conditions and treatments to study.

Rehab KQ3: **What are the relative merits of diverse rehabilitative treatments targeted at similar aspects of the disablement process in elderly patients?**

Hypothesis-generating studies are needed to develop a taxonomy for rehabilitation structure and process of care. Considerable work in geriatrics and rehabilitation has been devoted to developing outcome measures. However, measures of the input side are lacking, which causes difficulty in determining how to best improve rehabilitation outcomes. Theoretical models to measure rehabilitation treatment need to be developed, followed by a uniform terminology, so that multisite research to allow faster progress can be conducted. Multiple research methods could be used to identify the key measures of rehabilitation care, including focus groups, medical record review, and observational studies. Hypothesis-generating studies are needed to develop new treatments for disability in the older population. Animal and preliminary human studies are recommended. Emerging treatments of potential utility for the older population include interventions to facilitate neuroregeneration and novel assistive technologies for mobility limitations, vision and hearing impairments, and behavioral disorders.

Hypothesis-testing research is needed to examine the merits of differing rehabilitation interventions for the same condition. The results of hypothesis-generating studies in Rehab KQ1, Rehab KQ2, and this key question should be used to help identify conditions and interventions to be studied. The condition and the interventions to be studied should be tightly defined. For example, studies of musculoskeletal disorders should focus on a particular disease process (eg, tendinitis, fracture, osteoarthritis) and a particular joint (eg, shoulder, hip). Examples of interventions to be compared include differing methods of providing similar exercises (eg, exercise for rotator cuff tendonitis at home versus in clinic), types of exercise (eg, resistance versus functionally based exercise for cognitively impaired patients after acute hip fracture), or types of interventions (eg, cane versus exercise for osteoarthritis of the hip).

REFERENCES

1. Fried LP, Guralnik JM. Disability in older adults: evidence regarding significance, etiology, and risk. J Am Geriatr Soc 1997;45:92-100.
2. Hoenig H, Nusbaum N, Brummel-Smith K. Geriatric rehabilitation: state of the art. J Am Geriatr Soc 1997;45:1371-1381.
3. World Health Organization. International Classification of Functioning, Disability and Health (ICF). Geneva, Switzerland, 2001. [Online] Available: http://www3.who.int/icf/icftemplate. cfm.
4. Verbrugge LM, Jette AM. The disablement process. Soc Sci Med 1994;38:1-14.
5. Institute of Medicine (U.S.) Committee on a National Agenda for the Prevention of Disabilities. Executive summary. In Pope AM, Tarlov AR (eds): Disability in America: Toward a National Agenda for Prevention. Division of Health Promotion and Disease Prevention, Institute of Medicine. Washington, DC: National Academy Press, 1991. pp 1-15.
6. World Health Organization. 5. Model of functioning and disability. 5.1 Process of functioning and disability. In International Classification of Functioning, Disability and Health (ICF). Geneva, Switzerland, 2001.pp 18-19. [Online] Available: http://www.who.int/classification/icf/intros/ICF-Eng-Intro.pdf.
7. Ferrucci L, Guralnik JM, Simonsick E, et al. Progressive versus catastrophic disability: a longitudinal view of the disablement process. J Gerontol A Biol Sci Med Sci 1996;51:M123-M130.
8. Tinetti ME, Inouye SK, Gill TM, Doucette JT. Shared risk factors for falls, incontinence, and functional dependence: unifying the approach to geriatric syndromes. JAMA 1995;273:1348-1353.
9. Jagger C, Arthur AJ, Spiers NA, Clarke M. Patterns of onset of disability in activities of daily living with age. J Am Geriatr Soc 2001;49:404-409.
10. Hoenig H, Mayer-Oakes SA, Siebens H, et al. Geriatric rehabilitation: what do physicians know about it and how should they use it? J Am Geriatr Soc 1994;42:341-347.
11. Guralnik JM, Ferrucci L, Balfour JL, et al. Progressive versus catastrophic loss of the ability to walk: implications for the prevention of mobility loss. J Am Geriatr Soc 2001;49:1463-1470.
12. Morrison RS, Chassin MR, Siu AL. The medical consultant's role in caring for patients with hip fracture. Ann Intern Med 1998;128:1010-1020.
13. Hoenig H, Rubenstein LV, Sloane R, et al. What is the role of timing in the surgical and rehabilitative care of community-dwelling older persons with acute hip fracture? Arch Intern Med 1997;157:513-520.
14. Verbrugge LM, Lepkowski JM, Imanaka Y. Comorbidity and its impact on disability. Milbank Q 1989;67:450-484.
15. Boult C, Kane RL, Louis TA, et al. Chronic conditions that lead to functional limitation in the elderly. J Gerontol 1994;49:M28-M36.

16. Schoeni RF, Freedman VA, Wallace RB. Persistent, consistent, widespread, and robust? another look at recent trends in old-age disability. J Gerontol B Psychol Sci Soc Sci 2001;56: S206-S218.

17. Verbrugge LM, Patrick DL. Seven chronic conditions: their impact on US adults' activity levels and use of medical services. Am J Public Health 1995;85:173-182.

18. Keysor JJ, Jette AM. Have we oversold the benefit of late-life exercise? J Gerontol A Biol Sci Med Sci 2001;56:M412-M423.

19. Saboe LA, Darrah JM, Pain KS, Guthrie J. Early predictors of functional independence 2 years after spinal cord injury. Arch Phys Med Rehabil 1997;78:644-650.

20. Curt A, Keck ME, Dietz V. Functional outcome following spinal cord injury: significance of motor-evoked potentials and ASIA scores. Arch Phys Med Rehabil 1998;79:81-86.

21. Iezzoni LI, McCarthy EP, Davis RB, Siebens H. Mobility problems and perceptions of disability by self-respondents and proxy respondents. Med Care 2000;38:1051-1057.

22. Herrmann N, Black SE, Lawrence J, et al. The Sunnybrook Stroke Study: a prospective study of depressive symptoms and functional outcome. Stroke 1998;29:618-624.

23. Levine C. The loneliness of the long-term care giver. N Engl J Med 1999;340:1587-1590.

24. Covinsky KE, Goldman L, Cook EF, et al. The impact of serious illness on patients' families. SUPPORT Investigators. Study to Understand Prognoses and Preferences for Outcomes and Risks of Treatment. JAMA 1994;272:1839-1844.

25. Von Korff M, Gruman J, Schaefer J, et al. Collaborative management of chronic illness. Ann Intern Med 1997;127:1097-1102.

26. Evans RL, Matlock AL, Bishop DS, et al. Family intervention after stroke: does counseling or education help? Stroke 1988;19:1243-1249.

27. Evans RL, Connis RT, Bishop DS, et al. Stroke: a family dilemma. Disabil Rehabil 1994;16:110-118.

28. Glass TA, Dym B, Greenberg S, et al. Psychosocial intervention in stroke: Families in Recovery from Stroke Trial (FIRST). Am J Orthopsychiatry 2000;70:169-181.

29. Giacomini MK. The rocky road: qualitative research as evidence. ACP J Club 2001;134: A11-A13.

30. Fuhrer MJ. Overview of outcomes research in rehabilitation. In Fuhrer MJ (ed): Rehabilitation Outcomes: Analysis and Measurement. Baltimore MD: Paul H. Brookes, 1987. pp 1-15.

31. Fuhrer MJ. Comment on: Kramer AM. Rehabilitation care and outcomes from the patient's perspective. Med Care 1997;35:JS58-JS60.

32. Johnston MV, Stineman M, Velozo CA. Outcomes research in medical rehabilitation. In Fuhrer MJ (ed): Assessing Medical Rehabilitation Practices. Baltimore MD: Paul H. Brookes, 1997. pp 1-42.

33. Strasser DC, Falconer JA. Linking treatment to outcomes through teams: building a conceptual model of rehabilitation effectiveness. Top Stroke Rehabil 1997;4:15-27.

34. Kramer AM. Rehabilitation care and outcomes from the patient's perspective. Med Care 1997;35:JS48-JS57; discussion JS58-JS63.

35. Whyte J. Distinctive methodological challenges. In Fuhrer MJ (ed): Assessing Medical Rehabilitation Practices: The Promise of Outcomes Research. Baltimore MD: Paul H. Brookes, 1997. pp 43-59.

36. Henry SB, Holzemer WL. Achievement of appropriate self-care: does care delivery system make a difference? Med Care 1997;35:NS33-NS40.

37. Duncan PW, Hoenig H, Hamilton B, Samsa G. Characterizing medical rehabilitation interventions. In Fuhrer MJ (ed): Assessing Medical Rehabilitation Practices: The Promise of Outcomes Research. Baltimore MD: Paul H. Brookes, 1997. pp 307-317.

38. Hoenig H, Horner RD, Duncan PW, et al. New horizons in stroke rehabilitation research. J Rehabil Res Dev 1999;36:19-31.

39. Hoenig H, Sloane R, Horner RD, et al. A taxonomy for classification of stroke rehabilitation services. Arch Phys Med Rehabil 2000;81:853-862.
40. CARF Standards Manual and Interpretive Guidelines for Medical Rehabilitation. Tucson AZ: Commission on Accreditation of Rehabilitation Facilities, 1997.
41. Stroke Unit Trialists' Collaboration. Collaborative systematic review of the randomised trials of organised inpatient (stroke unit) care after stroke. BMJ 1997;314:1151-1159.
42. Stuck AE, Siu AL, Wieland GD, et al. Comprehensive geriatric assessment: a meta-analysis of controlled trials. Lancet 1993;342:1032-1036.
43. Cohen HJ, Feussner JR, Weinberger M, et al. A controlled trial of inpatient and outpatient geriatric evaluation and management. N Engl J Med 2002;346:905-912.
44. Buchanan JL, Rumpel JD, Hoenig H. Charges for outpatient rehabilitation: growth and differences in provider types. Arch Phys Med Rehabil 1996;77:320-328.
45. Duncan PW, Horner RD, Reker DM, et al. Adherence to postacute rehabilitation guidelines is associated with functional recovery in stroke. Stroke 2002;33:167-177.
46. Hoenig H, Rubenstein L, Kahn K. Rehabilitation after hip fracture–equal opportunity for all? Arch Phys Med Rehabil 1996;77:58-63.
47. McCue MJ, Thompson JM. The ownership difference in relative performance of rehabilitation specialty hospitals. Arch Phys Med Rehabil 1995;76:413-418.
48. Mitchell JM, Scott E. Physician ownership of physical therapy services: effects on charges, utilization, profits, and service characteristics. JAMA 1992;268:2055-2059.
49. Keith RA. The comprehensive treatment team in rehabilitation. Arch Phys Med Rehabil 1991;72:269-274.
50. Ottenbacher KJ, Jannell S. The results of clinical trials in stroke rehabilitation research. Arch Neurol 1993;50:37-44.
51. Ahlmen M, Sullivan M, Bjelle A. Team versus non-team outpatient care in rheumatoid arthritis. A comprehensive outcome evaluation including an overall health measure. Arthritis Rheum 1988;31:471-479.
52. Schned ES, Doyle MA, Glickstein SL, et al. Team managed outpatient care for early onset chronic inflammatory arthritis. J Rheumatol 1995;22:1141-1148.
53. Wieland D, Rubenstein LZ, Hedrick SC, et al. Inpatient geriatric evaluation and management units (GEMs) in the veterans health system: diamonds in the rough? J Gerontol 1994;49:M195-M200.
54. North Carolina Area Health Education Centers. North Carolina Health Careers. Chapel Hill, NC: University of North Carolina (Chapel Hill) School of Medicine, 1994. pp 98-99.
55. Hoenig H, Sloane R, Horner RD, et al. Differences in rehabilitation services and outcomes among stroke patients cared for in veterans hospitals. Health Serv Res 2001;35:1293-1318.
56. Hoenig H, Duncan PW, Horner RD, et al. Structure, process, and outcomes in stroke rehabilitation. Med Care 2002;40:1036-1047.
57. Hoenig H, Odom C. Rehabilitation. In Mezey MD, Bottrell MM, Siegler E, et al. (eds): Encyclopedia of Elder Care: The Comprehensive Resource on Geriatric and Social Care. New York, NY: Springer Publishing Company, 2001. pp 559-563.
58. Falconer J, Hayes KW, Chang RW. Therapeutic ultrasound in the treatment of musculoskeletal conditions. Arthritis Care Res 1990;3:85-91.
59. Puett DW, Griffin MR. Published trials of nonmedicinal and noninvasive therapies for hip and knee osteoarthritis. Ann Intern Med 1994;121:133-140.
60. van der Windt DA, van der Heijden GJ, van den Berg SG, et al. Ultrasound therapy for musculoskeletal disorders: a systematic review. Pain 1999;81:257-271.
61. Leveille SG, Guralnik JM, Ferrucci L, Langlois JA. Aging successfully until death in old age: opportunities for increasing active life expectancy. Am J Epidemiol 1999;149:654-664.

62. Murray MP, Duthie EH, Jr., Gambert SR, et al. Age-related differences in knee muscle strength in normal women. J Gerontol 1985;40:275-280.

63. Larsson L. Morphological and functional characteristics of the ageing skeletal muscle in man: a cross-sectional study. Acta Physiol Scand Suppl 1978;457:1-36.

64. Gibbs J, Hughes S, Dunlop D, et al. Predictors of change in walking velocity in older adults. J Am Geriatr Soc 1996;44:126-132.

65. Guralnik JM, Ferrucci L, Simonsick EM, et al. Lower-extremity function in persons over the age of 70 years as a predictor of subsequent disability. N Engl J Med 1995;332:556-561.

66. Fiatarone MA, O'Neill EF, Ryan ND, et al. Exercise training and nutritional supplementation for physical frailty in very elderly people. N Engl J Med 1994;330:1769-1775.

67. Yarasheski KE, Campbell JA, Kohrt WM. Effect of resistance exercise and growth hormone on bone density in older men. Clin Endocrinol (Oxf) 1997;47:223-229.

68. Lord SR, Menz HB. Physiologic, psychologic, and health predictors of 6-minute walk performance in older people. Arch Phys Med Rehabil 2002;83:907-911.

69. Bean JF, Kiely DK, Leveille SG, et al. The 6-minute walk test in mobility-limited elders: what is being measured? J Gerontol A Biol Sci Med Sci 2002;57:M751-M756.

70. Maffiuletti NA, Martin A. Progressive versus rapid rate of contraction during 7 wk of isometric resistance training. Med Sci Sports Exerc 2001;33:1220-1227.

71. Ewing JL, Jr., Wolfe DR, Rogers MA, et al. Effects of velocity of isokinetic training on strength, power, and quadriceps muscle fibre characteristics. Eur J Appl Physiol Occup Physiol 1990;61:159-162.

72. Green JS, Crouse SF. The effects of endurance training on functional capacity in the elderly: a meta-analysis. Med Sci Sports Exerc 1995;27:920-926.

73. Kelley GA, Sharpe Kelley K. Aerobic exercise and resting blood pressure in older adults: a meta-analytic review of randomized controlled trials. J Gerontol A Biol Sci Med Sci 2001;56:M298-M303.

74. Berard A, Bravo G, Gauthier P. Meta-analysis of the effectiveness of physical activity for the prevention of bone loss in postmenopausal women. Osteoporos Int 1997;7:331-337.

75. Leng GC, Fowler B, Ernst E. Exercise for intermittent claudication. Cochrane Database Syst Rev 2000:CD000990.

76. Jolliffe JA, Rees K, Taylor RS, et al. Exercise-based rehabilitation for coronary heart disease. Cochrane Database Syst Rev 2001:CD001800.

77. Lee PY, Alexander KP, Hammill BG, et al. Representation of elderly persons and women in published randomized trials of acute coronary syndromes. JAMA 2001;286:708-713.

78. Spirduso WW, Cronin DL. Exercise dose-response effects on quality of life and independent living in older adults. Med Sci Sports Exerc 2001;33:S598-S608; discussion S609-S610.

79. Norre ME, Beckers A. Benign paroxysmal positional vertigo in the elderly: treatment by habituation exercises. J Am Geriatr Soc 1988;36:425-429.

80. Province MA, Hadley EC, Hornbrook MC, et al. The effects of exercise on falls in elderly patients: a preplanned meta-analysis of the FICSIT Trials. Frailty and Injuries: Cooperative Studies of Intervention Techniques. JAMA 1995;273:1341-1347.

81. Wolf SL, Barnhart HX, Kutner NG, et al. Reducing frailty and falls in older persons: an investigation of Tai Chi and computerized balance training. Atlanta FICSIT Group. Frailty and Injuries: Cooperative Studies of Intervention Techniques. J Am Geriatr Soc 1996;44:489-497.

82. Wolfson L, Whipple R, Derby C, et al. Balance and strength training in older adults: intervention gains and Tai Chi maintenance. J Am Geriatr Soc 1996;44:498-506.

83. Tinetti ME, Baker DI, McAvay G, et al. A multifactorial intervention to reduce the risk of falling among elderly people living in the community. N Engl J Med 1994;331:821-827.

84. Krivickas LS. Training flexibility. In Frontera WR, Dawson DM, Slovik DM (eds): Exercise in Rehabilitation Medicine. Champaign, IL: Human Kinetics, 1999.pp 83-102.

85. Gehlsen GM, Whaley MH. Falls in the elderly: Part II, balance, strength, and flexibility. Arch Phys Med Rehabil 1990;71:739-741.

86. Girouard CK, Hurley BF. Does strength training inhibit gains in range of motion from flexibility training in older adults? Med Sci Sports Exerc 1995;27:1444-1449.

87. Alexander NB, Galecki AT, Grenier ML, et al. Task-specific resistance training to improve the ability of activities of daily living-impaired older adults to rise from a bed and from a chair. J Am Geriatr Soc 2001;49:1418-1427.

88. Schnelle JF, MacRae PG, Ouslander JG, et al. Functional Incidental Training, mobility performance, and incontinence care with nursing home residents. J Am Geriatr Soc 1995;43: 1356-1362.

89. Rogers JC, Holm MB, Burgio LD, et al. Improving morning care routines of nursing home residents with dementia. J Am Geriatr Soc 1999;47:1049-1057.

90. Morris JN, Fiatarone M, Kiely DK, et al. Nursing rehabilitation and exercise strategies in the nursing home. J Gerontol A Biol Sci Med Sci 1999;54:M494-M500.

91. Miltner WH, Bauder H, Sommer M, et al. Effects of constraint-induced movement therapy on patients with chronic motor deficits after stroke: a replication. Stroke 1999;30:586-592.

92. Pulvermuller F, Neininger B, Elbert T, et al. Constraint-induced therapy of chronic aphasia after stroke. Stroke 2001;32:1621-1626.

93. Ettinger WH, Jr., Burns R, Messier SP, et al. A randomized trial comparing aerobic exercise and resistance exercise with a health education program in older adults with knee osteoarthritis. The Fitness Arthritis and Seniors Trial (FAST). JAMA 1997;277:25-31.

94. Manton KG. Epidemiological, demographic, and social correlates of disability among the elderly. Milbank Q 1989;67 Suppl 2 Pt 1:13-58.

95. Shalala DE, Vladeck BC, Wolf LF, et al. Table 57. In Health Care Financing Review: Statistical Supplement. Washington DC: Health Care Financing Administration, Office of Research and Demonstrations, 1996. pp 320-321.

96. Russell JN, Hendershot GE, LeClere F, et al. Trends and differential use of assistive technology devices: United States, 1994. Adv Data 1997:1-9.

97. Cooper RA. A perspective on the ultralight wheelchair revolution. Technol Disabil 1996;5:383-392.

98. Cooper RA, Trefler E, Hobson DA. Wheelchairs and seating: issues and practice. Technol Disabil 1996;5:3-16.

99. Hoenig H, Taylor DH, Jr., Sloan FA. Does assistive technology substitute for personal assistance among the disabled elderly? Am J Public Health 2003;93:330-337.

100. Verbrugge LM, Rennert C, Madans JH. The great efficacy of personal and equipment assistance in reducing disability. Am J Public Health 1997;87:384-392.

101. Mann WC, Ottenbacher KJ, Fraas L, et al. Effectiveness of assistive technology and environmental interventions in maintaining independence and reducing home care costs for the frail elderly: a randomized controlled trial. Arch Fam Med 1999;8:210-217.

102. Rogers JC, Holm MB. Accepting the challenge of outcome research: examining the effectiveness of occupational therapy practice. Am J Occup Ther 1994;48:871-876.

103. Mann WC, Hurren D, Charvat B, Tomita. Problems with wheelchairs experienced by frail elders. Technol Disabil 1996;5:101-111.

104. Edwards NI, Jones DA. Ownership and use of assistive devices amongst older people in the community. Age Ageing 1998;27:463-468.

105. Gitlin LN, Levine R, Geiger C. Adaptive device use by older adults with mixed disabilities. Arch Phys Med Rehabil 1993;74:149-152.

106. Perks BA, Mackintosh R, Stewart CP, Bardsley GI. A survey of marginal wheelchair users. J Rehabil Res Dev 1994;31:297-302.

107. George J, Binns VE, Clayden AD, Mulley GP. Aids and adaptations for the elderly at home: underprovided, underused, and undermaintained. Br Med J (Clin Res Ed) 1988;296: 1365-1366.

108. Haworth RJ. Use of aids during the first three months after total hip replacement. Br J Rheumatol 1983;22:29-35.

109. Garber SL, Gregorio TL. Upper extremity assistive devices: assessment of use by spinal cord-injured patients with quadriplegia. Am J Occup Ther 1990;44:126-131.

110. O'Day BL, Corcoran PJ. Assistive technology: problems and policy alternatives. Arch Phys Med Rehabil 1994;75:1165-1169.

111. Chamberlain MA, Thornley G, Stowe J, Wright V. Evaluation of aids and equipment for the bath: II. a possible solution to the problem. Rheumatol Rehabil 1981;20:38-43.

112. Simmons SF, Schnelle JF, MacRae PG, Ouslander JG. Wheelchairs as mobility restraints: predictors of wheelchair activity in nonambulatory nursing home residents. J Am Geriatr Soc 1995;43:384-388.

113. Fuhrer MJ. Assistive technology outcomes research: challenges met and yet unmet. Am J Phys Med Rehabil 2001;80:528-535.

114. McDowell I, Newell C. Measuring Health: A Guide to Rating Scales and Questionnaires, 2nd ed. New York NY: Oxford University Press, 1996.

115. Patrick L, Knoefel F, Gaskowski P, Rexroth D. Medical comorbidity and rehabilitation efficiency in geriatric inpatients. J Am Geriatr Soc 2001;49:1471-1477.

116. Seel RT, Huang ME, Cifu DX, et al. Age-related differences in length of stays, hospitalization costs, and outcomes for an injury-matched sample of adults with paraplegia. J Spinal Cord Med 2001;24:241-250.

117. NIH Consensus Development Panel on Rehabilitation of Persons With Traumatic Brain Injury. Consensus conference: rehabilitation of persons with traumatic brain injury. JAMA 1999;282:974-983.

118. van Baar ME, Assendelft WJ, Dekker J, et al. Effectiveness of exercise therapy in patients with osteoarthritis of the hip or knee: a systematic review of randomized clinical trials. Arthritis Rheum 1999;42:1361-1369.

119. Vuori IM. Dose-response of physical activity and low back pain, osteoarthritis, and osteoporosis. Med Sci Sports Exerc 2001;33:S551-S586; discussion S609-S610.

120. Agency for Health Care Policy and Research. Post-stroke rehabilitation: assessment, referral, and patient management. Rockville, MD: U.S. Department of Health and Human Services, Public Health Service. AHCPR Publication No. 95-0663 (No. 16), 1995. pp 1-33.

121. VA/DoD Clinical Practice Guideline Working Group. Management of stroke rehabilitation in primary care. Veterans Health Administration, Department of Veterans Affairs and Health Affairs, Department of Defense [Online] Available: http://www.oqp.met.va.gov/cpg/STR/ STR_base.htm. 2003. Office of Quality and Performance publication 10Q CPG/STR-03.

122. Liepert J, Bauder H, Wolfgang HR, et al. Treatment-induced cortical reorganization after stroke in humans. Stroke 2000;31:1210-1216.

123. Goldstein LB. Effects of amphetamines and small related molecules on recovery after stroke in animals and man. Neuropharmacology 2000;39:852-859.

124. Kelly-Hayes M, Paige C. Assessment and psychologic factors in stroke rehabilitation. Neurology 1995;45:S29-S32.

125. Pohjasvaara T, Vataja R, Leppavuori A, et al. Depression is an independent predictor of poor long-term functional outcome post-stroke. Eur J Neurol 2001;8:315-319.

126. Kimura M, Robinson RG, Kosier JT. Treatment of cognitive impairment after poststroke depression : a double-blind treatment trial. Stroke 2000;31:1482-1486.

127. Sullivan DH, Walls RC. Impact of nutritional status on morbidity in a population of geriatric rehabilitation patients. J Am Geriatr Soc 1994;42:471-477.

128. Norton B, Homer-Ward M, Donnelly MT, et al. A randomised prospective comparison of percutaneous endoscopic gastrostomy and nasogastric tube feeding after acute dysphagic stroke. BMJ 1996;312:13-16.

129. Agency for Health Care Policy and Research. Cardiac Rehabilitation: Clinical Practice Guideline No. 17. Rockville, MD: U.S. Department of Health and Human Services, Public Health Service, 1995. AHCPR Publication No. 96-0672.

130. Swinne CJ, Shapiro EP, Lima SD, Fleg JL. Age-associated changes in left ventricular diastolic performance during isometric exercise in normal subjects. Am J Cardiol 1992;69:823-826.

131. Cameron ID, Lyle DM, Quine S. Cost effectiveness of accelerated rehabilitation after proximal femoral fracture. J Clin Epidemiol 1994;47:1307-1313.

132. Guccione AA, Fagerson TL, Anderson JJ. Regaining functional independence in the acute care setting following hip fracture. Phys Ther 1996;76:818-826.

133. Koval KJ, Friend KD, Aharonoff GB, Zukerman JD. Weight bearing after hip fracture: a prospective series of 596 geriatric hip fracture patients. J Orthop Trauma 1996;10:526-530.

134. Parker MJ, Handoll HH, Dynan Y. Mobilisation strategies after hip fracture surgery in adults. Cochrane Database Syst Rev 2000:CD001704.

135. Andrews KL. Rehabilitation in limb deficiency: 3. the geriatric amputee. Arch Phys Med Rehabil 1996;77:S14-S17.

136. Cutson TM, Bongiorni DR. Rehabilitation of the older lower limb amputee: a brief review. J Am Geriatr Soc 1996;44:1388-1393.

137. Hoenig HM, Rubenstein LZ. Hospital-associated deconditioning and dysfunction. J Am Geriatr Soc 1991;39:220-222.

138. Siebens H, Aronow H, Edwards D, Ghasemi Z. A randomized controlled trial of exercise to improve outcomes of acute hospitalization in older adults. J Am Geriatr Soc 2000;48:1545-1552.

139. Sullivan DH, Wall PT, Bariola JR, et al. Progressive resistance muscle strength training of hospitalized frail elderly. Am J Phys Med Rehabil 2001;80:503-509.

140. Roubenoff R, Hughes VA. Sarcopenia: current concepts. J Gerontol A Biol Sci Med Sci 2000;55:M716-M724.

141. Fried LP, Tangen CM, Walston J, et al. Frailty in older adults: evidence for a phenotype. J Gerontol A Biol Sci Med Sci 2001;56:M146-M156.

142. Oakley A, Dawson MF, Holland J, et al. Preventing falls and subsequent injury in older people. Qual Health Care 1996;5:243-249.

143. Gillespie LD, Gillespie WJ, Cumming R, et al. Interventions for preventing falls in the elderly. Cochrane Database Syst Rev 2000:CD000340.

144. Tinetti ME. Where is the vision for fall prevention? J Am Geriatr Soc 2001;49:676-677.

145. American Geriatrics Society, British Geriatrics Society, and American Academy of Orthopaedic Surgeons Panel on Falls Prevention. Guideline for the prevention of falls in older persons. J Am Geriatr Soc 2001;49:664-672.

146. American Geriatrics Society Panel on Persistent Pain in Older Persons. The management of persistent pain in older persons. J Am Geriatr Soc 2002;50:S205-S224.

147. Nguyen DM. The role of physical medicine and rehabilitation in pain management. Clin Geriatr Med 1996;12:517-529.

13

CROSS-CUTTING ISSUES

Joseph LoCicero III, MD, FACS, Chapter Editor, and Section Authors:
Arlene S. Bierman, MD, MS; Anne Louise Coleman, MD, PhD;
Marion Danis, MD; George W. Drach, MD; Lowell W. Gerson, PhD;
Laura C. Hanson, MD, MPH; Robert R. Karpman, MD, MBA;
Andrew G. Lee, MD; Steven M. Parnes, MD; Walter J. Pories, MD, FACS;
G. Alec Rooke, MD, PhD; Hilary C. Siebens, MD;
Morton A. Stenchever, MD

Conservative estimates in the United States predict that the number of persons aged 65 years and over will grow from 35 million in 2000 to 78 million in 2011, accounting for more than 20% of the overall population. [1] The number of those aged 85 years and over will grow from 4 million to 18.2 million. If life expectancy continues to increase at the same rate seen in the 1990s, the number of oldest old could balloon to 31.2 million by the year 2050.

Many of our older citizens will require hospitalization for medical and surgical conditions. In 1996, people over 65 years of age accounted for 35% of all of the inpatient and outpatient operations performed in this country. [2] In 1998, people over 65 years of age accounted for 39% of all hospital admissions. [3] Of the 39%, patients older than 85 years accounted for 11.6% of the procedures. For the twelve most common procedures chosen for each age group, elderly patients averaged 747 procedures per 100,000. Averages per 100,000 for the rest of the population were 75 for those under 15 years, 204 for those between 15 and 44 years, and 338 for those between 45 and 64 years.

In general, elderly patients are more susceptible to many perioperative problems and complications, including any or all of the following: acute renal failure, adverse drug events (incidence 10% to 15%), [4,5] functional decline due to deconditioning and immobility (incidence 32%), [6,7] dehydration (prevalence 7%), [8] delirium (10% to 50% in postoperative patients), [9] depression, [10] falls (incidence 4 to 11 per 1000 patient days), [11] incontinence (prevalence 11% on admission and 23% on discharge), [12] infection (especially pneumonia and urinary tract infection), malnutrition (prevalence as high as 61%), [13,14] pressure ulcers (incidence 3%), [15] and untreated or undertreated pain syndromes.

Because of the enormous public health burden imposed by the growing elderly population and the urgent need for research progress in this area, the American Geriatrics Society, with funding from the John A. Hartford Foundation, convened representatives from the following surgical and related medical subspecialties: anesthesiology, cardiac surgery, emergency medicine, general surgery, gynecology, ophthalmology, orthopedic surgery, otolaryngology, physical medicine and rehabilitation, thoracic surgery, and urology. This research agenda–setting group was charged with evaluating the current state of knowledge to identify critical gaps in our knowledge and to develop specific recommendations to promote research into the problems of older citizens having surgical procedures. One key point emerged during these discussions—many facets of aging processes influence the diagnosis and treatment of older patients in more than one specialty. It was decided to address these cross-cutting issues together, rather than addressing them repeatedly and separately in the specialty chapters. This chapter is a summary of the areas that cross multiple specialties and have impact on nearly all older surgical patients.

References

1. Statistical Abstract of the United States 1998: The National Data Book. Washington D.C.: Bernan Press. U.S. Department of Commerce, Bureau of Census, 1998.
2. Dennison C, Pokras R. Design and operation of the National Hospital discharge Survey: 1988 redesign. Vital Health Stat 2000;1(39).
3. Owings MF, Kozak LJ. Ambulatory and Inpatient Procedures in the United States, 1996. National Center for Health Statistics. Vital Health Stat 13(139), 1998.
4. Gray SL, Sager M, Lestico MR, Jalaluddin M. Adverse drug events in hospitalized elderly. J Gerontol A Biol Sci Med Sci 1998;53:M59-M63.
5. Leape LL, Brennan TA, Laird N, et al. The nature of adverse events in hospitalized patients. results of the Harvard Medical Practice Study II. N Engl J Med 1991;324:377-384.
6. Hansen K, Mahoney J, Palta M. Risk factors for lack of recovery of ADL independence after hospital discharge. J Am Geriatr Soc 1999;47:360-365.
7. Sager MA, Franke T, Inouye SK, et al. Functional outcomes of acute medical illness and hospitalization in older persons. Arch Intern Med 1996;156:645-652.
8. Warren JL, Bacon WE, Harris T, et al. The burden and outcomes associated with dehydration among US elderly, 1991. Am J Public Health 1994;84:1265-1269.
9. Inouye SK. Delirium in hospitalized elderly patients: recognition, evaluation, and management. Conn Med 1993;57:309-315.
10. Holmes J, House A. Psychiatric illness predicts poor outcome after surgery for hip fracture: a prospective cohort study. Psychol Med 2000;30:921-929.
11. Mahoney JE. Immobility and falls. Clin Geriatr Med 1998;14:699-726.
12. Palmer MH, McCormick KA, Langford A, et al. Continence outcomes: documentation on medical records in the nursing home environment. J Nurs Care Qual 1992;6:36-43.
13. Covinsky KE, Martin GE, Beyth RJ, et al. The relationship between clinical assessments of nutritional status and adverse outcomes in older hospitalized medical patients. J Am Geriatr Soc 1999;47:532-538.
14. Reuben DB, Greendale GA, Harrison GG. Nutrition screening in older persons. J Am Geriatr Soc 1995;43:415-425.
15. Williams S, Watret L, Pell J. Case-mix adjusted incidence of pressure ulcers in acute medical and surgical wards. J Tissue Viability 2001;11:139-142.

PHYSIOLOGIC CHANGES IN ORGAN SYSTEMS

The effects of aging on the cardiovascular, pulmonary, nervous, and renal systems are described in Chapter 2, Geriatric Anesthesia.

CELLULAR AND MOLECULAR CHANGES WITH AGING

The major principle underlying adverse changes with aging is that evolutionary pressure results in the selection of biochemical mechanisms that are beneficial in young organisms and that support reproduction, while it ignores their effects in older, postreproductive organisms. [1] Those effects are often deleterious. Important examples of "antagonistic pleiotropy" are apoptosis and cellular senescence. Another example is enhanced oxidative stress imposed by an increased rate of generation of reactive oxygen species (ROS) in aging mitochondria and decreased ROS-scavenging activity in the older organism. As a result, there is an age-related increase in cellular inflammatory components, including nuclear factor kappa B (NF-kappa B), activator protein-1 (AP-1), and hypoxia inducible factor (HIF-1). Further, ROS damage lipid membranes, proteins, the endoplasmic reticulum, and both nuclear and mitochondrial DNA, particularly the latter. Notably, all of these deleterious effects are less prominent in the calorie-restricted organism, and this is thought by many to be the mechanism for improvements in health and longevity in many calorie-restricted experimental animals.

The deleterious effects of accumulation of ROS are perhaps the most dramatic at neuronal synapses where nerve cell mitochondria are concentrated, leading to a focal accumulation of ROS bordering the synapse. On the other hand, the adverse changes accompanying brain aging are at least partially mitigated by adaptive mechanisms, especially increases in the production of neurotrophic factors, chaperones (heat-shock proteins), antioxidant enzymes, Bcl-2, and a protein that inhibits apoptosis. In *Caenorhabditis elegans,* heat-shock protein (HSF-1) and other molecular chaperones appear to foster longevity.

Another aspect of the biology of aging is impairment of angiogenesis in aged tissues. This is the result of poorly understood changes at molecular and cellular levels as well as at physiologic levels of regulation. Whatever the exact mechanism, endothelial cells, the hemostatic cascade, neurochemical mediators, and growth factors are all affected, and the ultimate result is delayed and impaired neovascularization and hence halting repair of injured tissues. [2]

Immunologic cellular mechanisms also change dramatically with aging. Graham et al have summarized the known changes in immunologic cellular mechanisms and the response to environmental changes. [3] Experiments include cultures of cells harvested from elderly volunteers and rodent models. There is evidence for T-cell and accessory-cell decline with age. Monocytes are clearly compromised in their function in the elderly specifically; they secrete less interleukin-1 and have decreased cytotoxicity and protein kinase translocation. [4] Disturbed signal transduction probably causes incomplete T-cell activation. Compromised T-cell activation in the elderly person is reflected in findings that cell surface alterations associated with activation are affected. For example, CD69 and CD71 upregulation does not take place. [5]

Damage to the cytoskeleton, paralleling aging may have profound effects on cell function. Cell cycle analyses of phytohemagglutinin (PHA)-stimulated cells from aged donors indicate a decreased frequency of cells entering S-phase with this age-related impairment of G1 progression correlating with decreased expression of c-jun, c-myc, c-myb, interleukin-2, and CD25. [6]

Aberrations in co-stimulatory pathways and receptors lead to compromised T-cell responses. Elderly cells, like certain other anergic (young) cells, may be able to actively suppress other cells in a mixed population, cells that otherwise would be capable of proliferation. [7] It has been long believed that a major dysfunction in T cells from elderly donors is a selectively decreased ability to secrete T-cell growth factors.

Many studies confirm that T cells from aged humans can also show defects in interleukin-2R expression, interleukin-2 secretion, and DNA synthesis after stimulation with mitogens like PHA.[3] Among the transcription factors of known importance for interleukin-2 production, CD3-stimulated induction of NF-kappa B was also found to be decreased in old mice and humans.[8,9] One reason for insufficient NF-kappa B activation may be that the natural inhibitor I-kappa B is not adequately degraded because of compromised proteosome function.[8] As well as altered cytokine levels in aging, altered levels of cytokine antagonists might also influence cytokine networks.

> **CCI 1 (Level B):** **Further basic scientific research should be carried out to better define the mechanisms and importance of cellular and molecular changes with aging, especially apoptosis, cellular senescence, the pathogenesis of nerve cell loss, the control over vascular repair and angiogenesis, and the impairment of immunologic cell function. Where possible, research should seek clues to the failure of older tissues to withstand stress as well as younger tissues.**

References

1. Campisi J. Cellular senescence and apoptosis: how cellular responses might influence aging phenotypes. Exp Gerontol 2003;38:5-11.
2. Edelberg JM, Reed MJ. Aging and angiogenesis. Front Biosci 2003;8:s1199-1209.
3. Pawelec G, Remarque E, Barnett Y, Solana R. T cells and aging. Front Biosci 1998;3:d59-d99.
4. Beckman I, Dimopoulos K, Xu XN, et al. T cell activation in the elderly: evidence for specific deficiencies in T cell/accessory cell interactions. Mech Ageing Dev 1990;51:265-276.
5. Lio D, Candore G, Cigna D, et al. *In vitro* T cell activation in elderly individuals: failure in CD69 and CD71 expression. Mech Ageing Dev 1996;89:51-58.
6. Pieri C, Recchioni R, Moroni F, et al. Phytohemagglutinin induced changes of membrane lipid packing, c-myc and c-myb encoded protein expression in human lymphocytes during aging. Mech Ageing Dev 1992;64:177-187.
7. Lombardi G, Sidhu S, Batchelor R, Lechler R. Anergic T cells as suppressor cells *in vitro*. Science 1994;264:1587-1589.
8. Trebilcock GU, Ponnappan U. Induction and regulation of NFkappaB during aging: role of protein kinases. Clin Immunol Immunopathol 1996;79:87-91.
9. Trebilcock GU, Ponnappan U. Evidence for lowered induction of nuclear factor kappa B in activated human T lymphocytes during aging. Gerontology 1996;42:137-146.

STRESS RESPONSE AS A FUNCTION OF AGING

At a clinical level, there have been innumerable observations, though no well-designed cohort studies, suggesting that older patients have a blunted response to stress and protracted recovery times. Many surgeons relate anecdotal stories of elderly patients who deteriorate for unclear reasons after what would have been a well-tolerated stress in a younger patient. On the other hand, some older patients seem to recover from major surgery with relatively little evidence of physiologic stress. The stress response is manifest in many organs and systems in the body and is accompanied by a complex interplay of adaptive and deleterious factors. Because the total organism is affected, it has been very difficult to explain why, on the average, the defense against stress is weaker in older patients than in younger ones.

Real proof that the stress response is detrimental remains elusive. Indirect evidence would be afforded if regional analgesia could be shown to attenuate the stress response and minimize complications and mortality as compared with systemic anesthesia. There have been many well-designed and well-executed studies of this type, with somewhat conflicting results, [1] but meta-analyses have led to the conclusion that there is very little if any benefit afforded by the lesser stress of regional analgesia. [2] (See also the section on regional versus general anesthesia in Chapter 2, Geriatric Anesthesia.)

Many studies discuss the aging process in relation to specific organs, but few address the aging process in detail for the whole organism. There is a complex interplay between systems that requires exposition. Since the aging process is not static, the response to surgical stress will change as a function of age. Studies need to address the dynamic changes in overall function with aging. Little is known about the changes in functional reserve and how the body responds, or not, to multiple challenges. Aged animals or animal models that mimic the aging process are necessary to quantify these responses.

ALLOSTATIS AND HOMEOSTENOSIS

McEwen has attempted to develop a framework for understanding the response to stress. [3] His concept is that an acute stress, such as a surgical operation, particularly activates the neuroendocrine system, the autonomic nervous system, and the immune system; this response is called *allostasis*, meaning "maintaining stability through change." In this response, epinephrine, cortisol, and several cytokines act on receptors in various tissues to initiate defenses against trauma to the body. These responses are adaptive in the short run but may become damaging if not terminated on time. If they continue, they may produce down-regulation of receptors and actual tissue damage; this process is called *allostatic load*, meaning "the cost of an overactive, prolonged, or inefficiently managed allostatic response." McEwen speculates that such abnormal responses might be characteristic of older persons. An example of damaging effects from stress turned chronic is the subtle increase in integrated daily plasma cortisol levels that is present in many older people. This is thought to contribute to the memory loss of aging as a result of the well-established adverse effects of extra cortisol on the hippocampus. This is the only reasonably firm evidence thus far that the stress reaction is harmful.

In addition, the acute allostatic response may be weaker in the aged patient because of impairments in various organ systems. Thus, deflections from the norm are often greater and the return to the norm slower. This phenomenon has been referred to as the *homeostenosis* of aging. Specific deficiencies that contribute to age-related homeostenosis in the fluid and electrolyte sphere include impaired thirst perception, decreased glomerular filtration rate, increased secretion of antidiuretic hormone and atrial natriuretic peptide, dysregulation of aldosterone secretion, decreased urinary concentrating ability, and impairment of renal excretion of water, sodium, potassium, and acid. [4]

A major surgical operation is a classic example of a stress with predictable deflections from the homeostatic norm. The metabolic characteristics of the postoperative state were described in a remarkable series of publications by Francis Moore and his colleagues in the period from 1948 to 1965. These findings have been confirmed and extended since then. [4] The key features of the postoperative state are sodium and water retention, potassium loss, catabolism, and rapid loss of dry weight.

Another important aspect of homeostasis is the maintenance of normal levels of intracellular calcium ions. Although there are age-related declines in various components of calcium movement systems, compensatory mechanisms seem to be capable of maintaining overall intracellular calcium ion homeostasis. The effect of surgical stress on the calcium content of various intracellular compartments has not been well studied.

ENDOCRINE AND METABOLIC RESPONSE

Sympathetic Nervous System and Catecholamines

An acute stress, such as a major operation, activates the sympathetic nervous system and the adrenal medulla. These responses are exaggerated in elderly patients, who carry higher levels of norepinephrine in the nonstressed state and show an overreaction after stress. To a greater extent, the elevated plasma levels are a compensatory response to impaired adrenergic receptor and postreceptor function throughout the body. However, this analysis does not apply to epinephrine, whose secretion is decreased in older patients, both in the nonstressed and stressed state. The sympathetic nervous system is similar to the norepinephrine part of the equation: its basal activity is greater and activation is more vigorous in older patients than in younger ones, but sympathetic nervous system effects are no greater because aged organs are hyporesponsive to sympathetic stimuli. Because of the reduced secretion of epinephrine and impaired β-adrenergic receptor function, receptor-mediated vasorelaxation is impaired in older patients, as is cardioacceleration in response to exercise or other stress. [5] In addition, arterial baroreceptor function is decreased in older people, a phenomenon correlated with increased arterial stiffness and resulting in impaired responses to hypertensive and hypotensive drugs in older patients. Interestingly, habitual exercise results in improvement by about 50% in the baroreceptor sensitivity in older persons, but tonic sympathetic nervous system activity is higher than in younger adults in those who exercise as well as in those who do not.

Adrenocortical Hormones

While plasma cortisol levels rise subtly and those of aldosterone fall slightly, the plasma level of dehydroepiandrosterone (DHEA) and its sulfate plummet with age to 10% to 20% of their levels in young adults. On the basis of research in rodents and observational correlation studies in the human, it seems that this fall might predispose the older patient to age-associated increases in the incidence of diabetes mellitus, cancer, heart disease, and immunologic deficiency. However, randomized controlled trials of DHEA replacement therapy in older men and women have yielded mixed results, so that recent authors have been forced to conclude that there is no scientific basis for recommending widespread use of DHEA replacement in older adults. [6] It is important to note, however, that DHEA is present in the brain in concentrations that do not correlate with plasma levels and accordingly is probably synthesized in the brain, where it may have beneficial effects on cognitive function.

The glucocorticoid system has a different setting in older humans (and other primates) than in youth. The hypothalamo-pituitary-adrenal axis is more resistant to suppression by dexamethasone in older than in younger adults. Also, adrenocorticotropic hormone administration causes a greater rise in plasma cortisol. Circadian variation is blunted; afternoon cortisol levels do not fall as they do in younger people. This pattern is similar to that which accompanies depression and also is suggestive of chronic stress (allostatic load).

Gonadal Steroids

Older women are severely deficient in both estrogen and testosterone, so any further fall that might occur as a result of surgical stress would probably have no significant effect. However, their chronic deficiency of anabolic hormones might set the stage for a greater catabolic response to surgery than would occur in older men. There are no published studies bearing on this speculation. On the other hand, older men actually have higher plasma estradiol than older women and have very much higher plasma testosterone and free testosterone levels, as a result of the slow pace of the andropause ("male menopause"). Some older men do have plasma testosterone levels in the frankly hypogonadal range, and these patients may be candidates for testosterone replacement therapy, although there is no consensus on this as yet.

Trauma leads to a short-term decline in estrogen and testosterone production. It is conceivable that older men and women would benefit from a short course of testosterone or other anabolic steroid to combat the postoperative catabolic state, but there is no firm evidence on this as yet.

Pituitary Growth Hormone

Older people experience a decline in growth hormone secretion and in plasma insulin-like growth factor-1 concentration. Because of the high frequency of significant sarcopenia and weakness in older patients, many seniors are treated with intramuscular growth hormone. There is no solid clinical evidence to support this practice, and, in fact, there is strong evidence that muscle strength does not improve with replacement doses of growth hormone. Acute stress leads to a further decline in growth hormone production, and short-term growth hormone therapy has been suggested. However, one randomized controlled trial of growth hormone treatment in supraphysiologic doses for intensive-care-unit medical patients actually showed increased mortality in the treated group. [7] No randomized controlled trials could be found in which one group of elderly postoperative patients was injected with placebo and one with human growth hormone.

For further information on the postoperative catabolic state, see Chapter 2 on anesthesia in older patients. To summarize our scanty knowledge: Major surgery leads to a profound catabolic state manifested by sarcopenia and weakness. Its severity is correlated with age, comorbid diseases, a sedentary lifestyle, and malnutrition. Management of the latter three factors preoperatively and postoperatively is helpful, but no such therapy has been shown to prevent catabolism completely. Pituitary hormone output is low in critical illness as a result of decreased hypothalamic output of releasing hormones. Administration of multiple releasing factors (growth hormone secretogogues, thyrotropin-releasing hormone, and gonadotropin-releasing hormone) induces anabolism and gives promise as a method to present the wasting syndrome. [8] Much research is needed to guide management of the elderly postoperative patient. Our knowledge to date indicates that early mobilization may be helpful in minimizing loss of muscle, weakness, and functional decline.

Immunologic Response

As described above, aging is associated with depressed immune function, and surgery causes a further depression at least as great in older patients as in younger patients. [9] General anesthesia and the stress of the operation independently depress the immune system. [1,10] Both humoral and cellular immune functions are affected, including suppression of natural killer cell function that may lead to an increased risk of metastases during tumor removal. Additionally, depressed immune function is associated with aging. [10] Presumably these effects contribute to higher infection rates in elderly patients, though a causal relationship has not been established between depressed cell counts or other isolated laboratory results and adverse postoperative outcomes. Attempts to enhance immune function in the perioperative period with nutritional supplements [11] or thymopentin [12] have demonstrated improved delayed-type hypersensitivity responses and other positive laboratory findings, but no study has examined the ability of such regimens to decrease postoperative infections.

> *CCI 2 (Level B)*: **There is urgent need for studies comparing cohorts of younger and older patients having the same operation, or at least operations of comparable stress, in which a vast array of measures would be made of components of the stress response and of clinical outcomes immediately postoperatively and serially over the next 2 months or more.**

> *CCI 3 (Level B)*: **In studies designed like those described in CCI 2, there should be a focus on identifying the mechanisms for ending the acute stress response and how they are altered with aging. This can be done by looking for correlates of the acute response, the turning off of the acute response, and the degree of allostatic load.**

> *CCI 4 (Level A)*: **Interventions designed to minimize the stress of surgery or maximize the defenses of older patients should be tested in randomized controlled trials of older patients (ideally stratified into frail and nonfrail) undergoing a common major operation, such as open colon resection or aortic aneurysm repair.**

> *CCI 5 (Level A)*: **The efficacy of long-term replacement doses of estrogen, androgen, dehydroepiandrosterone, and growth hormone aiming to prevent frailty in older people has been difficult to establish. Randomized controlled trials are needed on the short-term use of these hormones, singly or in combinations, preoperatively and postoperatively, in attempts to blunt the catabolic and other possibly deleterious aspects of the postoperative stress response.**

> *CCI 6 (Level A)*: **Randomized controlled trials with sufficient numbers of patients, especially elderly patients, are needed to establish firmly whether early or ultra-early ambulation programs improve postoperative recovery, complication rates, lengths of stay, and patient satisfaction. The effect of early ambulation needs to be dissected out from the package of accelerated rehabilitation programs. Later, the other components of these packages can be studied singly and in combination, again by randomized controlled trials wherever possible.**

> *CCI 7 (Level B)*: **Further exploratory work is necessary to evaluate general and specific stimulators and suppressors of the inflammatory and immune responses to stress.**

References

1. Liu S, Carpenter RL, Neal JM. Epidural anesthesia and analgesia: their role in postoperative outcome. Anesthesiology 1995;82:1474-1506.
2. Rodgers A, Walker N, Schug S, et al. Reduction of postoperative mortality and morbidity with epidural or spinal anaesthesia: results from overview of randomised trials. BMJ 2000;321: 1493.
3. McEwen BS. Interacting mediators of allostasis and allostatic load: towards an understanding of resilience in aging. Metabolism 2003;52:10-16.
4. Luckey AE, Parsa CJ. Fluid and electrolytes in the aged. Arch Surg 2003;138:1055-1060.
5. Schutzer WE, Mader SL. Age-related changes in vascular adrenergic signaling: clinical and mechanistic implications. Ageing Res Rev 2003;2:169-190.
6. Legrain S, Girard L. Pharmacology and therapeutic effects of dehydroepiandrosterone in older subjects. Drugs Aging 2003;20:949-967.
7. Ruokonen E, Takala J. Dangers of growth hormone therapy in critically ill patients. Curr Opin Clin Nutr Metab Care 2002;5:199-209.
8. Van den Berghe G. Endocrinology in intensive care medicine: new insights and therapeutic consequences. Verh K Acad Geneeskd Belg 2002;64:167-187; discussion 187-188.
9. Rinder CS, Mathew JP, Rinder HM, et al. Lymphocyte and monocyte subset changes during cardiopulmonary bypass: effects of aging and gender. J Lab Clin Med 1997;129:592-602.
10. Verhoef J. Transient immunodepression. J Antimicrob Chemother 1990;26 Suppl C:23-29.
11. Tepaske R, Velthuis H, Oudemans-van Straaten HM, et al. Effect of preoperative oral immune-enhancing nutritional supplement on patients at high risk of infection after cardiac surgery: a randomised placebo-controlled trial. Lancet 2001;358:696-701.
12. Faist E, Ertel W, Salmen B, et al. The immune-enhancing effect of perioperative thymopentin administration in elderly patients undergoing major surgery. Arch Surg 1988;123:1449-1453.

WOUND HEALING

Healing in the human body is a formidable process even in the young patient. In the older patient, minimal trauma may become a challenge for survival. Failure of wound healing in the elderly person is a chronic disabling condition; it occurs commonly in our society, requiring a major investment of medical care.

Wound healing may be impaired as a result of an inability to adequately express genes that facilitate escape from cell stasis by initiating cell division, thus commencing the healing process. [1] Many of the processes involved in wound healing are impaired in elderly persons. Using an animal model to study cellular proliferation, Marcus et al showed significantly higher proliferative indices in the young that were found to be sustained through 4 weeks while levels substantially declined in the aged. [2] However, in elderly patients not suffering from concomitant diseases, the rate of wound healing is normal or only slightly reduced. [3]

Although there have been many human, animal, and cell culture studies, no consensus exists on the ability of older organisms to heal an acute wound. Not only various systemic factors such as endocrine and hematologic diseases, nutritional deficiencies, and medications but also regional disorders such as vascular and neural diseases may impair wound healing. [4] These complicating conditions occur more commonly in aged subjects, thus rendering interpretation of human studies more difficult.

Nagy et al studied young and old patients who had sustained penetrating trauma and found that older patients have a poorer prognosis, longer stays in the hospital, and more protracted rehabilitation. [5] These researchers noted that elderly patients who sustain penetrating trauma have more comorbidities than their younger counterparts and concluded that this accounts for the older patients' longer hospital stay and lesser ability to be discharged home. However, the elderly patients studied were not found to have an increased complication rate. The findings suggest that improved wound healing for the elderly patient may require improved clinical approaches.

Specific tissues have been evaluated. One of the easiest to study is the skin. Age-related changes in the structure and function of the skin do occur. Some of these changes result from chronic solar radiation exposure rather than chronologic age alone. [3] The tensile strength of wounds, accumulation of wound-healing factors, and rate of wound closure have all been examined in relation to chronologic aging. However, the clinical impact of these changes in acute wound healing is small.

Poor healing in chronic wounds may be more often related to comorbid conditions than to age alone. The fact that the majority of chronic wounds occur in elderly populations has contributed to the conclusion that aging itself may influence healing. Holt et al made small epithelial defects on the legs of young and old volunteers and studied the rate of collagen production. [6] They found that in healthy humans, aging leads to delayed epithelialization. No effect of age on collagen synthesis was noted, although accumulation of wound noncollagenous protein was decreased. They postulated that this decrease might impair the mechanical properties of scarring in aged human beings. In studying the extracellular matrix of the skin, Meyer and Stern found that neither the concentration nor polymer size of hyaluronan changes as a function of age. [7] However, enhanced association with the tissue occurs, presumably through hyaluronan-binding proteins and alterations in the histolocalization of hyaluronan. Such observations may underlie some of the changes in human skin that occur with aging. Ballas and Davidson suggested that proteolysis might have a significant role in delayed wound healing in aged animals. They looked at fibroblasts from normal skin and from granulation tissue. [8] They noted that although granulation tissue fibroblasts from young and old rats show similar collagen gel contractility, skin fibroblasts from old rats display greater collagen gel contractile behavior than young skin fibroblasts. Greater gel contractility of fibroblasts from old rats appear to result, in large part, from the ability of those cells to cause generalized gel degradation. Gelatin zymography indicated a greater abundance of matrix metalloproteinase-2 in supernatants from gels containing skin fibroblasts from old rats. Taken together, these results suggest that the age-associated healing delay in the rat may not be related to the appearance or abundance of distinct myofibroblast or apoptotic cell populations

Other tissues have been studied. Following tooth extraction, alveolar bone was found to heal at the same rate in both young and old persons. [9] However, the chondrogenic potential of periosteal tissue from long bones declines significantly with age. [10] Even within certain healing tissues there may be a dual population of cells. Stanley and Osler took biopsies from venous ulcers and noted that the nonhealing ulcers had a higher percentage of cells that demonstrated in-vitro metabolic senescence. [11] But Serletti et al, treating musculoskeletal defects in patients with vascular disease, noted that free-tissue transfer in the elderly population demonstrates success rates similar to those of the general population. [12]

Local tissue oxygenation may be affected by age. Xia et al studied the effect of hypoxia on migration of keratinocytes isolated from human donors of increasing age. [13] The keratinocytes from elderly donors were found to have depressed migratory activity when exposed to hypoxia, as opposed to an increase in migration in young cells. This same group then studied enhancement of sluggish senescent healing by hyperbaric oxygen or transforming growth factor, or both. [14] They noted that the greatest improvement is from hyperbaric oxygen alone.

Over the years, it has been postulated that exogenous hormone therapy might be beneficial for improving well-being and possibly helping wound healing. Isolated reports have suggested that this might be true. The decrease in testosterone levels with age is both central (pituitary) and peripheral (testicular) in origin. [15] Because serum levels of sex-hormone-binding globulin increase with aging, the decrease in free testosterone is of even greater magnitude. Some have proposed that preoperative administration of exogenous testosterone should be routine, but the evidence supporting this is far from conclusive. [16] Exogenous administration of estrogen for women has not been effective. [16]

CCI 8 (Level B): **Clinical cohort studies should address whether it is possible to stimulate or accelerate wound healing by the use of hormones systematically or locally. Attention should also be paid to "overshoots," such as the occurrence of hyperplasia that may continue unabated, to the detriment of the organism.**

CCI 9 (Level A): **Depending on the findings in cohort studies about the use of hormones to stimulate wound healing (CCI 8), selective randomized controlled trials should be conducted to test the performance of the most promising interventions.**

References

1. Kudravi SA, Reed MJ. Aging, cancer, and wound healing. In Vivo 2000;14:83-92.
2. Marcus JR, Tyrone JW, Bonomo S, et al. Cellular mechanisms for diminished scarring with aging. Plast Reconstr Surg 2000;105:1591-1599.
3. Thomas DR. Age-related changes in wound healing. Drugs Aging 2001;18:607-620.
4. Van de Kerkhof PC, Van Bergen B, Spruijt K, Kuiper JP. Age-related changes in wound healing. Clin Exp Dermatol 1994;19:369-374.
5. Nagy KK, Smith RF, Roberts RR, et al. Prognosis of penetrating trauma in elderly patients: a comparison with younger patients. J Trauma 2000;49:190-193; discussion 193-194.
6. Holt DR, Kirk SJ, Regan MC, et al. Effect of age on wound healing in healthy human beings. Surgery 1992;112:293-297; discussion 297-298.
7. Meyer LJ, Stern R. Age-dependent changes of hyaluronan in human skin. J Invest Dermatol 1994;102:385-389.
8. Ballas CB, Davidson JM. Delayed wound healing in aged rats is associated with increased collagen gel remodeling and contraction by skin fibroblasts, not with differences in apoptotic or myofibroblast cell populations. Wound Repair Regen 2001;9:223-237.
9. Amler MH. Age factor in human alveolar bone repair. J Oral Implantol 1993;19:138-142.

10. O'Driscoll SW, Saris DB, Ito Y, Fitzimmons JS. The chondrogenic potential of periosteum decreases with age. J Orthop Res 2001;19:95-103.

11. Stanley A, Osler T. Senescence and the healing rates of venous ulcers. J Vasc Surg 2001;33:1206-1211.

12. Serletti JM, Higgins JP, Moran S, Orlando GS. Factors affecting outcome in free-tissue transfer in the elderly. Plast Reconstr Surg 2000;106:66-70.

13. Xia YP, Zhao Y, Tyrone JW, et al. Differential activation of migration by hypoxia in keratinocytes isolated from donors of increasing age: implication for chronic wounds in the elderly. J Invest Dermatol 2001;116:50-56.

14. Bonomo SR, Davidson JD, Tyrone JW, et al. Enhancement of wound healing by hyperbaric oxygen and transforming growth factor beta3 in a new chronic wound model in aged rabbits. Arch Surg 2000;135:1148-1153.

15. Basaria S, Dobs AS. Hypogonadism and androgen replacement therapy in elderly men. Am J Med 2001;110:563-572.

16. Shackelford DP, Lalikos JF. Estrogen replacement therapy and the surgeon. Am J Surg 2000;179:333-336.

PHARMACOLOGY

There is a lengthy history of original research, review articles, editorials, and textbook chapters focusing on use of pharmaceuticals by elderly patients. The body of work includes descriptions of the pharmacokinetics and pharmacodynamics of specific drugs in older people and inappropriate medication use . Most of this literature is descriptive; there are few analytic studies. The available experimental studies are mostly evaluations of the efficacy of therapeutics for specific conditions. Studies that examine the impact of organizational interventions, such as computerized patient order entry, to reduce prescribing errors, improve patient safety, and introduce systems to assure quality are new additions to the literature. The largest category of the pharmacologic literature in geriatrics focuses on suboptimal prescribing and adverse drug events; common topics include the misuse, overuse, or underuse of pharmaceuticals; polypharmacy; and drug-disease or drug-drug interactions. (For additional relevant discussion, see Chapter 2, Geriatric Anesthesia.)

MISUSE, OVERUSE, AND UNDERUSE OF MEDICATIONS

Inappropriate medication use by community-dwelling older persons is common. Hanlon et al analyzed information from the Duke Established Populations for Epidemiologic Studies of the Elderly, rounds two (1989–90) and three (1992–93). [1] They report rates of inappropriate drug use of 27% and 22.5%, respectively. Inappropriate use was determined by use of the Beers criteria. [2] One limitation of these criteria is the paucity of evidence on the use of many medications among elderly people since they commonly are excluded from clinical trials. The latest version of inappropriate drug use criteria was published in 1997 [3] and is used currently to measure quality of care. Chin et al showed that in one setting, 10.6% of patients were taking a potentially inappropriate medication on presentation to the emergency department. [4] Of these, 3.6% were given the inappropriate medication in the emergency department and 5.6% were prescribed one at discharge. Though not as common as potentially inappropriate medications, drug-disease interactions are not uncommon. As new drugs become available, a mechanism must be established to update the current criteria. Naranjo et al [5] proposed a method for estimating the probability of adverse drug reactions in 1981, but this work needs updating. Cluff as far back as 1965 recommended surveillance methods. [6] This, too, is an area of needed inquiry.

Overuse by elderly persons of both prescription and nonprescription drugs is seen with increasing frequency. Causes are multifactorial and include redosing because of forgetfulness or lack of perceived effect of prescribed doses and self-medication with over-the-counter remedies.

Underuse of effective medications by older patients—for example, angiotensin-converting enzyme inhibitors for congestive heart failure—has been well documented. Suboptimal management of chronic conditions potentially leads to worse perioperative and rehabilitation outcomes.

Adverse events associated with drug withdrawal are less well studied. Hanlon refers to earlier work he and colleagues did on adverse events associated with the withdrawal of prescription medications. [1] For 124 patients in the study, 238 medications were discontinued. Possible or probable adverse events were noted in 26% (62) of the withdrawn drugs; 41% of these were classed as major events. Kennedy et al found that withdrawal of drugs not related to the operation increased postoperative complications. [7]

Few studies are available that assess the impact of payment and policy changes on patient outcomes; ways to align financial incentives with desired outcomes are also little studied. System changes can, and should, facilitate medication use that maximizes therapeutic response and minimizes untoward events. A study from Montreal reported adverse events associated with drug costs. Tamblyn et al noted a 9% decrease in use of essential drugs, a 14% increase in emergency department visits, and a doubling of adverse events, all associated with the introduction of a 25% copayment. [8]

PERIOPERATIVE PHARMACEUTICALS

Studies of drugs in the perioperative period include investigations of the pharmacokinetics of specific drugs. Studies of premedication include evaluations of morphine by O'Sullivan et al, [9] fentanyl by Bentley et al, [10] and clonidine by Filos et al. [11] Bennett et al reviewed the literature to produce guidelines for prescribing perioperative medications to patients with renal failure. [12]

The use of patient-controlled analgesia by elderly patients has received limited attention. The few papers are small randomized controlled trials; two used morphine and one used propofol. [13–15] The morphine studies were for control of postoperative pain. [13,14] Herrick et al examined the use of patient-controlled propofol intraoperatively during cataract operation. [15] All three studies reported adequate pain control or sedation and increased patient satisfaction in comparison with standard fixed-dose and time-administered medications.

Postoperative cognitive impairment in older patients is a significant problem. A few descriptive or analytic studies have associated drug choice with cognitive impairment. [16–18]

Nausea and vomiting are unpleasant side effects. Tarkkila et al conducted a small randomized trial of three regimens to prevent nausea and vomiting in arthroplasty patients. [19] They reported superiority of premedication with oral promethazine (10 mg) and transdermal scopolamine (1.5 mg) in reducing nausea and vomiting over oral diazepam (5 to 15 mg) or oral promethazine alone. In one of the few studies involving older patients, Thune et al tested metoclopramide for laparoscopic cholecystectomy patients ranging in age from 21 to 79 years and found decreased postoperative nausea in comparison with the results of using no medication. [20]

COMPLEMENTARY (ALTERNATIVE) MEDICINE

There is an increasing use of complementary or alternative medicine in the United States population, including folk remedies. These medicines include substances that have a pharmacologic effect. Often, patients fail to report to surgeons their use of such substances, or they continue to take them throughout the surgical experience, assuming that they are of little importance. Virtually no reports exist concerning the effect of complementary or alternative medicines on the elderly surgical patient.

> *CCI 10 (Level B)*: **Clinicians in the specialties need support in their management during the perioperative period of the multiple medications that the typical older patient takes. Systems should be developed to routinely monitor inappropriate drug use and to provide methods to improve the quality of prescribing to older patients.**

> *CCI 11 (Level B)*: **Research is needed on the consequences of drug withdrawal in elderly surgical patients.**

> *CCI 12 (Level A)*: **Randomized controlled trials of system changes that might optimize medication use by older patients are needed.**

> *CCI 13 (Level A)*: **The short- and long-term effectiveness of interventions aimed at optimizing the management of chronic disease and comorbid conditions in older patients during the perioperative period should be assessed.**

> *CCI 14 (Level B)*: **New, easily usable guidelines for prescribing to patients with renal failure are needed.**

> *CCI 15 (Level B)*: **A meta-analysis is needed to obtain a more accurate estimate of the value of patient-controlled drug delivery for elderly surgical patients.**

> *CCI 16 (Level B)*: **The interaction of ethanol with other drugs and its effects on the elderly trauma victim need to be investigated.**

> *CCI 17 (Levels D, C)*: **The effects of complementary or alternative medicines on the incidence of complications in elderly surgical patients are unknown and should be investigated by observational cohort studies and ultimately for selected medications by randomized controlled trials.**

References

1.   Hanlon JT, Shimp LA, Semla TP. Recent advances in geriatrics: drug-related problems in the elderly. Ann Pharmacother 2000;34:360-365.

2. Cornoni-Huntley J, Ostfeld AM, Taylor JO, et al. Established populations for epidemiologic studies of the elderly: study design and methodology. Aging (Milano) 1993;5:27-37.

3. Beers MH. Explicit criteria for determining potentially inappropriate medication use by the elderly: an update. Arch Intern Med 1997;157:1531-1536.

4. Chin MH, Wang LC, Jin L, et al. Appropriateness of medication selection for older persons in an urban academic emergency department. Acad Emerg Med 1999;6:1232-1242.

5. Naranjo CA, Busto U, Sellers EM, et al. A method for estimating the probability of adverse drug reactions. Clin Pharmacol Ther 1981;30:239-245.

6. Cluff LE, Thornton G, Seidl L, Smith J. Epidemiological study of adverse drug reactions. Trans Assoc Am Physicians 1965;78:255-268.

7. Kennedy JM, van Rij AM, Spears GF, et al. Polypharmacy in a general surgical unit and consequences of drug withdrawal. Br J Clin Pharmacol 2000;49:353-362.

8. Tamblyn R, Laprise R, Hanley JA, et al. Adverse events associated with prescription drug cost-sharing among poor and elderly persons. JAMA 2001;285:421-429.

9. O'Sullivan G, Bullingham RE, McQuay HJ, et al. A comparison of intramuscular and sublingual buprenorphine, intramuscular morphine and placebo as premedication. Anaesthesia 1983;38:977-984.

10. Bentley JB, Borel JD, Nenad RE, Gillespie TJ. Age and fentanyl pharmacokinetics. Anesth Analg 1982;61:968-971.

11. Filos KS, Patroni O, Goudas LC, et al. A dose-response study of orally administered clonidine as premedication in the elderly: evaluating hemodynamic safety. Anesth Analg 1993;77:1185-1192.

12. Bennett WM, Aronoff GR, Morrison G, et al. Drug prescribing in renal failure: dosing guidelines for adults. Am J Kidney Dis 1983;3:155-193.

13. Wasylak TJ, Abbott FV, English MJ, Jeans ME. Reduction of postoperative morbidity following patient-controlled morphine. Can J Anaesth 1990;37:726-731.

14. Egbert AM, Parks LH, Short LM, Burnett ML. Randomized trial of postoperative patient-controlled analgesia vs intramuscular narcotics in frail elderly men. Arch Intern Med 1990;150:1897-1903.

15. Herrick IA, Gelb AW, Nichols B, Kirkby J. Patient-controlled propofol sedation for elderly patients: safety and patient attitude toward control. Can J Anaesth 1996;43:1014-1018.

16. Herrick IA, Ganapathy S, Komar W, et al. Postoperative cognitive impairment in the elderly: choice of patient-controlled analgesia opioid. Anaesthesia 1996;51:356-360.

17. Larson EB, Kukull WA, Buchner D, Reifler BV. Adverse drug reactions associated with global cognitive impairment in elderly persons. Ann Intern Med 1987;107:169-173.

18. Bowen JD, Larson EB. Drug-induced cognitive impairment: defining the problem and finding solutions. Drugs Aging 1993;3:349-357.

19. Tarkkila P, Torn K, Tuominen M, Lindgren L. Premedication with promethazine and transdermal scopolamine reduces the incidence of nausea and vomiting after intrathecal morphine. Acta Anaesthesiol Scand 1995;39:983-986.

20. Thune A, Appelgren L, Haglind E. Prevention of postoperative nausea and vomiting after laparoscopic cholecystectomy: a prospective randomized study of metoclopramide and transdermal hyoscine. Eur J Surg 1995;161:265-268.

CLINICAL OUTCOMES ASSESSMENT

Although independence is the usual endpoint for rehabilitation, older patients may value other goals more than independence or even in lieu of independence.[1] One study of outpatient geriatric assessment observed that geriatric assessment studies to date have measured primarily functional status, health services use, costs of care, caregiver stress, and patient and family satisfaction. [2] Interviews with patients and families indicated that the most common goals sought from geriatric assessment were obtaining education and referrals and improving social and family relationships. These goals have not systematically been measured in the assessment of health care outcomes of geriatric assessment programs.

MEASUREMENT CONSIDERATIONS AND FUNCTIONAL OUTCOMES

An important psychometric consideration is the relative responsiveness of condition-specific and generic health status measures in assessing outcomes. Condition-specific measures were used in one study of surgical outcomes for degenerative lumbar spinal stenosis. [3] Measurements were performed preoperatively and again at 6 months following operation. Questions about condition-specific symptoms were concerned with effects of the disease on the patient and included issues such as pain (frequency and location). Physical function questions asked about activities such as walking distance, walking for pleasure, and shopping. Generic measures used included the Sickness Impact Profile. Minimal clinically relevant improvement was estimated by the use of patient satisfaction as the external criterion. The condition-specific measures were found to be more sensitive and discriminating than the physical function questions and were therefore recommended as better primary endpoints for future studies. However, the effects of surgical procedures can be reflected in generic measures such as the Medical Outcomes Study Short Form 36-item health survey (SF-36) and those broader generic health measures. Health-related quality-of-life (HRQOL) measures permit a broader assessment of the impact of surgical procedures. [4]

Applying a common instrument across surgical or medical conditions, in addition to condition-specific measures, may help reveal shared risk factors for poorer clinical outcomes. The American Society of Anesthesiologists' Physical Status Score (ASA-PS) is one such global measure that could be applied to the preoperative assessment of the patient. [5] Since its development in 1961, multiple studies have demonstrated the strong correlation of poor physical status with higher rates of morbidity and mortality. The increasing information that has been assembled about older patients suggests that certain common measures also may predict outcomes across diagnoses and syndromes. For example, assessment of shared risk factors for falls, incontinence, and functional dependence has revealed that these different syndromes all have the same four independent predisposing factors: slow timed chair stands (lower-extremity impairment), decreased arm strength (upper-extremity impairment), decreased vision and hearing (sensory impairment), and either a high anxiety or depression score (affective impairment). [6]

The measurement of the outcomes of health care interventions—like emergency department visits, operations, and rehabilitation—will require the measurement of functional outcomes. HRQOL measures such as the SF-36 include physical function measures. Understanding the factors that contribute to poor functional outcomes will clarify which interventions may be harmful to function and which interventions could be modified to yield better functional outcomes. For instance, age and prefracture residence at a nursing home have been found to predict walking—not mortality—at 6 months after hip fracture. [7] However, functional measures have been found to predict both short-term and 2-year post-hospitalization mortality in a large study of nonsurgical patients. [8]

The measurement of hospitalization outcomes depends upon practicality, especially where some measures appear to be appropriate for routine clinical use to help physicians and others improve the care of older adults. For example, generic measures like the Nottingham Health Profiles have been presented as feasible for common hospital conditions. [9]

POSTOPERATIVE MORTALITY

Several large studies evaluated surgical outcomes in patients 80 years and older. Warner et al reported results of a retrospective cohort study of patients 100 years or older who were operated on between 1975 and 1994 with follow-up through 1995. [10] Eighty-eight percent of the patients were in American Society of Anesthesiologists (ASA) class III or worse. Only one major complication occurred, and the 48-hour, 30-day, and 1-year mortality rates were 0%, 16.1%, and 35.5%. These rates were comparable to the rate expected for age-matched controls.

Two reviews evaluated outcomes in patients 90 years and older. [11,12] An additional three case series evaluated outcomes in surgical cases involving persons 80 years and older. [13-15] In-hospital mortality rates (around 1 month mortality) were 13.4% (for major surgeries only), 1.6% (when cataract cases were included), and 5.2%, 4.6%, and 6.2% (overall, the three studies respectively). Overall, these findings fit with a trend of declining mortality rates following operations in octogenarians from greater than 20% in the 1960s to 10% in the 1970s, to under 10% in several more recent series. In these studies, ASA-PS status was found to be correlated with mortality. Additional risk factors included congestive heart failure, the presence of neurologic diseases, and a history of arrhythmias.

The literature on postoperative mortality in older adults covers two postoperative time periods for mortality. For nonorthopedic procedures, most series report mortality from the time during hospitalization to about 1 month after. The hip fracture literature, however, evaluates mortality at 3 months to 1 year and even later. For series on deaths during the index hospitalizations, risk factors for mortality have included advanced age, male gender, ASA-PS score, congestive heart failure, emergency surgery, renal disease, and major operations. One study evaluated cardiac ejection fraction, noting a mortality rate of 9.3% if ejection fractions were less than 50% but a 1.2% overall mortality rate. [16]

Recent studies of mortality focus on orthopedic fractures. Hamlet et al reported a 4.5 lower relative risk of mortality at 3 years in patients in ASA class I and II groups (N = 62) in comparison with class III and higher (10% mortality versus 50% mortality). [17] Zuckerman et al also reported increased mortality in the 12 months after hip fracture procedures with delay of 48 hours or more for operation. [18] However, when ASA-PS is added in calculating the adjusted hazard ratio, the timing of operation was no longer found to be statistically significant.

As the system of perioperative care improves, so do outcomes. Operative mortality was carefully examined in a Canadian study of older patients undergoing coronary artery bypass graft (CABG) procedures. [19] The risk-severity score and operative mortality were examined in 3330 consecutive patients aged 70 years and older who underwent isolated CABG procedures between 1982 and 1996. Operative mortality was found to have declined significantly from 17.2% to 8.9% despite an increase in prevalence of high-risk elderly patients from 16.2% to 26.9%. Poor ventricular function and repeat CABG procedures had the greatest impact on mortality.

PROCESS AND LENGTH-OF-STAY ISSUES

Hospitals are hazardous settings for older persons' care. [20] Health care costs can be reduced by shortening stays, provided adverse outcomes do not occur. Optimal methods for identifying factors that affect hospital length of stay may be a clustered model rather than stepwise regression models in which possible predictors are highly correlated. [21] However, most studies to date have used stepwise regression models. In addition, controlling for severity of disease is a difficult methodologic issue. In one evaluation, wide variations in hospital lengths of stay for hip fracture patients could not be explained by severity adjustments. [22]

Factors directly related to types of operation and modifications of surgical practice may account for some changes in length of stay. [23,24] Early and sufficient feeding postoperatively can reduce length of stay. [25] In studies of comorbidities, visual impairment was found to contribute 2.4 days ($P < .001$) to average length of stay in a series of multivariate models. [26] In another study, the use of sedative-hypnotic medications was found to be associated with longer hospital stays and higher hospital costs after controlling for severity of illness and comorbid conditions. [27] Several studies of medical patients showed that cognitive impairment and delirium can increase length of stay, as can prior impaired function. [20] These factors are likely to affect the outcomes of surgical patients as well. The role of age can be an independent risk factor for increased length of stay, controlling for other variables in surgical as well as medical patients. [28–32]

The Uniform Data System documents acute hospital and rehabilitation hospital lengths of stay along with functional status, using the Functional Independence Measure (FIM) for patients receiving inpatient rehabilitation. Comparison of data from 1990 to 1999 show substantial decreases in acute hospital lengths of stay (22 days to 11 days) and rehabilitation hospital lengths of stay (32 days to 20 days) for stroke survivors. There was no major change in rehabilitation admission median FIM (63 versus 64) or discharge median FIM (92 versus 91). [33,34] Most likely, unmeasured economic and administrative factors led to such significant decreases in length of stay at a national level.

PATIENT SATISFACTION

Patients' views of their care have been increasingly cited as important in the assessment of health care. [35–39] From patient focus groups and health care provider interviews, Gerteis et al identified seven primary dimensions of patient-centered care: respect for patients' values, preferences, and expressed needs; coordination and integration of care; information, communication, and education; physical comfort; emotional support and alleviation of fear and anxiety; involvement of family and friends (care partners); and transition and continuity (caring for self away from the health setting). [40]

The concept of patient satisfaction with care represents several aspects of these dimensions. Ware et al defined eight dimensions: interpersonal manner, technical quality, accessibility or convenience, financial aspects, physical environment, availability of providers and facilities, continuity of care, and efficacy or outcomes. [41] Some studies specifically examined patient satisfaction in relation to age and found that older patients generally were more satisfied. [38] In one national survey of acute hospital care, older patients reported fewer problems than younger patients did. [42,43] The reasons for this are unclear but may be related to the fact that elderly patients have acquired a tolerance for the health care system that has provided their care for so many years.

Studies of surgical and rehabilitation outcomes are evaluating dimensions of patient satisfaction as well as interventions that might improve satisfaction ratings. [44–47] Using the Picker Institute Consumer Satisfaction Survey, one study of hip and knee arthroplasty patients found increased patient satisfaction from 77% to 92% resulting from improvement of patient care processes between acute hospital and rehabilitation settings. [46] Higher satisfaction among stroke patients was found to be associated with higher function at discharge in a sample of 8900 patients evaluated at 80 to 180 days after discharge from inpatient rehabilitation. [47] Functions most associated with satisfaction were transfers, social cognition, and locomotion.

> *CCI 18 (Level B)*: **Observational cohort studies are needed to identify the most important preoperative predictors of functional outcome in elderly surgical patients.**

> *CCI 19 (Level A)*: **Interventional studies should be performed to help determine whether early identification and treatment of pre-existing risk factors leads to improved postoperative, posthospitalization, and rehabilitation outcomes in elderly surgical patients.**

> *CCI 20 (Level B)*: **Existing data from previous research studies on surgical outcomes should be re-examined for age-specific and age-stratified data to validate risk assessment and surgical complication rates in the older-old and oldest-old surgical patients.**

> *CCI 21 (Level A)*: **Prospective, age-specific, and age-stratified intervention studies are needed to help determine whether age is an independent risk factor for poorer surgical outcome for various specific surgical procedures and whether early identification and treatment of other risk factors lead to improved postoperative mortality rates and reduce hospital and intensive care unit lengths of stay for elderly surgical patients. These studies should be longitudinal to determine, among other outcomes, whether transfers out of acute-care facilities to other health care facilities actually decrease health care costs.**

> *CCI 22 (Level B)*: **Prospective patient satisfaction surveys are needed to identify the most important factors for elderly patients, including functional outcomes, quality of life, and return to independent living.**

> *CCI 23 (Level A)*: **Interventional studies are needed to determine whether early identification and treatment of comorbidities and postoperative complications in elderly surgical patients lead to improved patient satisfaction indices, functional outcomes, quality of life, and return to independent living.**

References

1. Spiro HM. Old doctors and old patients. Pharos Alpha Omega Alpha Honor Med Soc 1988;51:19-23.
2. Bradley EH, Bogardus ST, Jr., van Doorn C, et al. Goals in geriatric assessment: are we measuring the right outcomes? Gerontologist 2000;40:191-196.
3. Stucki G, Liang MH, Fossel AH, Katz JN. Relative responsiveness of condition-specific and generic health status measures in degenerative lumbar spinal stenosis. J Clin Epidemiol 1995;48:1369-1378.
4. Lieberman JR, Dorey F, Shekelle P, et al. Outcome after total hip arthroplasty: comparison of a traditional disease-specific and a quality-of-life measurement of outcome. J Arthroplasty 1997;12:639-645.
5. Dripps LA, Eckenhoff JE. The role of anesthesia in surgical mortality. JAMA 1961;178: 261-266.
6. Tinetti ME, Inouye SK, Gill TM, Doucette JT. Shared risk factors for falls, incontinence, and functional dependence: unifying the approach to geriatric syndromes. JAMA 1995;273: 1348-1353.
7. Browner WS, Li J, Mangano DT. In-hospital and long-term mortality in male veterans following noncardiac surgery. The Study of Perioperative Ischemia Research Group. JAMA 1992;268:228-232.
8. Inouye SK, Peduzzi PN, Robison JT, et al. Importance of functional measures in predicting mortality among older hospitalized patients. JAMA 1998;279:1187-1193.
9. O'Brien J, Bowie C. A methodology for collecting outcome measures for common hospital conditions. J Public Health Med 1992;14:380-384.
10. Warner MA, Saletel RA, Schroeder DR, et al. Outcomes of anesthesia and surgery in people 100 years of age and older. J Am Geriatr Soc 1998;46:988-993.
11. Adkins RB, Scott HW. Surgical procedures in patients aged 90 years and older. South Med J 1984;77:1357-1364.
12. Hosking MP, Warner MA, Lobdell CM, et al. Outcomes of surgery in patients 90 years of age and older [see comments]. JAMA 1989;261:1909-1915.
13. Liu LL, Leung JM. Predicting adverse postoperative outcomes in patients aged 80 years or older. J Am Geriatr Soc 2000;48:405-412.
14. Cheng KW, Wang CH, Ho RT, et al. Outcome of surgery and anesthesia in patients 80 years of age and older. Acta Anaesthesiol Sin 1994;32:37-43.
15. Djokovic JL, Hedley-Whyte J. Prediction of outcome of surgery and anesthesia in patients over 80. JAMA 1979;242:2301-2306.
16. Pedersen T. Complications and death following anaesthesia: a prospective study with special reference to the influence of patient-, anaesthesia-, and surgery-related risk factors. Dan Med Bull 1994;41:319-331.
17. Hamlet WP, Lieberman JR, Freedman EL, et al. Influence of health status and the timing of surgery on mortality in hip fracture patients. Am J Orthop 1997;26:621-627.
18. Zuckerman JD, Skovron ML, Koval KJ, et al. Postoperative complications and mortality associated with operative delay in older patients who have a fracture of the hip. J Bone Joint Surg Am 1995;77:1551-1556.
19. Ivanov J, Weisel RD, David TE, Naylor CD. Fifteen-year trends in risk severity and operative mortality in elderly patients undergoing coronary artery bypass graft surgery. Circulation 1998;97:673-680.
20. Calkins E. Care of older people in the hospital. In Calkins E, Wagner EH, Pacala JT (eds): New Ways to Care for Older People: Building Systems Based on Evidence. New York: Springer Publishing Company, 1999. p. 99-111.

21. Cohen YC, Rubin HR, Freedman L, Mozes B. Use of a clustered model to identify factors affecting hospital length of stay. J Clin Epidemiol 1999;52:1031-1036.

22. Shwartz M, Iezzoni LI, Ash AS, Mackiernan YD. Do severity measures explain differences in length of hospital stay? the case of hip fracture. Health Serv Res 1996;31:365-385.

23. Schwartz MH, Tartter PI. Decreased length of stay for patients with colorectal cancer: implications of DRG use. J Healthc Qual 1998;20:22-25.

24. Gardner TA, Bissonette EA, Petroni GR, et al. Surgical and postoperative factors affecting length of hospital stay after radical prostatectomy. Cancer 2000;89:424-430.

25. Neumayer LA, Smout RJ, Horn HG, Horn SD. Early and sufficient feeding reduces length of stay and charges in surgical patients. J Surg Res 2001;95:73-77.

26. Morse AR, Yatzkan E, Berberich B, Arons RR. Acute care hospital utilization by patients with visual impairment. Arch Ophthalmol 1999;117:943-949.

27. Yuen EJ, Zisselman MH, Louis DZ, Rovner BW. Sedative-hypnotic use by the elderly: effects on hospital length of stay and costs. J Ment Health Adm 1997;24:90-97.

28. Kalman PG, Johnston KW. Sociologic factors are major determinants of prolonged hospital stay after abdominal aneurysm repair. Surgery 1996;119:690-693.

29. Wong DT, Cheng DC, Kustra R, et al. Risk factors of delayed extubation, prolonged length of stay in the intensive care unit, and mortality in patients undergoing coronary artery bypass graft with fast-track cardiac anesthesia: a new cardiac risk score. Anesthesiology 1999;91:936-944.

30. Katz NM, Hannan RL, Hopkins RA, Wallace RB. Cardiac operations in patients aged 70 years and over: mortality, length of stay, and hospital charge. Ann Thorac Surg 1995;60:96-100; discussion 100-101.

31. Hirsch CH, Sommers L, Olsen A, et al. The natural history of functional morbidity in hospitalized older patients. J Am Geriatr Soc 1990;38:1296-1303.

32. Shah MR, Aharonoff GB, Wolinsky P, et al. Outcome after hip fracture in individuals ninety years of age and older. J Orthop Trauma 2001;15:34-39.

33. Granger CV, Hamilton BB. UDS report. The Uniform Data System for Medical Rehabilitation Report of First Admissions for 1990. Am J Phys Med Rehabil 1992;71:108-113.

34. Deutsch A, Fiedler RC, Granger CV, Russell CF. The Uniform Data System for Medical Rehabilitation report of patients discharged from comprehensive medical rehabilitation programs in 1999. Am J Phys Med Rehabil 2002;81:133-142.

35. Donabedian A. The quality of care. how can it be assessed? JAMA 1988;260:1743-1748.

36. Cleary PD, McNeil BJ. Patient satisfaction as an indicator of quality care. Inquiry 1988;25:25-36.

37. Ellwood PM, Jr., Lundberg GD. Managed care: a work in progress. JAMA 1996;276:1083-1086.

38. Laine C, Davidoff F. Patient-centered medicine: a professional evolution. JAMA 1996;275:152-156.

39. Kramer AM. Rehabilitation care and outcomes from the patient's perspective. Med Care 1997;35:JS48-JS57; discussion JS58-JS63.

40. Gerteis M, Edgman-Levitan S, Daley J, Delbanco TL. Medicine and health from the patient's perspective. In Gerteis M, Edgman-Levitan S, Daley J, Delbanco TL (eds): Through the Patient's Eyes: Understanding and Promoting Patient-Centered Care. San Francisco: Jossey-Bass, 1993. p. 1-18.

41. Ware JE, Davies AR, Stewart AL. The Measurement and Meaning of Patient Satisfaction: A Review of the Literature. Santa Monica, CA: RAND, 1977.

42. Cleary PD, Edgman-Levitan S, Roberts M, et al. Patients evaluate their hospital care: a national survey. Health Aff (Millwood) 1991;10:254-267.

43. Keith RA. Patient satisfaction and rehabilitation services. Arch Phys Med Rehabil 1998;79:1122-1128.
44. Anderson JG, Wixson RL, Tsai D, et al. Functional outcome and patient satisfaction in total knee patients over the age of 75. J Arthroplasty 1996;11:831-840.
45. Salmon P, Hall GM, Peerbhoy D, et al. Recovery from hip and knee arthroplasty: patients' perspective on pain, function, quality of life, and well-being up to 6 months postoperatively. Arch Phys Med Rehabil 2001;82:360-366.
46. Grissom SP, Dunagan L. Improved satisfaction during inpatient rehabilitation after hip and knee arthroplasty: a retrospective analysis. Am J Phys Med Rehabil 2001;80:798-803.
47. Ottenbacher KJ, Gonzales VA, Smith PM, et al. Satisfaction with medical rehabilitation in patients with cerebrovascular impairment. Am J Phys Med Rehabil 2001;80:876-884.

PREOPERATIVE RISK ASSESSMENT AND PREPARATION

Prior to undergoing an operative procedure, geriatric patients are often assumed to be at high risk for either bad outcomes or more severe complications. Assessing preoperative risk factors should allow for preoperative optimization when possible and provide a basis for appropriate perioperative intervention in urgent operations. (See also the section on age-related physiologic changes and preoperative care in Chapter 2, Geriatric Anesthesia.)

CARDIOPULMONARY FUNCTION

The large numbers of coronary artery bypass operations performed each year allow prospective evaluation of preoperative status with great statistical power. Such research includes the work by Elisheva et al (4835 patients),[1] John et al (19,224 patients),[2] Maharajah et al with 436 patients over 75 years of age,[3] Newman et al (2417 patients),[4] and Pederson et al (7305 patients).[5] Poor reserve with ST segment depression on exercise testing, prior history of myocardial infarction or cardiac operation, smoking, acute phase response with increased interleukin-6, and hypertension were associated with statistically greater complications with poor outcomes. Abnormal chest x-rays or decreased pulmonary function tests were associated with an increase in pulmonary complications following cardiac procedures.

In several studies, once risk had been identified, manipulations were used to determine the best method of reducing potential problems. In one study (Felding et al),[6] certain drugs were used to improve stress response, and in another (Kopp et al),[7] preemptive analgesia was implemented to modify postoperative pain response. Gotohda et al[8] applied a preoperative scoring system, and Newman et al[4] used a cluster scoring technique. Trzcieniecka-Green and Steptoe[9] attempted relaxation-based stress management for improvement in quality of life. Ashton et al[10] attempted self-hypnosis as a potential management strategy to reduce anxiety following bypass. (For further discussion of work on cardiac and pulmonary status preoperatively, see Chapter 2, Geriatric Anesthesia.)

NUTRITION

Himes reviewed the effects of poor nutrition on wound healing.[11] Protein-calorie malnutrition and involuntary weight loss continue to be prevalent among hospitalized and long-term care patients. Studies on nutritional intervention have established a correlation between nutritional status, body weight, and rate of wound healing. Nutritional intervention, however, must be provided early enough to prevent a catabolic-induced decline in lean muscle mass, which can further impair wound healing. Chronic, nonhealing wounds are particularly difficult to treat and contribute to significant morbidity, mortality, and hospitalizations. More aggressive nutritional management and a greater understanding of the role of nutrition and weight gain in wound healing can result in more effective patient care. Azad et al, using a variety of survey instruments, evaluated elderly patients for malnutrition at the time of admission. [12] They found that 44% of the older patients were at moderate risk for malnutrition and that 15% were malnourished upon admission. All physicians should be aware of this staggering fact and be prepared to act as early as possible in the patient's hospital course; most concur that the elderly patients were suffering from malnutrition. Linn et al in 1988 [13] noted that the malnourished patients had the poorest surgical outcomes of any group. More specifically, Covinsky et al [14] found that such patients risk greater mortality, have later functional recovery, and have higher rates of nursing-home usage.

The most effective method for screening patients for nutritional status appears to be serum albumin concentration. [15] Unfortunately, the threshold danger level calculated by different investigators varies, from 2.8 to 3.5 g/dL. Other screening measurements include total lymphocyte counts, serum transferrin, C-reactive protein, anergy to Candida and mumps skin testing, and abnormal serum globulin. Baker et al [16] indicated that good nutritional histories and the use of brief nutritional assessment instruments and of physical measurements such as skin fold thickness or body mass index are effective in defining malnutrition. Avenell et al [17] noted that patients having urgent surgical care are at greater risk, since any nutritional deficiency cannot be corrected readily. Although most accept that optimal preoperative nutrition is beneficial, no consensus has emerged for the type of nutritional enhancement or the route of administration. It is equally unclear which vitamin or mineral supplementations are best suited for malnourished elderly patients. (See also discussion of nutrition in Chapter 11, section on postoperative outcome.)

FLUID MANAGEMENT

Zawada et al [18] assumed that geriatric patients who arrive for a procedure after the traditional fast are in negative fluid balance and become volume contracted. This assumption is not proven, but Seymour at al [19] developed a dehydration score for patients 70 years and older and found that it correlated significantly with altered mental status. Garrison et al [20] proposed preoperative saline loading to expand blood volume, but the results were marginal. Arieff [21] estimated blood or extracellular fluid volumes but was unable to predict preoperatively which patients would develop severe overhydration or pulmonary edema. Another area of concern is preoperative serum sodium. Miller [22] performed an extensive review of this problem. The causes included inadequate dietary sodium, increased sodium loss from diarrhea or vomiting, overhydration from either oral or intravenous administration, impaired water excretion, overdiuresis, adrenal insufficiency (rare), and inappropriate ADH secretion. The more important surgical syndromes are hyponatremia due either to dilutional hyponatremia or low blood volume electrolyte loss. The optimal type of intravenous fluid placement for older patients still is not determined.

Preoperative low serum potassiums predicts serious postoperative arrhythmias. Wahr et al [23] and Bartholaw et al [24] noted that blood pressure measurement, spot urine chlorides, and serum renin and aldosterone measurements help to clarify hypokalemia and metabolic alkalosis. Kudoh et al [25] noted that concentrations of aldosterone and atrial natriuretic hormone in elderly patients with hyperkalemia are unresponsive to surgical stress and volume expansion. Antonelli et al [26] assessed 180 patients from admission to discharge or death and concluded that postoperative electrolyte imbalance is a marker for very frail medical status and a risk factor for poor outcome among elderly patients.

ETHICAL ISSUES

The most comprehensive research on ethics, advance directives, communication with medical patients and families, and informed consent is the Study to Understand Prognoses and Preferences for Outcomes and Risks of Treatment (SUPPORT), along with Hospitalized Elderly Longitudinal Project (HELP). [27] SUPPORT and HELP constituted a two-phase study. The observational phase was designed to describe patient preferences for care and to develop prognostic models. HELP was a supplemental study that enrolled patients aged 80 years and older.

Sixty-seven articles from the project were in print at the time our literature search was conducted. SUPPORT described a number of problems: physicians misunderstood patients' preferences, do-not resuscitate (DNR) orders were written shortly before death, the majority of patients died in intensive care units, and patients had substantial levels of pain during the hospital stay. The SUPPORT and HELP investigators produced a prognostic model for functional outcome in older patients [28] and survival in all patients. [29]

The SUPPORT intervention to change physician behavior was not successful. Lynn et al [30] reviewed reasons for the failure and concluded that individual physician instruction was insufficient and that a system-level intervention of innovation and quality improvement in routine care might be appropriate. The SUPPORT and HELP studies focused on severely ill patients and made little mention of surgical patients. Hamel et al [31] reported older age to be associated with higher rates of decisions to withhold an operation, ventilator support, and dialysis. This was found to be true even after adjustment for patients' prognoses and preferences.

Observational studies of surgical patients have described some of the processes studied by SUPPORT investigators. Brett and Rosenberg reviewed records of patients with gastrostomy tubes. [32] They reported that the patient's competence was documented only for two thirds of patients. A discussion with the patient about alternatives to the tube was charted in only one patient. Surrogates gave consent for over 90% of patients even though over 20% of patients were competent to give their own consent. In another record review, Trunkey et al [33] reported that 67% of geriatric trauma patients who died had documentation indicating that a decision had been made to withdraw therapy and that an early decision to provide comfort care had been made for only 10 patients. Llovera et al reported that older patients presenting to the emergency department are more likely than younger patients to have an advance directive, with an increase in the odds ratio of 0.03 for each year of age. [34] These researchers did not present the absolute frequency of advance directives for the elderly patients.

Outcomes of Surgical Management

A deficiency of data on outcomes for the elderly surgical patient limit the surgeon's ability to obtain informed consent. Most studies reporting surgical outcomes in older patients are case series that report the results of operations in patients above a specified age. [35] Geriatric patients in surgical case series are likely to be healthier than all patients with the disease, including some who do not have an operation. The selection bias introduced into descriptive studies by clinical decisions should be adjusted or described in future literature to yield more applicable information for surgeon-patient communication about surgical risks and benefits. Functional status and other severity-of-illness variables should be reported to allow the surgeon to determine when outcome data apply to an individual patient. [36] Often, geriatric patients are excluded from trials of new surgical procedures, again creating uncertainty about whether outcomes data are applicable to this population.

Conversely, there is insufficient literature available about the outcome of forgoing an operation, a choice that is more likely in the frail elderly population than in most other age groups. Frail older patients may refuse surgery or receive a recommendation against surgery when the physician believes that its risks outweigh potential benefits. [37] Outcomes for treatment and control groups of geriatric patients are rarely reported, despite their importance to informed decision making. Small studies have reported on the outcomes of nonoperative management of hip fractures in geriatric patients. [38,39] The results were uniformly poor.

Geriatric patients have shorter life expectancies than younger patients and therefore may value certain outcomes to a greater extent. An older patient may fear a permanently disabling stroke after cardiac bypass grafting more than he or she fears a lethal arrhythmia. Surgical outcomes studies should be expanded to include functional status and to consider other relevant outcome measures, such as residence in a nursing home, experience of delirium, and quality of life after surgery. [40,41]

Outcomes data on surgical versus nonsurgical management of common diseases have the potential to change ethical decision making at a societal level. Surgical management may be more costly than nonsurgical management, and the principle of distributive justice argues against the use of health care resources for minimal benefit.

Informed Consent

Although the ethics literature provides guidance about the ideal conduct of the consent process, [42] controversies remain concerning the normative requirements for decisional capacity, disclosure, comprehension, and voluntary choice. The clinical practice of informed consent for surgical procedures does not always achieve these ideals, particularly for older and more poorly educated patients. [32,43,44]

A prominent reality of informed consent for elderly patients is the prevalence of cognitive impairment. [45] Although there has been a great deal of research regarding advance directives for life-sustaining treatments, there has been virtually no research exploring advance directives for other types of treatment. Few living wills include preferences for or against major procedures, although frail older patients often elect to forgo surgical treatment. For surgical decisions for geriatric patients who have lost decisional capacity, appointing formal surrogate decision makers, for example, choosing someone to have a health care power of attorney or to be a legal surrogate under state law, may be more flexible and useful than relying on a living will. Morrison et al, for example, studied patients with end-stage dementia who nonetheless had surgery for hip fractures and found them to have a 6-month mortality rate of nearly 50%.[46] The problem is not only that demented patients have a short life expectancy but also that the surgery adds considerable expense, does little to enhance their quality of life since they cannot participate effectively in rehabilitation and thus do not walk, and also exposes them to potential prosthetic infection.

The Conduct of the Operation

One of the key ethical questions that arises once an operation is planned pertains to do-not-resuscitate orders in the operating room.[47,48] Practice guidelines from the American College of Surgeons and the American Society of Anesthesiologists recommend discussion of this issue prior to operation. Patients may feel strongly that they do not wish to receive life-sustaining treatments, regardless of the cause of the cardiac or respiratory arrest. Surgeons and anesthesiologists often feel ethically bound to treat an arrest or complication they perceive to be iatrogenic. Compromises concerning conduct of care should be reached before the patient goes to the operating room.

Postoperative Care

A critical postoperative ethical issue is the physician's obligation to ensure access to adequate rehabilitative care. Postoperative care can make a difference in the functional outcome of the surgical patient.[49] When prospective payment was linked to shorter length of hospital stay, it was found that hip fracture patients received less physical therapy, more frequent transfers to nursing homes, and fewer discharges to home, with more limited functional recovery.[50] Research shows that patients with more comprehensive insurance, better personal financial resources, and who receive intensive rehabilitative care do not suffer the adverse effects of early hospital discharge.[51]

PREOPERATIVE EDUCATION

Educating patients and their families improves outcomes and postoperative satisfaction. Patients and their families make the best advocates for the patient. Most patients want to take responsibility for playing their part in trying to optimize the outcome of their surgery, but many are frustrated by lack of information and support to allow them to fulfill this role to their satisfaction. Having patients as honorary members of the health care team may facilitate the development of a framework within which the potential contribution of patients to their own care could be valued and supported more effectively.[52] This would help optimize patient outcomes and increase patient satisfaction with care.

Implementing such a plan has significant problems. When questioned, patients have expressed pronounced individual preferences. Beresford et al found that three groups of patients having cardiac procedures emerged: those requesting little or no risk information, those requesting information about major risks, and those requesting full risk disclosure.[53] The patients were not generally concerned about the specific probabilities of any risk. These researchers concluded that clinicians counseling patients before operation should routinely discuss patient preferences before risk disclosure, distinguishing among a preference for "no risk information," "all potentially relevant risks," and "those risks considered significant or likely to occur." The fact of individual patient preferences may undermine the concept of the "reasonable patient" in determination of the legal requirements for risk disclosure. (A reasonable individual would be one who is well informed, and withholding information on preference would introduce bias.) In another study conducted by Stanley et al, patients undergoing femoral popliteal bypass or carotid surgery were randomized to obtain either routine consent only or consent after active participation by the patient in the consent process, with the patient receiving two forms of information, oral and written. [54] The authors found that additional written or verbal information did not improve a patient's understanding of the procedure or its risks and complications. Patients' anxiety levels were unaltered by the increase in the information they were given.

Some patients and families seek information on their own, hoping to expand on what the surgeon provides, often with no additional success. Publicly released performance reports ("report cards"), now available for cardiac surgery, are expected to foster competition on the basis of quality. Proponents frequently cite the need to inform a patient's choice of physicians and hospitals as a central element of this strategy. In a study by Schneider and Epstein, only 12% of patients surveyed reported awareness of a widely publicized report on cardiac surgery mortality before undergoing cardiac surgery. [55] Less than 1% knew the correct rating of their surgeon or hospital, and most reported that the data had only a moderate or minor impact on their selection of provider. Efforts to aid patient decision making with performance reports are unlikely to succeed without a tailored and intensive program for dissemination and patient education.

If the education of patients is to improve, they themselves must participate in the process of establishing the information used in the preoperative education. Taylor and Norton asked patients postoperatively what information they felt was required to help prepare someone for their experience (major bowel surgery). [56] The participants identified many issues that would not have been considered important by the surgeon. A survey concerning the preanesthetic visit showed that the general public considers anesthetic assessment prior to surgery to be an important part of preoperative preparation. [57] Fears of brain damage, death, and intraoperative awareness associated with general anesthesia remain prevalent, suggesting that preoperative education of patients should address these concerns. The general population was less concerned about realistic fears such as nausea, vomiting, and postoperative discomfort. Many surgeons and surgical groups develop materials on their own, some with good results. Extensive preoperative patient and family education with ample time for questions and follow-up calls should be provided by the surgeon's office. Trovar et al developed a clinical pathway that is based on patient education. [58]

> *CCI 24 (Level B)*: **Although the ASA-PS risk assessment has helped to stratify patients, more detailed work is needed to allow for better preoperative preparation. Large databases should be used to identify the age-specific risks in major surgical procedures. Stratification of the risk factors will help to determine the threshold for the elderly patient (as distinguished from the younger adult) for developing a poor outcome following major surgical procedure.**

> *CCI 25 (Level B)*: **A simplified, easily applied scoring system for an aggregate value as well as by specific outcome needs to be developed and validated to offer a predictor of both survival and postoperative function following major surgery.**

CCI 26 (Levels, B, A): On the basis of risk-factor identification (see CCI 24), we need to develop candidate preventive and therapeutic methods for elderly surgical patients and then test the most promising ones in controlled trials.

CCI 27 (Level B): We must anticipate common complications of major surgery for older patients—for example, stroke—and develop standard procedures to immediately limit damage.

CCI 28 (Level A): Antidelirium strategies for elderly patients undergoing operations need to be tested, using an approach analogous that that used by Inouye et al in older medical inpatients.

CCI 29 (Level B): Preoperative interventions designed to speed postoperative recovery and enhance functional outcomes for older surgical patients need to be developed and validated.

CCI 30 (Level B): We need to use available literature and new ideas to establish a preferred screening method for malnutrition and to plan nutritional supplementation for elderly patients who will have elective surgery.

CCI 31 (Levels B, A): A program of "preventive nutrition" for patients who are at high risk to need urgent surgical intervention should be studied in cohort studies and ultimately in randomized controlled trials.

CCI 32 (Level B): Cohort studies are needed to try to identify surgical patients who are especially likely to develop fluid and electrolyte problems.

CCI 33 (Levels, B, A): Having identified risk factors for fluid and electrolyte problems (see CCI 32), we should first perform cohort studies and ultimately randomized controlled trials wherein patients at high risk would receive various regimens of intensive fluid and electrolyte management to determine which are most effective.

CCI 34 (Level B): Observational studies are needed to describe older patients' preferences with regard to surgery, consent for resuscitation, and advance directives.

CCI 35 (Level B): Research is needed to provide more useful outcome measures to inform decisions about the advisability of surgery for the geriatric population. Studies of surgical and nonsurgical management should include data on comparative costs, in addition to data on patient-level outcomes such as survival duration, function, quality of life, and complication rates.

CCI 36 (Level B): Cohort studies are needed to determine what benefits would outweigh the risks of pain, aspiration, and delirium that often accompany major surgery for elderly patients with dementia.

CCI 37 (Level B): Studies are needed to examine the effect on outcomes and satisfaction of preoperative discussions of patients' or surrogates' preferences regarding resuscitation in the operating room in general and specifically resuscitation for complications thought to be iatrogenic.

CCI 38 (Level B): **Large surveys of patients' biases and preferences for information are needed to help clinicians determine the appropriate material to present in the preoperative preparation of patients and their families.**

CCI 39 (Level B): **Unbiased, procedure-specific, and age-specific data need to be generated with public input through each of the surgical specialty societies to give patients a reliable source of preoperative data.**

References

1. Elisheva S, Noya G, Yana ZG, et al. Sequential logistic models for 30 days mortality after CABG: pre-operative, intra-operative and post-operative experience–The Israeli CABG study (ISCAB): three models for early mortality after CABG. Eur J Epidemiol 2000;16:543-555.
2. John R, Choudhri AF, Weinberg AD, et al. Multicenter review of preoperative risk factors for stroke after coronary artery bypass grafting. Ann Thorac Surg 2000;69:30-35; discussion 35-36.
3. Maharajh GS, Masters RG, Keon WJ. Cardiac operations in the elderly: who is at risk? Ann Thorac Surg 1998;66:1670-1673.
4. Newman MF, Wolman R, Kanchuger M, et al. Multicenter preoperative stroke risk index for patients undergoing coronary artery bypass graft surgery. Multicenter Study of Perioperative Ischemia (McSPI) Research Group. Circulation 1996;94:II 74-80.
5. Pedersen T, Eliasen K, Henriksen E. A prospective study of mortality associated with anaesthesia and surgery: risk indicators of mortality in hospital. Acta Anaesthesiol Scand 1990;34:176-182.
6. Felding C, Mikkelsen AL, Clausen HV, et al. Preoperative treatment with oestradiol in women scheduled for vaginal operation for genital prolapse: a randomised, double-blind trial. Maturitas 1992;15:241-249.
7. Kopp A, Wachauer D, Hoerauf KH, et al. Effect of pre-emptive hydromorphone administration on postoperative pain relief–a randomized controlled trial. Wien Klin Wochenschr 2000;112:1002-1006.
8. Gotohda N, Iwagaki H, Itano S, et al. Can POSSUM, a scoring system for perioperative surgical risk, predict postoperative clinical course? Acta Med Okayama 1998;52:325-329.
9. Trzcieniecka-Green A, Steptoe A. Stress management in cardiac patients: a preliminary study of the predictors of improvement in quality of life. J Psychosom Res 1994;38:267-280.
10. Ashton C, Whitworth GC, Seldomridge JA, et al. Self-hypnosis reduces anxiety following coronary artery bypass surgery: a prospective, randomized trial. J Cardiovasc Surg (Torino) 1997;38:69-75.
11. Himes D. Protein-calorie malnutrition and involuntary weight loss: the role of aggressive nutritional intervention in wound healing. Ostomy Wound Manage 1999;45:46-51, 54-45.
12. Azad N, Murphy J, Amos SS, Toppan J. Nutrition survey in an elderly population following admission to a tertiary care hospital. CMAJ 1999;161:511-515.
13. Linn BS, Robinson DS, Klimas NG. Effects of age and nutritional status on surgical outcomes in head and neck cancer. Ann Surg 1988;207:267-273.

14. Covinsky KE, Martin GE, Beyth RJ, et al. The relationship between clinical assessments of nutritional status and adverse outcomes in older hospitalized medical patients. J Am Geriatr Soc 1999;47:532-538.

15. Kung SP, Tang GJ, Wu CW, Lui WY. Serum albumin concentration as a prognostic indicator for acute surgical patients. Chung Hua I Hsueh Tsa Chih (Taipei) 1999;62:61-67.

16. Baker JP, Detsky AS, Wesson DE, et al. Nutritional assessment: a comparison of clinical judgement and objective measurements. N Engl J Med 1982;306:969-972.

17. Avenell A, Handoll HH. Nutritional supplementation for hip fracture aftercare in the elderly. Cochrane Database Syst Rev 2000:CD001880.

18. Zawada ET, Horning JR, Jr., Salem AG. Renal, fluid, electrolyte, and acid-base problems during surgery in the elderly. In Katlic MR (ed): Geriatric Surgery. Comprehensive Care of the Elderly Patient. Baltimore: Urban & Schwarzenberg, Inc., 1990. p. 85-96.

19. Seymour DG, Henschke PJ, Cape RD, Campbell AJ. Acute confusional states and dementia in the elderly: the role of dehydration/volume depletion, physical illness and age. Age Ageing 1980;9:137-146.

20. Garrison RN, Wilson MA, Matheson PJ, Spain DA. Preoperative saline loading improves outcome after elective, noncardiac surgical procedures. Am Surg 1996;62:223-231.

21. Arieff AI. Fatal postoperative pulmonary edema: pathogenesis and literature review. Chest 1999;115:1371-1377.

22. Miller M. Fluid and electrolyte balance in the elderly. Geriatrics 1987;42:65-68, 71, 75-66.

23. Wahr JA, Parks R, Boisvert D, et al. Preoperative serum potassium levels and perioperative outcomes in cardiac surgery patients. Multicenter Study of Perioperative Ischemia Research Group. JAMA 1999;281:2203-2210.

24. Bartholow C, Whittier FC, Rutecki GW. Hypokalemia and metabolic alkalosis: algorithms for combined clinical problem solving. Compr Ther 2000;26:114-120.

25. Kudoh A, Sakai T, Ishihara H, Matsuki A. Renin-aldosterone in elderly patients with hyperkalaemia under anaesthesia. Eur J Anaesthesiol 1999;16:231-235.

26. Antonelli Incalzi R, Gemma A, Capparella O, et al. Post-operative electrolyte imbalance: its incidence and prognostic implications for elderly orthopaedic patients. Age Ageing 1993;22:325-331.

27. Phillips RS, Hamel MB, Covinsky KE, Lynn J. Findings from SUPPORT and HELP: an introduction. Study to Understand Prognoses and Preferences for Outcomes and Risks of Treatment. Hospitalized Elderly Longitudinal Project. J Am Geriatr Soc 2000;48:S1-S5.

28. Wu AW, Yasui Y, Alzola C, et al. Predicting functional status outcomes in hospitalized patients aged 80 years and older. J Am Geriatr Soc 2000;48:S6-S15.

29. Knaus WA, Harrell FE, Jr., Lynn J, et al. The SUPPORT prognostic model: objective estimates of survival for seriously ill hospitalized adults. Study to Understand Prognoses and Preferences for Outcomes and Risks of Treatment. Ann Intern Med 1995;122:191-203.

30. Lynn J, Arkes HR, Stevens M, et al. Rethinking fundamental assumptions: SUPPORT's implications for future reform. Study to Understand Prognoses and Preferences for Outcomes and Risks of Treatment. J Am Geriatr Soc 2000;48:S214-S221.

31. Hamel MB, Teno JM, Goldman L, et al. Patient age and decisions to withhold life-sustaining treatments from seriously ill, hospitalized adults. SUPPORT Investigators. Study to Understand Prognoses and Preferences for Outcomes and Risks of Treatment. Ann Intern Med 1999;130:116-125.

32. Brett AS, Rosenberg JC. The adequacy of informed consent for placement of gastrostomy tubes. Arch Intern Med 2001;161:745-748.

33. Trunkey DD, Cahn RM, Lenfesty B, Mullins R. Management of the geriatric trauma patient at risk of death: therapy withdrawal decision making. Arch Surg 2000;135:34-38.

34. Llovera I, Mandel FS, Ryan JG, et al. Are emergency department patients thinking about advance directives? Acad Emerg Med 1997;4:976-980.

35. Edmunds LH, Jr., Stephenson LW, Edie RN, Ratcliffe MB. Open-heart surgery in octogenarians. N Engl J Med 1988;319:131-136.

36. Concato J, Horwitz RI, Feinstein AR, et al. Problems of comorbidity in mortality after prostatectomy. JAMA 1992;267:1077-1082.

37. King SB, 3rd, Ullyot DJ, Basta L, et al. Task force 2: application of medical and surgical interventions near the end of life. J Am Coll Cardiol 1998;31:933-942.

38. Lyon LJ, Nevins MA. Management of hip fractures in nursing home patients: to treat or not to treat? J Am Geriatr Soc 1984;32:391-395.

39. Winter WG. Nonoperative treatment of proximal femoral fractures in the demented, nonambulatory patient. Clin Orthop 1987;(218):97-103.

40. Hannan EL, Magaziner J, Wang JJ, et al. Mortality and locomotion 6 months after hospitalization for hip fracture: risk factors and risk-adjusted hospital outcomes. JAMA 2001;285:2736-2742.

41. Marottoli RA, Berkman LF, Leo-Summers L, Cooney LM, Jr. Predictors of mortality and institutionalization after hip fracture: the New Haven EPESE cohort. Established Populations for Epidemiologic Studies of the Elderly. Am J Public Health 1994;84:1807-1812.

42. Seidman MD, Shapiro DP, Shirwany NA. Ethical issues for otolaryngology and surgery in the elderly. Ear Nose Throat J 1999;78:422, 424-426, 428.

43. Wenger NS, Lieberman JR. An assessment of orthopaedic surgeons' knowledge of medical ethics. J Bone Joint Surg Am 1998;80:198-206.

44. Sugarman J, McCrory DC, Hubal RC. Getting meaningful informed consent from older adults: a structured literature review of empirical research. J Am Geriatr Soc 1998;46:517-524.

45. Wenger NS, Lieberman JR. Achieving informed consent when patients appear to lack capacity and surrogates. Clin Orthop 2000;(378):78-82.

46. Morrison RS, Siu AL. Survival in end-stage dementia following acute illness. JAMA 2000;284:47-52.

47. Hoehner PJ. Ethical decisions in perioperative elder care. Anesthesiol Clin North America 2000;18:159-181, vii-viii.

48. Wenger NS, Greengold NL, Oye RK, et al. Patients with DNR orders in the operating room: surgery, resuscitation, and outcomes. SUPPORT Investigators. Study to Understand Prognoses and Preferences for Outcomes and Risks of Treatment. J Clin Ethics 1997;8:250-257.

49. Gerety MB, Soderholm-Difatte V, Winograd CH. Impact of prospective payment and discharge location on the outcome of hip fracture. J Gen Intern Med 1989;4:388-391.

50. Fitzgerald JF, Moore PS, Dittus RS. The care of elderly patients with hip fracture: changes since implementation of the prospective payment system. N Engl J Med 1988;319:1392-1397.

51. Palmer RM, Saywell RM, Jr., Zollinger TW, et al. The impact of the prospective payment system on the treatment of hip fractures in the elderly. Arch Intern Med 1989;149:2237-2241.

52. Edwards C. A proposal that patients be considered honorary members of the healthcare team. J Clin Nurs 2002;11:340-348.

53. Beresford N, Seymour L, Vincent C, Moat N. Risks of elective cardiac surgery: what do patients want to know? Heart 2001;86:626-631.

54. Stanley BM, Walters DJ, Maddern GJ. Informed consent: how much information is enough? Aust N Z J Surg 1998;68:788-791.

55. Schneider EC, Epstein AM. Use of public performance reports: a survey of patients undergoing cardiac surgery. JAMA 1998;279:1638-1642.

56. Taylor C, Norton C. Information booklets for patients with major bowel resection. Br J Nurs 2000;9:785-791.

57. Matthey P, Finucane BT, Finegan BA. The attitude of the general public towards preoperative assessment and risks associated with general anesthesia. Can J Anaesth 2001;48:333-339.
58. Tovar EA, Roethe RA, Weissig MD, et al. One-day admission for lung lobectomy: an incidental result of a clinical pathway. Ann Thorac Surg 1998;65:803-806.

PERIOPERATIVE CLINICAL PATHWAYS

Many common perioperative problems lend themselves to management by algorithms established through a consensus process. Although older patients may have conditions that alter the timing of diagnosis or require a deviation from the treatment protocol, the uniform application of standard management schemas permit the staff caring for these complex patients to remember to track and treat commonly occurring perioperative problems.

VENOUS THROMBOEMBOLISM

The diagnosis and treatment of deep-vein thrombosis (DVT) is relatively straightforward, but the prevention of DVT remains a controversial topic, particularly with regard to the elderly surgical patient. A well-designed clinical study to determine if any type of DVT prophylaxis is effective in decreasing the risk of fatal pulmonary embolism in elderly patients would require approximately 100,000 patients. To date, the largest studies have included fewer than 4000 patients.

The incidence of DVT in geriatric patients undergoing hip or knee replacement or hip fracture surgery varies, from 40% to 70%. Among those who do not have routine prophylaxis, fatal pulmonary embolism occurs in 0.37% to 3.3%. [1,2] Both mechanical and pharmacologic methods are used. Mechanical methods of prophylaxis include early mobilization, sequential compression stocking devices, foot pumps, and support stockings. Mechanical aids with or without pharmacologic methods decrease the incidence of DVT by approximately 50%. [3-5] Patients' tolerance of the mechanical devices, however, varies, and a patient who has decreased grip strength secondary to arthritis will find that support stockings are difficult to apply. Pharmacologic measures include aspirin, subcutaneous heparin, warfarin, dextran, and fractionated heparins. In a meta-analysis, Westrich et al found the best prophylactic method for safety and efficacy to be pneumatic compression and the least effective to be low-dose heparin. [6] For all of the pharmacologic agents, significant risks of bleeding complications occur, particularly with low-molecular-weight heparins and low-dose heparin. [7,8] Although promising, these agents may pose a significant risk in elderly patients. In joint-replacement patients, hematoma formation with the potential for infection can be a devastating complication.

Few studies actually demonstrate convincingly that any type of DVT prophylaxis decreases the rate of fatal pulmonary embolism. Ansari reported a risk of fatal pulmonary embolism following total knee replacement of 0.4% and suggested that prophylaxis was not warranted in patients undergoing unilateral total knee replacement. [9] Fender et al, utilizing a regional hip registry in England, found that the use of chemical prophylaxis did not seem to alter the very low rates of fatal pulmonary embolism. [10] Neither study had adequate power to rule out an effect.

The length of time of DVT prophylaxis also remains controversial. Several studies have shown that there are two peaks of increased incidence following an operation. The first peak of proximal DVT occurs at 7 days postoperatively (2.4%) and the second spike occurs at approximately 1 month (8.2%). [11-13] Current recommendations include continued prophylaxis for up to 6 weeks postoperatively.

For further discussion of DVT, see the section on joint replacement surgery in Chapter 11, Geriatric Orthopedics. Very little DVT research has focused on nonorthopedic surgical procedures.

POSTOPERATIVE DELIRIUM

Best described as an acute confusional state, delirium is a transient, often devastating phenomenon that may require months to disappear. Diagnosis can be based on the Confusion Assessment Method (CAM). [14] It requires the presence of an acute change in mental status with fluctuating course, inattention, and either disorganized thinking or an altered level of consciousness. Hallucinations may be present. Other guidelines exist. [15] It is also important to recognize that delirium may be the initial presentation of some systemic illness. It is essential to evaluate mental status preoperatively, not only to facilitate the subsequent diagnosis of delirium, but also because pre-existing dementia is the most potent predisposing factor for the development of delirium. This is most often done by means of the Mini–Mental State Examination. [16]

In hospitalized medical patients, the incidence of delirium runs between 15% and 50%. Among surgical patients, the incidence is highly dependent on procedure: only 1% to 3% after cataract procedures, 10% to 15% after general surgery, and 30% to 60% after major orthopedic procedures. [17-19] These rates are from studies designed to detect delirium. In clinical practice, physicians often miss the diagnosis. [19]

The enormous consequences of postoperative delirium include functional decline, increased length of hospital stay, increased need for nursing-home placement, and a several-fold increase in mortality. [17,20,21] The economic impact to the United States is estimated at $4 billion annually. [17] Effects on the family and friends have not been quantified.

The variety of predisposing and precipitating factors for delirium suggests that medical science has a long way to go before discovering the underlying mechanism. [22] All factors involve some degree of stress on the brain. Usually, multiple factors play a role. Important predisposing factors are pre-existing dementia, any severe illness (acute or chronic), major depression, poor social supports, vision impairment, and dehydration (high BUN-to-creatinine ratio). Precipitating factors include the stress of surgery, sleep and sensory deprivation, an unfamiliar environment, immobilization, metabolic derangements, malnutrition, pain, and perhaps most of all, psychoactive medications, especially those with anticholinergic effects and opioids and benzodiazepines. [23] Age is a nonmodifiable risk factor, and another risk factor, pre-existing dementia, is usually untreatable.

No study has ever demonstrated that the choice of anesthesia affects the incidence of delirium except for the first few hours after the operation. Smaller differences occur between general and regional anesthesia if sedation is utilized during the regional anesthetic. [18,24] (For further discussion of anesthesia and delirium, see Chapter 2, Geriatric Anesthesia.)

Since the cause of delirium is protean, there is no single treatment. Prevention and treatment require that all predisposing and precipitating factors be addressed, if possible. In an important study of prevention in one nonsurgical population, one ward received standard care and in another ward special efforts were made to maintain orientation, prevent sleep deprivation, encourage ambulation, manage visual and hearing impairment, and prevent dehydration. The incidence of new-onset delirium was 15% in the control ward and 10% in the other ward, a significant decrease. [25] When delirium did occur, however, its severity and duration were not different between the two groups. As encouraging as this study was, it was not possible to identify which parts of the intervention were effective and which were not. In a study of surgical patients with femoral neck fractures, the incidence of delirium was reduced by applying a program of geriatric consultation, subcutaneous heparin, supplemental oxygen, opiate analgesic, and aggressive treatment of hypotension and congestive heart failure. [26] The current trend of performing more and more procedures on an outpatient basis, even in elderly patients, may provide the unexpected benefit of decreasing the incidence of delirium. By getting back to a familiar environment quickly, the outpatient may not have time to suffer enough cumulative insults to make delirium likely.

In addition to delirium, an operation may also be associated with decrements in cognition. Building on anecdotal reports dating from the middle of the last century, new data confirm that some patients undergoing an operation under general anesthesia suffer permanent decrements in measurable cognition in comparison with nonhospitalized volunteers. [17,27] Significant cognitive decline was discovered in 10% of the patients 3 months after a procedure in comparison with only 3% of the volunteers 3 months after baseline measurement. Cognitive decline was associated with a higher degree of functional decline. Subject age was the only significant risk factor for cognitive decline at 3 months following a surgical procedure. (See also Chapter 2, Geriatric Anesthesia.)

POSTOPERATIVE DEPRESSION

Holmes and House summarized what little information is available on prevalence of postoperative depression. [28] Most studies from 1985 to 1996 were in patients following hip fracture. In the immediate postoperative period, an average of 13% of patients had evidence of a depressive disorder, although it is not known if they were depressed prior to having surgery.

Without testing for the presence of depression preoperatively, it is impossible to evaluate the impact of surgery on affect. One of the few studies with preoperative data on elderly patients having cataract extraction showed little evidence for increased depression postoperatively unless the patient was depressed preoperatively or had a poor outcome with respect to vision. [29]

FALLS PREVENTION

Instability and falls are important warning symptoms of underlying serious illness among elderly persons. Falls are a major source of injury in elderly people. Falls cause 90% of hip fractures. The current cost of hip fractures in the United States is estimated to be about 10 billion dollars. [30] The somatosensory, vestibular, and visual systems, which contribute to the maintenance of balance, deteriorate with age. These changes, coupled with age-related changes in muscles and bones, contribute to an increased risk of falls by elderly persons. The integrated rehabilitation-based model of risk factors for falls suggests that there are multiple opportunities for interventions that might reduce the risks. Little research exists on postsurgical patients, so inferences must be made from studies on community-dwelling older persons and older medical patients. (See also Chapter 11, Geriatric Orthopedics, for further discussion of issues related to falls.)

In the community, the incidence of falls can be reduced by a repeated campaign to alert older persons to the risk of falling. Assantachai et al used a leaflet for seniors containing information on important risk factors for falls within their community.[31] They noted a decreased fall rate with the educational efforts. It was found to be a cost-effective way to prevent falls by healthy elderly persons in the community.

Several studies have demonstrated that patients at risk of falls can be identified. Gunter et al used two scales to identify fallers: the "Get Up and Go" (a test involving lower-extremity strength and power, and mobility) and the Tandem Gait tests.[32] Those patients who were slow to get up were more likely to fall, which suggests that prevention strategies should concentrate on strength and mobility. In an analysis by Frels et al of falls among hospitalized elderly patients, most fallers were identified for risk of falling by ward staff.[33] Falls were least likely to occur during visiting hours, and peak incidence occurred during nighttime. Most significantly, these researchers observed that benzodiazepines were implicated in many of the falls, with an odds ratio of 5.6.

In the acute-care setting, Lane identified four risk factors for falls: age 60 and over, impaired memory, muscle weakness, and need of ambulatory assistance.[34] However, prevention strategies did not change the rate of falling. In a meta-analysis, Hill-Westmoreland et al found in 12 studies that intervention reduced risk of falling by only 4%.[35] At least one other evaluation shows better rates.[36] (See also Chapter 11, section on bone insufficiency and falls.)

PRESSURE ULCER PREVENTION

In 1992, the Agency for Health Care Policy and Research released a guideline on the prevention of pressure ulcers.[37] Although this was a seminal work, at the time there was very little evidence-based data available to its authors. Of the 26 recommendations made by the panel, only six (23%) had sufficient research data to warrant an A or B strength of evidence rating.[38] It was essentially an expert panel document. However, the guideline did provide physicians with five specific steps that can be used to prevent pressure ulcers in their patients:

- perform a risk assessment on all bed- and chair-bound patients,

- keep the pressure off the bony prominences of at-risk patients by using a turning schedule,

- use a pressure-reducing mattress in the treatment of all at-risk patients,

- avoid massage of bony prominences,

- encourage the development of institutional educational programs or skin care teams for the prevention and treatment of pressure ulcers.

Among medical patients, assessment at the time of admission identified that patients who were confused on arrival developed significantly more pressure ulcers than patients who were orientated to time and place.[39] However, there is limited information about pressure ulcer risk in the preoperative, intraoperative, and postoperative periods. Because the surgical period is defined temporally, in contrast to the protracted course of the chronically ill patient, the development of pressure ulcers must be examined using a time-based evaluation. Stotts called for the Agency for Health Care Policy and Research guideline for pressure ulcer prevention to be tested in surgical patients. [40] Surgical patients present a unique challenge in preventing pressure ulcers because the problem begins while the patients are immobile and unable to perceive the discomfort of prolonged pressure. Although the pathophysiology and etiology of pressure ulcers are well documented by years of research, the operating room as an etiologic factor is largely undefined. [41] The emphasis on the effect of intraoperative events on pressure ulcer occurrence has led to a quest for predictors of pressure ulcers in surgical patients. [42]

The prevention of pressure ulcers continues in the intensive care unit and on the ward. Few research studies address pressure ulcer prevention in the critical-care setting. Level of risk needs to be linked with intervention to assist the caregivers in managing the pressure-relief options that are available. While studies revolve around testing beds and other products, the prevention of pressure ulcers in critical care patients will continue to require vigilance and the best use of available knowledge in the field. [43]

> *CCI 40 (Level A)*: **To determine if deep-vein thrombosis prophylaxis should be instituted in all geriatric surgical patients or just a select few having certain procedures, a randomized controlled trial must be designed to determine for each common procedure what the likelihood is of getting deep-vein thrombosis, with or without prophylaxis.**

> *CCI 41 (Levels B, A)*: **The risks and complications of using vena cava filters in elderly patients to prevent pulmonary embolism as an alternative to other therapies should be evaluated by cohort studies and ultimately by a randomized controlled trial.**

> *CCI 42 (Level B)*: **Cohort studies are needed to determine if predisposing and precipitating factors for delirium in the older hospitalized surgical patient are the same as in the older hospitalized nonsurgical patient.**

> *CCI 43 (Level A)*: **Proof is needed that prevention of a given factor will lower the risk, or that treating a factor once delirium develops will lessen the adverse outcomes associated with delirium; this will require controlled, probably nonrandomized trials.**

> *CCI 44 (Level B)*: **Ultimately, the biochemical basis for delirium needs to be delineated in the hope that drug therapy will prove useful and cost-effective, not only for treatment but perhaps for prophylaxis as well.**

> *CCI 45 (Level A)*: **The likelihood of delirium after outpatient surgery needs to be compared by randomized controlled trials with that of inpatient surgery of comparable stress rating.**

> *CCI 46 (Level B)*: **In order to improve studies of postoperative cognitive decline, attempts should be made at developing methods of measuring cognition that can be applied serially and are sensitive to modest degrees of cognitive decline.**

CCi 47 (Level B): After development of improved measures of cognitive decline (see CCI 46), prospective cohort studies of surgical patients receiving general anesthesia should be designed that will assess the impact of postoperative cognitive decline on functional status and other long-term outcomes.

CCI 48 (Level B): The causal relationship between delirium and cognitive decline, if any, needs to be determined by longitudinal cohort studies.

CCI 49 (Levels B, A): The effect of successful versus unsuccessful outcomes of surgery on the incidence and ability to treat postoperative depression should be investigated by longitudinal cohort studies followed by case-control studies.

CCI 50 (Levels B, A): Treatment protocols that include behavioral and pharmacologic modalities should be developed for older patients who develop postoperative depression, and they should be tested first in cohort studies, followed ultimately by randomized controlled trials.

CCI 51 (Level A:) Simple, easily applied protocols have been validated to identify preoperatively those older patients who are at risk for falling. High-risk patients should be studied in randomized controlled trials to determine if an intervention program could significantly decrease the number of falls in the postoperative period. Cost analysis should accompany these studies.

CCI 52 (Levels B, A): Cohort studies are needed to determine the causative factors for pressure ulcers that occur in the operating room. Longitudinal evaluations are needed to determine if prevention strategies begun in the operating room make a difference in the incidence and severity of pressure ulcers in the elderly surgical population.

References

1. Wakefield TW, Proctor MC. Current status of pulmonary embolism and venous thrombosis prophylaxis. Semin Vasc Surg 2000;13:171-181.
2. White RH, Gettner S, Newman JM, et al. Predictors of rehospitalization for symptomatic venous thromboembolism after total hip arthroplasty. N Engl J Med 2000;343:1758-1764.
3. Donat R, Mancey-Jones B. Incidence of thromboembolism after transurethral resection of the prostate (TURP)—a study on TED stocking prophylaxis and literature review. Scand J Urol Nephrol 2002;36:119-123.
4. Warwick D, Harrison J, Whitehouse S, et al. A randomised comparison of a foot pump and low-molecular-weight heparin in the prevention of deep-vein thrombosis after total knee replacement. J Bone Joint Surg Br 2002;84:344-350.
5. Robertson KA, Bertot AJ, Wolfe MW, Barrack RL. Patient compliance and satisfaction with mechanical devices for preventing deep venous thrombosis after joint replacement. J South Orthop Assoc 2000;9:182-186.
6. Westrich GH, Haas SB, Mosca P, Peterson M. Meta-analysis of thromboembolic prophylaxis after total knee arthroplasty. J Bone Joint Surg Br 2000;82:795-800.

7. Palareti G, Leali N, Coccheri S, et al. Bleeding complications of oral anticoagulant treatment: an inception-cohort, prospective collaborative study (ISCOAT). Italian Study on Complications of Oral Anticoagulant Therapy. Lancet 1996;348:423-428.

8. Kakkar VV, Kakkar S, Sanderson RM, Peers CE. Efficacy and safety of two regimens of low molecular weight heparin fragment (Fragmin) in preventing postoperative venous thrombolism. Haemostasis 1986;16 Suppl 2:19-24.

9. Ansari S, Warwick D, Ackroyd CE, Newman JH. Incidence of fatal pulmonary embolism after 1,390 knee arthroplasties without routine prophylactic anticoagulation, except in high-risk cases. J Arthroplasty 1997;12:599-602.

10. Fender D, Harper WM, Thompson JR, Gregg PJ. Mortality and fatal pulmonary embolism after primary total hip replacement: results from a regional hip register. J Bone Joint Surg Br 1997;79:896-899.

11. Prandoni P, Bruchi O, Sabbion P, et al. Prolonged thromboprophylaxis with oral anticoagulants after total hip arthroplasty: a prospective controlled randomized study. Arch Intern Med 2002;162:1966-1971.

12. Kibel AS, Creager MA, Goldhaber SZ, et al. Late venous thromboembolic disease after radical prostatectomy: effect of risk factors, warfarin and early discharge. J Urol 1997;158:2211-2215.

13. Ricotta S, Iorio A, Parise P, et al. Post discharge clinically overt venous thromboembolism in orthopaedic surgery patients with negative venography–an overview analysis. Thromb Haemost 1996;76:887-892.

14. Inouye SK, van Dyck CH, Alessi CA, et al. Clarifying confusion: the confusion assessment method: a new method for detection of delirium. Ann Intern Med 1990;113:941-948.

15. O'Keeffe ST, Ni Chonchubhair A. Postoperative delirium in the elderly. Br J Anaesth 1994;73:673-687.

16. Folstein MF, Folstein SE, McHugh PR. "Mini-mental state": a practical method for grading the cognitive state of patients for the clinician. J Psychiatr Res 1975;12:189-198.

17. Ni Chonchubhair A, Valacio R, Kelly J, O'Keefe S. Use of the abbreviated mental test to detect postoperative delirium in elderly people. Br J Anaesth 1995;75:481-482.

18. Parikh SS, Chung F. Postoperative delirium in the elderly. Anesth Analg 1995;80:1223-1232.

19. Flacker JM, Marcantonio ER. Delirium in the elderly: optimal management. Drugs Aging 1998;13:119-130.

20. Inouye SK, Bogardus ST, Jr., Charpentier PA, et al. A multicomponent intervention to prevent delirium in hospitalized older patients. N Engl J Med 1999;340:669-676.

21. Marcantonio ER, Flacker JM, Michaels M, Resnick NM. Delirium is independently associated with poor functional recovery after hip fracture. J Am Geriatr Soc 2000;48:618-624.

22. Inouye SK. Delirium in hospitalized older patients. Clin Geriatr Med 1998;14:745-764.

23. Marcantonio ER, Juarez G, Goldman L, et al. The relationship of postoperative delirium with psychoactive medications. JAMA 1994;272:1518-1522.

24. Williams-Russo P, Urquhart BL, Sharrock NE, Charlson ME. Post-operative delirium: predictors and prognosis in elderly orthopedic patients. J Am Geriatr Soc 1992;40:759-767.

25. Inouye SK, Schlesinger MJ, Lydon TJ. Delirium: a symptom of how hospital care is failing older persons and a window to improve quality of hospital care. Am J Med 1999;106:565-573.

26. Gustafson Y, Brannstrom B, Berggren D, et al. A geriatric-anesthesiologic program to reduce acute confusional states in elderly patients treated for femoral neck fractures. J Am Geriatr Soc 1991;39:655-662.

27. Moller JT, Cluitmans P, Rasmussen LS, et al. Long-term postoperative cognitive dysfunction in the elderly ISPOCD1 study. ISPOCD investigators. International Study of Post-Operative Cognitive Dysfunction. Lancet 1998;351:857-861.

28. Holmes J, House A. Psychiatric illness predicts poor outcome after surgery for hip fracture: a prospective cohort study. Psychol Med 2000;30:921-929.

29. Billig N, Stockton P, Cohen-Mansfield J. Cognitive and affective changes after cataract surgery in an elderly population. Am J Geriatr Psychiatry 1996;4:29-38.

30. Carter ND, Kannus P, Khan KM. Exercise in the prevention of falls in older people: a systematic literature review examining the rationale and the evidence. Sports Med 2001;31:427-438.

31. Assantachai P, Chatthanawaree W, Thamlikitkul V, et al. Strategy to prevent falls in the Thai elderly: a controlled study integrated health research program for the Thai elderly. J Med Assoc Thai 2002;85:215-222.

32. Gunter KB, White KN, Hayes WC, Snow CM. Functional mobility discriminates nonfallers from one-time and frequent fallers. J Gerontol A Biol Sci Med Sci 2000;55:M672-M676.

33. Frels C, Williams P, Narayanan S, Gariballa SE. Iatrogenic causes of falls in hospitalised elderly patients: a case-control study. Postgrad Med J 2002;78:487-489.

34. Lane AJ. Evaluation of the fall prevention program in an acute care setting. Orthop Nurs 1999;18:37-43.

35. Hill-Westmoreland EE, Soeken K, Spellbring AM. A meta-analysis of fall prevention programs for the elderly: how effective are they? Nurs Res 2002;51:1-8.

36. Robertson MC, Campbell AJ, Gardner MM, Devlin N. Preventing injuries in older people by preventing falls: a meta-analysis of individual-level data. J Am Geriatr Soc 2002;50:905-911.

37. Agency for Health Care Policy and Research. Pressure ulcers in adults: prediction and prevention. Rockville, MD: U.S. Department of Health and Human Services, Public Health Service. AHCPR Publication No. 92-0050, 1992.

38. Xakellis GC. Guidelines for the prediction and prevention of pressure ulcers. The Agency for Health Care Policy and Research. J Am Board Fam Pract 1993;6:269-278.

39. Gunningberg L, Lindholm C, Carlsson M, Sjoden PO. Implementation of risk assessment and classification of pressure ulcers as quality indicators for patients with hip fractures. J Clin Nurs 1999;8:396-406.

40. Stotts NA. Risk of pressure ulcer development in surgical patients: a review of the literature. Adv Wound Care 1999;12:127-136.

41. Armstrong D, Bortz P. An integrative review of pressure relief in surgical patients. AORN J 2001;73:645-648, 650-643, 656-647 passim.

42. Byers PH, Carta SG, Mayrovitz HN. Pressure ulcer research issues in surgical patients. Adv Skin Wound Care 2000;13:115-121.

43. Glavis C, Barbour S. Pressure ulcer prevention in critical care: state of the art. AACN Clin Issues Crit Care Nurs 1990;1:602-613.

HEALTH-RELATED QUALITY OF LIFE

The Centers for Disease Control and Prevention defines HRQOL as a person's or group's perceived physical and mental health over time. Medical interest in measuring quality of life has evolved from the realization that "prolonging life may be a mixed blessing: patients want to live, not merely survive." [1]

Heyland et al in 1998 described a clear conceptual framework. [2] Only those domains of health status measurement that overlap with the quality-of-life domains constitute health-related quality of life. They include physical, psychologic, and social functioning. One of the most widely used measures is the Medical Outcomes Study Short Form 36-item health survey (SF–36), which has been validated in many chronic diseases. [3,4] The Sickness Impact Profile is another, but longer, general health questionnaire. Both of these measures were designed to apply generically, to any type of illness. However, measurement of outcomes for some interventions, for example, surgery, may require more disease-specific tools.

Despite the value of these general tools, new measurement tools have been developed. These new surveys can answer questions about speed and nature of recovery from surgical procedures for a group of patients. However, health status survey questions are designed to change practice over time and may not specifically help individual patients. [5]

Questions continue about the suitability of generic measures like the SF-36 in specific populations. [5–7] HRQOL may be affected by highly specific domain-sensitive criteria. For example, Terrell et al found that HRQOL after head and neck dissection for cancer depended greatly on whether cranial nerves V or XI were dissected, and that dissection of one or the other nerve produced different degrees of deterioration in HRQOL. [8]

Many older persons who have cognitive impairments from dementia are unable to answer questions relating to quality of life, but Brod et al suggest that persons with mild to moderate dementia can be considered good informants of their own subjective states. [9]

FUNCTIONAL PROBLEMS

Since the ability to perform daily functions changes one's perception of the quality of life, investigations have concentrated on common functions.

Sensory Disorders

The prevalence of sensory disorders in adults aged 70 years and older include 18% with self-reported vision impairments (4.4 million persons) and 33% (about 7 million) with hearing impairments; 8.6% report both vision and hearing impairments. [10] Numerous studies document the function-specific problems these patients experience. Because they have a variety of problems, some persons with severe vision problems and many with hearing problems do not get successful rehabilitation management. [11–14] Nonetheless, these services have proven benefits in specific populations. [14–16] (See also Chapter 7, Geriatric Ophthalmology, for a more detailed review of impaired vision, and Chapter 8, Geriatric Otolaryngology, for more a detailed review of impaired hearing.)

Sleep Problems

The NIH Consensus Conference on sleep disorders in 1990 mentions nothing about the sleep patterns of the surgical patient after operative intervention or during a stay in an intensive care unit (ICU). [17] Only two basic sleep problems were defined: obstructive sleep apnea and insomnia. Although postoperative pain clearly interferes with sleep, it may not be the only factor interfering with sleep after surgery or ICU experiences. Inouye et al included sleep enhancement in their overall Hospital Elder Life Program, but their intervention studies did not include postsurgical patients. [18]

Mobility

Many studies point to the fact that multiple factors contribute to decreased mobility in older adults. Immobility forms the third part of the triangle of evaluation of the elderly patient suggested by Katz. [19] (The other sides of the triangle are activities of daily living and instrumental activities of daily living.) Acute hospitalizations are associated with decreased independence in mobility and activities of daily living. [20] Some studies have shown that changes in acute hospital care systems may help improve functional outcomes. [21]

Most physicians and surgeons believe that early ambulation postoperatively is beneficial to patients, but proof is scarce. In one randomized controlled trial, 64 patients undergoing laparotomy and intestinal or rectal resection were randomized to usual care or to controlled rehabilitation with early ambulation and diet. The experimental group did better in time to discharge, complication and readmission rates, pain, and quality of life and patient satisfaction. Patients 70 years of age and over benefited from early ambulation but not quite as much as did patients younger than 70. [22] Other trials have confirmed benefit from accelerated rehabilitation but have not drawn distinctions that are based on age, usually because the number of patients in those trials was too small. [23]

Falls

Few studies have actually measured the HRQOL of older persons who fall in comparison with those who do not fall. Many risk factors for falls have been identified. Both vigorous and frail elderly persons are at risk for injurious falls. [24] Certain body characteristics such as underweight and osteoporosis clearly place one at increased risk of serious injury from falls. No studies specifically examined the risk for older adults of falling around the time of operation.

Sexuality

In a population survey, male erectile dysfunction was found to be significantly correlated with increasing age but to be less correlated with geographical location and to be independent of ethnicity. [25] Prostatic operations commonly interfere with erectile function. [26–28] Litwin noted that other types of procedures such as colon resection may affect erectile function. For cardiothoracic surgery, little information is available on postoperative sexual function. Litwin incorporated in his surveys of quality of life several "new" domains (sexual, urinary, and bowel). His survey instrument included measures of sexual function that had been excluded from many other measurement tools, for example, the Nottingham Health Survey [29] or the EuroQol measure. [30] Research on postoperative sexual dysfunction in women is almost nonexistent.

Urinary Incontinence

Many older adults alter their lives greatly to adjust to the problems of urinary incontinence. Women become incontinent more commonly than men do, and they most often respond by having less social interaction, especially with their families. [31] When incontinence occurs in women under age 60, they suffer greater deterioration of HRQOL than do older women. [32] In one group of women aged 70 years or more, 18% reported incontinence. They also reported more depressive feelings and a sense of decreased freedom of activity when incontinence hampers their lives. [33]

Pain

Chronic pain is common in older persons. Operations generally create acute pain on top of existing pain syndromes. Little literature specifically studies pain as a cause for or result of an operation in the elderly patient. Alteration of baseline pain and management of acute postoperative pain is a difficult problem in older patients, particularly because of the narrowing therapeutic range, which increases with age.

The relief of pain and suffering is a primary aim of medicine. Many geriatric patients fear the pain of surgery. Older patients can tolerate opioid medications with proper dosing and attention to side effects. In the postoperative setting, one of the pressing clinical issues is the need to balance adequate pain medication with the risks of delirium and excessive immobility. Assessment of pain in many patients with dementia is possible, but geriatric patients who are delirious or less verbal may not be asked about pain.

For further discussion of the management of acute and chronic pain along with research agenda items, see Chapter 2, Geriatric Anesthesia.

Procedure-Specific HRQOL

Some HRQOL assessments in cardiac, prostate, and cataract surgery demonstrate that many patients assess their results as worse than their preoperative states.[2] A sizable number of patients after cataract procedures do not show improved self-rated quality of life.[34] However, for larger operations such as coronary artery bypass, quality of life has been shown to generally improve.

Barriers to the Application of HRQOL Results

Newer types of outcomes measurements suggest that further research in HRQOL will provide useful data. However, barriers to studying HRQOL outcomes still persist. Clinicians often feel that HRQOL studies based on large patient databases do not reflect the unique problems of their own frail elderly patients. Results may point to unexpected outcomes that may suggest that certain procedures should not be performed on elderly patients or that physicians change their long-established behaviors. Despite the fact that value has been shown for some vision and incontinence rehabilitation programs, patients are not always referred for these services.

> **CCI 53 (Level B)**: **Generic health surveys to measure outcomes may not be adequate for use in the surgical population. However, disease- or syndrome-specific surveys have not been validated for this group. It is not known if health-related quality of life is domain-specific. Research therefore is needed to determine whether current measures require modification or new measures of health-related quality of life need to be developed.**

> **CCI 54 (Level B)**: **An instrument such as that for quality of life in dementia may help surgeons to make decisions about offering surgery to elderly demented patients, but such use requires validation.**

> **CCI 55 (Level B)**: **Measures of vision and hearing and of the effects of visual and auditory rehabilitation should be tested in the elderly surgical population by longitudinal cohort studies.**

> **CCI 56 (Level B)**: **The incidence, etiology, and severity of sleep disturbance in elderly postoperative patients should be evaluated, and longitudinal cohort studies should be performed to look for their temporary or long-lasting effects on health-related quality of life.**

> **CCI 57 (Level B)**: **Questions about sexuality should be included in all instruments used to measure health-related quality of life of elderly surgical patients.**

CCI 58 (Level B): **When instruments that include questions about sexuality become available (see CCI 57), then the ability to evaluate the effects of different operative procedures on the sexual aspects of quality of life should be tested and validated.**

CCI 59 (Level B): **Cohort studies or case-control studies should be performed to determine to what degree improvements or cure of incontinence improve health-related quality of life even in the presence of other negative quality-of-life factors, such as decreased mobility, chronic illness, or sleep disorders.**

CCI 60 (Level B): **It is necessary to continue to develop condition-specific instruments that will allow us to compare the health-related quality-of-life outcomes in operative and nonoperative therapies for the older population.**

References

1. Grunfeld E, Glossop R, McDowell I, Danbrook C. Caring for elderly people at home: the consequences to caregivers. CMAJ 1997;157:1101-1105.

2. Heyland DK, Guyatt G, Cook DJ, et al. Frequency and methodologic rigor of quality-of-life assessments in the critical care literature. Crit Care Med 1998;26:591-598.

3. Ware JE, Jr., Sherbourne CD. The MOS 36-item short-form health survey (SF-36): I. conceptual framework and item selection. Med Care 1992;30:473-483.

4. McHorney CA, Ware JE, Jr., Raczek AE. The MOS 36-Item Short-Form Health Survey (SF-36): II. psychometric and clinical tests of validity in measuring physical and mental health constructs. Med Care 1993;31:247-263.

5. Stadnyk K, Calder J, Rockwood K. Testing the measurement properties of the Short Form-36 Health Survey in a frail elderly population. J Clin Epidemiol 1998;51:827-835.

6. Hayes V, Morris J, Wolfe C, Morgan M. The SF-36 health survey questionnaire: is it suitable for use with older adults? Age Ageing 1995;24:120-125.

7. Dorman PJ, Waddell F, Slattery J, et al. Is the EuroQol a valid measure of health-related quality of life after stroke? Stroke 1997;28:1876-1882.

8. Terrell JE, Welsh DE, Bradford CR, et al. Pain, quality of life, and spinal accessory nerve status after neck dissection. Laryngoscope 2000;110:620-626.

9. Brod M, Stewart AL, Sands L, Walton P. Conceptualization and measurement of quality of life in dementia: the dementia quality of life instrument (DQoL). Gerontologist 1999;39:25-35.

10. Campbell VA, Crews JE, Moriarty DG, et al. Surveillance for sensory impairment, activity limitation, and health-related quality of life among older adults—United States, 1993-1997. MMWR CDC Surveill Summ 1999;48:131-156.

11. Rubin GS, Roche KB, Prasada-Rao P, Fried LP. Visual impairment and disability in older adults. Optom Vis Sci 1994;71:750-760.

12. Massof RW, Rubin GS. Visual function assessment questionnaires. Surv Ophthalmol 2001;45:531-548.

13. Parrish RK, Gedde SJ, Scott IU, et al. Visual function and quality of life among patients with glaucoma. Arch Ophthalmol 1997;115:1447-1455.

14. Scott IU, Smiddy WE, Schiffman J, et al. Quality of life of low-vision patients and the impact of low-vision services. Am J Ophthalmol 1999;128:54-62.

15. Swagerty DL. The impact of age-related visual impairment on functional independence in the elderly. Kans Med 1995;96:24-26.

16. Watson GR. Low vision in the geriatric population: rehabilitation and management. J Am
     Geriatr Soc 2001;49:317-330.
17. Drugs and insomnia. NIH Consensus Development Conference. Natl Inst Health Consens Dev
     Conf Summ 1984;4:1-9.
18. Inouye SK, Bogardus ST, Jr., Baker DI, et al. The Hospital Elder Life Program: a model of
     care to prevent cognitive and functional decline in older hospitalized patients. Hospital Elder
     Life Program. J Am Geriatr Soc 2000;48:1697-1706.
19. Katz S. Assessing self-maintenance: activities of daily living, mobility, and instrumental activi-
     ties of daily living. J Am Geriatr Soc 1983;31:721-727.
20. Mahoney JE, Sager MA, Jalaluddin M. Use of an ambulation assistive device predicts func-
     tional decline associated with hospitalization. J Gerontol A Biol Sci Med Sci 1999;54:
     M83-M88.
21. Iezzoni LI, McCarthy EP, Davis RB, Siebens H. Mobility impairments and use of screening
     and preventive services. Am J Public Health 2000;90:955-961.
22. Delaney CP, Zutshi M, Senagore AJ, et al. Prospective, randomized, controlled trial between a
     pathway of controlled rehabilitation with early ambulation and diet and traditional postopera-
     tive care after laparotomy and intestinal resection. Dis Colon Rectum 2003;46:851-859.
23. Basse L, Raskov HH, Hjort Jakobsen D, et al. Accelerated postoperative recovery programme
     after colonic resection improves physical performance, pulmonary function and body compo-
     sition. Br J Surg 2002;89:446-453.
24. Speechley M, Tinetti M. Falls and injuries in frail and vigorous community elderly persons. J
     Am Geriatr Soc 1991;39:46-52.
25. Jonler M, Moon T, Brannan W, et al. The effect of age, ethnicity and geographical location on
     impotence and quality of life. Br J Urol 1995;75:651-655.
26. Litwin MS. Health related quality of life in older men without prostate cancer. J Urol
     1999;161:1180-1184.
27. Litwin MS. Measuring quality of life after prostate cancer treatment. Cancer J Sci Am
     1999;5:211-213.
28. Schover LR, Fouladi RT, Warneke CL, et al. Defining sexual outcomes after treatment for
     localized prostate carcinoma. Cancer 2002;95:1773-1785.
29. Lukkarinen H, Hentinen M. Assessment of quality of life with the Nottingham Health Profile
     among patients with coronary heart disease. J Adv Nurs 1997;26:73-84.
30. EuroQol—a new facility for the measurement of health-related quality of life. The EuroQol
     Group. Health Policy 1990;16:199-208.
31. Bernstein I, Sejr T, Able I, et al. Assessment of lower urinary tract symptoms in women by a
     self-administered questionnaire: test-retest reliability. Int Urogynecol J Pelvic Floor Dysfunct
     1996;7:37-47.
32. Dugan E, Cohen SJ, Robinson D, et al. The quality of life of older adults with urinary incon-
     tinence: determining generic and condition-specific predictors. Qual Life Res 1998;7:337-344.
33. Kutner NG, Schechtman KB, Ory MG, Baker DI. Older adults' perceptions of their health and
     functioning in relation to sleep disturbance, falling, and urinary incontinence. FICSIT Group. J
     Am Geriatr Soc 1994;42:757-762.
34. Lundstrom M, Stenevi U, Thorburn W. Quality of life after first- and second-eye cataract
     surgery: five-year data collected by the Swedish National Cataract Register. J Cataract Refract
     Surg 2001;27:1553-1559.

MODELS OF CARE DELIVERY

Most older patients receiving surgical and rehabilitation care are living with one or, commonly, several chronic illnesses. Improving care for these complicated patients involves interventions aimed at the multiple components of the health care system, described by Donabedian as care by practitioners and other providers, patient- and family-initiated care, and community services. [1]

Comorbidities often impede older persons from helping themselves to heal. Arthritis and immobility make them vulnerable to additional postoperative complications and prevent them from properly caring for their wounds. Boynton suggests that systems will be necessary to assist them to take appropriate steps in the healing process. [2] This is true even in the ICU, where resources must be brought together to assist the older patient through the period of maximum vulnerability. [3]

INTERDISCIPLINARY TEAMS AND PROCESS OF CARE

Teamwork and interdisciplinary care play important roles in the care of older patients. [4,5] A large Veterans Affairs study of more than 1600 stroke patients demonstrated that some measures of team function predict patient recovery and decreased length of stay. [6] Continence improvement correlated with the attributes of team organization, order, and quality management. [7] Another approach in health care emphasizes teamwork by applying W. Edwards Deming's management principles; Deming espoused collaborative work environments that used the skill and knowledge of all workers. This approach was found to lead to improved patient outcomes and decreased health care costs when applied to ICU care. [8] Team or collaborative care leads to improved outcomes in outpatient management of chronic illnesses like diabetes mellitus. [9] These approaches often involve changes in care processes using personnel already involved in patient care but may require additional team members. Such team behavior is not necessarily an intrinsic skill of health care professionals. [10] Methods are available to teach and measure interdisciplinary team building with specific application to the care of older patients. [11,12]

THE FAMILY'S CONTRIBUTION TO CARE

Family and caregiver health can be adversely affected by many illnesses like dementia, stroke, and hip fracture. The psychologic and financial burdens families face when patients survive with severe chronic disability are huge and a source of significant animosity toward the health care system. [13–16] Some studies point to unmet needs identified by families. [17] Little is known about the effects of different types of caregiving on patients' outcomes from surgical and rehabilitation treatments. Some studies suggest that, in the setting of chronic disease, training family and friends in methods of assisting patients improves patient outcomes and prevents caregiver burnout. [18–20] The types and goals of family interventions are subjects of ongoing research. [21,22]

SYSTEMS INTERVENTIONS TO IMPROVE QUALITY

There exists a mismatch between the health needs of older patients and the way health care systems are organized to deliver care. Research has identified elements of care needed to promote improved health outcomes. For example, in the Chronic Care Model, productive interactions between physicians and patients requires decision support, clinical information systems, self-management support for patients, delivery system redesign, and linkages to community services, all operating within a health system supportive of these objectives. [23]

Quality Improvement Methodologies

Physicians and health systems require tools and methods to improve patient outcomes and the quality of care. Quality improvement efforts may be conducted to offer new ways to gain knowledge relevant to the care of older adults. [24] Methods used in industrial quality improvement are applicable to specific problems in health care delivery. [25–27] Through close collaboration of clinicians, the Northern New England Cardiovascular Disease Study Group improved outcomes and reduced mortality among patients undergoing coronary artery bypass grafting. [28] For years, surgeons have analyzed individual complications through surgical morbidity and mortality conferences. [29] In the past, these conferences focused on clinical decisions alone, but including analysis of process and systems issues in the conferences could clarify other sources of error in hospital care. [30–32]

Evidence-Based Medicine

Applications of evidence-based medicine for older patients is another approach that may improve outcomes. [33,34] Practicing evidence-based medicine requires the acquisition of new skills by physicians. [35] However, many studies lack inclusion of older subjects, thereby limiting the amount of evidence available to guide clinical decisions regarding the care of older patients. Wenger at al summarized the literature on many of the clinical conditions where data are available for the management of the vulnerable elderly. [36] Difficulties in conducting research to produce adequate evidence may include conflicts of interest, ethical contraindications to including older patients in clinical research, the presence of many comorbidities, and interference by medications for chronic illnesses. [37]

Postoperative Planning and Coordination

Inefficiencies in discharge planning may play a role in longer lengths of stay since some, but not all, studies with targeted discharge planning processes have reduced hospital lengths of stay. [38] Rigorous use of evidence-based clinical pathways in hip fracture patients did reduce length of stay by 1 day for nursing-home patients but not for other patients. [39] This lack of reduction in average length of stay after hip fracture was found in another study in which care managers were used for "low-risk" patients. [40] This latter study did achieve decreased lengths of stay for total hip and knee replacement cases without significant changes in patient outcomes but may have just shifted the cost of health care, because more short-stay total hip replacement patients went to nursing homes or rehabilitation facilities. Total cost of care may actually have been increased through such transfers rather than having patients remain 1 or 2 more days in the acute-care hospital. For ICUs, decreased lengths of stay were achieved through team care and implementation of protocols. [41]

Settings for Post-Hospital Care

An increasing number of studies have evaluated the most appropriate settings for post-hospital care and rehabilitation. Many of these suggest that care of older adults can be improved by changes in how care is organized and delivered. [42] One study evaluated patient satisfaction and functional outcomes by following elective hip and knee replacement patients after a 7-day surgical hospitalization. Patients were discharged to either an inpatient rehabilitation stay or home, primarily on the basis of patient preference. There were no differences in outcomes. [43] In a study of high-risk individuals after these elective joint procedures, patients were found to do better if they were transferred to a rehabilitation facility on postoperative day 3 rather than 7. [44] Another large national study showed better functional outcomes at 6 months for stroke survivors but no difference in hip fracture outcomes for patients treated in acute rehabilitation hospitals rather than in skilled nursing facilities. [45] Tinetti et al examined a multicomponent home-based rehabilitation program for older persons after hip fracture, comparing it with usual care, and found no differences in final outcomes. [46]

Continuity of Care

A single older patient may receive care for a single illness event, like stroke or complicated surgical procedure, from many different treatment teams, including ones in an acute-care hospital, a rehabilitation hospital, a subacute-care facility, then an outpatient rehabilitation facility and their physicians' offices. If patients have suboptimal function after a rehabilitation hospital stay, they may go to a nursing facility or may use home health services as well as services offered by their primary care physician.

Patients are at increased risk when information that is transferred from one institution to another is not complete or correct. [47] Receiving teams are known to repeat tests and procedures. [48] Quality indicators for continuity of care have been suggested to improve continuity as well as to integrate quality assurance across settings of care. [36,49] The Domain Management Model and the use of patient care notebooks kept by patients and families are possible tools to standardize information transfer among sites of care. [50,51]

Measuring and Improving Access to Necessary Care

Barriers in access to care and disparities in health care quality can lead to poorer health outcomes among vulnerable subgroups of older people, such as those with lower socioeconomic status, from racial and ethnic minority groups, or those with disabilities. Administrative databases can provide critical information about Medicare patient access to well-defined and appropriate services. [52,53] Asch et al studied 345,253 randomly selected elderly Medicare beneficiaries in 1994–1996. [52] They examined 26 indicators for necessary care and documented that these patients in fact were receiving that care. However, using 16 different indicators, Hannan found that fewer than 66% of beneficiaries were receiving the care. [53] In this study, patients in poverty areas were found to have poorer access. Among the first steps for improving quality of care for older surgical and rehabilitation patients is the assessment of access to care. [54]

> *CCI 61 (Level B)*: **Observational studies are needed to learn where errors occur and where established evidence for best practice improves perioperative care.**

> *CCI 62 (Level A)*: **Interventional studies are needed to test methods to improve outcomes by reducing errors and applying relevant evidence for best practices.**

CCI 63 (Level B): Observational studies are needed to suggest which components of post-hospital care are associated with better outcomes.

CCI 64 (Level A): Interventional trials of different post-hospital care treatments and management strategies are needed to test hypotheses of ways to improve outcomes.

CCI 65 (Level B): Observational studies are needed to document specific problems in communication among settings of care that lead to medical errors, duplication of staff work, and patient and family confusion and lack of compliance.

CCI 66 (Level A): Interventional studies are needed to assess the effectiveness of strategies that foster communication and coordination among settings of care.

CCI 67 (Level B): Observational studies are needed to identify specific barriers to and disparities in the quality of care for vulnerable elderly subgroups.

CCI 68 (Level A): Interventional studies are needed to assess the effectiveness of specific targeted interventions designed to reduce barriers to and disparities in quality of care for older persons.

CCI 69 (Level B): Descriptive studies are needed to assess the relationship of team function and organizational characteristics to outcomes in older surgical patients.

CCI 70 (Level A): Interventional studies are needed to determine the optimal composition and structure of interdisciplinary teams as well as to determine how to improve team function to economically improve outcomes for elderly surgical patients in different care settings.

CCI 71 (Level B): Prospective studies are needed to assess the effects of various types of family caregiving on the outcomes for older patients who require surgery, emergency department visits, and rehabilitation care.

CCI 72 (Level B): Observational studies are needed to assess family or caregivers' identification of unfulfilled needs during the course of an elderly patient's recovery.

CCI 73 (Level A): Interventional trials will ultimately be needed to determine if patient and caregiver outcomes can be improved with targeted interventions.

References

1. Donabedian A. The quality of care: how can it be assessed? JAMA 1988;260:1743-1748.
2. Boynton PR, Jaworski D, Paustian C. Meeting the challenges of healing chronic wounds in older adults. Nurs Clin North Am 1999;34:921-932, vii.
3. Tullmann DF, Dracup K. Creating a healing environment for elders. AACN Clin Issues 2000;11:34-50; quiz 153-154.

4. Counsell SR, Kennedy RD, Szwabo P, et al. Curriculum recommendations for Resident Training in Geriatrics Interdisciplinary Team Care. J Am Geriatr Soc 1999;47:1145-1148.

5. Keith RA. The comprehensive treatment team in rehabilitation. Arch Phys Med Rehabil 1991;72:269-274.

6. Strasser DC, Falconer JA, Herrin J, Bowen SE. Team functioning and patient outcomes in stroke rehabilitation in VA hospitals (poster). Arch Phys Med Rehabil 2000;81:1291.

7. Strasser DC, Falconer JA, Herrin J, Bowen SE. The relation of rehabilitation team functioning and urinary continence for Veterans Administration stroke patients (abstract). Arch Phys Med Rehabil 2001;82:1491.

8. Clemmer TP, Spuhler VJ, Oniki TA, Horn SD. Results of a collaborative quality improvement program on outcomes and costs in a tertiary critical care unit. Crit Care Med 1999;27:1768-1774.

9. Wagner EH. More than a case manager. Ann Intern Med 1998;129:654-656.

10. Fulmer T. Curriculum recommendations for Resident Training in Geriatrics Interdisciplinary Team Care. J Am Geriatr Soc 1999;47:1149-1150.

11. Hyer K, Fairchild S, Abraham I, et al. Measuring attitudes related to interdisciplinary training: revisiting the Heinemann, Schmitt and Farrell 'attitudes toward health care teams' scale. J Interprof Care 2000;14:249-258.

12. Siegler EL, Hyer K, Fulmer T, Mezey M (eds): Geriatric Interdisciplinary Team Training. New York: Springer Publishing Company, 1998.

13. Levine C. The loneliness of the long-term care giver. N Engl J Med 1999;340:1587-1590.

14. Somers AR. Long-term care at home (letter). N Engl J Med 1999;341:1005.

15. Levine C. Long-term care at home (reply). N Engl J Med 1999;341:1005.

16. Covinsky KE, Goldman L, Cook EF, et al. The impact of serious illness on patients' families. SUPPORT Investigators. Study to Understand Prognoses and Preferences for Outcomes and Risks of Treatment. JAMA 1994;272:1839-1844.

17. Greveson G, James O. Improving long-term outcome after stroke—the views of patients and carers. Health Trends 1991;23:161-162.

18. Von Korff M, Gruman J, Schaefer J, et al. Collaborative management of chronic illness. Ann Intern Med 1997;127:1097-1102.

19. Evans RL, Matlock AL, Bishop DS, et al. Family intervention after stroke: does counseling or education help? Stroke 1988;19:1243-1249.

20. Evans RL, Connis RT, Bishop DS, et al. Stroke: a family dilemma. Disabil Rehabil 1994;16:110-118.

21. Glass TA, Dym B, Greenberg S, et al. Psychosocial intervention in stroke: Families in Recovery from Stroke Trial (FIRST). Am J Orthopsychiatry 2000;70:169-181.

22. Lenz ER, Perkins S. Coronary artery bypass graft surgery patients and their family member caregivers: outcomes of a family-focused staged psychoeducational intervention. Appl Nurs Res 2000;13:142-150.

23. Wagner EH, Austin BT, Von Korff M. Improving outcomes in chronic illness. Manag Care Q 1996;4:12-25.

24. Casarett D, Karlawish JH, Sugarman J. Determining when quality improvement initiatives should be considered research: proposed criteria and potential implications. JAMA 2000;283:2275-2280.

25. Berwick DM. Continuous improvement as an ideal in health care. N Engl J Med 1989;320:53-56.

26. Berwick DM. Developing and testing changes in delivery of care. Ann Intern Med 1998;128:651-656.

27. Langley G. The Improvement Guide: A Practical Approach to Enhancing Organizational Performance. San Francisco: Jossey-Bass, 1996.

28. O'Connor GT, Plume SK, Olmstead EM, et al. A regional intervention to improve the hospital mortality associated with coronary artery bypass graft surgery. The Northern New England Cardiovascular Disease Study Group. JAMA 1996;275:841-846.

29. Gordon L. Gordon's Guide to the Surgical Morbidity and Mortality Conference. Philadelphia: Hanley & Belfus Inc., 1994. p. 1-88.

30. Feldman SE, Roblin DW. Medical accidents in hospital care: applications of failure analysis to hospital quality appraisal. Jt Comm J Qual Improv 1997;23:567-580.

31. Pearse RM, Dana EC, Lanigan CJ, Pook JA. Organisational failures in urgent and emergency surgery: a potential peri-operative risk factor. Anaesthesia 2001;56:684-689.

32. Neale G, Woloshynowych M, Vincent C. Exploring the causes of adverse events in NHS hospital practice. J R Soc Med 2001;94:322-330.

33. Sackett DL, Straus SE, Richardson WS, et al. (eds): Evidence-based Medicine: How to Practice and Teach EBM, 2nd ed. Edinburgh: Churchill Livingstone, 2000.

34. Duncan PW, Horner RD, Reker DM, et al. Adherence to postacute rehabilitation guidelines is associated with functional recovery in stroke. Stroke 2002;33:167-177.

35. Cabana MD, Rand CS, Powe NR, et al. Why don't physicians follow clinical practice guidelines? a framework for improvement. JAMA 1999;282:1458-1465.

36. Wenger NS, Rosenfeld K. Quality indicators for end-of-life care in vulnerable elders. Ann Intern Med 2001;135:677-685.

37. Rosenstock L, Lee LJ. Attacks on science: the risks to evidence-based policy. Am J Public Health 2002;92:14-18.

38. Heseltine D. Community outreach rehabilitation. Age Ageing 2001;30 Suppl 3:40-42.

39. March LM, Cameron ID, Cumming RG, et al. Mortality and morbidity after hip fracture: can evidence based clinical pathways make a difference? J Rheumatol 2000;27:2227-2231.

40. Weingarten S, Riedinger MS, Sandhu M, et al. Can practice guidelines safely reduce hospital length of stay? results from a multicenter interventional study. Am J Med 1998;105:33-40.

41. Young MP, Gooder VJ, Oltermann MH, et al. The impact of a multidisciplinary approach on caring for ventilator-dependent patients. Int J Qual Health Care 1998;10:15-26.

42. Calkins E, Boult C, Wagner EH, Pacala JT (eds): New Ways to Care for Older People: Building Systems Based on Evidence. New York: Springer Publishing Company, 1999.

43. Mahomed NN, Koo Seen Lin MJ, Levesque J, et al. Determinants and outcomes of inpatient versus home based rehabilitation following elective hip and knee replacement. J Rheumatol 2000;27:1753-1758.

44. Munin MC, Rudy TE, Glynn NW, et al. Early inpatient rehabilitation after elective hip and knee arthroplasty. JAMA 1998;279:847-852.

45. Kramer AM, Steiner JF, Schlenker RE, et al. Outcomes and costs after hip fracture and stroke: a comparison of rehabilitation settings. JAMA 1997;277:396-404.

46. Tinetti ME, Baker DI, Gottschalk M, et al. Home-based multicomponent rehabilitation program for older persons after hip fracture: a randomized trial. Arch Phys Med Rehabil 1999;80:916-922.

47. Byington M. Ensuring patient safety from care site to care site. Harvard Risk Manage Found Forum 1997;18:12-13.

48. Boult C, Pacala JT. Integrating care. In Calkins E, Boult C, Wagner EH, Pacala JT (eds): New Ways to Care for Older People: Building Systems Based on Evidence. New York: Springer Publishing Company, 1999. p. 196-209.

49. Coleman EA, Besdine RW. Integrating quality assurance across sites of geriatric care. In Calkins E, Boult C, Wagner EH, Pacala JT (eds): New Ways to Care for Older People: Building Systems Based on Evidence. New York: Springer Publishing Company, 1999. p. 185-195.

50. Siebens H. Applying the domain management model in treating patients with chronic diseases. Jt Comm J Qual Improv 2001;27:302-314.

51. Siebens H, Weston H, Parry D, et al. The Patient Care Notebook: quality improvement on a rehabilitation unit. Jt Comm J Qual Improv 2001;27:555-567.
52. Asch SM, Sloss EM, Hogan C, et al. Measuring underuse of necessary care among elderly Medicare beneficiaries using inpatient and outpatient claims. JAMA 2000;284:2325-2333.
53. Hannan EL. The continuing quest for measuring and improving access to necessary care. JAMA 2000;284:2374-2376.
54. Bierman AS, Magari ES, Jette AM, et al. Assessing access as a first step toward improving the quality of care for very old adults. J Ambulatory Care Manage 1998;21:17-26.

INDEX

Page references followed by *t* and *f* indicate tables and figures, respectively. Page references in **bold** indicate agenda items and key research questions.